Handbook of
Health Behavior Research III
Demography, Development, and Diversity

Handbook of
Health Behavior Research III
Demography, Development, and Diversity

Edited by

David S. Gochman
University of Louisville
Louisville, Kentucky

Plenum Press • New York and London

Library of Congress Cataloging-in-Publication Data

Handbook of health behavior research / edited by David S. Gochman.
        p.   cm.
     Includes bibliographical references and indexes.
     Contents: I. Personal and social determinants -- II. Provider
determinants -- III. Demography, development, and diversity --
IV. Relevance for professionals and issues for the future.
     ISBN 0-306-45443-2 (I). -- ISBN 0-306-45444-0 (II). -- ISBN
0-306-45445-9 (III). -- ISBN 0-306-45446-7 (IV)
     1. Health behavior. 2. Health behavior--Research.   I. Gochman,
David S.
     [DNLM: 1. Health Behavior--handbooks. 2. Research--handbooks.   W
49 H236 1997]
RA776.9.H363   1997
613--dc21
DNLM/DLC
for Library of Congress   97-14565
                                                                     CIP

ISBN 0-306-45445-9

© 1997 Plenum Press, New York
A Division of Plenum Publishing Corporation
233 Spring Street, New York, N. Y. 10013

http://www.plenum.com

Printed in the United States of America

DEDICATION

Throughout my career I have been helped and encouraged by many persons. There are a few whose help was so special that my debt to them is enormous. It is in recognition of what I owe them that this *Handbook* is dedicated to Zelda S. Ackerman, O. J. Harvey, and D. Eldridge McBride, and to the memories of John H. Russel, William A. Scott, and John P. Kirscht. Mrs. Ackerman, my advisor in New York City's High School of Music and Art (now LaGuardia High School), facilitated my early entrance into academia. "Mac" McBride and John Russel, inspired and committed teachers, advisors, and counselors during my formative years at Shimer College, served as role models and continued as my friends over the decades. Bill Scott and O. J. Harvey were encouraging and supportive advisors during my graduate training at the University of Colorado. Bill taught me methodological rigor and innovation, and O. J. encouraged me to think in new and divergent ways. Both of them maintained high standards for their own performance, and demanded no less from me and others.

Jack Kirscht was a pioneer in health behavior research, a community activist, and a person of great wit, humor, and charm. In 1967 he convinced me to come to the University of Michigan's School of Public Health and to bring my research interests in cognitive development and structure to the area of health behavior. He was also a contributor to my 1988 book. Health behavior research lost a giant with his untimely death. He is very much missed by many as a friend and colleague and as a teacher and scholar.

Contributors

B. Jaye Anno, Consultants in Correctional Care, Santa Fe, New Mexico 87505

Patricia J. Bush, Department of Family Medicine, Georgetown University School of Medicine, Washington, DC 20007

Peter E. Campos, Department of Psychiatry and Behavioral Sciences, Emory University School of Medicine, Atlanta, Georgia 30308

Melissa A. Clark, Department of Community Health Sciences, School of Public Health, University of Illinois at Chicago, Chicago, Illinois 60612

Jeannine Coreil, Department of Community and Family Health, College of Public Health, University of South Florida, Tampa, Florida 33612

Julia Muennich Cowell, Department of Public Health, Mental Health, and Administrative Nursing, University of Illinois at Chicago, Chicago, Illinois 60612-7350

Paul N. Duckro, Department of Community and Family Medicine, School of Medicine, St. Louis University Health Sciences Center, St. Louis, Missouri 63104

Eugene B. Gallagher, Department of Behavioral Science, University of Kentucky School of Medicine, Lexington, Kentucky 40536-0086

David S. Gochman, Kent School of Social Work, University of Louisville, Louisville, Kentucky 40292

Timothy Hawley, Seven Counties Services, Louisville, Kentucky 40203

Laurie M. Joyner, Department of Sociology, Loyola University, New Orleans, Louisiana 70118

Michael R. Kauth, Psychology Service, Veterans Affairs Medical Center, New Orleans, Louisiana 70146

Philip Magaletta, Department of Community and Family Medicine, School of Medicine, St. Louis University Health Sciences Center, St. Louis, Missouri 63104

Beth A. Marks, Department of Public Health, Mental Health, and Administrative Nursing, University of Illinois at Chicago, Chicago, Illinois 60612-7350

Robert W. O'Brien, The CDM Group, Inc., Chevy Chase, Maryland 20815

Louis G. Pol, Department of Marketing, University of Nebraska at Omaha, Omaha, Nebraska 68182

Joseph Prejean, Department of Psychology, Louisiana State University, Baton Rouge, Louisiana 70803

Thomas R. Prohaska, Department of Community Health Sciences, School of Public Health, University of Illinois at Chicago, Chicago, Illinois 60612

William Rakowski, Department of Community Health and Center for Gerontology and Health Care Research, Brown University, Providence, Rhode Island 02912

Terry D. Stratton, Department of Behavioral Science, University of Kentucky School of Medicine, Lexington, Kentucky 40536-0086

Richard K. Thomas, Medical Services Research Group, Memphis, Tennessee 38104

Bradley T. Thomason, Department of Family and Preventive Medicine, Emory University School of Medicine, Atlanta, Georgia 30308

Holly C. VanScoy, Academic Research Associates, Inc., Grand Rapids, Michigan 49506

Ann Wolf, Department of Community and Family Medicine, School of Medicine, St. Louis University Health Sciences Center, St. Louis, Missouri 63104

James D. Wright, Department of Sociology, Tulane University, New Orleans, Louisiana 70118

Lore K. Wright, Department of Mental Health/Psychiatric Nursing, School of Nursing, Medical College of Georgia, Augusta, Georgia 30912-4220

Preface to All Volumes

THE STATE OF THE ART

The *primary* objective of this *Handbook* is to provide statements about health behavior research as a basic body of knowledge moving into the 21st century. It is expected that the *Handbook* will remain in use and current through 2005, at least. The *Handbook* presents a broad and representative selection of mid-1990s health behavior findings and concepts in a single work. While texts and books of readings are available in related areas, such as health psychology (e.g., DiMatteo, 1991; Stone et al., 1987), medical anthropology (e.g., McElroy & Townsend, 1989; Nichter, 1992), medical sociology (e.g., Cockerham, 1995; Helman, 1990; Wolinsky, 1988), behavioral health (e.g., Matarazzo, Weiss, Herd, Miller, & Weiss, 1984), behavioral risk factors (e.g., Hamburg, Elliott, & Parron, 1982), and changing health behaviors (Shumaker et al., 1990), none of these works was intended to address basic research-generated knowledge of health behavior, and none was intended to transcend individual disciplines. Accordingly, none of these works presents a broad and representative spectrum of basic health behavior research reflecting multidisciplinary activities. One work with a title identical to this one but for one word, the *Handbook of Health Behavior Change* (Shumaker et al., 1990), deals almost exclusively with applications. This *Handbook* thus presents the reader with the "state of the art" in health behavior research, something not found elsewhere.

In the context of this primary objective, it was not intended that the chapters be journal articles. Authors were encouraged to provide extensive coverage of their topics and to provide original findings to the degree that such findings were relevant. They were not encouraged to write research reports, and the reader should not expect the chapters to read as though they were journal articles.

HEALTH BEHAVIOR AS BASIC RESEARCH

Health behavior is not a long-established, traditional area of inquiry, comparable to chemistry or psychology, but a newly emerging interdisciplinary and multidisciplinary one. Health behavior is still establishing its identity as a domain of scientific research.

Although the earlier work (Gochman, 1988) that helped define it is now nearly a decade old, there are still relatively few institutional or organizational structures, i.e., departments and programs, that reflect the field, and few books and no journals are directed at it.

A *second* objective of the *Handbook* is to reaffirm the identity of health behavior and help secure its position as an important area of basic research, worthy of being studied in its own right. In the context of their discussion of the emergence of medical anthropology, Foster and Anderson (1978, pp. 2–3) stated: "When a sufficient number of researchers focus on the same, or related, topics, and as significant new data begin to appear, the stage is set for the emergence of a new discipline or subdiscipline. But some spark is essential to coalesce these emerging interests around a common focus; usually, it seems, an appropriate name supplies this spark." It is hoped that this *Handbook* will provide such a spark.

LEVELS OF ANALYSIS

Personal, Social, and Provider Determinants

A *third* objective, very much related to the first two, is to view health behavior research as transcending particular behaviors, specific illnesses or health problems or strategies for intervention, or single sets of determinants. One major way of achieving this objective is to look at health behavior in transaction with a range of personal, social systems: as an outcome or product, as well as a factor that affects these systems (in this context, the term *system* is often used interchangeably with *unit* or *entity*), rather than primarily as a set of risk factors or as targets for interventions directed at behavioral change. Volumes I and II of this *Handbook* thus deal largely with characteristics of the system of concern, and focus on specific health behaviors, or specific health problems or conditions, as ways of demonstrating the impact of these systems.

Volume I begins with conceptualizations of health and health behavior and then moves from smaller to larger systems, demonstrating how health behavior is determined by—and often in transaction with—personal, family, social, institutional and community, and cultural factors. These levels of analysis cannot be neatly differentiated, and at times the distinctions between them are arbitrary: Families, organizations, and institutions are all social systems. Moreover, although all individuals differ in their responses to and interpretations of family, social, and cultural norms, personalities and cognitive structures nonetheless reflect family, social, and cultural factors; additionally, families, social groupings, and organizations all reflect elements of the culture in which they exist. Furthermore, the categorizing and sequencing of sections and chapters in no way reflect an attempt to exclude material that deals with other levels of determinants; they serve primarily to facilitate focusing more on one of these determinants than on others. Volume I concludes with an integration that relates categories of health behaviors to characteristics of personal and social systems, identifies common themes, and suggests future research directions.

Since so much of health behavior is determined by providers—the health professionals and institutions that comprise the care delivery system—Volume II examines the way encounters with health providers determine health behaviors, and how health behaviors and the providers reciprocally affect one another. Volume II begins with an overview section on communication, continues with a section on interactional and structural determinants, i.e., professional characteristics, perceptions, power, and role relations, and organizational, locational, and environmental factors; and then presents major sections on the impact of provider characteristics on adherence to and acceptance of both disease-focused and lifestyle regimens.

Populations and Professional Applications

Volume III begins with an overview section on the demography of health behavior and continues with an examination of health behaviors in a range of populations selected on the basis either of the life-span continuum; of a health status risk due to an existing condition, a socially constructed label, or restrictive economic and environmental conditions; or of membership in defined communities. Volume IV examines the relevance of knowledge generated by health behavior research for the training and clinical (and other) practice activities of health professionals; for health services management and health policy; and for planned applications in school, family, community and workplace settings, and the media. Volume IV aims to position health behavior research in the 21st century through a discussion of the four major disciplines that inform health behavior research: health psychology, medical anthropology, medical geography, and medical sociology. Volume IV also presents a working draft of a taxonomy of health behavior and of a matrix framework for organizing health behavior knowledge.

Glossary and Index

Each of the volumes concludes with a glossary of health behavior concepts and definitions, and an index. Both of these reflect the contents of the entire *Handbook*.

A FRAMEWORK FOR ORGANIZING HEALTH BEHAVIOR KNOWLEDGE: A WORK IN PROGRESS

A Taxonomy for Health Behavior

Reviewing the contributed chapters in a volume with the editorial objective of integration led to the development of a "work in progress" taxonomy of health behaviors that became a primary organizing principle for the final chapter of each of the first three volumes. The taxonomy continued to evolve from Volume I to Volume III. The integration of Volume I would have been modified and organized slightly differently had it been written *after* those for Volumes II and III, but the fundamentals remained the same. Virtually all of the health behavior findings reported could be subsumed under one of six categories: health cognitions; care seeking; risk behaviors; lifestyle; responses to illness, including adherence; and preventive, protective, and safety behaviors.

A Matrix Framework

The working taxonomy appears in a different way in Volume IV. With one minor modification—the distinction between nonaddictive and addictive risk behaviors—it combines with the range of personal and social systems used as organizing principles in Volumes I and II, and in the integration chapters for Volumes I through III, to become part of a matrix framework for organizing health behavior knowledge. This framework is presented in Chapter 20 of Volume IV, entitled "Health Behavior Research, Cognate Disciplines, Future Identity, and an Organizing Matrix: An Integration of Perspectives."

DIVERSITY OF PERSPECTIVES

A *fourth* objective is to assure that the reader is exposed to varied perspectives in conceptual models, disciplines, populations, and methods, as well as to nonmedical frames of reference. The *Handbook* exposes the reader to a range of theories and models. The contributors bring expertise from their training or professional involvements in varied disciplines, including (in alphabetical order) anthropology, biology, communications, dentistry, education, engineering, ethics, geography, health management and policy, health promotion and health education, medicine, nursing, psychiatry, psychology, public health, social work, and sociology.

DIVERSITY OF READERS

A *fifth* objective is to assure the relevance of the *Handbook* for persons in a number of fields who are interested in issues related to research in health behavior. The potential readership includes researchers in the social and behavioral sciences who want to know more about health behavior in general, or particular aspects of it, or who want to develop their own health behavior research; students in courses that integrate social and behavioral science and health, in disciplines such as anthropology, psychology, and sociology, and in professional programs in dentistry, medicine (including psychiatry), nursing, public health, and social work; professionals who provide, plan, implement, and evaluate health services and programs: fitness and exercise physiologists; family planners; health educators and promoters; health managers; health planners; hospital administrators; nutritionists; pharmacists; physicians in community and family practice; physiatrists; public health dentists, nurses, physicians; rehabilitation therapists; social workers; and so forth.

THE PRACTICAL RELEVANCE OF HEALTH BEHAVIOR RESEARCH

The practical value of increasing knowledge and understanding of health behavior through rigorous, systematic research is implicit in the grave concern with health status in many contemporary societies. Solutions to an appreciable number of health problems require large-scale efforts at local, regional, and national levels to develop and enforce policies to control, minimize, and ultimately reduce air, land, and water pollution; the hazards of transportation; and the risks of the workplace environment. Many of these solutions transcend individual health behaviors. Solutions to other health problems, however, involve policies, programs, and processes that interact with the personal health behavior of individuals and the population at large, in their family, social, workplace, institutional, and community milieus.

As material in Volume IV demonstrates, attempts to change individual health behaviors, either through individual therapeutic interventions or through larger-scale health promotion or health education programs, have been less than impressive. Many attempts are purely programmatic, hastily conceived, and lacking in theoretical rationale or empirical foundation. A major reason for this is the lack of *basic* knowledge about the target behaviors, about the contexts in which they occur, and about the factors that determine and stabilize them. Basic research in health behavior, aside from being worthy of study in its own right, may very well increase the effectiveness of interventions and programs designed to bring about behavioral change.

DELIBERATE OMISSIONS

Notably absent from the *Handbook* are chapters devoted to topics such as "Type A" personality, psychosomatics, and stress. While these considerations may be linked to health status, and sometimes to health behavior, they have been omitted because they are more generally models for understanding the etiology of disease and illnesses. Furthermore, while "holism" has become a catchword among many who disavow the traditional medical model, the term has come to include charlatanism and cultism, as well as some impressive approaches to treatment. At present, it remains more a statement of faith suggesting future research alternatives than a body of well-thought-through, rigorously conducted research. Moreover, caution against a reverse "ethnocentrism" and overly romanticized views of non-high-technological medicine is cogently provided by Eisenberg and Kleinman (1981). In their words (Eisenberg & Kleinman, 1981, p. 10): "Healing ceremonies can be efficacious, but hardly substitute for antibiotics or surgery." Accordingly, there is no section on "holism" or "holistic medicine" or "holistic health" in the *Handbook*.

REFERENCES

Cockerham, W. C. (1995). *Medical sociology* (6th ed.). Englewood Cliffs, NJ: Simon & Schuster.

DiMatteo, M. R. (1991). *The psychology of health, illness, and medical care: An individual perspective.* Belmont, CA: Brooks/Cole.

Eisenberg, L., & Kleinman, A. (Eds.). (1981). *The relevance of social science for medicine.* Dordrecht, Netherlands: Reidel.

Foster, G. M., & Anderson, B. G. (1978). *Medical anthropology.* New York: Wiley.

Gochman, D. S. (Ed.). (1988). *Health behavior: Emerging research perspectives.* New York: Plenum Press.

Hamburg, D. A., Elliott, G. R., & Parron, D. L. (Eds.). (1982). *Health and behavior: Frontiers of research in the biobehavioral sciences.* Washington, DC: National Academy Press.

Helman, C. G. (1990). *Culture, health and illness* (2nd ed.). London: Wright/Butterworth.

Matarazzo, J. D., Weiss, S. M., Herd, J. A., Miller, N. E., & Weiss, S. M. (Eds.). (1984). *Behavioral health: A handbook of health enhancement and disease prevention.* New York: Wiley.

McElroy, A., & Townsend, P. K. (1989). *Medical anthropology in ecological perspective* (2nd ed.). Boulder, CO: Westview.

Nichter, M. (Ed.). (1992). *Anthropological approaches to the study of ethnomedicine*. Amsterdam, Netherlands: Gordon and Breach Science Publishers.

Shumaker, S.A., Schron, E. B., Ockene, J. K., Parker, C. T., Probstfield, J. L., & Wolle, J. M. (Eds.). (1990). *The handbook of health behavior change*. New York: Springer.

Stone, G. C., Weiss, S. M., Matarazzo, J. D., Miller, N. E., Rodin, J., Belar, C. D., Follick, M. J., & Singer, J. E. (Eds.). (1987). *Health psychology: A discipline and a profession*. Chicago: University of Chicago Press.

Wolinsky, F. D. (1988). *The sociology of health: Principles, practitioners, and issues* (2nd ed.). Belmont, CA: Wadsworth.

Preface to Volume III

HEALTH BEHAVIOR AND POPULATION CHARACTERISTICS

Unlike Volumes I and II, which focus on selected determinants of health behavior, Volume III deals with health behaviors in defined populations. The volume is organized into five parts: Part I, an overview, defines and focuses on health demography and deals with population changes and concomitant changes in health behaviors. Part II, on development, deals with health behavior and the human life span—with changes in health behavior related to human growth and maturation, particularly in children, adolescents, and the elderly, the life-span categories that have been most frequently studied. Part III considers population groups "at risk," those populations or segments of a population whose health status may be threatened because of an existing condition, a socially constructed label, or restrictive economic and environmental conditions. Part IV, on structured communities, deals with health behavior in populations living in defined and somewhat closed communities, such as prisons and religious orders. The volume concludes with Part V, an integrating chapter that relates categories of health behaviors to personal and social characteristics within different population groups, identifies common themes, and suggests future research directions.

Acknowledgments

Many persons provided greatly valued assistance during the nearly four years from the time the *Handbook of Health Behavior Research* was conceptualized until its publication, and I owe all of them my thanks. The substantial help I received from some of them merits special recognition. Among the support staff at the Raymond A. Kent School, I especially wish to thank Shannon R. Daniels and Kelley E. Davis for their expeditious and careful photocopying of what must have seemed like tons of manuscripts, Jane Isert for her dedication in assuring that calls and mail from contributors and from the publisher reached me in a timely way, and Sally Montreuil-Palmarini for expediting mailings of material to contributors.

Among the highly professional and committed staff at the University of Louisville's Ekstrom Library, special thanks go to all of the reference librarians, and particularly to Carmen Embry (now at Barrier Islands Art Center) for some insightful content suggestions; Sharon Edge for her expediting access to materials; and S. Kay Womack (now at the University of Oklahoma) for her astute and knowledgeable guidance through computer and other literature searches, particularly in areas in which little had been written that was adequately indexed.

Thomas R. Lawson, Director of the Kent School, deserves recognition for his continued encouragement of my scholarly activities, his efforts in securing a sabbatical leave for me to assure the *Handbook*'s timely completion, and his generosity in providing necessary supplies and personnel resources.

A great debt is owed to all of the authors whose scholarly chapters grace the *Handbook*, and add immeasurably to its value, for the care they devoted to their work, and for their receptivity and constructive responses to the high density of editorial suggestions made throughout the *Handbook*'s progress. A number of authors and others also provided suggestions about potential contributors for several topics. Among those whose help in this quest was exceptional were M. Robin DiMatteo, Eugene B. Gallagher, Russell E. Glasgow, Michael R. Kauth, Jeffrey Kelley, James E. Maddux, Lillian C. Milanof, R. Prasaad Steiner, and David P. Willis.

Gene Gallagher, along with Zeev Ben-Sira (whose untimely death occurred prior to the final revision of his chapter), John G. Bruhn, Patricia J. Bush, Henry P. Cole, Reed Geertsen, Marie R. Haug, Richard R. Lau, Alexander Segall, and Ingrid Waldron had all contributed to the 1988 book. Their willingness to contribute anew to this one is most appreciated.

Finally, Richard Millikan merits special recognition for the excellence of his copyediting work, his ability to perceive issues that cross-cut the four volumes, and for his skill in helping me clarify my own thinking; and Eliot Werner, Executive Editor at Plenum Publishing Corporation, deserves special thanks for his vision and encouragement in the area of health behavior research, for his faith in the value of the *Handbook*, and for being laid back and calming in the face of my "overfunctioning" and obsessive-compulsivity.

Contents

Chapter 8.   Health Behavior in Persons with HIV and AIDS 163

Bradley T. Thomason and Peter E. Campos

Chapter 9.   Health Behavior in Developing Countries 179

Jeannine Coreil

David S. Gochman

I
OVERVIEW

HEALTH DEMOGRAPHY

Health demography is a newly emerging discipline, closely related to epidemiology—the study of how illnesses are distributed, i.e., where they originate, and how they progress, within a population (Pol & Thomas, 1992, p. 4). It is especially related to social epidemiology, which examines the socially relevant factors related to illness origins and progressions. Health demography combines the traditional biosocial epidemiological variables of age, sex, race, and ethnicity with sociocultural characteristics such as marital status, income, education, occupation and employment status, and religion and religiosity to predict health-relevant variables. Health demography has focused essentially on utilization of health services, including hospital admissions, patient hospital days, length of stay, nursing home admissions, admission to other facilities, physician utilization, dentist utilization, utilization of other health care personnel, treatment rates, insurance coverage indicators, and drug utilization (Pol & Thomas, 1992, chapt. 11). Some of those focuses—utilization of physicians, dentists, druggists, other health care personnel; and carrying insurance coverage—are clearly health behaviors; others, such as treatment rates and lengths of hospital stay, are not. Health demography also examines risk behaviors and perceived health status as predictors of need for services.

Although an abundant epidemiological literature links *health status* with population characteristics, the distribution of a wide range of *health behaviors* throughout a population has been poorly documented. While there is evidence of a nonrandom distribution of risk and care-seeking behaviors, there is little in the way of rigorous evidence of the distribution of responses to illness, sick role enactments, preventive behaviors, and a large number of health cognitions within a population and across subpopulations within that population. Krick and Sobal's (1990) analysis of protective and health-promoting behaviors in a national sample is one of the few studies to have analyzed such matters. Much as such analyses are needed to increase understanding, unless they are thoughtfully developed and appropriately conducted, there is a risk that they will only increase the amount of unusable, unassimilable bits of information already available (Feinleib, 1993).

The characteristics of human populations change dynamically over time as a result of factors such as fertility and mortality rates, diseases, wars, internal migrations, emigrations, and economics and politics. Such changes often affect health behaviors, particularly those related to use of services. Evidence suggests, however, that the impact of such changes is not always predictable. For example, migration, with its ensuing acculturation, does not necessarily increase demand for preventive care (Van der Stuyft, De Muynck, Schillemans, & Timmerman, 1989).

FRAMES OF REFERENCE

A cluster of related questions provides major conceptual frames of reference for thinking about the topics and materials in this volume:

1. How are health behaviors (or a particular type of health behavior) and their determinants and correlates distributed within a population?
2. What accounts for changes in health behaviors within a population?
3. What accounts for demographic differences within a population?
4. How are health behaviors and their determinants and correlates distributed across different populations (or population subgroups)?
5. What accounts for differences in health behaviors between populations (and population subgroups)?

The research literature provides little in the way of definitive answers to these questions. Rarely, if ever, have a wide range of health behaviors been studied in a population, let alone in a systematic comparison of two or more populations. This volume therefore attempts to provide some insights into what is known about some specific types of behaviors in some population groupings.

In Chapter 1, on the demography of health behavior, Pol and Thomas provide a conceptual framework for understanding how changing population characteristics such as age and gender can be linked to a variety of health behaviors. The chapter projects some changes in health behavior, especially those related to planning for future health services, through the early years of the 21st century.

REFERENCES

Feinleib, M. (1993). From information to knowledge: Assimilating public health data. *American Journal of Public Health, 83*, 1205-1207.

Krick, J. P., & Sobal, J. (1990). Relationships between health protective behaviors. *Journal of Community Health, 15*, 19-34.

Pol, L. G., & Thomas, R. K. (1992). *The demography of health and health care*. New York: Plenum Press.

Van der Stuyft, P., De Muynck, A., Schillemans, L., & Timmerman, C. (1989). Migration, acculturation and utilization of primary health care. *Social Science and Medicine, 29*, 53-60.

1

Demographic Change and Health Behavior

Louis G. Pol and Richard K. Thomas

INTRODUCTION

Demographic change has been a major contributor to altered patterns of health services demand, health services supply, health status, and health behavior throughout the history of modern medicine; nevertheless, the implications of current patterns of demographic change for health behavior are not as yet clearly understood. Researchers in general have focused on the most basic relationships between demographics and health care, often overlooking the more subtle and indirect implications of these connections. Moreover, little attention has been paid to the dynamics of demographic change, which often occurs over a very short period of time.

The applications of demography to health care can be placed into two general categories. First, a number of contributors to the literature

Louis G. Pol • Department of Marketing, University of Nebraska at Omaha, Omaha, Nebraska 68182.   Richard K. Thomas • Medical Services Research Group, Memphis, Tennessee 38104.

Handbook of Health Behavior Research III: Demography, Development, and Diversity, edited by David S. Gochman. Plenum Press, New York, 1997.

have focused on the implications of aggregate demographic change for the markets for health-related goods and services. For example, Braus (1994) addressed the impact of population aging in the United States on the need for nursing homes and nursing-home-related services. Sherer (1993) analyzed the aging of the Florida population with respect to the growing demand for a host of health care services. Herbig and Koehler (1993) studied the consequences that aging baby busters (the age cohorts born after the baby boom) will bring to the need for and delivery of health care services. Thomas (1993) described a variety of changes in the demand for health care that can be attributed to society-wide demographic trends.

Second, many health researchers have utilized a number of demographic variables among their predictors of health service needs and health behavior. Bean and Talaga (1991), for example, found that sex, marital status, race, and social class are associated with appointment-breaking behavior. McDaniel, Gates, and Lamb (1992) concluded that in rural communities, the likelihood of utilizing a local rather than a regional hospital increases with age but decreases with income.

There is no common theme, set of methods, or consistent approaches that lead to a clear understanding of the relationship between demographic events and health behaviors. A body of relevant research literature is only now beginning to take shape. This chapter should be relevant to those interested in demographic implications for health behavior, whether their focus is on short- or long-term consequences or on the local, regional, or national level.

The health behavior issues that emerge in the context of changing demographic conditions are part of a relatively new area of study, *health demography* (Pol & Thomas, 1992; Thomas & Pol, 1993). Health demography emerged in the 1980s as a subdiscipline within demography. While the relationship between health and demography in such fields as epidemiology predates the emergence of health demography, research in those areas has not focused on the implications for health services management and has almost entirely ignored the marketing implications (e.g., Crimmins, Hayward, & Saito, 1994; Manton, Corder, & Stallard, 1993). Health demography, as defined in this chapter, has a vital connection to managerial, marketing, and other private-sector issues in health care.

Health demography is best defined as the application of the content and methods of demography to the study of health status and other health-related phenomena. Health demography concerns itself with the manner in which factors such as age, marital status, and income influence both the health status and the health behavior of populations and, in turn, how health-related phenomena affect the demographic attributes of a population. The major focus of health demography, however, is on the dynamic nature of population change and the implications of such change for health care.

Health demography has become the focal point in health care marketing for the development of data sources and of the techniques and methodologies necessary for the formulation of marketing strategies. At the macro level, demographic data and analyses are critical for market area delineation, market segmentation, growth potential estimation, and strategy development. At the micro level, customer demographic characteristics have proven useful in better understanding who the customers are, as well as how well they are being served. Day-to-day operational concerns such as case mix, payer mix, patient origin, and staffing levels all have significant demographic components. Health demographers are now driving the assembly of the elements necessary for the development of a mature marketing function within the industry.

Health demography has relevance for health behavior, in that a number of correlates between demographic characteristics and patterns of health behavior have been identified through research. Health behavior refers to actions taken in response to the onset of health problems, to prevent health problems, or to maintain or enhance health status. Health behavior can be viewed as the actions of individuals, groups, or even organizations. Most of the discussion in this chapter will focus on the behavior of individuals, although, as will be seen, membership in various demographic *groups* is often a determinant of individual patterns of health behavior.

Health behavior can be categorized as *formal* or *informal*. Formal health behavior refers to the use of "structured" health services, including physician visits, hospital admissions, emergency room use, and so forth. Use of these services is also considered formal in that these events are typically recorded in some official manner. Most health care costs are accounted for by formal health behavior.

Informal health behavior involves actions taken for the prevention or treatment of health conditions, or for the maintenance or enhancement of health, that do not involve the use of formal services. These actions could be directly related to health conditions, involving such "self-care" activities as the use of over-the-counter pharmaceuticals, home diagnostic devices, and self-prescribed physical therapy. Informal health behavior would also include preventive actions taken that are related to health, such as oral hygiene and breast self-examination. Increasingly, health behavior has come to include actions that are even less directly related to health problems, but reflect the health implications of lifestyles. Thus, healthy diets, adequate exercise, adequate sleep, and moderate alcohol use are seen as actions that contribute to the maintenance or enhancement of health. Most of the examples in this article are related to the health implications of lifestyle patterns.

Although health behavior, as a distinct topic for analysis, has yet to attract the attention in Europe that it has in the United States, it is beginning to receive more interest from both research and intervention perspectives. There appear to be different approaches to these issues, for example, between continental western Europe, the British Isles, and the Scandinavian countries, although the move toward European unity appears to have engendered some convergence (Visser, 1993).

In the contemporary literature, a number of articles involve broad-scale community studies focusing on knowledge of health information and actual health behavior (O'Reilly & Shelley, 1991; Wardle & Steptoe, 1991). These include studies intended to measure factors that influence health behavior (Backett & Davidson, 1995; Peters & Robling, 1995; Steptoe & Wardle, 1992). Others are more focused in their research, targeting such areas of health concern as smoking (Piha, Besselink, & Lopez, 1993) and cancer education (Austoker, 1994). Another category of research reports on intervention strategies vis-à-vis health behavior and their impact (EURO Report Studies, 1988). In Italy, for example, several studies conducted by the National Institute of Statistics contain questions on smoking and alcohol consumption. The RIFLE (Risk Factors and Life Expectancy) project, which comprises a series of studies, focuses in part on health behaviors related to life expectancy.

This chapter begins by presenting six demographic predictions or forecasts for the United States for the year 2010. The discussion describes the factors that underlie these predictions and examines their implications for health behavior at the national (United States) level. These six demographic trends represent the major changes in the United States population that are likely to occur over the next 15 years. These trends are clearly interwoven with the social, economic, and political forces that are driving the future level of health services utilization, and with the manner in which health services are delivered.

The data used in this paper are based on the United States Census Bureau's 1994 middle-series population projections. The projections were produced by the cohort-component methodology, utilizing the 1992 population estimates by age, race, and sex as the base population. Projections were derived by varying the assumptions regarding future fertility rates, survival rates, and net immigration (Campbell, 1994, pp. xx–xxxiii). The middle-series projection assumed middle projections for all three components of change. Although in most ways the middle series is regarded as the "most likely" scenario, unforeseen events could alter these figures. Minor fluctuations in any or all of birth, death, and migration patterns (the only processes that can change the size and age structure of the population) have a relatively small impact on the national trends being described in the short term. At the local level, however, the short-term impact of such changes may be much greater. Today, health behaviorists must be able to make accurate distinctions between local and national trends if the dynamics of local conditions are to be clearly understood.

DEMOGRAPHIC TRENDS

Population Growth and Age Composition

Projecting population change is always a challenge for demographers. Recent fluctuations in the birth rate and increases in the number of immigrants make it even more challenging to forecast the size and age structure of the United States population. During the mid-1980s, birth rates and immigration flows were generally stable and demographers could feel reasonably confident about the accuracy of short-term population projections. At that time, many demographers projected a cessation of population growth for the United States, with a situation of zero population growth expected by around the middle of the 21st century. Immigration reform in the mid-1980s, however, which resulted in increased immigration flows, and an unexpected increase in fertility rates in the latter 1980s have made demographers much less confident about these projections (Ahlburg, 1993; Ahlburg & Vaupel, 1990). There is now a general consensus that the cessation-of-growth scenario envisioned by forecasters in the 1980s is no longer attainable in the near-term future (Pollard, 1994).

Table 1 presents population projections by age cohort for 2000 and 2010. Data from the 1990 Census of Population serve as a base for comparison. Although the United States population is projected to increase by 10.5% and 8.5%, respectively, during the 1990s and 2000s, these figures reflect the continued slowing of United States population growth rates. Growth rates during the 1960s, 1970s, and 1980s, in contrast, were 13.4%, 11.4%, and 9.8%, respectively.

Variations in the age structure of the population over time are much more marked than changes in population size or rate of growth. In general, population growth within the older age cohorts (age 55 and above), and particularly among the oldest old (age 85 and over), will be faster than that for the younger cohorts. Several younger cohorts, in fact, are likely to experience a net loss of or little increase in population. In the 20-year period covered, the population of age 85 years and over is expected to grow by 2.7 million (or by nearly 89%). At the leading edge of the baby boom, persons age 45–54 will increase by 18.7 million (or by 75%). Absolute losses are projected for the age group 25–34, showing a decline of 4.8 million persons (or 11%). Little numerical change will be experienced in the age cohorts under 5 years and 35–44.

As a result of these differential growth rates, the age structure in 2010 will be noticeably different from that observed in 1990. Persons age 55 and over made up 21% of the population (52 million persons) in 1990. By the year 2010, per-

Table 1. Most Recent Census Data and Population Projections for the United States: 1990, 2000, and 2010[a]

Age group	Population (in 1000s)					
	1990		2000		2010	
Under 5	18,758	(7.5%)	18,908	(6.9%)	19,730	(6.6%)
5–13	31,826	(12.8%)	36,051	(13.1%)	35,425	(11.9%)
14–17	13,340	(5.4%)	15,734	(5.7%)	16,908	(5.7%)
18–24	26,942	(10.8%)	26,117	(9.5%)	30,007	(10.1%)
25–34	43,161	(17.4%)	37,416	(13.6%)	38,367	(12.9%)
35–44	37,435	(15.1%)	44,662	(16.3%)	38,853	(13.0%)
45–54	25,057	(10.0%)	37,054	(13.5%)	43,737	(14.7%)
55–64	21,112	(8.5%)	23,988	(8.7%)	35,378	(11.9%)
65–74	18,045	(7.3%)	18,258	(6.6%)	21,235	(7.1%)
74–84	10,012	(4.0%)	12,339	(4.5%)	12,767	(4.3%)
85 and over	3,021	(1.2%)	4,289	(1.6%)	5,702	(1.9%)
TOTALS:	248,709		274,816		298,109	

[a]From Day (1992, Table 2).

sons in this age range will comprise over 25% of the population (75 million persons). The baby boom cohorts, age 25–44, comprised 32.5% of the population in 1990. In 2010, persons age 25–44 will constitute only 25.9% of the population. For those age 17 and younger, the decrease in representation will be from 25.7% to 24.2%.

Overall, the United States population may well grow by nearly 50 million persons between 1990 and 2010 and, at the same time, undergo considerable aging. As baby boomers move into the older ages after 2010, the momentum toward an increasingly older age structure will increase. Cohort-to-cohort differentials in growth rates will persist, however, as the result of fluctuating fertility rates, the effect of large cohorts moving through their childbearing years, and changes in immigration patterns.

Racial and Ethnic Composition

Population projections by race and ethnicity are presented in Table 2, utilizing approximately the same age categories as in Table 1. The racial and ethnic categories utilized adhere to Federal Statistical Directive No. 15, issued by the Office of Management and Budget. Anglos are non-Hispanic whites who are any of the original peoples of Europe, North Africa, or the Middle East. African-Americans (non-Hispanic) are persons

Table 2. Percentage of Population by Age and Race/Ethnicity: 2000 and 2010[a]

Age group		Anglo		African-American		Hispanic		Other		Total
				2000						
<18		23.1		32.0		33.9		29.6		25.7
18–24		8.8		11.1		11.6		10.7		9.5
25–34		12.8		14.3		17.0		16.6		13.6
35–44		16.4		15.7		15.7		16.5		16.3
45–54		14.5		11.6		9.9		12.0		13.5
55–64		9.6		6.9		5.7		7.2		8.7
65–74		7.6		4.8		3.7		4.6		6.6
75–84		5.3		2.6		1.9		2.2		4.5
85+		1.9		1.0		0.6		0.7		1.6
MEDIAN AGE:		38.4 yr		30.1 yr		28.1 yr		30.9 yr		35.6 yr
TOTAL POPULATION (1000s):	196,701	(71.6 %)	33,834	(12.3%)	30,602	(11.1%)	13,678	(5.0%)		274,816
				2010						
<18		21.0		30.6		32.0		28.4		24.2
18–24		9.4		11.6		11.9		10.8		10.0
25–34		12.1		13.3		14.9		15.3		12.9
35–44		12.7		12.8		14.2		15.1		13.0
45–54		15.6		13.2		12.2		12.6		14.7
55–64		13.4		9.6		7.6		8.9		11.9
65–74		8.3		5.2		4.1		5.2		7.1
75–84		5.1		2.6		2.3		2.7		4.3
85+		2.4		1.1		0.8		1.0		1.9
MEDIAN AGE:		40.9 yr		31.0 yr		29.2 yr		32.0 yr		37.5 yr
TOTAL POPULATION (1000s):	201,668	(67.6 %)	38,201	(12.9%)	39,312	(13.2%)	18,928	(8.3%)		298,109

[a]From: Day (1992, Table 2).

having origins in any of the black race groups of Africa. Hispanics (either white or black) are persons of Mexican, Puerto Rican, Cuban, Central or South American, or other Spanish culture or origin. "Other" refers to American Indians, Eskimos or Aleuts, and Asian and Pacific Islanders. Again, these are middle-series projections and are subject to the same caveats applicable to the data Table 1. Instead of presenting the raw numbers, Table 2 provides percentage breakdowns within each race/ethnicity category along with total population figures.

Although Anglos will remain the largest racial category in 2010, racial and ethnic minority populations are growing at a much faster rate. Between 2000 and 2010, the Anglo, African-American, Hispanic, and Other (mostly Asian) populations are projected to increase by 2.5%, 12.9%, 28.5%, and 38.4%, respectively. As a result of these differentials in growth rates, the Anglo proportion of the population will decline from 71.6% to 67.6%, while all other groups will increase their shares. By 2010, the three minority populations shown in Table 2 will comprise nearly one third of the total United States population; for certain age cohorts (e.g., the school-age population), their representation will exceed 40%.

These data also indicate substantial variation in age structure among the racial/ethnic groups. The Anglo population is by far the oldest and the Hispanic the youngest, with a projected difference of more than 10 years in median age in 2000 (38.4 versus 28.1 years). The differential widens to 11.7 years between 2000 and 2010 (40.9 versus 29.2). About one third of the African-American and Hispanic populations will be under age 18 in 2000, while fewer than 25% of the Anglo population will fall into this category. Although the percentage of population under age 18 will decline for all four racial/ethnic groups between 2000 and 2010, the rate of decline for Anglos will be greatest. Conversely, in 2000, over 24% of the Anglo population will be age 55 and over, compared to 15%, 12%, and 15% for African-Americans, Hispanics, and Others, respectively. By 2010, the gap in the proportion of age 55 and over widens:

Anglo, 29%; African-American, 19%; Hispanic, 15%; and Other, 18%. The Anglo population is not only the oldest of the four groups, but also is aging at a faster pace than the others.

Households and Families

A *household* is defined as one or more persons living in a housing unit; a *family* is composed of two or more persons living together in a housing unit who are related by blood, marriage, or adoption. All families are therefore also households, but not all households are families. Table 3 presents projections of households and families through 2010 based on the middle population projections series. The projections were produced by multiplying householder rates by age, sex, and race/ethnicity from the 1990 census by the age, sex, and race/ethnicity population projections produced by the United States Bureau of the Census. That is, the householder rates for 1990 are assumed to prevail for the entire population.

The total number of United States households is expected to increase of 22.6 million (or 25%) between 1990 and 2010. Differential rates of growth are seen, however, among the various household types. Overall, the number of family households will grow faster than that of nonfamily households (26% versus 22%). The fastest-growing household type will be single-parent households (DaVanzo & Rahman, 1993). Father-only or mother-only families (children present in both) are projected to grow by more than 34% over the 20-year interval. The absolute increase in mother-only families will exceed 2 million.

By the year 2010, nonfamily households will comprise about 28% of all households, down nearly one-half percentage point from 1990. As might be expected, the largest increase is projected to be among male-only or female-only households (no spouse present, with or without children). In 1990, these households made up nearly 15% (14 million) of all households. By 2010, this category is projected to make up about 16% (18 million) of all households. Although there will be significant growth in the number of

**Table 3. Number and Percent of Households by Type:
1990, 2000, and 2010[a]**

Household type	Households (in 1000s)			Change
	1990	2000	2010	
Family households:	65,329	73,899	82,099	25.7%
Married couple:				
With own children	24,512	27,909	31,199	27.3%
Without own children	27,156	30,110	32,825	20.9%
Male householder with no spouse present				
With own children	1,331	1,558	1,785	34.1%
Without own children	1,729	2,014	2,297	32.9%
Female householder with no spouse present				
With own children	6,031	7,061	8,086	34.1%
Without own children	4,570	5,247	5,907	29.3&
Nonfamily households	26,617	29,660	32,487	22.1%
TOTAL HOUSEHOLDS:	91,946	103,559	114,586	24.6%

[a]Unpublished data supplied by Steven Murdock, Texas A&M University. The data were produced by multiplying middle-series population projections by the current family/household structure (in percentage form) for the United States.

households over the 20-year period, the distribution by type of household is not expected to change markedly.

Fertility Variation

Fertility levels in the United States since World War II, can best be described as "variable." Year-to-year differences in the number of births are a consequence of the number of women in their childbearing years and the fertility rate characterizing these women. Table 4 presents the fluctuation in births in the United States from 1945 to 2010 in 5-year intervals. A relatively long historical perspective is taken because it captures the large post–World War II birth cohorts that have influenced so many demographic and nondemographic developments in the United States.

As can be seen, the annual number of births in the United States was relatively small in 1945, marking a continuation of the low Depression-era fertility rate. The data for 1950 show the beginning stage of the baby boom, which continued until 1964, the last year in which there were 4

**Table 4. Births to Women in the United States:
1945–2010[a]**

Year	Births (in millions)	Year	Births (in millions)
1945	2.9	1980	3.6
1950	3.6	1985	3.7
1955	4.1	1990	4.1
1960	4.3	1995	4.0
1965	3.8	2000	3.9
1970	3.7	2005	4.0
1975	3.1	2010	4.2

[a]From Pol and Thomas (1992, p. 157) and Day (1992, Figure 13).

million or more annual births in the postwar era. The baby boom reflected the large increase in birth rates resulting in part from the increased economic prosperity (Easterlin, 1968, 1976). The data from the later 1960s and the 1970s represent the period labeled the "baby bust." Both birth rates and the number of women in their childbearing years declined during this period. By 1975, the number of births had declined to 3.1 million annually (or 28%) from the peak of 4.3

million in 1960. The number of annual births increased, however, during the later 1970s. The 1980s were marked by "echo effect" fertility; that is, an increase in annual births resulted from the increase in the number of women in their child-bearing years without any increase in birth rates. The increase in annual births in the late 1980s was generated by an unexpected increase in birth rates.

Birth projections to the year 2010 show considerable variation as well. Although annual births are likely to continue to decrease during the 1990s decade, there will be an increase in annual births after the turn of the century. By 2010, there could well be as many births annually as there were at the peak of the baby boom. Moreover, projections beyond 2010 show a continued increase in births to as many as 5 million per year by the middle of the 21st century.

Life Expectancy

Life expectancy refers to the average number of years a group of persons can expect to live given current rates of mortality. Most often, life expectancy is expressed as years from birth, although calculations from any age can be useful. Table 5 presents data on life expectancy at birth for the United States population by sex and race. Overall, life expectancy is increasing and is projected to rise, albeit slowly, through 2010. Males

experienced a life expectancy increase of 4.7 years (from 67.1 to 71.8) between 1970 and 1990. The increase for males from 1990 to 2010 is projected to be only 2.4 years. African-Americans experienced the greatest increase, 5.0 years between 1970 and 1990, and are projected to show an increase of 3.1 years between 1990 and 2010.

In 1970, there were wide sex and age differentials in life expectancy: 7.6 years between males and females and 6.4 years between African-Americans and Anglos (data not shown in the table). Females and whites exhibited significantly greater life expectancy than males and African-Americans, respectively. As the decade draws to a close, these large differentials will persist, though the gap will have narrowed somewhat. Over the entire 40-year span (1970–2010), the African-American/Anglo differential for males is projected to decrease slightly, from 8.0 to 7.8 years; that for females is projected to decline more sharply, from 7.2 to 4.5 years.

While life expectancy at birth is an important measure of increased longevity, health demographers often study life expectancy at older ages. An examination of life expectancy at age 65, for example, contributes to a better understanding of the impact of developments in medical science and other factors on the life expectancy of the adult population. Between 1990 and 2010, life expectancy at age 65 is expected to increase from 15.4 to 17.4 years for white males (data not shown); i.e., 2.0 years of the 2.4-year increase in life expectancy at birth for white males shown in Table 5 will be due to increases at age 65 and above (Day, 1993, Table B-2). The same pattern is seen over this 20-year interval for white females (19.5 to 20.8 years). The increase for African-American males (14.0 to 14.9 years) and African-American females (18.0 to 18.9 years) is smaller, however, than the increase for white males and white females, respectively.

In sum, life expectancy at birth is projected to increase slowly through the year 2010. Large African-American/Anglo differences will persist, due largely to greater mortality among infants and young males within the African-American

Table 5. Life Expectancy at Birth by Race and Sex: 1970–2010[a]

	Total		White		African-American	
Year	Male	Female	Male	Female	Male	Female
1970	67.1	74.7	68.0	75.6	60.0	68.3
1980	70.0	77.4	70.7	78.1	63.8	72.5
1990	71.8	78.8	72.7	79.4	64.5	73.6
2000	73.0	80.0	73.9	80.5	66.5	75.8
2010	74.2	81.1	75.1	81.5	67.3	77.0

[a]From Day (1992, Table B-1) and U.S. Bureau of the Census (1993, Table 115).

population. The vast majority of anticipated life expectancy increases can be attributed to improved longevity at age 65 and over.

Regional Differentiation in Population Growth

The final projection involves differential growth rates among regional and divisional populations within the United States. Differences in projected growth are the product of variations in the initial size and age structure of the population (i.e., 1990), as well as variations in rates of fertility, mortality, and migration (both internal and international). The numbers of births and deaths fluctuate primarily as a result of variations in age structures. Table 6 presents population projections for the four regions and nine divisions of the United States for 2000 and 2010, beginning with the base-year population (1990). The Northeast region comprises two divisions: New England (Maine, Vermont, New Hampshire, Massachusetts, Connecticut, Rhode Island) and Middle Atlantic (New York, New Jersey, Pennsylvania). The Midwest region is made up of two divisions: East North Central (Wisconsin, Michigan, Illinois, In-

diana, Ohio) and West North Central (North Dakota, South Dakota, Minnesota, Iowa, Nebraska, Kansas, Missouri). Three divisions make up the South region: South Atlantic (Florida, Georgia, South Carolina, North Carolina, Virginia, West Virginia, Maryland, Delaware, District of Columbia), East South Central (Kentucky, Tennessee, Mississippi, Alabama), and West South Central (Oklahoma, Texas, Arkansas, Louisiana). The West region comprises two divisions: Mountain (Montana, Idaho, Wyoming, Nevada, Utah, Colorado, Arizona, New Mexico) and Pacific (Alaska, Hawaii, Washington, Oregon, California).

Overall, the population is projected to grow fastest in the South and West regions during the 20-year time interval, or by 21.6 million (25.3%) in the South and 20.3 million (38.4%) in the West. By comparison, the Northeast region is projected to increase by only 2.5 million (4.8%). The regional differences shown here are the result of significant growth rate variations by division and state (data not shown in table). For example, the New England division is projected to grow by only 550,000 persons (4.2%) over the 20-year interval compared to 5.4 million (39.0%) for the Mountain division.

Table 6. Populations Projections by Region and Division: 1990, 2000, and 2010[a]

Region and divisions	Population (in 1000s)					
	1990		2000		2010	
Northeast	50,837	(20.4%)	51,885	(18.8%)	53,301	(17.8%)
New England	13,204	(5.3%)	13,217	(4.8%)	13,754	(4.6%)
Middle Atlantic	37,663	(15.1%)	38,668	(14.0%)	39,547	(13.2%)
Midwest	59,781	(24.0%)	63,837	(23.1%)	66,332	(22.1%)
East North Central	42,091	(16.9%)	44,806	(16.2%)	46,258	(15.4%)
West North Central	17,690	(7.1%)	19,031	(6.9%)	20,074	(6.7%)
South	85,733	(34.3%)	97,242	(35.2%)	107,386	(35.7%)
South Atlantic	43,732	(17.5%)	50,004	(18.1%)	55,321	(18.4%)
East South Central	15,210	(6.1%)	16,762	(6.1%)	17,941	(6.0%)
West South Central	26,791	(10.7%)	30,476	(11.0%)	34,124	(11.3%)
West	53,039	(21.3%)	63,287	(22.9%)	73,412	(24.4%)
Mountain	13,734	(5.5%)	16,899	(6.1%)	19,094	(6.4%)
Pacific	39,305	(15.8%)	46,388	(16.8%)	54,318	(18.0%)

[a]From Campbell (1994, Table 1).

State differentials for population change are greater than regional/divisional differences and range from 47,000 (+2.6%) for West Virginia and 30,000 (+3.0%) for Rhode Island to 11.2 million (+37.5%) for California and 5.8 million (+34.0%) for Texas. Other high-growth states include Nevada (+58.9%) and Idaho (+43.5%).

The growth patterns shown in Table 6 are also driving a marked redistribution of the population. The Northeast and Midwest regions together are expected to decline from 44.4% of the total population to 39.8% between 1990 and 2010. The largest percentage losers will be the Middle Atlantic (−1.9%) and East North Central (−1.5%) divisions. The greatest percentage increases will be seen in the Pacific (2.2%), Mountain (0.9%), and South Atlantic (0.9%) divisions.

In summary, the growth rate of the United States population has slowed, though zero population growth is no longer in sight. The population is aging and becoming more diverse with respect to race/ethnicity and living arrangements. Regional and divisional variations in growth are evident, and although none of these geographic units is projected to lose population over the 20-year span, the populations of several individual states are likely to decrease.

The connection between health care issues and population size is clear: A larger population requires more health services, all other factors being equal. Everything else is not equal, however, and older and more racially/ethnically diverse populations have very different health services needs than younger, racially/ethnically homogeneous populations. Moreover, changing household structure (i.e., smaller households and more diverse household types) has serious implications for health care support services (e.g., in-home), as well as insurance provisions under our current system of health insurance coverage.

Conclusions

Much of the research in health demography and related fields such as epidemiology has fo-cused on the relationship between demographic characteristics and health status. The correlation between demographic variables such as age, sex, and race, on one hand, and the types and number of health conditions within a population, on the other, has been well documented. Thus, if one can determine the age and sex composition of a population group, for example, it becomes possible to estimate the prevalence of various conditions.

Less attention has been paid to the relationship between demographic characteristics and health behavior, although in many ways the ability to predict health behavior has more clear-cut practical implications than does the ability to predict the existence of health conditions. The ability to predict health behavior—particularly the use of formal health services— is critical for any health planning or marketing activities.

Health demographers and other researchers have identified associations between health behaviors of various types and a number of demographic variables (Pol & Thomas, 1992). The likelihood of utilizing formal health services is correlated with such variables as sex, age, and income, and this correlation applies to both the type and the level of health services utilization. Similarly, informal health behavior (e.g., use of over-the-counter remedies) can be linked to individuals in certain demographic categories. The same thing can be said of health-enhancing behaviors, such as diet and exercise. Lifestyle-related health behaviors are not randomly distributed within a population, but are more likely to occur among certain demographically defined groups than among others. The next section examines the link between demographic change, health behavior, and health care services in a more precise manner.

IMPLICATIONS FOR HEALTH BEHAVIOR AND HEALTH SERVICE PROVISION

As interesting as these trends may be, the important question becomes: What are the implications of these trends for health behavior? All of these factors have important implications for one aspect or another of health behavior. It is obvious that the elderly exhibit different patterns of health behavior than the young, that women exhibit different patterns of health behavior than men, that members of various racial and ethnic groups exhibit different patterns of health behavior than white Anglo-Saxon Protestant Americans, and that the rich and better educated exhibit different patterns of health behavior than the poor and uneducated. In fact, the married have different health behavior patterns than the unmarried, and those living in traditional households have different behavior patterns than those living in nontraditional household situations.

The changing age distribution is going to result in significant shifts in the demand for health services. The elderly obviously require and utilize more intensive services and a different set of medical specialists than do the nonelderly. Members of this age cohort are already driving the demand for specialized services in the areas of cardiology, oncology, and rheumatology. The large and aging baby boom cohort is beginning to demand "older adult services," including urology, gynecology, and chronic disease management.

It has been suggested, in fact, that the population is clearly divided in terms of health behavior on the basis of age (Thomas & Sehnert, 1989). A clear dividing line has been posited between the population born prior to World War II and the postwar age cohorts. The environment in which the older, prewar cohort developed was very traditional, emphasizing security, authority, and the sanctity of societal institutions, including the health care system. This population purchased indemnity insurance, followed doctor's orders, and did not ask too many questions. This generation had been convinced that individuals could do little to care for themselves or to control their destinies with regard to health. The only route to health was held to be through the formal health care system (Thomas & Sehnert, 1989).

The backgrounds of the postwar age cohorts are quite different, and this difference is reflected in health behavior. This age category, epitomized by the large baby boom cohort, grew up in unprecedented prosperity. It had many advantages that previous generations did not have. This postwar generation came to believe that it was in control of its destiny, and its members became convinced that they should have input into all aspects of their lives—including health care. This population has been responsible for changing behavior in terms of both the formal and the informal aspects of health care. Postwar generations have led the transformation from traditional forms of care to innovative forms, making possible the shift from indemnity insurance to health maintenance organizations, from inpatient care to ambulatory care, and from hospital emergency rooms to minor emergency centers. This population has also led the revolution in informal health behavior. Convinced that they could indeed control their destinies, baby boomers in particular have reasserted themselves in the management of their own bodies, forcing a shift toward more preventive care, and dramatically demonstrating the manner in which a change in lifestyles can affect health status (Thomas & Sehnert, 1989).

Females will increasingly dominate the patient population. For whatever reason, women are sick more often than men, and they use health services more frequently (Verbrugge, 1989). They already make most of the decisions with regard to health care, and the treatment of women will be a major issue within the health care system of the future. Increasingly, women want services tailored to their problems, needs, and lifestyles, and as female baby boomers emerge as a major patient population, these demands are going to intensify.

The dramatic shifts in fertility levels over the past three decades and those forecast into the 21st century have significant implications for the demand for health services. The United States has experienced a progression from modern-day record lows in the number of births in the 1960s and 1970s, to record highs in the late 1980s and early 1990s, to an anticipated decline through the first few years of the new century. The demand for obstetricians, which boomed in the 1980s, will drop dramatically (for at least 10 years). The demand for pediatric care, on the other hand, will remain high past the turn of the century and then drop off rapidly as the demand for obstetrical care increases again. Of course, the health services implications of a very irregular age structure have been noted above, since that irregularity is in part a function of fluctuating birth rates.

Perhaps the trend that is becoming most important in terms of its implications for health care is changing family and household structures. Individuals who are not married and do not live in traditional households tend to have more health problems and exhibit different health behaviors than do those who are married and live in traditional households (Umberson, 1987). This difference holds true for both physical and mental illness. Further, the unmarried not only get sick more often, but also suffer from more serious conditions and more complications than the married. The unmarried and members of nontraditional households tend to be less efficient utilizers of the system (health behavior) and are less likely to get the appropriate care at the appropriate time (Umberson, 1987). Perhaps even more important in these days of financial retrenchment, unmarried individuals and those in nontraditional households have much less ability to pay for health care. They tend to have lower incomes (meaning they are less able to pay out of pocket), and they are less likely to have employer-sponsored insurance. Most private insurance is predicated upon the existence of employed individuals with family insurance coverage. A lack of insurance affects health behavior in that uninsured persons are less likely to seek preventive care and more likely to seek care in the most expensive environments, hospital emergency rooms.

Members of various ethnic and racial groups offer a wide diversity in terms of their needs. Immigration has contributed to the variety of ethnic groups in United States society, and this variety has added another dimension to the health care demand picture. Because of nutritional practices and cultural preferences, these populations often suffer from conditions different from those usually treated by the present United States health care system (Pol & Thomas, 1992). Members of some of these groups are likely to display considerable apprehension toward a health care system that does not understand their cultures and lifestyles, and many may be openly hostile to any formal institution in society. The United States system must adapt itself to the needs of an increasingly diverse population and repackage its services to be responsive to the cultural backgrounds of many different groups (Thomas, 1993).

Some of these trends suggest higher levels of health services utilization; other trends suggest lower levels. As a result, the constellation of services demanded in the future will be quite different from that of the past, as will the type of patient. Patients will be older, more likely to be female, more ethnically diverse, less likely to live in a traditional family, and perhaps less able to pay for health care.

Changes in health behavior will have myriad implications for health care. New "products" (e.g., menopause management) must be developed and existing products (e.g., geriatric services) modified in keeping with the changing nature of the patient population. A new approach to the marketing of health care must emerge. Packaging will become critical, as products must be tailored to the diverse needs of the evolving patient population. "Price" will be an issue for the large segment of the population with an interest in elective procedures (i.e., the baby boomers); managed care programs will increasingly comparison shop for providers of health services. Distribution channels will become increasingly important with the continuation of trends to redistribute the population and restructure its composition. Various components of an increasingly diverse patient population are going to demand different settings and locales.

The promotion component of the marketing mix may be the most affected by changing demographic trends. The marketing approaches utilized will have to become more differentiated to accommodate a diversifying population. Market segmentation analysis will have to be refined in view of these trends, and the message as well as the medium will become critical for the future marketing of health services.

DEMOGRAPHIC CHANGE AND HEALTH BEHAVIOR

Health Behavior

This section explores the relationships between demographic change and specific health behaviors. First, nine selected health behaviors are presented with respect to a limited number of demographic correlates. The majority of the behaviors are related to some aspect of lifestyle, either in a positive (e.g., trying to lose weight) or a negative (e.g., smoke cigarettes) regard. Following this introduction, population-based projections of the aggregate number of behaviors are presented. The projections were generated by linking current incidence/prevalence rates for the nine selected behaviors with population projections such as those presented in Table 1. The population projections utilized are from the Census Bureau's middle series for 2000 and 2010 and are subject to the same caveats discussed earlier.

Demographic Correlates of Nine Health Behaviors

Table 7 contains estimates of the number of dental visits by age of person in 1989. The data were derived from the National Health Interview Survey (NHIS), a sample survey designed to be representative of the United States civilian, non-institutionalized population. The age categories in the table reflect usage differentials while retaining a significant level of age detail. As can be seen, the number of annual visits varies considerably by age, starting with 0.9 visits per year for ages 2–4 and rising to 2.8 for ages 12–17. A

Table 7. Average Annual Dental Visits by Age: 1989[a]

Age group	Average annual visits	Age group	Average annual visits
2–4	0.9	35–44	2.2
5–11	2.1	45–54	2.3
12–17	2.8	55–64	2.4
18–24	1.6	65–74	2.2
25–34	1.9	75 and over	1.8

[a]From Bloom, Gift, and Jack (1992).

decline follows, then another increase at ages 35–44, and another decline at ages 65 and over.

Table 8 presents data on smokers by age and sex, for three annual periods, 1965, 1985, and 1991. The age categories in the table are those available in published reports. The data come from the NHIS. Clearly, there has been a reduction in the prevalence of smoking since 1965 among all ages and both sexes. Since 1965, more

Table 8. Percentages of Persons Who Were Cigarette Smokers by Age and Sex: 1965, 1985, and 1991[a]

Age and sex	Smokers (%)		
	1965	1985	1991
Male			
12–17	NA	NA	11.8
18–24	54.1	28.0	23.5
25–34	60.7	38.2	32.8
35–44	58.2	37.6	33.1
45–64	51.9	33.4	29.3
65 years and over	28.5	19.6	15.1
Female			
12–17	NA	NA	9.8
18–24	38.1	30.4	22.4
25–34	43.7	32.0	28.4
35–44	43.7	31.5	27.6
45–64	32.0	29.9	24.6
65 years and over	9.6	13.5	12.0

[a]From U.S. Bureau of the Census (1993, Tables 209 and 210). A cigarette smokers is defined as a person who has smoked at least 100 cigarettes and currently smokes. (NA) Data not available.

over, there has been a significant narrowing in the prevalence of smoking between females and males. Despite these changes, there continue to be large differentials in smoking prevalence by age and sex. Male percentages are greater than female percentages at all ages. Both sexes show a rise in incidence from the youngest ages to a peak between the ages of 25 and 44, followed by a decrease at the oldest ages.

The percentages of persons who in 1991 were current users of alcohol, marijuana, and cocaine, cross-classified by age and sex, are presented in Table 9. The National Household Survey on Drug Abuse is the source of the data. In addition to the large prevalence rate differences across drug categories, there are wide intradrug variations by age and sex. In all categories, females show lower prevalence rates than males. Moreover, the highest prevalence is for the ages 18–25 or 26–34. For example, marijuana use is seen in 5.0% of the male population aged 12–17, peaks at 15.7% at ages 18–25, and declines to 3.0% of the population aged 35 and over.

Table 10 provides data for 1990 on four additional health behaviors (one is a combination of health behavior and health status): percentage of persons who are at least 20% over desired body weight, percentage of overweight persons trying to lose weight, percentage of persons who exercise or play sports regularly, and percentage of persons who in the last year drove their car at least once when they thought that they had too much to drink. The data come from the National Household Survey on Drug Abuse.

Once again, there are wide differentials in behavior by age and sex. For example, while 46% of the overweight male population age 18–29 were trying to lose weight, 65% of the overweight female population age 18–29 were trying to lose weight. In general, males were more likely to be overweight, less likely to be trying to lose weight, more likely to exercise or play sports regularly, and more likely to have driven a car at least once when they thought they had too much to drink. There are, however, significant intrasex-age differentials in the percentages as well.

Behavior Projections

Tables 11–14 provide projections of aggregate behaviors derived by multiplying the age-/sex-specific numbers and percentages seen in Tables 7–10 by the age/sex population projections presented in Day (1992). The behavior projections assumed that behavior incidence/prevalence measures would remain constant and that the population projections are accurate. Given that neither of these assumptions is likely to hold, the health behavior projections should be seen as illustrative of the effect that demographic change can have on the total number of persons engaging in various types of health behavior.

Table 11 presents projections for dental visits. The 62.7 million increase in the number of visits (12.6%) is the result of the changing size and age composition of the United States population between 1990 and 2000. The 52.8 million increase in visits between 2000 and 2010 (9.4%) marks a decline in the percentage rise in visits due to a slowing of population growth. In fact, if the population were to retain the 1990 age distribution for the years 2000 and 2010, there would be a reduction in visits of 6.9 and 10.6 million, respec-

Table 9. Percentages of Persons Who Were Current Users of Alcohol, Marijuana, and Cocaine by Age and Sex: 1991[a]

	Current users (%)		
Age and sex	Alcohol	Marijuana	Cocaine
Male			
12–17	22.3	5.0	0.5
18–25	69.7	15.7	2.8
26–34	70.8	9.5	2.6
35 years and over	57.4	3.0	0.6
Female			
12–17	18.2	3.7	0.3
18–25	57.8	10.5	1.3
26–34	52.8	4.5	1.1
35 years and over	42.5	1.3	0.3

[a]From U.S. Bureau of the Census. (1994).

Table 10. Selected Health Behaviors by Age and Sex: 1990[a]

| Behavior | Manifesting the behavior (%) | | | | | | | |
| | Male | | | | Female | | | |
	18–29	30–44	45–64	65+	18–29	30–44	45–64	65+
At least 20% over desired body weight[b]	20.1	32.0	37.8	26.3	15.9	24.7	34.2	28.2
Overweight persons trying to lose weight	45.6	45.8	44.7	40.1	65.0	66.9	63.6	48.8
Exercise or play sports regularly	56.1	44.3	35.6	36.9	44.2	40.1	34.6	29.1
Drove a car at least once in the past year when they thought they had too much to drink	24.5	17.0	9.7	3.7	13.4	8.0	2.7	2.0

[a]From Schoenborn and Schoenborn (1993).
[b]By Metropolitan Life Insurance standards for height and sex.

tively. In other words, not only would population growth increase the number of visits, but also a favorable change in age structure would lead to an additional increase. In 2000, 11% of the projected increase from 1990 is due to the favorable change in age structure; in 2010, the age structure effect over the decade accounts for 20% of the increase.

Projections of current smokers are presented in Table 12. As can be seen, increases are pro-

Table 11. Projected Dental Visits by Age: 1990, 2000, and 2010[a]

| Age group | Number of visits (in 1000s) | | |
	1990	2000	2010
2–4	10,069	10,560	10,715
5–11	52,937	60,207	58,642
12–17	56,118	66,326	71,893
18–24	42,781	41,458	48,352
25–34	82,034	72,650	72,540
35–44	82,674	99,271	87,250
45–54	58,013	83,191	101,428
55–64	50,755	56,856	82,925
65–74	39,835	40,812	46,152
75 and over	23,643	30,188	34,427
TOTALS:	498,859	561,519	614,324

[a]The projections were produced by multiplying age-specific visit figures from Table 7 by age-specific population projections from Day (1992).

jected for both sexes and all ages, although the increase between 2000 and 2010 is somewhat slower than for the previous decade. Total male smokers increase from 26.0 to 28.9 million (2.9 million, or 11.1%) between 1990 and 2000 and from 28.9 to 31.9 (3.0 million, or 10.4%) in the following decade. In this instance, however, the changing age structure is "unfavorable" to the total number of smokers. That is, were the 1990 age structure to stay constant through 2000 and 2010, there would be 2.0 and 0.6 million more male smokers, respectively, than the figures projected in Table 12. As the result of the changing age structure, there is a reduction of 6.9% and 1.8%, respectively, in the number of male smokers.

CONCLUSIONS

Although population growth rates are slowing, the absolute increases anticipated in the number of persons and households portend significant demographic change over the next 15 years. Moreover, shifts in the compositional characteristics of the population will assure even greater demographic diversity. The relatively rapid aging of the population, increasing racial and ethnic diversity, and continued household restructuring are but three of the trends contributing to marked shifts in health behavior. All

Table 12. Projected Number of Current Cigarette Smokers by Age and Sex: 1990, 2000, and 2010[a]

| Age and sex | Number of smokers (in 1000s) | | | | | |
| | 1990 | | 2000 | | 2010 | |
	Male	Female	Male	Female	Male	Female
12-17	1,213	956	1,435	1,130	1,557	1,223
18-24	3,200	2,939	3,097	2,853	3,615	3,324
25-34	7,076	6,135	6,251	5,447	6,229	5,449
35-44	6,155	5,240	7,423	6,264	6,494	5,530
45-64	6,536	5,920	8,501	7,588	11,448	9,943
65 and over	1,897	2,241	2,205	2,486	2,593	2,752
TOTALS:	26,077	23,431	28,912	25,768	31,936	28,221

[a]The projections were produced by multiplying age/sex-specific percentages from Table 8 (1991) by age/sex-specific populations from Day (1992).

Table 13. Projected Numbers of Alcohol, Marijuana, and Cocaine Users by Age and Sex: 1990, 2000, and 2010[a]

| Age and sex | Users (in 1000s) | | | | | |
| | 1990 | | 2000 | | 2010 | |
	Male	Female	Male	Female	Male	Female
	Alcohol					
12-17	2,293	1,776	2,712	2,099	2,942	2,271
18-25	9,490	7,584	10,369	8,336	12,101	9,709
26-34	15,274	11,406	12,291	9,235	12,044	9,096
35 and over	30,689	26,234	37,908	31,562	43,546	35,440
TOTALS:	57,746	47,000	63,280	51,232	70,633	56,516
	Marijuana					
12-17	514	361	608	427	660	462
18-25	2,138	1,378	2,336	1,514	2,726	1,764
26-34	2,049	972	1,649	787	1,616	775
35 and over	1,604	802	1,981	965	2,276	1,084
TOTALS:	6,305	3,513	6,574	3,693	7,278	4,085
	Cocaine					
12-17	51	29	61	35	66	37
18-25	381	171	417	187	486	218
26-34	561	238	451	192	442	190
35 and over	321	185	1,325	637	1,449	695
TOTALS:	1,314	623	2,254	1,051	2,443	1,140

[a]The projections were produced by multiplying age/sex-specific percentages from Table 9 by age/sex-specific populations from Day (1992).

Table 14. Projected Numbers Manifesting Selected Behaviors by Age and Sex: 1990, 2000, and 2010[a]

| Age and sex | Numbers (in 1000s) | | | | | |
| | 1990 | | 2000 | | 2010 | |
	Male	Female	Male	Female	Male	Female
At least 20% over desired body weight						
18–29	4,887	3,774	4,493	3,486	5,075	3,932
30–44	9,431	7,403	10,338	8,073	9,198	7,246
45–64	8,432	8,230	10,967	10,549	14,769	13,823
65 and over	3,304	5,267	3,841	5,843	4,516	6,467
TOTALS:	26,054	24,674	29,639	27,951	33,558	31,468
Overweight and trying to lose weight						
18–29	2,229	2,454	2,050	2,267	2,315	2,557
30–44	4,321	4,951	4,736	5,399	4,214	4,846
45–64	3,772	5,234	4,906	6,709	6,607	8,790
65 and over	1,324	23,115	1,539	25,643	1,810	28,382
TOTALS:	11,646	35,754	13,231	40,018	14,946	44,575
Exercise or play sport regularly						
18–29	13,639	10,492	12,542	9,690	14,164	10,931
30–44	13,056	12,018	14,311	13,106	12,734	11,763
45–64	7,941	8,326	10,329	10,673	13,909	13,984
65 and over	4,636	5,435	5,388	6,030	6,337	6,674
TOTALS:	39,272	36,271	42,570	39,499	47,144	43,352
Drive a car at least once in the past year when they thought they had too much to drink						
18–29	5,956	3,181	5,477	2,938	6,186	3,314
30–44	5,010	2,398	5,492	2,615	4,887	2,347
45–64	2,164	650	2,814	833	3,790	1,091
65 and over	465	373	540	414	635	459
TOTALS:	13,595	6,602	14,323	6,800	15,498	7,211

[a]The projections were produced by multiplying age/sex-specific behavior rates from Table 10 by age/sex-specific populations from Day (1993).

components of the health care delivery network will have to respond to these shifts if the needs of the "new" health care market are to be met.

National-level trends are important, but most health planning decisions are made at the local level. Demographic change at the local level is much faster and more dramatic than the patterns observed for the nation as a whole. In the last decade, shortages in the availability of health services have been observed in rapidly growing states such as Florida, as well as in rural areas that have undergone depopulation. In other instances, e.g., many suburban areas, shifts in population, real or expected, or both real and expected, have resulted in an overreaction on the part of the medical community, with a subsequent oversupply of health care services.

Health care researchers, planners, and marketers made significant progress in incorporating demographic change into their conceptual models during the last decade. In the future, however, health professionals must be able to anticipate demographic shifts in order to more accurately predict service needs. Health professionals need to better understand how demographic change is produced, so as to improve predictions of health behaviors and subsequent determination of health care needs at the local market level. With no in-depth knowledge of how and why demographic change occurs, health professionals will have to rely on predictions they cannot explain. A broad understanding of how and why demographic change occurs will assist in the evaluation of data that are purchased from vendors (e.g., population projections) and assist in the conceptual development of information systems for the support of planning and operational functions. In the future health care environment, this knowledge will no longer be in the nice-to-know category. An in-depth understanding of complex demographic processes will be essential for survival.

From a health care provider perspective, three important issues emerge. First, changes in some aggregated health behavior, e.g., the number of persons who visit the dentist in a year, are products of the propensity to visit a health service provider and changing demographic conditions (e.g., size and age structure). While promotional efforts may increase the incidence of dental visits, the force of demographic change is substantial and irrespective of promotional efforts may change a market in a positive or negative way. As discussed earlier, demographic changes at the local level may have an even greater marketplace impact than those at the national level.

Second, not all persons who engage in particular types of health behaviors are the same. In particular, differences by age—e.g., of persons who visit the dentist—have serious ramifications for the types of services provided. The increasingly old dental visit population seen in Table 11 is likely to have a lesser need for preventive services, as compared to younger patients, and a

greater emphasis on dental surgeries to address the chronic problems seen in an older population.

Third, a combination of health-related behavior propensities and shifting demographic structure can produce a substantial market for other health services. For example, the data seen in Table 10 showing an increase by age in the percentage of persons at least 20% over desired body weight are clearly linked to the recent surge in the market for a number of diet plans ranging from physically safe to dangerous. Given that this percentage peaks at ages 45–64, and that this age cohort is projected to increase substantially in size over the next two decades, one can expect a booming market for diet plans for some time to come.

ACKNOWLEDGMENTS. The authors wish to thank Jackie Lynch for her assistance in the preparation of this chapter. The authors would also like to thank Steven Murdock for providing data on projections of households and families.

REFERENCES

Ahlburg, D. A. (1993). The census bureau's new projections of the U.S. population. *Population and Development Review*, *19*(1), 159–174.

Ahlburg, D., & Vaupel, J. (1990). Alternative projections of the U.S. population. *Demography*, *27*(4), 639–652.

Austoker, J. (1994). Cancer prevention: Setting the scene. *British Medical Journal*, *308*(May), 1415–1420.

Backett, K. C., & Davison, C. (1995). Lifecourse and lifestyle: The social and cultural location of health behaviours. *Social Science and Medicine*, *40*(5), 629–638.

Bean, A., & Talaga, J. (1991). Appointment breaking: Causes and solutions. *Journal of Health Care Marketing*, *12*(4), 14–25.

Bloom, B., Gift, H. C., & Jack, S. S. (1992). Dental services and oral health: United States, 1989. *Vital and health statistics*, Series 10, No. 183. Hyattsville, MD: National Center for Health Statistics.

Braus, P. (1994). Nursing homes: The hard facts. *American Demographics*, *16*(3), 46–47.

Campbell, P.C. (1994). Population projections for states, by age, sex, race and Hispanic origin: 1993 to 2050. *Current population reports*, Series P-25, No. 1111. Washington, DC: U.S. Government Printing Office.

Crimmins, E. M., Hayward, M. D., & Saito, Y. (1994). Changing mortality and morbidity rates and the health status and life expectancy of the older population. *Demography, 31*(1), 159-175.

DaVanzo, J., & Rahman, O. (1993). American families: Trends and correlates. *Population Index, 59*(3), 350-386.

Day, J. C. (1992). Population projections of the United States, by age, race and Hispanic origin: 1992-2050. *Current population reports*, Series P-25, No. 1092. Washington, DC: U. S. Government Printing Office.

Day, J. C. (1993). Population projections of the United States, by age, race and Hispanic origin: 1993-2050. *Current population reports*, Series P-25, No. 1104. Washington, DC: U.S. Government Printing Office.

Easterlin, R. (1968). *Population, labor force and long swings in economic growth*. New York: National Bureau of Economic Research.

Easterlin, R. (1976). What will 1984 be like? Socioeconomic implications of recent twists in age structure. *Demography, 15*(4), 397-432.

EURO Report Studies. (1988). *Comprehensive cardiovascular community control programmes in Europe, 106*, 1-91.

Herbig, P., & Koehler, W. (1993). Implications of the baby bust generation upon the health care market. *Health Marketing Quarterly, 10*(3/4), 23-29.

Manton, K., Corder, L. S., & Stallard, E. (1993). Estimates of change in chronic disability and institutional incidence and prevalence rates in the U.S. elderly population from the 1982, 1984 and 1989 National Long Term Care Survey. *Journal of Gerontology, 48*(5), 170-182.

McDaniel, C., Gates, R., & Lamb, C. (1992). Who leaves the service area? Profiling the hospital outshopper. *Journal of Health Care Marketing, 12*(3), 2-9.

O'Reilly, O., & Shelley, E. (1991). The Kilkenny post-primary schools survey: A survey of knowledge, attitudes and behaviour relevant to non-communicable diseases. *Irish Journal of Medical Science, 160*(Supplement 9), 40-44.

Piha, T., Besselink, E., & Lopez, A. D. (1993). Tobacco or health. *World health statistics*. Copenhagen: WHO Regional Office for Europe.

Pill, R., Peters, T. J., & Robling, M. R. (1995). Social class and preventive health behaviour: A British example. *Journal of Epidemiology and Community Health, 49*(1), 28-32.

Pol, L. G., & Thomas, R. K. (1992). *The demography of health and health care*. New York: Plenum Press.

Pollard, K. M. (1994). Population stabilization no longer in sight for U. S. *Population Today, 22*(5). Washington, DC: Population Reference Bureau.

Schoenborn, A., & Schoenborn, C. A. (1993). Health promotion and disease prevention: United States, 1990. *Vital and health statistics*, Series 10, No. 185. Hyattsville, MD: National Center for Health Statistics.

Sherer, J. (1993). Age wave. *Hospitals and Health Networks, 67*(15), 40, 54.

Steptoe, A., & Wardle, J. (1992). Cognitive predictors of health behaviour in contrasting regions of Europe. *British Journal of Clinical Psychology, 31*(4), 485-502.

Thomas, R. K. (1993). *Health care consumers in the 1990s*. Ithaca, NY: American Demographic Books.

Thomas, R. K., & Pol, L. G. (1993). Health demography comes of age. *Health Marketing Quarterly, 10*(3/4), 67-82.

Thomas, R. K., & Sehnert, W. F. (1989). The dual health care market. *American Demographics, 11*(April), 46-47.

Umberson, D. (1987). Family status and health behaviors: Social control as a dimension of social integration. *Journal of Health and Social Behavior, 30*(September), 306-319.

U. S. Bureau of the Census. (1993). *Statistical abstract of the United States, 1993*. Washington, DC: U.S. Government Printing Office.

U.S. Bureau of Census. (1994). *Statistical abstract of the United States, 1994*, Table 209. Washington, DC: U.S. Government Printing Office.

Verbrugge, L. M. (1989). The twain meet: Empirical evidence of sex differences in health and mortality. *Journal of Health and Social Behavior, 30*(September), 282-304.

Visser, A. P. (1993). Patient education in health psychology: A pan-European perspective. *Patient Education Counselor, 22*(3), 115.

Wardle, J., & Steptoe, A. (1991). The European health and behaviour survey: Rationale, methods, and initial results from the United Kingdom. *Social Science and Medicine, 33*(8), 925-36.

II

HEALTH BEHAVIOR AND
THE HUMAN LIFE SPAN

HEALTH BEHAVIOR AND
HUMAN DEVELOPMENT

While there are abundant studies of health beliefs and health behaviors at different age periods from very early childhood through senescence, issues of developmental and life-span change have been underemphasized in health behavior research (e.g., Bruhn & Parcel, 1982; Drotar et al., 1989; Susman, Dorn, Feagans, & Ray, 1992). Although there is some evidence of expected developmental changes in cognitions about the causes of disease (Nagy, 1953), body parts (Gellert, 1962), definitions and conceptions of health and illness (Natapoff, 1982; Rashkis, 1965; Simeonsson, Buckley, & Monson, 1979), and perceived vulnerability to health problems and health motivation (Gochman, 1986), there remain large gaps in understanding of the origins, determinants, and developmental changes of broad ranges of health beliefs and behaviors. Burbach and Peterson (1986) remark that in contrast to the abundance of research over a long period of time on the dynamics of illness, there have been far fewer studies—and they are much more recent in origin—of the developmental studies of health-related cognitions. Block, Block, and Keyes (1988), making note of the longitudinal developmental studies already reported in the literature, comment that these studies do not begin early enough

in life—rarely with respondents younger than 13—and that they follow respondents for only relatively short periods of time.

Much of the research done on "developmentally" defined populations attempts to define correlates of health behavior rather than their developmental foundations. A major portion of the research conducted on young populations deals with the acquisition of risk behaviors, such as drug and alcohol consumption, smoking, unprotected sex, and inappropriate eating, and with injury and safety behaviors. In contrast, a major portion of the research conducted in older populations deals with perceptions of health status and use of services. Critical issues in developmental research on health behavior are risk perceptions, complexity of influences, and mechanisms that underlie change.

RISK PERCEPTIONS

In the context of the great risks faced by young persons from use of drugs, smoking, sexual behavior, and vehicular injuries, perceptions of risk in young persons have emerged as an important area of health behavior research. Yet, in one series of cross-sectional and longitudinal assessments of health-related expectations in a young population aged between 8 and 17 derived from the health belief model (e.g., Gochman, 1986; Gochman & Sauçier, 1982), beliefs about vulnerability were seen to be remarkably consistent and stable during the years of childhood and adolescence. Average levels of perceived vulnerability hovered around a point of neutrality, indicating that young populations do not see themselves as either vulnerable or invulnerable to a range of health problems. Nor do other data suggest that adolescents demonstrate either a healthy or a risky lifestyle (Terre, Ghiselli, Taloney, & DeSouza, 1992).

Although evidence based on different calculations of risk suggests that adolescents are unrealistically optimistic about health-threatening risks, it is unclear that they differ greatly from adults in this attitude (Cohn, Macfarlane, Yanez, & Imai, 1995). Like adults, adolescents may exhibit an optimistic bias. The dynamics of perceived risks in relation to HIV/AIDS among adolescents may involve nonrational tendencies to deal with threat by denial or avoidance (Gladis, Michela, Walter, & Vaughn, 1992).

Adolescent perceptions of risk for HIV/AIDS are also influenced by social and cultural factors. Strunin (1991) notes ethnic and racial differences in levels of risk perception: The results of both telephone and school surveys suggest that Asian and Hispanic adolescents had higher levels of perceived risk than whites or blacks. Strunin urges more research on the nature of the social environment in which adolescents live, including economic and ideological contexts, to improve understanding of their risk perceptions.

COMPLEXITY OF INFLUENCES

Initiation of drug use is complexly determined. In adolescents, it is related to prior use of licit substances, such as tobacco and alcohol (Bailey, 1992), as well as to peer and parental factors. The relative impact of parental and peer factors, however, changes developmentally; parental attachment influences initiation among younger adolescents, while peer pressure exerts greater effects on older ones (Bailey & Hubbard, 1990).

Studies of the interactive effect of social influences on drug use (e.g., Stacy, Newcomb, & Bentler, 1992) reveal the importance of certain mediating or buffering variables. The degree to which an adolescent is susceptible to social influence is an important factor that mediates the initiation of drug usage, as is the congruence between ideological beliefs and social norms; liberal beliefs, which attenuated the importance of social conformity, acted as a buffer against peer influences to cocaine and marijuana use (Stacy et al., 1992).

Flay and his colleagues (e.g., Flay et al., 1994) have developed a structural model of smoking escalation that analyzes parental, peer, and ethnic influences on initiation and maintenance of smoking. Ennett and Bauman (1993) examine the interplay between social isolation and social networks as determinants of smoking and identify the need to examine social networks beyond the immediate school environment.

Adolescents engage in high levels of sexual behavior that puts them at risk for AIDS/HIV, other sexually transmitted diseases, and pregnancy. Both parental monitoring and peer perceptions were related to adolescent use of condoms, and while knowledge about risks increased with age, it is apparently unrelated to risk activity (Romer et al., 1994). Cultural factors also influence adolescent sexual risk behaviors. For example, Mexican-American teenage females are less likely to have had intercourse than their non-Hispanic white counterparts, but more likely to have a live birth if they become pregnant (Aneshensel, Fielder, & Becerra, 1989).

The complexity of influences can also be seen in eating, dieting, and nutritional behaviors, which are major focuses in health behavior research in young populations. A large-scale study of more than 30,000 adolescents revealed that problem eating behaviors such as binging and purging were linked to body image and that eating problems in general were linked to use of tobacco and alcohol, suicide risk, and peer acceptance, and negatively related to family connectedness (French, Story, Downes, Resnick, & Blum, 1995).

Safety and injury-related activities are also a major health focus of health behavior research in young populations. The interactions of parental education, other family and community characteristics, and personal factors in injury risk have been explored by Pless, Verreault, and Tenina (1989). Peterson and her colleagues (e.g., Peterson, Farmer, & Kashani, 1990; Peterson, Gillies, Cook, Schick, & Little, 1994) have examined parental, developmental, and cognitive factors underlying childhood injury and injury-related risk behavior.

A multiplicity of factors also underlie some protective behaviors. Sunscreen use among a random sample of more than 15,000 Norwegian high school students was found to have multiple predictors, including risk perceptions, opportunities to sunbathe, appearance motivation, gender, peer influences such as friends' use of sunscreens, and friends' tanning behavior (Wichstrøm, 1994).

Among older populations, the complexity of influences on health behaviors can be seen in the participation rates in health promotion programs for "seniors," which are apparently influenced by mental and social status more than by physical health indices (Buchner & Pearson, 1989). Those elderly who participated apparently had lower mental and social status ratings than nonparticipants, but did not differ in physical health. Data suggesting that the elderly tend to underestimate the importance of nervousness, headaches, depression, and nausea also reveal the complex interactions between perceptions of risk, degree of physician contact, use of alternative sources of care, family discussion, and the media involved in perception and reporting of symptoms in the elderly (Stoller, Forster, Pollow, & Tisdale, 1993).

MECHANISMS THAT UNDERLIE CHANGE

The mechanisms that underlie the acquisition of health behaviors and their changes with development have not yet been clearly identified, nor is there any emerging consensus about these mechanisms. Several productive frameworks, however, have been proposed.

On the basis of data gathered in Norway and Wales under World Health Organization auspices, Nutbeam, Aarø, and Catford (1989) propose a framework for understanding the developmental changes in young people's health behavior. Their framework includes the health belief model as well as social learning theory, behavioral intention theory, and environmental opportunities and constraints, including concepts such as the supply and demand for health-enhancing versus health-damaging goods.

Chassin and her colleagues (e.g., Chassin, Presson, Sherman, & Edwards, 1992) highlight the importance of role issues, such as being a student, married, or employed, in the emergence of smoking behavior, and introduce concepts of role incompatibility and "pseudomaturity"—acquiring marital and occupational roles as a result of attenuating the student role. Other role issues are introduced by Peterson and her colleagues (e.g., Peterson et al., 1990), who demonstrate the importance of parental beliefs in relation to parents engaging in the role of health educator in injury prevention.

The concepts of *enduring family socialization*, *lifelong openness*, and *windows of vulnerability* have been proposed by Lau, Quadrel, and Hartman (1990) to explain the development of, and changes in, health-related cognitions. Enduring family socialization suggests that health cognitions are learned within the family during childhood, that parents have primary influence on these cognitions, and that the cognitions remain relatively stable throughout adulthood. Lifelong openness suggests that health cognitions change over a lifetime and are influenced by a range of socializing agents. The concept of windows of vulnerability suggests that parental influence will continue in the absence of other potent socializing agents during critical developmental periods.

In Chapter 2, Prohaska and Clark employ the concept of developmental and life transitions as a framework for discussing the prevalence and stability of a range of health behaviors across the life span, noting the differential importance at different ages of selected theoretical models.

In Chapter 3, O'Brien and Bush emphasize the implications for health behavior of the developmental differences between the cognitive processes of children and adults. The chapter further stresses the importance of the personal, family, social, and institutional determinants in the development of preventive and risk behaviors and in responses to treatment.

In Chapter 4, Cowell and Marks integrate conceptually derived and clinically derived observations on health behavior in adolescents and show the complex relationships between developmental transitions and personal, family, social, and economic factors in a range of health behaviors.

In Chapter 5, Rakowski emphasizes the critical role of both behavioral and psychosocial epidemiology in understanding health behaviors in the elderly and stresses the importance of information seeking as a mediating factor.

REFERENCES

Aneshensel, C. S., Fielder, E. P., & Becerra, R. M. (1989). Fertility and fertility-related behavior among Mexican-American and non-Hispanic white female adolescents. *Journal of Health and Social Behavior*, *30*, 56–76.

Bailey, S. L. (1992). Adolescents' multisubstance use patterns: The role of heavy alcohol and cigarette use. *American Journal of Public Health*, *82*, 1220–1224.

Bailey, S. L., & Hubbard, R. L. (1990). Developmental variation in the context of marijuana initiation among adolescents. *Journal of Health and Social Behavior*, *31*, 58–70.

Block, J., Block, J. H., & Keyes, S. (1988). Longitudinally foretelling drug usage in adolescence: Early childhood personality and environmental precursors. *Child Development*, *59*, 336–355.

Bruhn, J. G., & Parcel, G. S . (1982). Current knowledge about the health behavior of young children: A conference summary. In D. S. Gochman & G. S. Parcel (Eds.), *Children's health beliefs and health behaviors. Health Education Quarterly*, *9*, 142–166.

Buchner, D. M., & Pearson, D. C. (1989). Factors associated with participation in a community senior health promotion program: A pilot study. *American Journal of Public Health*, *79*, 775–777.

Burbach, D. J., & Peterson, L. (1986). Children's concepts of physical illness: A reward and critique of the cognitive-developmental literature. *Health Psychology*, *5*, 307–325.

Chassin, L., Presson, C. C., Sherman, S. J., & Edwards, D. A. (1992). The natural history of cigarette smoking and young adult social roles. *Journal of Health and Social Behavior*, *33*, 328–347.

Cohn, L. D., Macfarlane, S., Yanez, C., & Imai, W. K. (1995). Risk-perception: Differences between adolescents and adults. *Health Psychology*, *14*, 217–222.

Drotar, D., Johnson, S. B., Iannotti, R., Krasnegor, N., Matthews, K. A., Melamed, B. G., Millstein, S., Peterson, R. A., Popiel, D., & Routh, D. K. (1989). Child health psychology. In A. Baum (Ed.), *Proceedings of the National Working Conference on Research in Health and Behavior* [Special Issue]. *Health Psychology*, *8*, 781–784.

Ennett, S. T., & Bauman, K. E. (1993). Peer group structure and adolescent cigarette smoking: A social network analysis. *Journal of Health and Social Behavior*, *34*, 226–236.

Flay, B. R., Hu, F. B., Siddiqui, O., Day, L. E., Hedeker, D., Petraitis, J., Richardson, J., & Sussman, S. (1994). Differential influence of parental smoking and friends' smoking on adolescent initiation and escalation of smoking. *Journal of Health and Social Behavior*, *35*, 248–265.

French, S. A., Story, M., Downes, B., Resnick, M. D., & Blum, R. W. (1995). Frequent dieting among adolescents: Psychosocial and health behavior correlates. *American Journal of Public Health*, *85*, 695–701.

Gellert, E. (1962). Children's conceptions of the content and functions of the human body. *Genetic Psychology Monographs*, *61*, 293–405.

Gladis, M. M., Michela, J. L., Walter, H. J., & Vaughn, R. D. (1992). High school students' perceptions of AIDS risk: Realistic appraisal or motivated denial? *Health Psychology*, *11*, 307–336.

Gochman, D. S. (1986). *Youngsters' health cognitions: Cross-sectional and longitudinal analyses*. Louisville, KY: Health Behavior Systems.

Gochman, D. S., & Saucier, J.-F. (1982). Perceived vulnerability in children and adolescents. In D. S. Gochman & G. S. Parcel (Eds.), *Children's health beliefs and health behaviors. Health Education Quarterly* [Special Issue]. *9*(2–3), 46–59.

Lau, R. R., Quadrel, M. J., & Hartman, K. A. (1990). Development and change of young adults' preventive health beliefs and behavior: Influence from parents and peers. *Journal of Health and Social Behavior*, *31*, 240–259.

Nagy, M. H. (1953). The representation of "germs" by children. *Journal of Genetic Psychology*, *83*, 227–240.

Natapoff, J. N. (1982). A developmental analysis of children's ideas of health. In D. S. Gochman & G. S. Parcel (Eds.), *Children's health beliefs and health behaviors. Health Education Quarterly* [Special Issue], *9*(2–3), 34–45.

Nutbeam, D., Aarø, L., & Catford, J. (1989). Understanding children's health behaviour: The implications for health promotion for young people. *Social Science and Medicine*, *29*, 317–325.

Peterson, L., Farmer, J., & Kashani, J. H. (1990). Parental injury prevention endeavors: A function of health beliefs? *Health Psychology*, *9*, 177–191.

Peterson, L., Gillies, R., Cook, S. C., Schick, B., & Little, T. (1994). Developmental patterns of expected consequences for simulated bicycle injury events. *Health Psychology*, *13*, 218–223.

Pless, I. B., Verreault, R., & Tenina, S. (1989). A case–control study of pedestrian and bicyclist injuries in childhood. *American Journal of Public Health*, *79*, 995–998.

Rashkis, S. R. (1965). Children's understanding of health. *Archives of General Psychiatry*, *12*, 10–17.

Romer, D., Black, M., Ricardo, I., Feigelman, S., Kaljee, L., Galbraith, J., Nesbit, R., Nornik, R. C., & Stanton, B. (1994). Social influences on the sexual behavior of youth at risk for HIV exposure. *American Journal of Public Health*, *84*, 977–985.

Simeonsson, R. J., Buckley, L., & Monson, L. (1979). Conceptions of illness causality in hospitalized children. *Journal of Pediatric Psychology*, *4*, 77–84.

Stacy, A. W., Newcomb, M. D., & Bentler, P. M. (1992). Interactive and higher-order effects of social influences on drug use. *Journal of Health and Social Behavior*, *33*, 226–241.

Stoller, E. P., Forster, L. E., Pollow, R., & Tisdale, W. A. (1993). Lay evaluation of symptoms by older people: An assessment of potential risk. *Health Education Quarterly*, *20*, 505–522.

Strunin, L. (1991). Adolescents' perceptions of risk for HIV infection: Implications for future research. *Social Science and Medicine*, *32*, 221–228.

Susman, E. J., Dorn, L. D., Feagans, L. V., & Ray, W. J. (1992). Historical and theoretical perspectives on behavioral health in children and adolescents: An introduction. In E. J. Susman, L. V. Feagans, & W. J. Ray, (Eds.), *Emotion, cognition, health, and development in children and adolescents* (pp. 1–8). Hillsdale, NJ: Erlbaum.

Terre, L., Ghiselli, W., Taloney, L., & DeSouza, E. (1992). Demographics, affect, and adolescents' health behaviors. *Adolescence*, *27*, 13–24.

Wichstrøm, L. (1994). Predictors of Norwegian adolescents' sunbathing and use of sunscreen. *Health Psychology*, *13*, 412–420.

2

Health Behavior and the Human Life Cycle

Thomas R. Prohaska and Melissa A. Clark

INTRODUCTION

Research in health behavior has shown considerable growth since the mid-1970s. During this growth, researchers and practitioners have focused primarily on health practices and interventions within age-specific groups and special "at-risk" populations. Researchers and practitioners have addressed health behaviors associated with maternal and child health (Boyd & Windsor, 1993), adolescent populations (Cowell & Montgomery, 1993), young adult and college-age populations (Gottlieb & Baker, 1986) and middle-age, and more recently, older adults in community settings (Gliden, Hendryx, Casia, & Singh, 1989) and nursing homes (Fiatarone et al., 1990). Even with this emphasis on special populations, noted Gottlieb and Green (1987), much of the research to date has concentrated primarily on younger, white, motivated, middle-class populations.

Thomas R. Prohaska and Melissa A. Clark • Department of Community Health Sciences, School of Public Health, University of Illinois at Chicago, Chicago, Illinois 60612.

Handbook of Health Behavior Research III: Demography, Development, and Diversity, edited by David S. Gochman. Plenum Press, New York, 1997.

There are situations in which it is quite appropriate to investigate health practices and to design health promotion interventions for specific populations across limited age ranges of the life span. First, there are critical periods in the life of an individual when health risk factors are particularly harmful. For example, inappropriate health behaviors by a woman during pregnancy, especially during the first trimester, can have serious consequences for prenatal development of the child (Prager, Malin, Spiegler, Van Natta, & Placeck, 1984). Also, there are specific time periods for an individual when inappropriate health practices are likely to develop and prevention is a priority. Initiation of smoking during childhood or adolescence, for example, results in a higher likelihood that tobacco use will continue into adulthood (Flay, d'Avernas, Best, Kersell, & Ryan, 1983). Finally, it is appropriate to target health education interventions to catchment areas in which specific age groups are likely to predominate, such as schools (Kolbe & Iverson, 1984), worksites (Nathan, 1984), and senior centers (Rubenstein, Josephson, Nichol-Seamons, & Robins, 1986).

There are benefits, however, to adopting a life-span approach to health behaviors and health education. The life-span perspective is defined in terms of individual development as measured by chronological age and experiences of biological and social role transitions (e.g., puberty, parenthood, caregiving, and loss of spouse). This perspective allows an examination of how transitions in various developmental life stages may account for changes in health practices. Bulcroft, Bulcroft, and Borgotta (1994) noted that current health education intervention strategies give little consideration to family role transitions as facilitators of self-initiated changes in health practices. They argue that health practices are most heavily influenced in the context of developing and changing family roles over the life course.

The adoption of a life-span perspective on health practices provides an opportunity to examine not only the incidence and prevalence of health risk factors over the entire life span, but also the continuity and discontinuity of these practices. Unfortunately, while there is some information on the stability of health practices across limited ranges of the life span (Breslow & Engstrom, 1980; Rakowski, 1987), there is little knowledge of the personal history of the individual in terms of initiation and maintenance of specific health practices. It is possible that while a health practice may remain stable, the factors that control a specific health or risk behavior may change over the life span of the individual (Leventhal, Prohaska, & Hirschman, 1985).

A life-span perspective allows examination of the utility of theoretical constructs influencing health practices across age groups and over the life course. For example, the health belief model has been shown to predict preventive health behaviors and sick role behaviors across a wide age range (Janz & Becker, 1984). It is unclear, however, whether the health belief model and other cognitively based models of health behavior have differential predictive power at various points in the life span. Also, the validity of theoretical constructs that comprise models of health behavior change has not been well documented across all segments of the life span. It is therefore not well known whether constructs such as peer pressure, perception of stress, and social support operate exactly the same way across the entire life span. A life-span perspective may facilitate the application of successful age-specific models or health education programs to other age groups.

A life-span approach allows examination of the relative success of health education interventions across age groups and over the life course. Leventhal et al. (1985) noted that little is known about differences between various age groups (e.g., young versus old) in successfully completing health promotion programs. Health education interventions such as community-based smoking cessation programs have provided evidence that older individuals show success (quit rates) comparable to that of other age groups (Clark, Kuiz, Prohaska, Crittenden, & Warnecke, 1992). There are still few reported findings, however, regarding the relative impact of health promotion programs across wide age ranges and during life transitions.

This chapter examines life-span topics and issues associated with health practices. The issues are organized around four basic questions that guide much of the research in health promotion:

1. What is the incidence and prevalence of health practices across the life span?
2. Do major life transitions influence the stability of health practices?
3. How do health practices affect the health and well-being of individuals across the life span?
4. What are the mechanisms that control health practices at various points in the life span?

PREVALENCE AND STABILITY OF HEALTH PRACTICES THROUGHOUT THE LIFE SPAN

Health Practices Survey Methodology

What is known about incidence and prevalence rates of health practices is primarily based on large national surveys and smaller regional and local surveys using both cross-sectional and longitudinal methods. Findings on health practices from national surveys typically rely on self-reported health practices and often focus on broad segments of the life span. For example, the National Health Interview Survey of Health Promotion and Disease Prevention (U.S. Department of Health and Human Services [USDHHS], 1986) included adults age 18 and older, and the Behavioral Risk Factor Survey (BRFS) was based on heads of household 18 years of age and older (Frazier, Franks, & Sanderson, 1992). There are also national surveys of health practices for younger populations (Johnston, O'Malley, & Bachman, 1989; Kann et al., 1993). These surveys of health practices for younger populations are often based on school rosters and sample the population by grade levels.

National surveys frequently are cross-sectional in design and usually report only current health practices, and therefore, report findings on prevalence rather than incidence rates of health practices. Furthermore, prevalence rates from these national surveys are frequently aggregated by basic demographic characteristics such as age, gender, and race, with little attention to life transitions (e.g., puberty, parenthood, becoming a caregiver, loss of spouse).

The majority of the regional surveys are also cross-sectional and inquire only about current health practices. A number of such surveys, however, are longitudinal. These surveys are helpful in providing insight into changes in health practices over time and the relationships between health practices and subsequent health status. Two of the most widely known regional surveys of this type are the Alameda County Population Studies (Berkman & Breslow, 1983) and the Framingham Heart Study (Dawber, 1980). The duration of these longitudinal surveys (beginning in 1965 for Alameda County and 1950 for the Framingham Study) has allowed them to provide considerable information about health practices over extended periods of time and for a wide age range.

Prevalence of Health Practices across Age Groups

National data on prevalence rates (and incidence rates) of health practices in younger children are scarce. A conference review of the state of knowledge on health practices in young children acknowledged the paucity of information on the early development of health practices in young children (Bruhn & Parcel, 1982). The conference identified four major areas in which gaps in knowledge of health behavior in young children need to be addressed: (1) family influences, (2) developmental and psychological characteristics of the child, (3) children's health behavior, and (4) indicators of children's health status (Bruhn & Parcel, 1982).

The 1991 Youth Risk Behavior Survey provides national data on the prevalence of health risk behavior among adolescents age 12–19 years. While this survey is based on a restricted age range, age patterns are evident. Exercise, as measured by enrollment in physical education classes and self-reported moderate physical activity, significantly decreased between the 9th and 12th grades (Kann et al., 1993). Conversely, cigarette smoking and use of other addictive substances were positively associated with increasing grade level. Self-reported regular cigarette use (1 cigarette per day for 30 days) increased from 17% of the 9th-grade students to 24% of the 12th-grade students. On the positive side, the prevalence of fighting decreased with increase in grade such that 12th-grade students were significantly less likely to carry a weapon than 9th- and 11th grade students. Regular use of seat belts remained relatively constant across grades at 23–29% (Kann et al., 1993). Results from this same data source show that the adolescents who did not attend school, 9% of the total sample, were more likely to engage in inappropriate health behaviors such as carrying a weapon, cigarette smoking, and alcohol use (*Morbidity and Mortality Weekly Report*, 1994).

Estimates from the National Health Interview Survey of Health Promotion and Disease

Prevention (USDHHS, 1986), the National Survey of Personal Health Practices and Consequences (USDHHS 1981a,b), and regional surveys have shown considerable variation among adult age groups in the performance of specific health practices. The list of health practices varies considerably across surveys, although many are based on seven health risk behaviors developed for the Alameda County Population Survey: never smoking cigarettes, regular physical activity, moderate or no use of alcohol, 7–8 hours of sleep per night, maintaining weight, eating breakfast, and not eating between meals (Berkman & Breslow, 1983).

Prevalence rates for heath practices reported in the National Health Interview Survey (Supplement on Health Promotion and Disease Prevention) are reported by adult age groups (18–29 years, 30–44 years, 45–64 years, and 65 years and older). Many of the appropriate health practices show a general increase in prevalence rates with age. Compared to persons age 30–64 years, those age 65 years and older are more likely to report never having smoked cigarettes and are less likely to be heavy smokers (25 cigarettes per day). Older adults are also more likely than younger adults to abstain from alcohol, drink in moderation, eat breakfast regularly, and obtain general medical exams (Thornberry, Wilson, & Golden, 1986). In contrast, younger persons are more likely to participate in regular physical activity, especially vigorous activity, and are more likely to report a recent medical screening such as a Pap smear or a breast examination. Age patterns in exercise activities in the NHIS sample are in agreement with other sources showing that 43% of older adults reportedly engage in no leisure time activity, while one third of America's older adult population participates in moderate physical activity (e.g., walking gardening) and fewer than 10% participate in vigorous physical activity (USDHHS, 1990; *Healthy People, 2000*, 1991).

In general, the prevalence rates of health practices by age reported in the National Health Interview Survey are in agreement with findings from the National Survey of Personal Health Practices and Consequences (Rakowski, 1988). Preva-

lence rates of various health practices from regional surveys are also in general agreement with the national surveys. For example, Prohaska, Leventhal, Leventhal, and Keller (1985) found that compared to younger respondents (18–64 years), community-residing elderly (65 years and older) from a Midwest city reported higher frequencies of health-promoting actions (avoidance of salt, regular sleep, and eating a balanced diet), but were less likely to exercise regularly.

Stability of Health Practices across the Life Span

What is known about the stability of health practices over the life course of an individual? A life-span perspective on this question can be helpful in determining key transitions in the individual's life when changes in health practices are likely to occur. These transitions may provide windows of opportunity for intervention. Also, stability of a negative health behavior does not necessarily imply inability to change; rather, it suggests the necessity for additional efforts in health education.

Childhood and adolescent years are times for considerable changes in health behaviors, including development of specific health practices and experimentation with risk behaviors. Although based on a cross-sectional design, findings from the 1991 Youth Risk Behavior Survey suggested considerable instability in adolescent health practices (Kann et al., 1993). Tschann et al. (1994) also provided evidence on the extent of instability of health practices in the adolescent years. They followed 6th- and 7th-grade students (mean age 12.4 years) to examine the initiation of substance use and found that 25% of their student sample tried one or more substances (cigarettes, alcohol, marijuana) at first assessment and that within 1 year, 81% had used one or more substances. Research on the stability of health practices in childhood and adolescent populations over longer periods of time suggests a weak association with health practices in young adulthood. Mechanic (1979) examined the stability of health practices including smoking, exercise, alcohol use, and risk taking in children (1st-, 4th-, and 7th-grade students) over a 16-year period and reported a low level of continuity over time. Unfortunately, the 16-year interval and inconsistency in defining health practices over the two assessments makes it difficult to draw strong conclusions about the stability of health practices during the transition from childhood to early adulthood.

In one of the few national studies to address the stability of health behaviors across age groups in an adult population over a 1-year period, Rakowski (1987) examined data from Wave 1 (1979) and Wave 2 (1980) of the National Survey of Personal Health Practices. Considerable consistency was found between the two assessment periods for most of the nine activities studied (recency of seeing a dentist, physician, and having an eye exam; limiting red meat; use of seat belts; taking long walks; use of dental floss or water pick; number of free-time activities; and a composite score based on items from the Alameda County Population Study health practice index). Compared to the demographic and social psychological predictors, self-reported behaviors in Wave 1 were by far the strongest predictors of the corresponding measures at Wave 2. Little evidence was found for age differences in the stability of health activities over the 1-year period.

Findings from the Alameda County Population Study on behavioral risk factors also provide evidence for stability of health practices for adults over extended periods of time (Breslow & Engstrom, 1980). The seven health practices were combined into a composite score (0 to 7) and were assessed at two time periods, 9½ years apart (1965–1974). The authors concluded: "Although no information is available for the intervening years, it does seem that the extent to which the health habits are practiced is reasonably stable. People seemed to maintain about the same number of health habits in 1974 as they did in 1965, the average being 4.9 in both surveys" (p. 472). It is difficult to draw conclusions about the stability

of *specific* health practices over time, since health practices were combined into a composite score (0 to 7 health practices). Therefore, although the number of health habits may have remained relatively constant, some types of health behaviors may have been replaced by others during the duration of the study. Also, the considerable time between interviews (9½ years) makes it difficult to provide insight into short-term stability of health practices in individuals. Although the authors sampled adults age 20 years and older (younger than age 20 years if married), they did not report this stability of health practices for specific age groups. Finally, the Alameda County Population Study contains information on life transitions such as marital status, employment status, change in household composition, and widowhood, but no findings have been reported to date on the relationship between these transitions and health practices.

Research and Methodological Issues

Issues such as selective survival, cohort effects, and historical influences confound knowledge of age patterns in health practices. It is not appropriate to conclude that age *differences* in health practices based on cross-sectional findings reflect age *changes* in these health practices. Clearly, selective survival may account for some of the apparent improvement in self-reported health practices with age. The relationship between health practices and mortality is not constant across the life span. The loss of those with poor health practices through selective survival is less likely in the childhood and young adulthood years than it is in middle-age and older adults. The length of time individuals perform inappropriate health practices is also a factor in determining risk, and this duration is not equally distributed across the life span. For instance, in a community-based study of smokers aged 18–29, 30–49, and 50 years or older, the mean number of smoking years reported by subjects was 8, 20, and 41 years, respectively (Kviz, Clark, Crittenden, Freels, & Warnecke, 1994). Age differences in the association between inappropriate health practices and poor health may therefore be confounded with the length of time the individual has been engaging in health risk behavior.

Historical influences and cohort effects may also contribute to the patterns of health practices observed in both cross-sectional and longitudinal surveys of health practices. For example, the low prevalence of cigarette smoking by the current cohort of older women may be due, in part, to the social norms that deterred women from smoking at the time many would have adopted the behavior. Cohort and historical factors may also influence the patterns we currently see in childhood and adolescent health practices.

Another source of difficulty in determining age patterns in health practices stems from methodological and conceptual differences between surveys of health practices. These are inconsistencies in the time between health practice assessments and differences in the operational definitions of health practices. The period between health behavior assessments can vary considerably, and lengthy time intervals between assessments make it difficult to draw conclusions about short-term stability in health practices. Researchers have often concluded that the best predictor of performance of a health activity is past performance (e.g., Mullen, Hersey, & Iverson, 1987; Rakowski, 1987). Findings from the 1991 Youth Risk Behavior Survey, however, demonstrate how greatly health practices can vary over a short period of time during specific segments of the life span (Kann et al., 1993). Sequential strategies designed to disentangle age, period, and cohort effects may be necessary to determine developmental life-span changes in health practices (Baltes, Reese, & Nesselroade, 1977).

Conclusions

There is a complicated pattern of stability and instability of health practices over the life span. Early childhood and adolescent years appear to be times of health practice development, experimentation, and considerable change. Health practices in the adult years appear to be more stable. There is clearly a lack of information, however, on how life transitions within age groups account for observed changes in health practices. For example, observed changes in diet in an older adult may be due to the loss of a spouse rather than an age-associated change per se. There are also major gaps in knowledge regarding individual health behavior over specific segments of the life span. For instance, there is very little information on individual health practices during the transition from high school to young adulthood. This lack could be due to differences in methodology when conducting survey research in school-based populations and community-based samples. That is, selection methods for surveying health practices in children are frequently based on school rosters, while community-based surveys of adults use strategies such as random digit dialing and household surveys. Finally, there is a paucity of knowledge regarding the development of health practices in the early childhood years.

Previous research on health practices across the life span has primarily examined age patterns and difference in health practices. It has neglected to consider changes in health practices *within* age groups as they experience biological and social role transitions. Next, this chapter addresses how health practice patterns may be associated with these life-span transitions.

HEALTH PRACTICES AND LIFE TRANSITIONS

There are major transitions throughout the life span. These transitions often mark turning points in the life course of the individual and may include both biological and social role changes. Theoretical perspectives describing life stages and transitions throughout the life course include Erikson's theory of identity development (Erikson, 1959) and family role development (Bulcroft et al., 1994; Duval, 1971). Rather than discuss how these models may be used to address health practices, this chapter will select major transition points in the life span and discuss the influence of these transitions on health practices. The life transitions discussed include the onset of puberty, transition to parenthood, becoming a caregiver for an older relative, and loss of spouse. While these transitions are not all of the major biological and social role transitions across the life span, they are life transitions shared by large proportions of the population.

Puberty

The major biological and social role transition during adolescence is puberty. The timing of and transition through puberty have been associated with changes in health practices. Tschann et al. (1994) reported an association between smoking and the timing of puberty in that early pubertal maturers reported more substance use (cigarettes, alcohol, marijuana) within the year following puberty compared with later-maturing adolescents. This association held for both males and females. Smoking patterns during this transition may result from both biological and social factors. For instance, Bauman, Foshee, and Haley (1992) reported an association between adolescent smoking activity, testosterone level, and peer and parent smoking behavior. The positive association between the smoking status of adolescents and the smoking status of their same-gender parent was greater for individuals with higher testosterone levels. Regardless of testosterone level, however, the positive association between adolescent's smoking status and the smoking status of their friends remained high.

Sexual risk-taking behavior is weakly associated with the transition of puberty. For males, increases in testosterone are associated with sexual behavior (Udry, 1988), while the association between sexual behavior and hormonal levels has not been found to be linked in females (Udry, Talbert, & Morris, 1986). Based on a review of determinants of adolescent initiation of sexual behaviors, Morris (1992, p. 121), concluded: "Within the normal range of hormone levels, it is

not currently possible to predict which individuals are those who will exhibit a high frequency of sexual behaviors or the opposite." She suggests that a biosocial integration model may be more appropriate than any one model for understanding sexual risk-taking behavior in adolescent populations.

Parenthood

The time of pregnancy and parenthood is one of the most researched areas regarding health practices and life transitions. Most of the research on modifications of health practices, however, has focused on the mother rather than the father. Prevalence rates of inappropriate health practices are often high in women just prior to pregnancy. Over 50% of women report drinking alcohol in the 3 months prior to becoming pregnant, and 30% of women are cigarette smokers when they become pregnant (Bruce, Adams, Shulman, & Martin, 1993; Prager et al., 1984).

There is evidence that a substantial proportion of women quit or cut back on cigarette smoking during their pregnancy. O'Campo, Faden, Brown, and Gielen (1992) examined the impact of pregnancy on women's prenatal and postpartum smoking behavior. They reported that 32% of the women were smoking before becoming pregnant, and 41% of these women quit smoking during pregnancy. Three of four mothers who quit smoking during the pregnancy cited fear of adverse pregnancy outcomes and infant health problems as the main reason for quitting. The majority of those who continued to smoke through the pregnancy reported reducing cigarette consumption by smoking fewer cigarettes or changing to cigarettes lower in tar or nicotine). A total of 39% of the mothers who had quit during their pregnancy relapsed by 6–12 weeks postpartum.

Dramatic reductions in alcohol use during pregnancy have also been reported. Bruce et al. (1993) noted that over half of the pregnant women surveyed reported drinking alcohol in the 3 months prior to their pregnancy, but over three quarters of them had stopped drinking by the last 3 months of their pregnancy.

Very little is known about how the transition into parenthood influences health practices of fathers. Richmond, Rospenda, and Kelly (in press) examined alcohol abuse across the transition to parenthood in married couples. They reported that while only 2% of the fathers reported problems with alcohol prior to learning of the pregnancy, 13% of fathers self-reported problems with alcohol in the 6-month period following childbirth. In contrast to non–problem drinkers, problem drinkers reported feeling less comfortable sharing their feelings about parenthood. The authors cautioned that these findings are based on a small nonrepresentative sample and suggest future directions for research. It would be of value to examine multiple health practices and follow both parents prospectively through the transition of parenthood.

Caregiving

Caring for a frail older member of the family is a life transition that is experienced by a considerable proportion of the population (Glick, 1977). Perhaps as much as 80% of the care provided to the frail elderly is provided by family and other informal sources (Shanas, 1979). The number of years a primary caregiver (usually a wife or daughter) devotes to the care of a frail relative is comparable to the number of years parents devote to raising their own families (Watkins & Kligman, 1993). Often, the caregiver has the responsibility of simultaneously caring for children and an older relative (Brody, 1990). While the burden and health consequences for the caregiver during this life transition are well documented, relatively little is known about the effect of this transition on health practices of middle-aged or older caregivers. In one study, Burton, Schulz, German, Hirsch, and Mittlemark (1994) investigated the effect of caring for a spouse on lifestyle health practices of the caregiver. Using data from the National Caregiving Health Effects Study, they compared married adults who were caring for a spouse with impairments in activities of daily living to married individuals who were not caring for a spouse. A larger proportion of the caregivers reported significantly less time for exercise, rest, or their own health concerns.

Loss of Spouse

The loss of a spouse is a major life transition experienced by a significant proportion of the population, especially older married couples. Older women are much more likely than older men to lose a spouse, with nearly half of all women age 65 and older being widowed (U.S. Bureau of the Census, 1988). Loss of a spouse can have severe psychological, social, and economic consequences (Gallager, Thompson, & Peterson, 1981–1982). A primary focus of the research regarding loss of spouse has been on the subsequent health status of the widowed person (Murrell, Himmelfarb, & Phifer, 1988). While there have been suggested explanations for changes in health of the widowed person, such as stress reaction and joint unfavorable health environments, few studies have proposed that modifications in health practices may account for the deteriorating health of widowed persons.

Loss of spouse and the bereavement process have been linked with changes in nutritional intake. Rosenbloom and Whittington (1993) used recorded dietary intakes to compare changes in eating behaviors in adults age 60 years and older who had recently been widowed to same-age adults whose spouses were still living. Compared to individuals with spouses still living, widows reported a loss of appetite and a lack of enjoyment for eating meals. Widowed subjects were more likely to show unintentional weight loss and were less likely to use vitamin and mineral supplements. The authors noted that greater levels of grief were associated with adverse eating behaviors. These findings are compatible with those of other studies demonstrating that decreases in caloric intake and body weight follow stressful life events in older adults (Willis, Thomas, Garry, & Goodwin, 1987).

Closely associated with the life transition of losing one's spouse are the consequences that living alone has for health practices. Over 80% of the elderly living alone are likely to be widowed (Louis Harris and Associates, 1986). More than 31% of older adults age 65 and older residing in the community live alone, and over 20% of them report difficulties with basic and instrumental activities of daily living, such as difficulties with mobility, meal preparation, and eating (Prohaska, Mermelstein, Miller, & Jack, 1993). These activities of daily living are basic to the independence of the individual, and the inability to conduct these self-care activities is associated with nursing home placement. The loss of one's spouse may result in an older individual's losing an assistant for activities of daily living. For example, the older husband who has difficulty with meal preparation and mobility may eat a proper diet and remain active with assistance provided by his wife. The death of his wife may deprive him of assistance; as a result, his diet and activity levels may be compromised.

Conclusions

The studies described suggest that life transitions may be occasions for both voluntary and involuntary changes in health practices, focusing on four representative life transitions: puberty, transition to parenthood, becoming a caregiver, and the loss of a spouse. Other life transitions such as a young adult's leaving home, menopause, and retirement may also influence health practices.

Other life-stage approaches have been proposed to explain influences on health practices. For example, Bulcroft et al. (1994) proposed that transitions in the individual in relation to the family cycle provide occasions for changes in health practices. They asserted that stages in the family cycle such as being young and married without children or being married with preschool children impose on the individual demands that may reduce the likelihood that the individual will engage in positive health practices.

Timing of the life transition may be a major factor contributing to changes in health practices. Tschann et al. (1994) demonstrate that early pubertal maturers reported more substance abuse. Similarly, Richmond et al. (in press) suggested that fathers who are not ready to accept their new role as parent may increase their use of alcohol. Neugarten's concept of "on-time" and "off-time" of life events may be useful in determining how the timing of life transitions influences health practices (Neugarten, Moore, & Lowel, 1975). It may be that life transitions that are early in onset or unexpected face individuals with challenges they may not be prepared to meet. For example, assuming the role of caregiver early in life when demands of children and career are high may be particularly challenging and may result in changes in self-care activities and health practices. Life transitions have been associated with changes in health-promoting practices and health risk behaviors. These life transitions should be viewed as opportunities for health education interventions to promote and support positive changes in health practices and to focus prevention strategies for health risk behaviors.

The chapter next turns to the third area of health behavior across the life span, the association between health practices and health status.

EFFECTS OF HEALTH PRACTICES ON HEALTH THROUGHOUT THE LIFE SPAN

Conceptual Underpinnings

The definition of health behaviors implies that these practices are either directly or indirectly associated with health outcomes. That is, the relationships between health practices and health can be inferred from their associations with measures of health, as in the outcomes of observational studies. On the other hand, associations can be directly linked through controlled trials of health practices, with the outcomes of an intervention being subsequent changes in health. While many of the associations between health practices and health make intuitive sense, looking at these associations across the life span demonstrates how complicated these relationships can be.

Basic questions about the relationship between health practices and health throughout the life span have yet to be fully addressed. For example, does a health risk behavior for a younger adult have the same or greater health consequences for an older adult? Do inappropriate health practices by individuals in life transitions such as pregnancy or while providing care for a frail relative have greater adverse effects on health than such practices have on the health of persons of similar age not experiencing the life transition?

Determining the relationships between health practices and health status typically involves population-based epidemiological and behavioral science research designs. In observational studies, individuals who exhibit the health practice are compared to a group who do not (e.g., exercisers and nonexercisers; cigarette smokers and nonsmokers). Health status characteristics such as morbidity and mortality of the two groups are then compared. If the health practice does not have a significant association with the health measures, the rates of adverse health problems should be comparable between those who do and do not engage in the health behavior. If, however, the behavior is associated with a greater likelihood of poor health, then the group with the inappropriate behavior should have a greater percentage of people with health problems, leading to the conclusion that the behavior is a risk factor contributing to the health of the general population. The ratio of adverse health consequences between groups who do and do not manifest the health behavior is often referred to as the *relative risk* associated with the health practice. Often, the association between health practices and health status is not consistent when relative risks are examined

across the life span (Kaplan, Seeman, Cohen, Knudsen, & Guralnik, 1987).

It is also important to examine the association between *multiple* health practices (or health practice indices) and health outcomes throughout the life span. The advantage of studying multiple health practices is the opportunity it provides to assess their potential additive impact on the individual's health, given that health consequences are often additive for multiple health risk behaviors (Breslow & Engstrom, 1980). Another advantage of examining multiple health practices within a population is that it allows making direct comparisons of health risks across health practices. For example, findings from the Alameda County Study provide estimates of risk for all-cause mortality associated with multiple health behaviors including cigarette smoking and maintaining relative weight within a community sample age 60 years and older (Kaplan et al., 1987). Given that multiple health practices were assessed in the same population, estimates of relative risk for mortality across health practices are possible. The authors reported that the relative risk for mortality was greater for current smoking than it was for not maintaining moderate weight.

The concept of attributable risk is also particularly important in understanding the association between health risk behaviors and health outcomes across the life span. Attributable risk measures the amount of disease (disability or mortality) in a high-risk group that could be eliminated if that risk factor were eliminated. A measure of attributable risk can be made by taking the incidence rate of the health outcome in the group performing the health behavior and comparing it to the group not performing the behavior (Duncan, 1988). The remaining rate is the rate of disease due to the health practice. Since chronic illness and mortality increase with age, it is very possible that relative risk for a health practice may remain constant and the attributable risk associated with the practice may increase across the life span (Prohaska & Clark, 1994).

Research and Methodological Issues

The most important health outcomes are not always identical across the life span. An examination of the health objectives for the nation (*Healthy People, 2000,* 1991) reveals the diversity of health concerns across age groups and life transitions. For example, low birth weight and short gestation are important foci for pregnant women, while injuries, unwanted pregnancy, sexually transmitted diseases, and the development of lifelong health risk behaviors are important for adolescents. Finally, the ability to carry out activities of daily living, functional status, and use of health services are health objectives for older adults.

The association between health practices and subsequent health is further complicated by selective survival. That is, there are changes in the composition of the population because individuals who engage in risk behaviors experience higher mortality rates with advancing age. Also, deteriorating health and chronic diseases that are not associated with health practices are more likely with advancing age. Health practices may therefore have a greater impact on individuals whose health is already compromised (particularly older adults). Even with these methodological problems, clear and consistent patterns between health practices and health status across the life span are evident. The following section provides a summary of some of these associations.

Health Practices and Health Consequences

In a review of risk factors associated with mortality, McGinnis and Foege (1993) concluded that approximately half of all deaths that occurred among United States residents in 1990 could be attributed to identifiable external factors including health risk behaviors. Among the leading behavioral health risk factors contributing to death in the United States are tobacco use, diet/activity patterns, alcohol, firearms, and sex-ual behavior. They concluded that tobacco accounts for approximately 400,000 deaths each year in the United States, while poor diet and sedentary activity account for at least 300,000 deaths each year. Misuse of alcohol was estimated to account for 100,000 deaths per year. These behavioral risk factors are linked to deaths from cancers, cardiovascular disease, lung disease, low birth weight, motor vehicle fatalities, and injuries. These findings demonstrate the extent to which health practices are associated with health outcomes.

The association between health risk behaviors and health outcomes in adolescence can be both immediate and long-term. Immediate health risks for this age group include the association between driving while under the influence of alcohol and traffic fatalities (Brewer et al., 1994) and between sex risk practices and unwanted pregnancy (Hayes, 1987). Health practices in adolescent populations that have serious health consequences later in life include sedentary lifestyle and obesity. Finally, cigarette smoking during adolescence is an example of a health behavior with both immediate and long-term health consequences. The health risk of cancer and cardiovascular disease in later ages posed by cigarette smoking is well documented (USDHHS, 1989). Research, however, has demonstrated relatively immediate health consequences of smoking, including adverse changes in pulmonary function and lipid proteins among adolescent smokers (Dwyer, Lippert, Reiger-Ndakorewa, & Semmer, 1987).

The association between health practices and health consequences has also been documented in the adult population. For example, the association between driving while under the influence of alcohol and automobile fatalities remains strong in the adult population. Brewer et al. (1994) compared driver-history files for drivers who died in motor vehicle crashes with blood alcohol levels of at least 20 mg per deciliter with those who had blood alcohol levels below 20 mg per deciliter. Those with the higher blood alcohol levels were more likely to have a history of being arrested for driving while under the influence of alcohol. Also, the benefits of exercise for adults is significant in helping to prevent and treat chronic conditions such as coronary heart disease, diabetes, hypertension, and osteoporosis (Louis Harris and Associates, 1989).

Many of the health practices associated with adverse health outcomes in younger adults also have an impact on morbidity and mortality in older adults. Cigarette smoking is associated with mortality and morbidity well into the 7th decade of life (Hirdes, Brown, Vigoda, Forbes, & Crawford, 1987; Rimer, Orleans, Keintz, Cristinzio, & Fleisher, 1990). Among those 60 years of age and older, current smokers have 1.5 times the mortality risk of those who never smoked and 1.2 times the mortality risk of past smokers (Kaplan et al., 1987). Older adults are at high risk from continued smoking because they are more likely to have chronic health problems and disabilities in activities of daily living that may be exacerbated by smoking.

Positive health consequences from exercise for older adults are also well documented (for a review, see Edward & Larson, 1992). The cardiovascular effects of aerobic exercise training as measured by maximal oxygen consumption have been shown to improve in healthy older adults (Blumenthal et al., 1989) as well as older coronary patients (Ades, Hanson, Gunther, & Tonino, 1987). Weight-bearing and resistance training has improved muscle strength and increased bone mass in older populations (Fiatarone et al., 1990). The psychological benefits of exercise for older adults are mixed, with some programs showing minimal psychological benefits (Gitlin et al., 1992), and others showing significant improvements in depression (Perlman et al., 1990) and enhanced self-confidence and self-efficacy (Blumenthal et al., 1989; Hughes, 1984).

Extensive research has linked health risk behaviors to health outcomes during pregnancy. Cigarette smoking during pregnancy increases the risk for a low-birth-weight infant and for infant mortality (Kleinman, Pierre, Madaus, Land, & Schwann, 1988). Cocaine abuse has also been

linked to perinatal complications, fetal death, and low birth weight (Little, Snell, Klein, & Gilstrap, 1989). Maternal alcoholism during pregnancy is associated with fetal alcohol syndrome. Unfortunately, there is very little research regarding the association between health practices engaged in by individuals during other life transitions and subsequent health status.

There is some evidence that health practices associated with measures of health in younger adults maintain their association into later adulthood. For example, Kaplan et al. (1987) examined the association between multiple health practices and 17-year mortality in four age groups: age 38–49 years, 50–59 years, 60–69 years, and 70 years and older. Relative risks for 17-year mortality were estimated for the four age groups while simultaneously adjusting for all seven health practices (smoking, physical activity, relative weight, alcohol consumption, hours slept, eating breakfast, and snacking). These researchers found that for some health practices such as current versus never smoking, and maintaining physical activity, the relative risk remained significant across all age groups. The health practice of maintaining versus not maintaining moderate relative weight, however, was not consistent across all age groups. While maintaining moderate relative weight was a significant protective factor for mortality in the 38–49 age group, there was little association between relative weight and mortality in the 60–69 age group. Similarly, sleeping 7–8 hours per night was a significant protective factor for mortality in individuals 50–59 years, but hours of sleep was not significantly associated with mortality for the other age groups (Kaplan et al., 1987). These findings suggest that while health behaviors are associated with health outcomes across the adult life span, the associations are not always consistent.

Multiple Health Practices and Risk

A number of investigations have examined the association between multiple health behaviors and health outcomes across the adult life span. Breslow and Engstrom (1980) combined 7 health practices into a health index (0 to 7) and examined the association between health index scores and mortality over a 9½-year period. They found that for adults, the number of positive health practices showed an inverse relationship with age-adjusted mortality rates. For example, men who followed all 7 health practices had a mortality rate of only 28% that of men following 0–3 health practices.

Kaplan et al. (1987) examined the additive effects of the same 7 health practices on mortality rates over 17 years across four adult age groups. Even after simultaneous adjustment for all 7 health practices, the majority of the health practices were significantly associated with mortality for all four age samples. This finding demonstrates the additive and unique contribution of various health practices to mortality throughout the adult life span.

The ability to carry out activities of daily living is associated with health practices. Physical functioning is an important health outcome for older adults and is often measured in terms of ability to accomplish instrumental and basic activities of daily living (e.g., dress and bathe oneself, prepare meals and do shopping). Activities of daily living are an indication of the individual's ability to live independently and are associated with institutional placement and use of health care services (Branch & Jette, 1982; Shapiro & Tate, 1988). Guralnik and Kaplan (1989) examined the relative contribution of six health behaviors to the ability of older adults to maintain high functional status over a 19-year period. They reported that individuals who quit or never smoked cigarettes, maintained relative weight, and reported moderate use of alcohol were more likely to maintain high functional status at the 19-year follow-up period. This association between health practices and functional status held after adjusting for chronic diseases and conditions (e.g., high blood pressure, arthritis, and back pain) as well as demographic characteristics such as age, gender, race, and marital status (Guralnik and Kaplan, 1989).

Conclusions

There is considerable evidence of the association between health practices and health throughout the life span. It is clear that health practices influence health outcomes in much the same way across the life span. Other than pregnancy, however, there seems to be a paucity of data on the association between health practices and measures of health for life transitions. Given the potential burden and stress associated with some of these life transitions, it would be of value to examine the role of health practices on health during these transitions.

Research shows that the effects of multiple health practices on measures of health are additive, at least for the outcomes of all-cause mortality (Breslow & Engstrom, 1980; Kaplan et al., 1987). This additive consequence of inappropriate health practices seems to be common across the adult life span, including adults age 70 years and older. In fact, for older adults, the additive effect of multiple health risk behaviors influences functional disability as well as mortality.

Research on the association between health practices and measures of health frequently examines the presence of the behavior (smoking versus nonsmoking) or levels of the health practice (moderate use of alcohol versus heavy use of alcohol). Additional characteristics of the health practice may also influence the association between health practices and measures of health. For example, the amount of time the individual has been performing the health practice may also contribute to health outcomes.

COGNITIVELY BASED THEORETICAL MODELS OF HEALTH PRACTICES

While important differences in health and risk behaviors have been identified among multiple age groups, an understanding of why these differences exist is only beginning to be reached. The majority of research on reasons that individuals perform specific health practices has focused on cognitive rational decision-based models such as the health belief model (Maiman & Becker, 1974; Rosenstock, 1974), the theory of reasoned action and theory of planned behavior (Ajzen, 1985, 1991; Ajzen & Fishbein, 1980), social cognitive theory or social learning theory (Bandura, 1977, 1986, 1989; Bandura & Adams, 1977), and the transtheoretical model of behavior change (Prochaska & DiClemente, 1983; Prochaska, DiClemente, & Norcross, 1992). These theoretical approaches to health practices have not been equally applied across the life span. There is sufficient application of three of these models in a variety of age groups, however, to discuss the utility of the three models across the life span: the health belief model, social cognitive theory, and the transtheoretical model.

Health Belief Model

The health belief model (HBM), one of the most widely used theoretical frameworks to understand health behavior, has been used to predict a variety of behaviors in many different types of populations, such as college students, mothers of children receiving health services, clinic patients, and senior citizens (Janz & Becker, 1984). Few studies, however, have used the health belief model to predict health behaviors during life transitions. Also, few studies have determined the effectiveness of the health belief model in predicting a specific behavior across multiple cohorts as well as over the life course of the individual.

There is some indication that components of the health belief model may not adequately predict health behaviors *across* age groups. For instance, in a community sample of young, middle-aged, and elderly adults by Prohaska et al. (1985), elderly respondents reported higher frequencies of health-promoting practices. All three age groups agreed, however, about the benefits and barriers associated with performing the health practices as well as the effectiveness of the health practices in preventing illnesses. This finding suggests that there were other unmeasured motiva-

tions such as symptom reduction that may have predicted the age differences in self-reported health behaviors. Also, *within* an age group such as adolescence, mechanisms that control behavior may change. For instance, in a study of safer-sex intentions among adolescents, Potasa and Jackson (1991) found that the HBM accounted for 43% of the variance in safer-sex intentions among 7th-grade students, 27% of the variance among 9th-grade students, and 17% among 11th-grade students. Thus, the HBM was not helpful in understanding sexual intentions of 11th grade students. The authors suggested that forces other than health concerns, such as need for acceptance, esteem, and affection, may more strongly influence the intentions of older adolescents.

Unfortunately, the health belief model has a number of limitations that may decrease its utility in predicting health behaviors across the life span. First, cognitive models predict a small amount of the variance in behaviors regardless of the type of population studied (Mullen et al., 1987). Second, the HBM has limited predictive value when there is little disagreement in the health belief. For instance, most individuals, regardless of age, agree on the severity of illnesses such as lung and colon–rectal cancer (Prohaska et al., 1985). Therefore, in attempting to determine if the mechanisms that control health practices differ over the life span, perceived severity as a factor in the HBM loses its predictive value. Finally, the HBM has been found to be more adequate at predicting the initiation of a behavior than at predicting continuation and termination of behaviors (Janz & Becker, 1984). Although initiation of a behavior is important, the more important information, when assessing behavior over the life course of an individual, is why the person maintained, relapsed, or terminated health behaviors at various times.

Perceptions of Efficacy (Social Cognitive Theory)

The HBM has been modified to accommodate components of social cognitive theory, also referred to as social learning theory (Rosenstock, Strecher, & Becker, 1988). According to social cognitive theory, a behavior change process such as the adoption of exercise or cessation of smoking is a function of setting personal goals based on outcome expectations associated with the behavior change, the tasks required to achieve those goals, and self-efficacy expectations for performing those tasks (Bandura, 1977, 1986, 1989; Bandura & Adams, 1977). These concepts of self-efficacy and outcome efficacy are based on the recognition that if individuals are to engage in specific behaviors, they must first believe that they have the necessary skills to engage in the behaviors. This perception of competence is particularly important for complex activities such as lifestyle behaviors and long-term changes in health practices. Self-efficacy can be developed through a variety of sources of information, such as past performance accomplishments, vicarious experiences, social and verbal persuasion, and physical or emotional arousal (Bandura, 1977, 1986).

Like other cognitively based perspectives, the ability of the social learning theory to predict behavior changes across the life span has not been adequately addressed. Most often, outcome behaviors are treated as either present or absent with the result that there is no discussion of the association between efficacy and (1) strength of the activity, (2) the transition from nonperformance to performance, or (3) maintenance of the activity at multiple time intervals. It may be speculated, however, that efficacy may be lower in younger persons with limited experience with behavior performance as well as in older individuals with multiple failed attempts at the behavior as well as loss of physical or mental abilities (Rodin & Timko, 1992).

Not only is it necessary to gain more information about the association of efficacy and health behaviors across the life span, but also perceived efficacy during the course of a behavior must be addressed. For instance, more positive experiences with condom use may be necessary for adolescents to maintain safer sex practices as compared to other age groups. The necessity of multiple positive experiences at particular ages may be due not only to the gradual development of competence but also to the expectations that health behaviors will have desired results. Thus, older adults may be less likely than young and middle-age adults to quit smoking because they perceive that smoking cessation cannot modify symptoms associated with a long history of tobacco use. Finally, outcome efficacy may be especially important at various ages because positive health outcomes from appropriate health practices do not occur at the same rate across the life span.

Transtheoretical Model of Behavior Change

The transtheoretical model of behavior change (Prochaska & DiClemente, 1983; Prochaska et al., 1992), or stages of change model, when combined with other cognitively based models, may provide a useful perspective to address health practices across the life span. Although the original model and the majority of early research were designed to address the termination of addictive behaviors such as tobacco use, the model has recently been applied to the adoption or cessation of multiple health practices. The basic construct of the transtheoretical model is that persons change behaviors by proceeding through stages. The stages of change model proposes that individuals move through a cycle of precontemplation, contemplation, preparation, action, and maintenance stages. Precontemplation is the stage at which there is no apparent intention to change behavior. Contemplation is the stage at which people are aware that a problem exists and are seriously thinking about overcoming it. Preparation is the stage at which persons have taken small steps to engaging in the behavior but have not yet taken effective action. Action is the stage at which persons have modified their behavior and are participating in the appropriate health practice. Maintenance is the stage at which persons have begun to stabilize the behavior and it has become routine. A relapse is viewed as movement from one stage to a previous stage.

Using the transtheoretical model, a health behavior can be viewed in terms of readiness for its adoption (precontemplation, contemplation, and preparation stages) and its strength once it is performed (action and maintenance stages), rather than as being simply present or absent. The utility of this model is the ability to predict individual movement from one stage to the next. Given this stage approach, there are a number of alternatives with which individuals may be deemed successful in behavior change modification. Any movement of an individual from one stage to the next can be considered a success. For example, individuals whose intentions change from not considering adoption of a low-fat diet (precontemplation) to considering a low-fat diet in the near future (contemplation stage) are considered successful. Thus, in this model, a target behavior is not viewed as a strictly "all-or-none" event.

Another advantage of a stage-based model is that it provides a framework for determining which psychosocial and perceptual factors are most critical for moving an individual from one stage to the next. For example, self-efficacy and outcome efficacy may be important in health practices in general, but they may be most important in the successful transition from the contemplation to the action stage or from the action to the maintenance stage. Furthermore, perceptions of outcome efficacy may be important in the transition from contemplation to action stage, while actual demonstration of outcome efficacy may be critical in the transition from action to maintenance stage. This model allows one to determine not only *whether* a psychosocial factor is important in adoption of health practices but also *when* it is important. This time dimension is a critical factor when considering health behavior changes throughout the life span.

Although studies using a stages of change perspective have thus far primarily consisted of samples of college students and participants in worksite health programs (Marcus, Rossi, Selby, Niaura, & Adams, 1992; Prochaska et al., 1994),

the model has also been applied to middle-aged and older adults (Clark, Kviz, Prohaska, Crittenden, & Warnecke, 1995; Orleans, Rimer, Cristinzio, Keintz, & Fleisher, 1991). Unfortunately, few studies have used a life-span approach to determine the usefulness of the model in predicting behavior change across multiple cohorts. Kviz and colleagues (Kviz et al., 1994; Kviz, Clark, Crittenden, Warnecke, & Freels, 1995) examined smoking cessation behaviors during a 3-month period among smokers in three age groups: 18–29, 30–49, and 50 or older. They found that smokers in the two youngest age groups were most likely to have been in the contemplation stage, while those age 50 or older were most likely to have been in the preparation stage (Kviz et al., 1994). There were no significant differences by age, however, in the percentage who tried to quit or actually quit smoking during the study period (Kviz et al., 1995).

Summary

The value of the transtheoretical model of behavior change in combination with the health belief model may be in their capacity to quantify readiness to adopt health practices across the life span. It may be that differences in performing health practices across the life span and at life transitions represent different stages of change. For example, older adults who have recently lost their spouse may be challenged in ways that make it difficult to maintain positive health practices, especially activities requiring considerable effort such as proper diet. Due to new challenges, they may relapse into a contemplation stage for proper nutrition. It my not be until self-efficacy is regained that the individual moves from contemplation to action. Alternatively, the transition to parenthood may be a cue to action that disposes the individual to consider or contemplate current inappropriate health practices. Issues such as self-efficacy may not contribute to behavior change *until* an individual is seriously considering or contemplating adoption of the health practice.

It may be that during certain life transitions, rational cognitively based models may have little utility in predicting behavior change. For example, health practices during puberty may be influenced by emotional or psychological factors. Alternatively, if the onset of puberty is "on time," cognitively based models may predict health practices. If puberty is "off time," however, emotional factors may have a more influential role in health behavior changes.

There are a number of reasons that it may be difficult to identify the controlling factors for health practices in individuals across the life span. It is possible that different factors control the same health or risk behavior for different age groups. Thus, young adults may use condoms in order to avoid unwanted pregnancies, while middle-aged and older adults may practice the same behavior in order to prevent sexually transmitted diseases. Second, factors that control specific health or risk behaviors may change over the natural history of the behavior. Third, factors that control behavior may change over the life span of the individual. For example, a younger adult may start a program of regular physical activity (running) to be a part of a group in school (peer pressure); the person may then continue the exercise activity throughout young adulthood and middle age for weight control or other health reasons. Fourth, the natural history of a behavior may change across the life span of the individual. It may be that part of the natural history of health practices includes life transitions. These life transitions may influence the stability of health practices. If common factors associated with these life transitions can be identified, their identification may lead to finding opportunities to promote positive health practices and to prevent negative changes in these behaviors.

REFERENCES

Ades, P., Hanson, J., Gunther, P., & Tonino, R. (1987). Exercise conditioning in the elderly coronary patient. *Journal of the American Geriatrics Society, 35,* 121–124.

Ajzen, I. (1985). From intentions to actions: A theory of planned behavior. In J. Kuhl & J. Beckman (Eds.), *Action control: From cognition to behavior* (pp. 11–39). New York: Springer.

Ajzen, I. (1991). The theory of planned behavior. *Organizational Behavior and Human Decision Process, 50,* 179–211.

Ajzen, I., & Fishbein, M. (1980). *Understanding attitudes and predicting social behavior.* Englewood Cliffs, NJ: Prentice-Hall.

Baltes, P., Reese, H., & Nesselroade, J. (1977). *Life-span developmental psychology: Introduction to research methods.* Belmont, CA: Wadsworth.

Bandura, A. (1977). Self-efficacy: Toward a unifying theory of behavioral change. *Psychological Review, 84,* 191–215.

Bandura, A. (1986). *Social foundations of thought and action.* Englewood Cliffs, NJ: Prentice-Hall.

Bandura, A. (1989). Human agency in social cognitive theory. *American Psychologist, 44,* 1175–1184.

Bandura, A., & Adams, N. (1977). Analysis of self-efficacy theory of behavioral change. *Cognitive Therapy and Research, 1,* 287–308.

Bauman, K., Foshee, V., & Haley, N. (1992). The interaction of sociological and biological factors in adolescent cigarette smoking. *Addictive Behaviors, 17,* 459–467.

Berkman, L., & Breslow, L. (1983). *Health and ways of living: The Alameda County study.* New York: Oxford University Press.

Blumenthal, J., Emery, C., Madden, D., George, L., Coleman, R., Riddle, M., McKee, D., Reasoner, J., & Williams, R. (1989). Cardiovascular and behavioral effects of aerobic exercise training in healthy older men and women. *Journal of Gerontology, 44,* 147–157.

Boyd, N., & Windsor, R. (1993). A meta-evaluation of nutrition education intervention research among pregnant women. *Health Education Quarterly, 20,* 327–345.

Branch, L., & Jette, A. (1982). A prospective study of long-term care institutionalization among the aged. *American Journal of Public Health, 72,* 1373–1379.

Breslow, L., & Engstrom, J. (1980). Persistence of health habits and their relationship to mortality. *Preventive Medicine, 9,* 469–483.

Brewer, R., Morris, P., Cole, T., Watkins, S., Patetta, M., & Popkin, C. (1994). The risk of dying in alcohol-related automobile crashes among habitual drunk drivers. *New England Journal of Medicine, 331,* 513–517.

Brody, E. (1990). *Women in the middle: Their parent care years.* New York: Springer.

Bruce, F., Adams, M., Shulman, H., & Martin, M. (1993). Alcohol use before and after pregnancy. *American Journal of Preventive Medicine, 9,* 267–273.

Bruhn, J., & Parcel, G. (1982). Current knowledge about the health behavior of young children: A conference summary. *Health Education Quarterly, 9,* 238–261.

Bulcroft, K., Bulcroft, R., & Borgatta, E. (1994). *Family devel-*

opment theory as a basis for identifying potential points of adult health behavior change. Unpublished manuscript. University of Washington, Seattle.

Burton, L., Schulz, R., German, P., Hirsch, C., & Mittlemark, M. (1994). *Effects of caregiving on life-style health behaviors and preventive health seeking: A multi-site national caregiving health effects study, an ancillary study of the cardiovascular health study.* Paper presented at the Annual Meeting of the Gerontological Society of America, Atlanta.

Clark, M., Kviz, F., Prohaska, T., Crittenden, K., & Warnecke, R. (1992). *Older smokers' participation in a community-based smoking cessation intervention.* Paper presented at the Annual Meeting of the Gerontological Society of America, Washington, DC.

Clark, M., Kviz, F., Prohaska, T., Crittenden, K., & Warnecke, R. (1995). Readiness of older adults to quit smoking in a televised intervention. *Journal of Aging and Health, 7,* 119–138.

Cowell, J., & Montgomery, A. (1993). *Patterns of physical activity among school aged children.* Paper presented at the Annual Meeting of the American Public Health Association, San Francisco.

Dawber, T. (1980). *The Framingham study: Epidemiology of atherosclerotic disease.* Cambridge, MA: Harvard University Press.

Duncan, D. (1988). *Epidemiology: Basis for disease prevention and health promotion.* New York: Macmillan.

Duval, E. (1971). *Family development* (4th ed.). Philadelphia: J. B. Lippincott.

Dwyer, J., Lippert, P., Reiger-Ndakorewa, G., & Semmer, G. (1987). Some chronic disease factors and cigarette smoking in adolescents: The Berlin–Bremen study. *Morbidity and Mortality Weekly Report, 36,* 35–40.

Edward, K., & Larson, E. (1992). Benefits of exercise in older adults: A review of existing evidence and current recommendations for the general population. *Clinics in Geriatric Medicine, 8,* 35–50.

Erickson, E. (1959). *Identity and the life cycle.* New York: International Universities Press.

Fiatarone, M., Marks, E., Ryan, N., Meredith, C., Lipsitz, L., & Evans, W. (1990). High-intensity strength training in nonagenarians. *Journal of the American Medical Association, 263,* 3029–3034.

Flay, B., d'Avernas, J., Best, J., Kersell, M., & Ryan, K. (1983). Cigarette smoking: Why young people do it and ways of preventing it. In P. J. McGrath & P. Firestone (Eds.). *Pediatric and adolescent behavioral medicine: Issues in treatment* (pp. 132–182). New York: Springer.

Frazier, A., Franks, A., & Sanderson, L. (1992). Behavioral risk factor data. *Using chronic disease data: A handbook for public health practitioners* CDC. 4-14-4-17. Atlanta: Centers for Disease Control and Prevention, Public Health Service, U.S. Department of Health and Human Services.

Gallager, D., Thompson, L., & Peterson, J. (1981–1982). Psy-

chosocial factors affecting adaptation to bereavement in the elderly. *International Journal of Aging and Human Development, 14,* 79–95.

Gitlin, L., Lawton, M., Windsor-Landsberg, L., Kleban, M., Sands, L., & Posner, J. (1992). In search of psychological benefits: Exercise in healthy older adults. *Journal of Aging and Health, 4,* 174–192.

Glick, P. (1977). Updating the life cycle of the family. *Journal of Marriage and the Family, 39,* 5–13.

Gliden, J., Hendryx, M., Casia, C., & Singh, S. (1989). The effectiveness of diabetes education programs for older patients and their spouses. *Journal of the American Geriatrics Society, 37,* 1023–1030.

Gottlieb, N., & Baker, J. (1986). The relative influence of health beliefs, parental and peer behaviors and exercise program participation on smoking, alcohol use and physical activity. *Social Science and Medicine, 22,* 915–927.

Gottlieb, N., & Green, L. (1987). Ethnicity and lifestyle health risk: Some possible mechanisms. *American Journal of Health Promotion, 2,* 37–45.

Guralnik, J., & Kaplan, G. (1989). Predictors of healthy aging: Prospective evidence from the Alameda County Study. *American Journal of Public Health, 79,* 703–708.

Hayes, C. (1987). *Risking the future: Adolescent sexuality, pregnancy, and childbearing.* Washington, DC: National Academy Press.

Healthy People, 2000. (1991). *National health promotion and disease prevention objectives.* DHHS Publication No. PHS 91-50213. Washington, DC: U.S. Government Printing Office.

Hirdes, J., Brown, K., Vigoda, D., Forbes, W., & Crawford, L. (1987). Health effects of cigarette smoking: Data from the Ontario longitudinal study on aging. *Canadian Journal of Public Health, 78,* 13–17.

Hughes, J. (1984). The psychological effect of habitual aerobic exercise: A critical review. *Preventive Medicine, 13,* 66–78.

Janz, N., & Becker, M. (1984). The health belief model: A decade later. *Health Education Quarterly, 11,* 1–47.

Johnston, L., O'Malley, P., & Bachman, J. (1989). *Drug use, drinking, and smoking: National survey results from high school, college and young adult populations, 1975–1988.* DHHS Publication No. (PHS) 89-1638. Washington, DC: U.S. Government Printing Office.

Kann, L., Warren, W., Collins, J., Ross, J., Collins, B., & Kolbe, L. (1993). Results from the National School-Based 1991 Youth Risk Behavior Survey and progress toward achieving related health objectives for the nation. *Public Health Reports, 108*(Suppl. 1), 47–55.

Kaplan, G., Seeman, T., Cohen, R., Knudsen, L., & Guralnik, J. (1987). Mortality among the elderly in the Alameda County study: Behavioral and demographic risk factors. *American Journal of Public Health, 77,* 307–312.

Kleinman, J., Pierre, M., Madaus, J., Land, J., Schwann, W. (1988). The effects of maternal smoking on fetal and infant mortality. *American Journal of Epidemiology* 127, 274-282.

Kolbe, L., & Iverson, D. (1984). Comprehensive school health education programs. In J. Matarazzo, S. Weiss, J. Herd, N. Miller, & S. Weiss, (Eds.), *Behavioral health: A handbook of health enhancement and disease prevention* (pp. 1094-1116). New York: Wiley.

Kviz, F., Clark, M., Crittenden, K., Freels, S., & Warnecke, R. (1994). Age and readiness to quit smoking. *Preventive Medicine, 23*, 211-222.

Kviz, F., Clark, M., Crittenden, K., Warnecke, R., & Freels, S. (1995). Age and smoking cessation behaviors. *Preventive Medicine, 24*, 297-307.

Leventhal, H., Prohaska, T., & Hirschman, R. (1985). Preventive health behaviors across the life span. In J. C. Rosen & L. J. Solomon (Eds.), *Prevention in health psychology* (pp. 191-235). Hanover, NH: University Press of New England.

Little, B., Snell, L., Klein, V., Gilstrap, L. (1989). Cocaine abuse during pregnancy: Maternal and fetal implications. *Obstetrics and Gynecology, 73*, 157-160.

Louis Harris and Associates, Inc. (1986). *Problems facing elderly Americans living alone: A national survey*. No. 854010. New York: Author.

Louis Harris and Associates, Inc. (1989). *The Prevention index '89: Summary report*. Emmaus, PA: Rodale.

Maiman, L., & Becker, M. (1974). The health belief model and sick role behavior. *Health Education Monographs, 2*, 387-408.

Marcus, B., Rossi, J., Selby, V., Niaura, R., & Adams, D. (1992). The stages and processes of exercise adoption and maintenance in a worksite sample. *Health Psychology, 11*, 386-395.

McGinnis, J., & Foege, W. (1993). Actual causes of death in the United States. *Journal of the American Medical Association, 270*, 2207-2212.

Mechanic, D. (1979). The stability of health practices: Results from a 16-year follow-up. *American Journal of Public Health, 69*, 1142-1145.

Morbidity and Mortality Weekly Report. (1994). Health risk behaviors among adolescents who do and do not attend school—United States, 1992. *Morbidity and Mortality Weekly Report, 43*(8), 129-132.

Morris, N. (1992). Determination of adolescent initiation of coitus. *Adolescent Medicine: State of the Art Reviews, 3*, 165-180.

Mullen, P., Hersey, J., & Iverson, D. (1987). Health behavior models compared. *Social Science and Medicine, 24*, 973-981.

Murrell, S., Himmelfarb, S., & Phifer, J. (1988). Effects of bereavement/loss and pre-event status on subsequent physical health in older adults. *International Journal of Aging and Human Development, 27*, 89-107.

Nathan, P. (1984). The worksite as a setting for health promotion and positive lifestyle change. In J. Matarazzo, S. Weiss, J. Herd, N. Miller, & S. Weiss (Eds.), *Behavioral health: A*

handbook of health enhancement and disease prevention (pp. 1061-1064). New York: Wiley.

Neugarten, B., Moore, J., & Lowel, J. (1975). Age norms, age constraints, and adult socialization. In B. Neugarten (Ed.), *Middle age and aging* (pp. 22-28). Chicago: University of Chicago Press.

O'Campo, P., Faden, R., Brown, H., & Gielen, A. (1992). The impact of pregnancy on women's prenatal and postpartum smoking behavior. *American Journal of Preventive Medicine, 8*, 8-13.

Orleans, C., Rimer, B., Cristinzio, S., Keintz, M., & Fleisher, L. (1991). A national survey of older smokers: Treatment needs of a growing population. *Health Psychology, 10*, 343-351.

Perlman, S., Connell, K., Clark, A., Robinson, M., Conlon, P., Gecht, M., Caldron, P., & Sinacore, J. (1990). Dance-based aerobic exercise for rheumatoid arthritis. *Arthritis Care and Research, 3*, 29-35.

Potasa, R., & Jackson, K. (1991). Using the health belief model to predict safer sex intentions among adolescents. *Health Education Quarterly, 18*, 463-476.

Prager, K., Malin, H., Spiegler, D., Van Natta, P., & Placeck, P. (1984). Smoking and drinking behavior before and during pregnancy of married mothers of live-born infants and stillborn infants. *Public Health Reports, 99*, 117-127.

Prochaska, J., & DiClemente, C. (1983). Stages and processes of self-change in smoking: Toward an integrative model of change. *Journal of Consulting and Clinical Psychology, 5*, 390-395.

Prochaska, J., DiClemente, C., & Norcross, J. (1992). In search of how people change: Applications to addictive behaviors. *American Psychologist, 47*, 1102-1114.

Prochaska, J., Velicer, W., Rossi, J., Goldstein, M., Marcus, B., Rakowski, W., Fiore, C., Harlow, L., Redding, C., Rosenbloom, D., & Rossi, S. (1994). Stages of change and decisional balance for 12 problem behaviors. *Health Psychology, 13*, 39-46.

Prohaska, T., & Clark, M. (1994). The interpretation and misinterpretation of health status and risk assessments. *Generations, 18*, 57-61.

Prohaska, T., Leventhal, E., Leventhal, H., & Keller, M. (1985). Health practices and illness cognition in young, middle aged, and elderly adults. *Journal of Gerontology, 40*, 569-578.

Prohaska, T., Mermelstein, R., Miller, B., & Jack, S. (1993). Functional status and living arrangements. In J. Van Nostrand, S. Furner, & R. Suzman (Eds.), *Health data on older Americans: United States, 1992*. National Center for Health Statistics. *Vital Health Statistics, 3*(27), 23-39.

Rakowski, W. (1987). Persistence of personal health practices over a one year period. *Public Health Reports, 102*, 483-493.

Rakowski, W. (1988). Age cohorts and personal health behavior in adulthood. *Research on Aging, 10*, 3-35.

Richmond, J., Rospenda, K., & Kelley, M. (in press). Gender

roles and alcohol abuse across the transition to parenthood. *Journal of Studies on Alcohol.*

Rimer, B., Orleans, C., Keintz, M., Cristinzio, S., & Fleisher, L. (1990). The older smoker: Status, challenges and opportunities for intervention. *Chest, 97,* 547-553.

Rodin, J., & Timko, C. (1992). Sense of control, aging and health. In M. Ory, R. Abeles, & P. Lipman (Eds.), *Aging, health and behavior* (pp. 174-206). Newbury Park, CA: Sage.

Rosenbloom, C., & Wittington, F. (1993). The effects of bereavement on eating behaviors and nutrient intakes in elderly widowed persons. *Journal of Gerontology, 48,* S223-S229.

Rosenstock, I. (1974). Health belief model and preventive health behavior. *Health Education Monographs, 2,* 354-386.

Rosenstock, I., Strecher, V., & Becker, M. (1988). Social learning theory and the health belief model. *Health Education Quarterly, 15,* 175-183.

Rubenstein, L., Josephson, K., Nichol-Seamons, M., & Robins, A. (1986). Comprehensive health screening for well elderly adults: An analysis of a community program. *Journal of Gerontology, 41,* 342-352.

Shanas, E. (1979). The family as a social support system in old age. *Gerontologist, 19,* 169-174.

Shapiro, E., & Tate, R. (1988). Who is really at risk of institutionalization? *Gerontologist, 28,* 237-245.

Thornberry, R., Wilson, W., & Golden, P. (1986). Health promotion and disease prevention: Provisional data from the National Health Interview Survey: United States, Jan.-June 1985. In *Advance data from vital and health statistics.* No. 119. DHHS Publication No. (PHS) 86-1250. Hyattsville, MD: National Center for Health Statistics.

Tschann, J., Adler, N., Irwin, C., Millstein, S., Turner, R., & Kegeles, S. (1994). Initiation of substance use in early adolescence: The roles of pubertal timing and emotional distress. *Health Psychology, 13,* 326-333.

Udry, J. (1988). Hormonal and social determinants of adolescent initiation. In J. Bancroft (Ed.), *Adolescence and puberty.* New York: Oxford University Press.

Udry, J., Talbert, L., & Morris, N. (1986). Biosocial foundations for adolescent female sexuality. *Demography, 23,* 217-230.

U.S. Bureau of the Census. (1988). Marital status and living arrangement: March 1989. *Current population reports,* P-20, No. 445. Washington, DC: U.S. Government Printing Office.

U.S. Department of Health and Human Services. (1981a). *Basic data from wave 1 of the national survey of personal health practices and consequences: United States, 1979.* National Center for Health Statistics, DHHS Publication No. (PHS) 81-1162. *Vital and Health Statistics,* Series 15, No. 2.

U.S. Department of Health and Human Services. (1981b). *Highlights from wave 1 of the national survey of personal health practices and consequences: United States, 1979.* National Center for Health Statistics, DHHS Publication No. (PHS) 81-1162. *Vital and Health Statistics,* Series 15, No. 1.

U.S. Department of Health and Human Services. (1986). *Health promotion data for the 1990 objectives: Estimates from the national health interviews survey of health promotion and disease prevention: United States, 1985.* National Center for Health Statistics. *Advance Data,* No. 126, September 19.

U.S. Department of Health and Human Services (1989). Office of the Surgeon General. *Reducing the health consequences of smoking; 25 Years of progress: A report to the Surgeon General.* DHHS Publication No. (PHS) 89-8411. Washington, DC: U.S. Government Printing Office.

U.S. Department of Health and Human Services. (1990). *The health beliefs of smoking cessation.* DHHS Publication No. (CDC) 90-8416. Office on Smoking and Health. Center for Chronic Disease Prevention and Health Promotion, Centers for Disease Control, Public Health Service, U.S. Department of Human Services.

Watkins, A., & Kligman, E. (1993). Attendance patterns of older adults in a health promotion program. *Public Health Reports, 108,* 86-91.

Willis, L., Thomas, P., Garry, P., & Goodwin, J. (1987). A prospective study of response to stressful life events in initially healthy elders. *Journal of Gerontology, 42,* 627-630.

3

Health Behavior in Children

Robert W. O'Brien and Patricia J. Bush

Most researchers, when viewing childhood, have focused on issues such as learning, school performance, emotional development, and family and peer relationships. Childhood is now coming to be perceived, however, as a critical period in the overall development of the individual for the acquisition of appropriate health behaviors and the assumption of a healthful lifestyle. During childhood, health behaviors develop as a function of the interaction among an individual's developmental levels, personal characteristics, social environment, and experiences. The intent of this chapter is to provide a framework for understanding why studying children's health behaviors is important and for recognizing that children's health behaviors need to be considered separately from those of adults.

INTRODUCTION

It is essential that children's health behaviors be addressed separately from adults' health

Robert W. O'Brien • The CDM Group, Inc., 5530 Wisconsin Avenue, Chevy Chase, Maryland 20815.   **Patricia J. Bush** • Department of Family Medicine, Georgetown University School of Medicine, Washington, DC 20007.

Handbook of Health Behavior Research III: Demography, Development, and Diversity, edited by David S. Gochman. Plenum Press, New York, 1997.

behaviors because of the qualitative differences between children's and adults' thinking processes and actual behaviors. The stability seen in many health behaviors by the time of adolescence shows that the health behaviors an individual exhibits as an adult are determined, in many ways, during childhood.

The influences on child health behaviors are quite different from those that confront adults, the reason being that personal experiences and information are perceived differently by children and adults. First, children's reasoning and logical thinking skills are qualitatively different from those of adults, as is readily apparent in the decisions that children make, including those regarding their health. Unfortunately, many adults in a position to influence the development of positive health behaviors fail to recognize these differences and assume that a child's primary problem is quantitative, i.e., a lack of factual knowledge.

Another false assumption is that the ongoing status of children's health is primarily the responsibility of a parent. Many parents assume the responsibility for their children's health. Typically, they tell their children what to do, rather than give them an opportunity to make choices about their behavior, as adults do. This chapter presents concepts of individual development, including personal autonomy, and discusses how they relate to children's health behavior.

THEORIES APPLIED TO CHILDREN'S HEALTH BEHAVIORS

Three theoretical approaches have been predominant in the literature attempting to explain the development of children's health behaviors: cognitive developmental theory, social learning theory, and behavioral intention theory. The children's health belief model was adapted from the health belief model by incorporating aspects of these learning theories.

Cognitive Developmental Theory

Cognitive developmental theory (CDT) is based on the stage theory proposed by Piaget regarding the nature of how children think. This theory proposes that children are not just products of their environment. Rather, it assumes that children take an active role in the construction of their own knowledge and behavior (Inhelder & Piaget, 1964). Specific cognitive skills develop over time in a universally recognized sequence; consequently, the logical thought processes applied to health and health behaviors are constantly developing. Children's interpretations of significant events and information are also constantly growing and changing. Perspectives that consider the acquisition and modification of health behaviors among children must take this developmental process into account. This chapter covers differences among children and how such differences may affect thinking about health and illness.

Social Learning Theory

Social learning theory (SLT), originally proposed by Bandura (1977a, 1977b), considers social influences on the development of behavior. The learning aspect of SLT reflects the belief that behaviors are shaped by the positive and negative consequences that the behaviors elicit from the environment. The social aspect is the intrinsic value of specific behaviors that are drawn from others and is a factor in whether a behavior is continued and in what form it continues. The social environments in which behaviors develop include family, school, peers, media, and also the various settings in which children interact with health care providers.

Social cognitive theory (SCT), adapted from SLT by Bandura (1986), emphasizes that behaviors are acquired and shaped through attention, retention, production, and motivation operating in these personal, behavioral, and environmental domains. Personal factors include the child's own value system; expectations derived from observation and experience; behavioral factors, including performance skills; and environmental factors, including modeling and the expressed opinions of peers, family, and media. SCT supports the notion that children learn and evaluate health behaviors by observing and interacting with those around them. This view suggests, for example, that parents who have a healthful lifestyle are able to pass their lifestyle on to their children. Some health educators have adopted SLT, and more recently SCT, as a theoretical base for interventions recognizing the importance of addressing all three domains to produce behavior change (Parcel & Baranowski, 1981).

Behavioral Intention Theory

Behavioral intention theory (BIT) explains health behavior in terms of the attitudes and norms that individuals apply to specific behaviors (Fishbein & Ajzen, 1975). BIT proposes that behaviors have a personal and a social aspect. (More recent forms of BIT are the theory of reasoned action and the theory of planned behavior.) The personal aspect is one's beliefs about a particular behavior and what the consequences of that behavior might be. The social aspect is seen in others' perceptions of the behavior and how these perceptions affect the individual's motivation to engage in the behavior. For example, in a study of bicycle helmet use among school-children, respondents knew why they should wear their helmets, yet helmet use was low and children expressed concern for the teasing they anticipated from their peers (Howland et al.,

1989). In this case, perceived social outcomes were weighed against the factual knowledge to decide behavioral practices.

Children's Health Belief Model

Finally, the children's health belief model (CHBM) proposes a comprehensive view that incorporates aspects of the other theories into an explanation of children's health behaviors. Bush and Iannotti (1990) were able to explain medicine use among children using a model that included cognitive and affective variables (e.g., knowledge, autonomy, health locus of control), environmental variables (e.g., caretaker motivation and perceptions related to medicine use), and specific readiness factors (e.g., child motivation, perceived illness threat, and perceived benefit of medicines).

Throughout this chapter, references are made to these theories, and a discussion at the end summarizes their role in child health behavior research.

DEVELOPMENTAL CHARACTERISTICS

Individual characteristics change and progress along well-defined and well-studied developmental curves regarding health-related abilities. While developmental differences across children are important, behaviors also provide an indication of development *within* individuals. Two characteristics serve as focal points for this chapter: (1) children's understanding of health and illness and (2) autonomy in children's health behaviors.

Cognitive Understanding of Health and Illness

General Cognitive Development. Understanding cognitive development in children requires recognition of two facts about how children think. First, the thinking processes of children are *qualitatively* different from those of adults;

second, children advance through *qualitatively* different stages of thinking as they develop from infancy through childhood and into adolescence. The sequence of development is the same for all, but individuals vary in the rate at which they develop their cognitive skills (Ginsburg & Opper, 1979).

Although cognitive development is often described in terms of stages, children do not advance in discernible steps. Rather, a gradual and continuous transition occurs across the stages as children build upon existing skills to develop abilities associated with successively higher stages. An individual is considered to be in a particular stage when he or she exhibits thinking that is generally characteristic of that stage.

The four stages applied in CDT are (1) sensory motor (age: birth to 2 years); (2) preoperations (age: 2–7 years); (3) concrete operations (age: 7–11 years); and (4) formal operations (age: 12 years and up). Given that there are individual differences in rates of development, these age ranges are only estimates.

Early in their cognitive development, children interpret the world in terms of familiar events and experiences. Their thoughts are simple, and they attend to only one aspect of a problem or situation at a time (preoperations). This level of logical skills makes young children poor evaluators and gives them a limited attention span. Gradually, physiological, social and mechanical explanations become integrated, but presented or considered in observable terms (concrete operations).

Finally, many individuals develop the capacity for logical and systematic speculation about processes and possibilities without concrete prompts (formal operations). This ability to consider problems in increasingly complex ways reflects the new capacity for abstract thinking. Individuals who reach this level do not do so fully until adolescence or later, and it may not be a skill easily generalizable across different domains (e.g., thinking about health is different from thinking abut history or about geography). For the purposes of this chapter, this summary, although brief, provides a basis for understanding how children are different from adults. The summary introduces more specific discussion about how children approach the issue of health and health behaviors.

Concepts of Health and Illness. Because it follows a pattern of systematic development in a predictable sequence of stages, the development of children's understanding of health and illness is consistent with Piaget's theory (Bibace & Walsh, 1979, 1980; Burbach & Peterson, 1986). This concordance was first shown by Bibace and Walsh (1979, 1980) through content analyses of open-ended interviews with children. Similar interview techniques have been used to study children's conceptions of death (Koocher, 1981), birth and sexuality (Bernstein & Cowan, 1981), physiology (Crider, 1981), and specific diseases (Obeidallah et al., 1993; Walsh & Bibace, 1991).

The six stages proposed by Bibace and Walsh (1979, 1980) are consistent with preoperations, concrete operations, and formal operations as outlined by Piaget. These workers proposed that understanding of illness follows the progression of phenomenism (inferring a relationship where none exists), contagion, contamination, internalization, and physiological and psychophysiological conceptions of illness, and this progression can be observed through open-ended interviews.

Developmental studies suggest that to understand children's conceptions of illness and health, it is necessary to go beyond the simple knowledge of facts (Bibace & Walsh, 1980; Obeidallah et al., 1993). Unfortunately, most health-related surveys focus on knowledge of facts, not on understanding of physiological processes. To understand the decisions that drive health-related behavior, it is necessary to have a sense of the cognitive skills of the child. Examples of cognitive concepts that may affect a child's understanding of health and disease are conceptions of time and space, understanding of short-term and long-term consequences of actions, and the ability to consider unobservable actions (e.g., the entry and impact of germs inside the body). Nei-

ther socioeconomic status (SES) nor gender effects were found in two developmental studies of children's understanding of the cause, prevention, and treatment of AIDS and other health problems (Johnson et al., 1994; Schonfeld, Johnson, Perrin, O'Hare, & Cicchetti, 1993).

Autonomy in Health Actions

The growth of behavioral autonomy during childhood is important to the acquisition of preventive health behaviors as well as appropriate compliance behaviors for treatment of acute or chronic health problems.

What Children Can Do and When They Can Do It. Few investigations have examined autonomy and children's health behaviors, especially between infancy and adolescence, despite the obvious importance of autonomy and factors associated with it for health education. Instead, most autonomy research has taken a developmental perspective, looking in infancy at issues of willfulness or self-control (Erikson, 1968) and in adolescence at individuation (Blos, 1979), resistance to control by parents or peers (Kandel & Lesser, 1972), and self-reliance or competence (Greenberger, 1984). In the area of health behavior, with few exceptions, children are typically viewed as passive, with parents making decisions for them and answering for them to health care providers and researchers. Exceptions are research undertaken by Pratt (1973), by the Lewises (Lewis, Lewis, Lortimer, & Palmer, 1977), by Bush and colleagues (Bush & Davidson, 1982; Bush & Iannotti, 1985, 1988, 1990), and most recently by a group of collaborative researchers from Europe and the United States (Bush et al., 1996). All these researchers gathered information about health behavior, including information about autonomy, directly from children.

In the early 1970s, Pratt (1973) showed that 9- to 13-year-old children whose parents encouraged autonomy and responsibility, provided reasons and information, and rewarded good behavior to a greater extent than they punished misbehavior had better health behaviors than other children. Autonomy was identified as the extent to which the child performed a variety of activities without a parent's help or reminder. In regression analyses, autonomy was the most important child-rearing variable with respect to dental, sleep, exercise, and smoking behavior. When the parenting style included all of the three hypothesized behaviors, the children's health behaviors were better than when the parenting style was disciplinarian.

Lewis and Lewis (Lewis & Lewis, 1982a,b; Lewis et al., 1977) investigated the determinants of illness-related behavior of elementary-school children and evaluated interventions designed to give children the opportunity to make decisions about health- and illness-related behaviors. These decisions included whether to participate in an influenza vaccine trial, whether to visit the school nurse, and whether to participate in the treatment of the problem leading to the visit. The researchers concluded that for child-initiated care to be maximally effective, interventions should involve children before the 3rd grade, mothers (or primary caregivers) and children's physicians should be involved, school programs should stimulate children's decision-making, and programs should be directed at children's self-concepts. Parents who ignore their children or who deal with them in an authoritarian way produce children with poor health-care-related beliefs and behaviors. "Health care behaviors are communicated best by individuals who model the desired behaviors and simultaneously explain the reasons they are taking certain actions.... Children are far more competent in a variety of dimensions, including decision making, than adults perceive (or want) them to be" (Lewis & Lewis, 1983, pp. 280–281).

Autonomy in nutrition, in medicine use, and in preventive health care has been investigated in a series of studies among District of Columbia families. Relative to nutrition, informal observations of children eating their school lunches suggested that the traditional dietary measures for children that relied on the caregivers' report of their children's nutritional intake were seriously flawed, especially when the children reached school age (Davidson & Kandel, 1981). Ethnographic methods were employed in various schools and neighborhoods to observe what children ate and the contexts in which they ate. Eating patterns of schoolchildren were described as "grazing" (snacking throughout the day), and the influence of peers was best described as a process of "let's make a deal." Much of what schoolchildren ate was seen to be outside the purview of their caregivers; children traded food, purchased food, and discarded food. Thus, caregivers could hardly be accurate informants on the subject of what their children ate.

A similar situation was found when mothers and children were interviewed about medicine use, particularly vitamins and mineral supplements (Bush, Iannotti, & Davidson, 1985). The mothers reported that their children had been directed to take a daily vitamin supplement, but in fact the children's reports did not always substantiate the mothers' reports.

When parents themselves have had little opportunity to learn sensible health behaviors, they have limited ability to model appropriate behavior or to provide adequate reasons for their behavior. Medicine use is such an area. Parents are largely influenced by the media concerning the purchase and use of proprietary medicines and are under physicians' orders concerning prescription medicines. Thousands of medicines are available, many with the same active ingredients but different brand names. Many are combination products. It is not surprising that parents rarely receive adequate information to educate themselves, let alone their children, about medicines or about when it is safe for children to assume some responsibility for their own medicine use. Considering the pervasiveness of medicine use in society, however, all children have been exposed to medicines, either through personal use or by observing others, including through the media. By the time children are school age, they have developed some beliefs, attitudes, and expectations about medicines.

In 1980, a series of studies was begun among primary-grade children and their mothers to investigate how children are socialized into medicine use, what they know about medicines, and how much autonomy they have in medicine use (Bush & Davidson, 1982; Bush & Iannotti, 1985, 1988, 1990; Bush et al., 1985). Areas of exploration included taking medicines without asking an adult, accessibility of household medicines, buying medicines, giving medicines to younger children, and taking medicines to school. Results indicated that although children are generally regarded as passive recipients of medicines, children perceive themselves to be quite involved in the medicine use process (Table 1). One indicator of autonomy was that on the day the children were interviewed, 8.3% of them had one or more medicines with them at school. When the mothers were asked in a follow-up telephone call if their children ever took a medicine to school, more than half the mothers of children with medicines at school denied that their children ever took a medicine to school. This finding again suggests that children are better informants about their own health behaviors than their mothers.

From kindergarten to the 7th grade, most or all of the household medicines (75–90%) were physically accessible to most of the children by

Table 1. Medicine-Related Activities Reported by Children in the 3rd, 5th, and 7th Grades of Washington, DC, Public Schools[a]

Behavior	Grade 3	Grade 5	Grade 7
Requested a medicine	67%	72%	78%
Took medicine independently	23%	28%	51%
Gave medicine to another child	9%	9%	25%
Independently picked up a prescription	38%	34%	44%
Independently purchased medicine[b]	14%	29%	29%

[a]From Bush et al. (1985).
[b]Medicine purchase was confirmed through visits to neighborhood stores and pharmacies.

the age of 6 or 7. This accessibility was replicated in other studies in Chapel Hill, North Carolina, and in studies conducted in Europe (Greece, Spain, Germany, Finland, Yugoslavia, and the Netherlands) (Sanz, Bush, & Garcia, 1996).

PERSONAL CHARACTERISTICS

As with adults, individual characteristics may be linked with subsequent children's health behaviors. These characteristics include variables of two quite different types. First are sociodemographic characteristics, such as gender, parent education, and income, which may not be open for intervention. Second, personal health beliefs and attitudes are characteristics that reflect how an individual views his or her position in the world relative to health concerns. The latter are typically outcomes associated with educational interventions.

Predisposing Sociodemographic Variables

Evidence supporting the contribution of sociodemographic variables to the development of patterns of health behaviors is still inconsistent. SES and mothers' education may potentially be the most useful. Bush and Iannotti (1988, 1990) found that SES, as a function of caregiver education, family income (relative to the child's school census tract), race, and the child's parental status (e.g., single parent, two parents), contributed to regression models predicting expected medicine use for both mothers and children. Glik, Greaves, Kronenfeld, and Jackson (1993) also found that SES was important, because the occurrence of environmental risks to safety increased in lower-SES homes. Maternal education may affect some health attitudes that come into play in the making of decisions regarding whether or not to engage in health behaviors (Farrand & Cox, 1993).

Some research has noted gender differences in children's health behaviors. With a sample of 9- to 10-year-old schoolchildren, Farrand and Cox

(1993) found that girls reported a greater number of positive health behaviors than boys. This finding was supported by a corresponding difference in positive health self-concepts. Cohen, Brownell, and Felix (1990) completed a study of health behaviors and beliefs among a broad age range of schoolchildren. With gender as one of the main independent variables, they reported that healthful foods were chosen more often by girls than by boys. They also noted, however, that girls reported more smoking and less exercise than boys (Cohen et al., 1990).

Some older studies noted that girls made more visits to school nurses (Rogers & Reese, 1965; Van Arsdell, Roghmann, & Nader, 1972). Such behaviors, however, may not necessarily reflect the rate of more preventive health behaviors, such as eating healthful foods or keeping fit. Bush and Iannotti (1990) found that gender was not a contributing variable when evaluating the CHBM as a means of predicting medicine use among children.

Race and ethnicity were determined to influence participation in fitness activities. In a study of activity and obesity, Hispanic and Asian children had lower activity levels than children from other racial groups (Wolf et al., 1993). Obesity was highest for the African-American and lowest for the Asian children. Before racial or ethnic differences on an outcome such as obesity can be validated, however, efforts must be made to account for the relationship between sociocultural attitudes and beliefs regarding health behaviors (Wolf et al., 1993).

Children's Health Beliefs and Motivations

Personal Control. While knowledge is sometimes a prerequisite for behavior change, it does not cause change (DiClemente, 1989). SLT or SCT and CDT are most often used to explain health behavior and health behavior change, but these theories have shown only moderate success (Bush & Iannotti, 1985). Theorists coming from various perspectives have suggested that personal control or self-regulation may be the key motivating factor in health promotion efforts (C. Peterson & Stunkard, 1989). This position is perhaps best articulated by C. Peterson and Stunkard, who incorporated the Bandura (1977b) concept of self-efficacy into a theory of personal control. Research by Bush and colleagues (Bush & Iannotti, 1985, 1988, 1990; O'Brien, Bush, & Parcel, 1989) highlights the importance of one's interpretation of health and illness and of the role of health locus of control in a child's intentions to take action in response to health problems. Personal control increases in importance as a child's autonomous action in his or her own health care becomes increasingly evident (Iannotti & Bush, 1992a,c; Iannotti, O'Brien, Cowen, & Wilson, 1990; O'Brien & Iannotti, 1993).

Health locus of control (HLOC) reflects one's beliefs regarding the source of reinforcement and control one has over the status of one's own health. Beliefs range from the notion that individuals maintain internal control of their own health to external beliefs that the self is helpless in controlling health status. In this case, good or bad health is due to uncontrollable factors (good or bad luck) under the control of a more powerful or knowledgeable individual (e.g., a parent, physician, or nurse). Internal control may be associated with greater responsibility for personal health (Hackworth & McMahon, 1991).

HLOC has been established as a measurable construct in children (O'Brien et al., 1989; Parcel & Meyer, 1978; Thompson, Butcher, & Berenson, 1987) that may peak during transition to adolescence. At that point, a locus of control measure more specific to particular health concerns, such as weight control (O'Brien, Smith, Bush, & Peleg, 1990), may be preferable. Cohen et al. (1990) noted that the 6th grade was an optimal point for HLOC and that the preadolescent period is an optimal one for health education because of behavioral and attitudinal fluctuations during adolescence.

Similar to HLOC, self-efficacy is considered by some to be an indicator of an individual's belief that he or she could execute particular behaviors. Such a belief is closely related with HLOC, although measuring self-efficacy, for specific health behaviors in adults and in children, has been difficult.

Vulnerability to Health Problems. One of the factors in CDT and SLT or SCT is understanding the consequences of behavioral action or inaction. Individuals base their behaviors, health or other, on what they anticipate will happen in the future. The evidence for impact of perceived vulnerability on health behaviors is still unclear. Gochman and Saučier (1982) suggested that anxiety in childhood may be exhibited through perceived vulnerability, making perceived vulnerability a construct without high reliability among children.

Perceived vulnerability is a major factor in an adult health belief model (Becker, 1974; Maiman & Becker, 1974), but has not typically been a strong predictor in tests of the CHBM (Bush & Iannotti, 1985, 1988; Gochman, 1971). Bush and Iannotti (1988, 1990) suggested that vulnerability was a weak predictor of children's medicine use because of its link with children's cognitive skills. Perceptions of vulnerability are dependent on one's ability to anticipate future events or ones not previously experienced—skills that are significantly limited during early stages of development.

Perceived Benefits of Health Behaviors. In their work on the CHBM, Bush and Iannotti (1988, 1990) also explored the effects of perceived benefits of health actions on health behaviors. They found that children's perceptions of the benefits of medicine use were significantly associated with expected medicine use. Perceptions may be based on experience or on information provided by an adult, such as a parent or a health care provider. Additional work is needed to explore further how these perceptions affect motivations and behavioral patterns.

Risk-Taking Behavior. In certain circumstances, children's behaviors increase their risk

for serious health problems. For example, riding a bicycle without a helmet may reflect a choice by the rider. This behavior, however, also increases the risk for a serious head injury. Approximately 300,000 injuries serious enough to warrant emergency room attention were suffered by bicycle riders in the 5- to 15-year-old age group, and about one third of the injuries were head injuries (Centers for Disease Control [CDC], 1987). Surveys of schoolchildren show, however, that even when students know why they should wear a helmet, they are likely to report not using a helmet, even if they own one. Their reasons for not wearing a helmet may include fear of being teased and mocked by peers for doing so (Howland et al., 1989).

Peer pressure has a large impact on whether children and adolescents engage in risk behaviors. Lewis and Lewis (1984) found that as children progressed from the 5th to the 8th grade, there was a corresponding increase in reported peer pressure to engage in problem behaviors. They also found an increase in actual engagement and in how much risk was associated with the behavior as the child got older. Risks included substance use and behaviors that increased the risk of personal injury. The increasing tendency to risk behavior is now being characterized as a developmental process (Levitt, Selman, & Richmond, 1991). The formation of health beliefs and attitudes during childhood, and the impact of environmental and social factors, play a large part in whether or not an individual engages in risk behaviors during childhood, adolescence, or adulthood. Baumrind (1987) emphasized that as an individual moves into adolescence, an understanding of risk behavior goes beyond cognitive and moral explanations. Increased weight must be attributed to the influence of the current youth culture on risk behavior.

SOCIALIZATION

Experiences across varying domains affect the development of child health behaviors. These domains range from very specific settings, such as the family, to the broader categories of culture and media. This section briefly explores the influence of various social contexts.

Family

A strict application of SLT presumes that the role modeling experienced by children at home would be a powerful influence on the development of health behaviors, but the data have not provided a strong case for this argument. For example, Bush and Iannotti (1988) found the case for supporting SLT in the development of medicine use to be mixed, at best. No consistent pattern of correlations between child and parent behaviors has supported this link.

In the area of fitness and activity, Sallis et al. (1993) found that physical activity in a class of 4th-grade children was not significantly associated with activity or fitness reported by parents. Factors such as availability of appropriate activities (Alpert, Field, Goldstein, & Perry, 1990) and parental support (e.g., transportation) (Sallis et al., 1993) might be more important in determining physical activity and improved fitness levels in children.

Parents do seem to engage in discussions about health and health behaviors with children, particularly girls (Cohen et al., 1990; Iannotti & Bush, 1992a). The effects of these conversations, however, have not yet been documented. Tinsley (1992) noted an association between parental health attitudes and the health status of children. Earlier work (Parke & Tinsley, 1987) found that the child-rearing methods parents used were related to child health behaviors. The more use parents made of rationales and assigned responsibility, the more appropriate were the children's health behaviors. Remy and Power (1995) found that increased use of rationales by parents was associated with higher HLOC in children.

Sallis and Nader (1988), emphasizing the effects of the family environment, felt that health behaviors tend to aggregate within families. They cited evidence for this view in exercise, smoking, and dietary behaviors. Overall, continued work is needed to learn just how families influence the development of health behaviors in children. The mixed findings noted earlier may reflect the need for a greater focus on how families transmit information about health behaviors in the context set by an individual's developmental level and the relevant social and cultural conditions. Familial patterns may influence the child's future health-related beliefs, attitudes, behaviors, and health status, but a great deal more longitudinal research is needed to understand possible causal pathways.

Schools

Aside from investigating peer pressure, little research has been completed on the influence of peers on health behaviors. Schools, however, have been noted for the educational programs on prevention they present to children. Unfortunately, health is not usually given a major place in the curriculum during the preschool and elementary years. In light of the autonomy in health behaviors shown by young children (Iannotti & Bush, 1992a), it makes sense to develop programs for children before the onset of problem behaviors. More programs are usually available for older children, particularly as the likelihood of certain risk behaviors increases. School health programs are available, however, for a range of ages (Tinsley, 1992). These programs can cover general preventive behaviors or present guidelines for preventing specific health problems (e.g., AIDS, cardiovascular disease). Head Start programs, with their emphasis on the health component, demonstrate how preventive health behaviors can be incorporated into the daily activities of preschool classrooms (Keane, O'Brien, Connell, & Close, 1996).

Media

From television and radio to newspapers and magazines, most children are exposed to a constant barrage of media information. Observers have noted the influences of the media and social factors (e.g., gender roles) on children's health behaviors, particularly related to foods. Jeffrey, McLellarn, and Fox (1982) noted that television advertising for low-nutrient foods increased the recall, purchase, and consumption of these foods. Evidence linking food advertising and increased consumption of unhealthful foods was also reviewed by Tinsley (1992).

One area that is drawing considerable attention for older children is media information regarding behaviors associated with the spread of HIV and AIDS. Media attention, including attention from several sources that address children directly, has helped spread information to certain segments of the population. This information takes on additional importance when it deals with a topic that many parents may feel uncomfortable discussing with their children. A recent study investigated sources of information about AIDS and related behaviors for school-age children (Mitchell, O'Brien, Semansky, & Iannotti, 1995). Electronic media, along with family members, were the two major sources of such information reported by these children and their parents. Interestingly, neither of these sources was among the top choices of children or parents for preferred sources of additional AIDS information. Children indicated that they thought health professionals were preferable as appropriate sources of that information; parents were more likely to look to print media (Mitchell et al., 1995).

The Health Care System

In a series of studies of doctors' interactions with families, Korsch and colleagues (Korsch, Gozzi, & Francis, 1968; Korsch & Negrete, 1972) found that provider communication with children was very limited. Less than 15% of physicians' communication was child-directed, and less than 1% consisted of actual health information. More recent studies (Pantell, Stewart, Dias, Wells, & Ross, 1982; Perlman & Abramovitch, 1987) showed that only about 50% of physicians'

statements during pediatric visits were related to the child's health, and fewer than 10% of these statements were directed to the children.

Children attentively listen to and accurately recall statements regarding their own health that providers make to their parents and are very interested in receiving more direct information about their own health (McCarthy, 1974; Perlman & Abramovitch, 1987). Because health information tends to be very technical, even for adults (Hunt, Jordan, Irwin, & Browner, 1989; Korsch & Negrete, 1972) it creates the potential for problems when children overhear statements they may or may not understand. Because the development of knowledge and understanding of health and illness goes through a progression (Bibace & Walsh, 1979, 1980), children attempt to make sense of the complex information they hear with the cognitive tools at hand, which are simple and not always logical. Misinformation, incomplete information, or no information at all may increase children's anxiety regarding their health (Vaughn, 1957) and have a negative impact on their health behaviors.

These studies investigating the effects of health-related communication with children have led to the suggestion that improvements in this area should improve child health behaviors, such as compliance with medicine taking (Haight, Black, & DiMatteo, 1985; Pantell & Lewis, 1986; Pantell et al., 1982). Improved perceptions of health care providers should also improve participation by children in their own health care (Falvo & Tippy, 1988).

HEALTH BEHAVIORS

Preventive Behaviors

The primary areas in which children's behaviors affect their health status are exercise, hygiene, nutrition, safety, and use of abusable substances. Some behaviors in these areas have short-term impact, but most have long-term effects. Behaviors may be a matter of commission (e.g., exercise and hygiene), a matter of omission (e.g., abusable substance use), or a combination (e.g., nutrition and safety). All may be viewed developmentally within a model of environmental facilitation, caregiver responsibility, and children's autonomy. As shown in Figure 1, at any age, children have more autonomy for one behavior than for another. For any behavior, as the child grows and develops, the level of autonomy shifts from the caregiver to the child. For example, the first area that the average child begins to take some responsibility for is hygiene; a great deal of responsibility in this area, however, lies with the caregiver. With an increase in age, almost total responsibility in this area shifts to the child. At the other end of the age continuum lies the use of abusable substances. For this behavior, the young child has no autonomy. An adolescent, however, has begun to assume responsibility for use of abusable substances.

Moreover, the child's environment may promote or impede each behavior both instrumentally and by social sanctions. For example, if the child is to have a healthful diet, healthful food must be available in the various places where the child eats. Significant others must convey the importance of good nutrition to the child through words and actions. Since increasing autonomy over food intake is a fact of development, and the child is likely to be faced with food choices throughout life, it is important that the child acquire the decision-making skills and associated motivations to make healthful choices.

Hygiene. Hygiene-related behavior among young children has not stimulated recent research. In early years, however, health messages from mothers may emphasize hygiene and associated behaviors. Two-year-olds and their mothers participated in one study of child-rearing patterns that provided information on maternal–child interactions related to hygiene (Iannotti & Bush, 1992a). The mothers' behaviors in a laboratory setting resembling a three-room apartment with a kitchen and bath were examined for references to illness, their children's physical needs, attributions of responsibility, and recommendations for health behaviors. Although messages concerning nutrition were most frequent (e.g., "That's for after we've had our body-building food"), hygiene was a close second (e.g., "When's the last time you brushed your teeth?"). Very few mothers made any recommendations regarding exercise, fitness, or medicines. The third most frequently mentioned area was injury, but mothers' recommendations concerning injury numbered only about one third as many as those for nutrition and hygiene.

Nearly 50% of the mothers made one or more statements regarding attributions of responsibility or cause for health or illness. Mothers varied in how much they encouraged and discouraged autonomy and personal control in health behavior, attributing about 40% to themselves, 40% to their children, and the remainder to others or to chance. Although mothers varied considerably, clearly mothers in this study de-

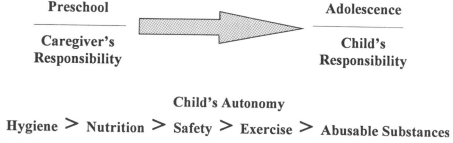

Figure 1. Relationships among child's autonomy for health behaviors, relative parent and child responsibilties, and child's age.

voted considerable time to teaching their children about hygiene.

Nutrition. In an affluent society, it is not surprising that the major causes of death are associated with "stuffing, sitting, smoking, and sipping." These activities account for the excesses in total energy, saturated fats, cholesterol, sugars, salt, tobacco, alcohol, and lack of exercise associated with hypertension, hyperlipidemia, obesity, diabetes mellitus, and many kinds of cancer.

Cohen et al. (1990) found evidence of gender differences in that girls reported more healthful eating habits than boys. These researchers noted that while snacking behavior increased with age, this increase was less evident for girls, and boys were more likely to have eaten fast food recently. A study of 4th graders by Gustafson-Larson and Terry (1992) found that girls had greater weight-related concerns than boys and that these concerns increased with age. These researchers even noted that 40% of the students had reported some dieting activity. Clearly, nutrition and associated factors (e.g., weight) are important factors to many children.

Informal observations of children eating school lunches led to the conclusion that traditional dietary measures for children that relied on mothers' recalls of their children's dietary intake were inadequate (Davidson & Kandel, 1981). For 4 years, beginning with students in the 4th, 5th, and 6th grades, Bush and colleagues (Smith, Zuckerman, & Bush, 1990) had the students report their snack consumption by checking off on a list any of the 25 snack foods they had eaten in the preceding 24 hours. A 20% random sample of the students participated in a 24-hour dietary recall interview, while a cohort of 200 subjects completed dietary questionnaires asking about food consumption and the time, preparer, and place of its preparation. The primary findings of this research were as follows:

- Even in the youngest group (4th–6th grades), well over 80% of the children stated that they sometimes cooked for themselves and others at home.
- All of the children stated that they engaged in some food-related activity, including cooking, shopping, or assisting with meal preparation, and most reported purchasing a snack at least once every day either at school or in neighborhood stores.
- In each year, the greatest percentage of daily calories was derived from food prepared or selected by the child. Similar relationships were found for other dietary components, including fats.
- Subjects were responsible for between 39% and 52% of their total daily caloric intake.
- Potato chips and chocolate candy were the number one contributors of fat to subjects' diets; the remainder of the ten most frequently consumed contributors of total fat were also snacks and fast foods.

Results from this study show an increase in autonomy with age and a tendency toward the consumption of high-fat, high-sodium foods as subjects increased their autonomy. Girls were more likely to self-select food, while higher-SES children were less likely to select or to prepare their own foods.

In summary, by 9 to 10 years of age, children are largely responsible for what they eat. Food likes and dislikes are determined early, and increasing autonomous behavior overall is correlated with greater control over food choice. It is also clear that children play a role in influencing what is prepared and the way it is prepared by others in the home and in determining what foods they are served. These facts suggest that children can and should be the targets of interventions designed to improve their nutritional status and to modify health risk behavior. Such interventions may carry over into the home, especially if children exert these types of control over their diet.

Safety. Childhood injuries remain one of the most critical areas in need of intervention.

CDC reports show that in one year, approximately 16 million children under age 20 suffer injuries serious enough to be seen in emergency rooms (CDC, 1990). Because many of these injuries occur in predictable patterns, the CDC (1990) also suggests that many injuries are preventable, particularly through proper adult supervision. Common causes of childhood injuries include motor vehicle accidents (including those in which the child was either occupant or pedestrian), homicide, drowning, burns, and falls (CDC, 1990).

As noted earlier, a developmental perspective on risk taking includes the cognitive aspect of children's decisions to engage in risk behaviors. Young children, for example, are generally unable to anticipate the future consequences of many of their actions, particularly when they have not previously experienced or observed the consequences of these actions. Even during adolescence, a sense of invincibility is pervasive due to an inability to assess the possible immediate or short- or long-term impact of particular behaviors. While this misperception may result from the incomplete development of cognitive skills, such thinking remains a concern in the risk behaviors shown by many adults as well.

Environmental changes may be the most effective method of modifying behavior and facilitating decreases in injury rates. Such changes could reduce the opportunities for children to engage in risky activities. Among the steps that could be taken are the use of safety caps on medicine bottles, reducing the temperature of hot water, using stair gates with young children, putting reflectors on bicycles and clothing, using bicycle helmets, covering pools, and even X-raying children's Halloween candy. Glik et al. (1993) recommended that adults take both active and passive steps in establishing a safe environment for children. This approach involves both environmental changes and education as appropriate methods for preventing childhood injuries.

Unfortunately, parents are not always active in injury prevention. L. Peterson, Farmer, and Kashani (1990) reported that the mean of parents' reports regarding how much they worry about their children sustaining each of a variety of injuries was less than "occasional worry, some stress" (less than 5 on a scale of 10, with 10 being the greatest level of worry). Worry increased as children got older, and some types of injuries or activities were more worrisome on the basis of the child's age and gender (e.g., cars generated more worry about older children, bicycles about younger children). As a result, parents need to be convinced of the efficacy of change before there can be any hope of success in undertaking change.

Children need to take an active role in their own health and safety. One example is the use of bicycle helmets by school-age children. Kimmel and Nagel (1990) found that only 6% of a school-age sample (grades 4–8) even owned bicycle helmets, and only one half of these children reported wearing the helmet at least 50% of the time. In the same sample of children, more than one third of the respondents said they had experienced a bicycle accident in the previous year. Clearly, the composite experiences of many of these children were insufficient to motivate them to engage in this preventive behavior following the experiences.

Similar research, already cited, reported that social perceptions among children were more powerful than knowledge of bicycle safety issues in predicting bicycle helmet use among schoolchildren (Howland et al., 1989; Kimmel & Nagel, 1990). Over time, psychosocial factors that increase risk for injury may be modifiable, but modification often requires a change in cultural perceptions, not just individual perspectives, to change these factors.

Exercise and Fitness. Besides nutrition, lack of exercise is increasingly targeted as a health risk. The relationships among nutrition, fitness, and several chronic diseases, particularly cardiovascular disease, are well enough established in adults that exercise has been targeted by the federal government as among the top-priority health promotion areas (DHHS, 1990).

The evidence for promoting fitness in children is less convincing than in adults. Fitness in children 10–14 years old has been negatively associated with obesity and systolic and diastolic blood pressures and positively associated with high-density lipoprotein/total cholesterol ratios (Hofman & Walter, 1989; Zuckerman et al., 1989). All of these factors have been shown to track into adulthood and to exhibit intrafamilial correlations (Bush, Iannotti, Zuckerman, O'Brien, & Smith, 1991).

In a study involving the cardiovascular risk factors of mothers with two sibling children of ages about 3 and 9 years, step tests to measure cardiovascular fitness were conducted for the older sibling and the mother, and an activity history was taken for both children and their mother (Bush et al., 1991). Mothers in the highest quartile of fitness were more likely to have children who were also in the highest quartile than to have children in the lowest quartiles. Similarly, mothers in the lowest quartile of fitness were more likely to have children who also ranked in the lowest quartiles. Although the older children were the most fit and reported the most activity, 15% could not complete or could not keep up the pace of the fitness step test.

Information on the state of children's exercise was measured in the National Children and Youth Fitness Studies (NCYFS I and II). In NCYFS I, 59% of 5th- to 12th-grade children reported exercising at an appropriate level during all four seasons, and 47% reported engaging in activities with potential for "carryover" (into adulthood). More than 84% of the time devoted to exercise was reported as being outside school. Beyond supporting most of the findings in NCYFS I, NCYFS II found a positive correlation between parent and child physical activity and between the child's fitness and the amount of physical exercise, and a negative correlation between fitness and time spent watching television.

Activity may be an area well suited for parents to have an impact. Moore et al. (1991) reported that children's activity level was related to that of their parents. These observations suggested that families should share certain activities

and that parents can serve as role models who give values to fitness-related activities.

Conditions that promote exercise include motivation, selecting activities, scheduling time, finding a place (including transportation if necessary) and possibly equipment, and having support or encouragement from others. Managing these requirements is generally easier for an adult than it is for a child. Consequently, schools have been increasingly viewed as places to be targeted for increasing children's fitness levels.

Recent trends that have raised concern among health providers include a generational increase in same-age children's weight over time (Shear, Freedman, & Burke, 1988) and an increase in sedentary activities, including hours of viewing television and playing computer games. Opposing these trends is the promotion of sports for girls and an attempt to promote sports as enjoyable lifetime activities that are not primarily about teams and competition, but have potential for the carryover of benefits into adulthood.

Although the school is an obvious target because more than three fourths of students in the 5th through 12th grades are enrolled in physical education (PE) classes an average of 3.6 times per week, the range of classes is unevenly distributed. More important, most of the time spent in PE is not spent in vigorous physical activity, but is usually devoted to organizing for competitive sports, playing competative sports, and participating in informal play that includes inactivity (Simons-Morton, Parcel, O'Hara, Blair, & Pate, 1988). PE classes have been found lacking, with many children not getting very much high-level activity during the limited time they are in class (Simons-Morton, Taylor, Snider, & Huang, 1993).

As noted by Simons-Morton et al. (1988), normative data alone do not permit qualitative judgments about children's fitness levels. The evidence for developing exercise goals for children is not as compelling as for adults. In fact, little information is available about children's orientations toward exercise and whether participation in childhood will increase the probability of exercise in adulthood. There is therefore a growing consensus that cognitive and attitudinal aspects of exercise, in addition to skills building and goal setting, need to be addressed in childhood. A population-based public health approach should be taken, rather than putting the focus on short-term gains in limited numbers of children.

Behavioral Responses to Treatment Instructions

Compliance during Acute Health Conditions. Estimates of noncompliance vary depending on whether the health problem being treated is chronic or acute. For acute illnesses in children, current estimates of compliance are usually below 50% across a 10-day treatment period (Williams et al., 1986). The National Council on Patient Information and Education (NCPIE) reported that children are receiving prescribed medicines at a very high rate; however, there are many barriers to successful treatment of both acute and chronic illnesses, including improper medicine use (NCPIE, 1989). A recent report by the NCPIE (1989) lists four major concerns in this area: (1) stopping a medicine too soon, (2) not taking enough of a medicine, (3) refusing to take a medicine, and (4) taking too much of a medicine. All of these concerns relate directly to the problem of noncompliance.

Problems associated with noncompliance have both health and economic implications. These implications include recurrence of the health problem, unnecessary continued diagnosis and treatment, side effects from stopping medicines too soon, the development of resistant strains of bacteria, and the potential for misuse of medicines that may remain in the home because they were not completed as prescribed (NCPIE, 1989).

Predictors of Compliance or Noncompliance. For many years, studies were carried out testing personality variables as predictors of compliance behavior. There is growing evidence, however, that these variables are not very helpful (Cromer & Tarnowski, 1989; Kaplan & Simon, 1990). Wil-

liams (1989) suggested that focusing on health beliefs may not be an effective strategy, either.

Patient satisfaction may be more salient in striving for successful outcomes. Satisfaction is based on several variables that affect patient performance, including patient perceptions of the physician (Korsch et al., 1968; Rapoff & Christopherson, 1982), characteristics of the physician–patient interaction (Haynes, Taylor, & Sackett, 1979), and physician sensitivity to the patient's needs (Falvo & Tippy, 1988; Rapoff, Purviance, & Lindsley, 1988).

Approaches to Effecting Change in Compliance. It is typical, in cases of childhood infection, for treatment interventions to be directed toward the individuals deemed most responsible for assuring proper home care, typically parents (Finney, Friman, Rapoff, & Christopherson, 1985; Williams et al., 1986). The efficacy of working directly with children remains to be tested in cases of acute infections, although children have been given a role in the home treatment of their own chronic illnesses (Taggart et al., 1991).

In concurrence with CDT, any interaction with children regarding compliance should occur at a developmentally appropriate level (NCPIE, 1989; O'Brien & Bush, 1993; Pantell & Lewis, 1986; Pantell et al., 1982). Unfortunately, such training is rare in medical education (Pantell & Lewis, 1986). A variety of strategies have been tried with varying degrees of success. Strategies for improving the exchange of information between physicians and patients include reminders from physicians' offices (Casey, Rosen, Glowasky, & Ludwig, 1985) and follow-up for appointment keeping (Friman, Finney, Rapoff, & Christopherson, 1985).

Compliance during Chronic Health Conditions. Many factors that affect compliance for treatment of acute conditions, such as patient satisfaction, also affect compliance with treatment for chronic health conditions. In the latter case, additional barriers come from family stress and the burden of constantly engaging in treatment.

Children's compliance behaviors improve with increased support from families (Tebbi, 1992). The notion of families as a key factor was supported by other studies. Gordis, Markowitz, and Lilienfeld (1969) found that variables indicative of parent involvement with the ill child were associated with improved compliance by the child. The impact of psychosocial factors on compliance was the focus of research by Cummings, Becker, and Kirscht (1982). They reported that as stress related to the illness increased within the family, compliance behavior decreased. Interventions in this area clearly need to be directed toward families, not just the ill children.

Harmful Health Behaviors

Abusable Substances. The topic of children's health behaviors relative to the use of abusable substances cannot be afforded justice here. As noted by Perry and Kelder (1992), most current models of abusable substance use prevention are implemented in junior high and high school and address risk factors in three domains: environment, personality, and behavior. The programs attempt to modify the student's interaction with the social environment that provides the conditions for drug use in the form of passive observation, role models, and availability of drugs.

Problem behavior theory (Jessor & Jessor, 1977) posits that specific deviant behavior is a product of exposure, behavior modeling, and social support in the adolescent's immediate environment. Therefore, as argued by Elliott, Huizinga, and Ageton (1985), the clustering and sequencing of deviant behaviors are more a product of the environment than of psychological predispositions.

The environmental influence of peer substance use is among the most consistent correlates of abusable substance use in adolescence (Kandel, 1986; Needle et al., 1986; Newcomb & Bentler, 1986) and preadolescence (Gillmore et al., 1990; Iannotti & Bush, 1992b). Moreover, Glynn (1981) concluded, after reviewing the literature, that while the influence of parents never

completely disappears, it recedes relative to the influence of peers as children move into adolescence.

Consistent positive correlations have been observed between use by family members and children's use and expectations to use abusable substances. For example, Bush and Iannotti (1985) found that the number of family users of alcohol, marijuana, and cigarettes was correlated with elementary schoolchildren's use and use intentions. In earlier research, Shute, Pierre, and Burke (1981) showed that half of a sample of preschool children exposed to smoking at home indicated that they intended to smoke in the future, compared with only 11% who were not exposed. For adolescents, the influence of parental drug use has been less than the influence of use by older siblings and peers (Brook, Nomura, & Cohen, 1989; Needle et al., 1986). Family modeling and parental bonding may operate indirectly through peer factors to influence adolescent drug use (Hansen et al., 1987).

Beginning in 1988–1989, 4th-grade students attending District of Columbia public schools participated in annual abusable substance use surveys through the 7th grade in 1991–1992. In an extension of the study, the 8th grade, in addition to the 7th grade, was surveyed in the last year. This additional survey facilitated a comparison of drug use by District 8th graders with that by 8th graders who participated in the national "Monitoring the Future" study (*NIDA Notes*, 1992).

Compared with the national sample, alcohol use was more prevalent among District students, and a higher proportion of District students reported having been drunk. District student cigarette smoking rates, at 43.4%, were almost identical to those measured nationally at 44.0%. Except for crack cocaine use, for which District rates were higher, the rates from the "Monitoring the Future" sample for all other comparable substances (i.e., marijuana, LSD, inhalants, steroids, tranquilizers, stimulants, and other forms of cocaine) were higher than among District 8th graders.

The comparisons of drug use among District 8th graders—who were predominantly African-American—with those surveyed in the national sample are consistent with other surveys. These findings indicate that African-American students tend to have higher rates of alcohol use and proceed to heavier use at younger ages than other students, but have lower rates of use of most illegal substances. Indeed, the greatest risk to District students, and especially boys, may come from a home and community environment that exposes them to involvement in illegal drug use and sales that can end in violence, incarceration, and even death.

In each year of the District of Columbia study, environmental and attitudinal factors were associated with abusable substance use, and in each year the majority of the students reported that they had witnessed drug sales. The percentage of students reporting that they had witnessed a drug sale by a family member or a family friend remained stable at about 17% during the survey years (Bush & Iannotti, 1994). If a student helped sell drugs, the odds of that student's being a drug user increased from 4 to 14 times, depending on the substance. The elevated risk was especially great for boys because boys were more than 4 times more likely than girls to be involved in drug sales.

The proportion of students who perceived that their friends used drugs increased each year from the 4th to 7th grades for alcohol, cigarettes, and marijuana (Bush, 1994). Conversely, the proportion of students reporting that friends offered them alcohol, cigarettes, and marijuana, and the amounts of perceived peer pressure to use these substances, fell from the 4th to 7th grades.

There was an inverse relationship between perceived pressure to use a substance and its social acceptability. In every year, the amount of perceived peer pressure to use marijuana was greater than for cigarettes, with alcohol ranking between the two. Thus, the amount of perceived peer pressure to use a particular substance is dependent on the child's age and the social acceptability of the substance. The relative ranks remained the same, but perceived peer pressure for all substances declined as the student moved up in grade level.

The percentage of 6th graders admitting to having been drunk and the magnitude of the increase from 5th to 6th grade in both cigarette experimentation and the use of alcohol without the mother's permission suggested that interventions for alcohol and cigarettes should be implemented before the 6th grade. The largest increase in use of other substances was from the 6th to the 7th grade, suggesting that interventions targeted toward substances other than cigarettes and alcohol should begin before the 7th grade.

Whether earlier or later, school-based programs seek to improve bonding to the conventional norms of society and often seek to strengthen family bonds (Hansen, Johnson, & Flay, 1988; Hawkins, Catalano, & Miller, 1992). Certainly, the conventional norms of society do not condone selling drugs. Little information is available, however, on how children deal with the mixed messages they receive when there is a conflict between those presented by teachers, the media, and the wider community and those presented by the behavior of families, family friends, and neighbors. Is it possible that those preadolescents with the strongest bonds to family members are likely to acquiesce to those members' requests even when the requests are in conflict with conventional norms? The theoretical perspective taken has implications for intervention. Essentially, one of these perspectives says that children are simply socialized into deviant behaviors because they are normative within the child's environment. The other view is that some children develop psychological traits that attract them to whatever deviant opportunities are at hand (Jessor & Jessor, 1977). If the latter view is taken, a goal of intervention should be to attempt to prevent formation of those traits associated with proneness to problem behavior. If the former view predominates, then the primary goal should be to change the children's social environments.

Either of these perspectives poses problems for school-based programs. A school-based program that teaches resistance skills will have a difficult time implementing a program to help students resist the urging of their family members and family friends. Most resistance curricula focus on the influences of media, peers, and perceptions of peers rather than those of family members, family friends, or neighbors (Perry & Murray, 1985). Social skills curricula may have some success in teaching resistance to peers and neighbors; families were the weakest influence on being asked to help sell drugs only, but simply being asked was associated with an elevated risk of drug use. The greater risk of sales involvement may not be amenable to school-based education because of its association with family users and sellers. Early adolescents need a program to identify high-risk students and arm them with skills that would protect them in the very homes and neighborhoods where they derive love, support, socialization, and identification. Broad community-based education that does not address the underlying social problems may have limited effect on adolescent involvement.

SUMMARY

The utility of using models of health behaviors with children is still unresolved. Three theories were described at the beginning of the chapter, but the evidence for any of the three remains mixed, at best. Bush and Iannotti (1990) attempted to integrate the theories into the children's health belief model, and while the initial results were encouraging, the results are based on reports of expected behaviors. The model remains to be tested on actual health behaviors. Such an effort may be a major contribution to the study of children's health behaviors.

The most important considerations in predicting children's health behaviors are parent and child attitudes and how they fit with the current sociocultural conditions. Future directions in research should focus on these areas in the effort to develop future interventions for children.

FUTURE RESEARCH DIRECTIONS

The methodologies currently used in health behavior research with children are subject to certain limitations. In response to interviews, surveys, or individual questionnaires, the predominant sources of information are parents, peers, and the children themselves. Unfortunately, as children get older, they spend less and less time with their parents, decreasing the reliability of the latter as reporters of their children's health behaviors. Because some adults will feel that their reports about their children's health behaviors reflect the job they are doing as parents, there is the potential for inaccurate reports (Weinfurt & Bush, 1996). Children may be the best source of information on their own behaviors, but certain limitations in understanding, memory, and expressive skills may also put in question the reliability of their answers. As children get older, peers may be in a better position than parents to comment on certain health behaviors, particularly those related to health risks. The reliability and validity of these peer reports, however, must also be viewed with some caution.

A major consideration in soliciting information from parents or children is the quality of the research instrument and its effectiveness in communicating to the respondent what information is being sought. Limited-choice instruments allow individuals to respond, even when they do not understand the question. Extensive pilot testing and evaluation of research instruments is certainly a requirement to determine the reliability and validity of these instruments. Use of well-established standardized instruments is recommended wherever possible.

Well-trained, sensitive interviewers are an important prerequisite for any type of personal data collection, but may be even more critical when working with children of varying developmental stages. Such individuals can communicate to respondents the importance of their answers with the hope of fostering truthfulness in responses. A good interviewer can also tell when a respondent does not understand a question and is able to assist the respondent without prompting certain answers.

In most cases, research reports are based on a single methodology. Future research will be more useful if built on a combination of methodologies. Possible methodologies include observations, ethnography, self-reports of behaviors, and reports from parents. The latter two are the easiest to use and provide insights into beliefs, attitudes, and motivations. Observational methods, which attempt to unobtrusively catch individuals in the course of behavior, is certainly the most costly in terms of time, financial resources, and personnel. It can be used, however, to address the lack of objective information on children's activities regarding their health. Ethnographic studies will provide understanding of the physical and social contexts within which behaviors occur. The blending of observational and ethnographic perspectives may also provide additional insights into how health behaviors develop.

Longitudinal research is another approach that is needed in understanding development of children's health behaviors. Solid longitudinal research, which incorporates self-reports and parent reports in combination with broader use of available methodologies, may improve validity and lead to great steps that will further the study of children's health behaviors.

The key here may be to increase the focus on children and on what children do in their parents' absence. It is recognized that parents are very involved in many areas because of the level of responsibility certain health behaviors require (e.g., purchasing food, taking medicines, treating injuries). The evidence is clear, however, that children are making a significant number of health decisions on their own, including many that parents never know about. Research on children's health behaviors is best when it considers the contributions of both parents and children, but particularly recognizes the unique and variable contributions of children.

REFERENCES

Alpert, B., Field, T., Goldstein, S., & Perry, S. (1990). Aerobics enhances cardiovascular fitness and agility in preschoolers. *Health Psychology, 9,* 48–56.

Bandura, A. (1977a). *Social learning theory.* Englewood Cliffs, NJ: Prentice-Hall.

Bandura, A. (1977b). Toward a unifying theory of behavioral change. *Psychological Review, 84,* 191–215.

Bandura A. (1986). *Social foundations of thought and action.* Englewood Cliffs, NJ: Prentice-Hall.

Baumrind, D. (1987). A developmental perspective on adolescent risk taking in contemporary America. In C. E. Irwin, Jr. (Ed.), *New Directions in Child Development: Adolescent Social Behavior and Health,* No. 37, 93–125.

Becker, M. H. (1974). The health belief model and personal health behavior. *Health Education Quarterly, 2,* 324–508.

Bernstein, A. C., & Cowan, P. A. (1981). Children's conceptions of birth and sexuality. In R. Bibace & M. E. Walsh (Eds.), *New Directions in Child Development: Children's Conceptions of Health, Illness and Bodily Function, 14,* 9–29.

Bibace, R., & Walsh, M. (1979). Developmental stages in children's conceptions of illness. In G. Stone, F. Cohen, & N. Adler (Eds.), *Health psychology* (pp. 285–301). San Francisco: Jossey-Bass.

Bibace, R., & Walsh, M. (1980). Development of children's concepts of illness. *Pediatrics, 66,* 913–917.

Blos, P. (1979). *The adolescent passage.* New York: International Universities Press.

Brook, J. S., Nomura, C., & Cohen, P. (1989). A network of influences on adolescent drug involvement: Neighborhood, school, peer, and family. *Genetic Society General Psychological Monographs, 115,* 123–145.

Burbach, D. J., & Peterson, L. (1986). Children's concepts of physical illness: A review and critique of the cognitive-developmental literature. *Health Psychology, 5,* 307–325.

Bush, P. J. (1994). *Black children's substance use: Longitudinal influences.* Final Report (Grant No. RO1 DA04497). Submitted to the National Institute on Drug Abuse.

Bush, P. J., & Davidson, F. R. (1982). Medicines and "drugs": What do children think? *Health Education Quarterly, 9,* 209–224.

Bush, P. J., & Iannotti, R. J. (1985). The development of children's health orientations and behaviors: Lessons for substance abuse prevention. In C. L. Jones & R. J. Battjes (Eds.), *Etiology of drug abuse* (pp. 45–54). National Institute on Drug Abuse Monograph 56, DHHS Publication No. (ADM)85-1335. Washington, DC: U.S. Government Printing Office.

Bush, P. J., & Iannotti, R. J. (1988). Origins and stability of children's health beliefs relative to medicine use. *Social Science and Medicine, 27,* 345–352.

Bush, P. J., & Iannotti, R. J. (1990). A children's health belief model. *Medical Care, 28,* 69–86.

Bush, P. J., & Iannotti, R. J. (1993). Differences in the use of alcohol, cigarettes, and marijuana among fourth grade urban schoolchildren in 1988–89 and 1990–91. *American Journal of Public Health, 83,* 111–114.

Bush, P. J., & Iannotti, R. J. (1994). *Drug sales involvement in early adolescence.* Paper presented at the annual meeting of the Society for Behavioral Medicine, Boston.

Bush, P. J., Iannotti, R. J., & Davidson, F. R. (1985). A longitudinal study of children and medicines. In D. D. Breimer & P. Speiser (Eds.), *Topics in pharmaceutical sciences* (pp. 391–403). New York: Elsevier.

Bush, P. J., Iannotti, R. J., Zuckerman, A. E., O'Brien, R. W., & Smith, S. (1991). Relationships among black families' cardiovascular disease risk factors. *Preventive Medicine, 20,* 447–461.

Bush, P. J., Trakas, D. J., Sanz, E. J., Wirsing, R., Vaskilampi, T., & Prout, A. (1996). *Children, medicines and culture.* Binghamton, NY: Haworth.

Casey, R., Rosen, B., Glowasky, A., & Ludwig, S. (1985). An intervention to improve followup of patients with otitis media. *Clinical Pediatrics, 24,* 149–152.

Centers for Disease Control. (1987). Bicycle-related injuries: Data from the national electronic injury surveillance system. *Morbidity and Mortality Weekly Report, 36,* 269–270.

Centers for Disease Control, Division of Injury Control. (1990). Childhood injuries in the United States. *American Journal of Diseases of Children, 144,* 627–646.

Cohen, R. Y., Brownell, K. D., & Felix, M. R. (1990). Age and sex differences in health habits and beliefs of schoolchildren. *Health Psychology, 9,* 208–224.

Crider, C. (1981). Children's conceptions of body interior. In R. Bibace & M. E. Walsh (Eds.), *New Directions in Child Development: Children's Conceptions of Health, Illness and Bodily Function, 14,* 49–65.

Cromer, B. A., & Tarnowski, K. J. (1989). Noncompliance in adolescents: A review. *Journal of Developmental and Behavioral Pediatrics, 10,* 207–215.

Cummings, K. M., Becker, M. H., & Kirscht, J. P. (1982). Psychosocial factors affecting adherence to medical regimens in a group of hemodialysis patients. *Medical Care, 20,* 567–580.

Davidson, F. R., & Kandel, R. F. (1981). The individualization of food habits. *Journal of the American Dietetic Association, 72,* 341–348.

Department of Health and Human Services. (1990). *Healthy People, 2000.* Washington, DC: U.S. Government Printing Office.

DiClemente, R. J. (1989). Prevention of human immunodeficiency virus infection among adolescents: The interplay of health education and public policy in the development and implementation of school based AIDS education programs. *AIDS Education and Prevention, 1,* 70–78.

Elliott, D. S., Huizinga, D., & Ageton, S. S. (1985). *Explaining delinquency and drug use.* Beverly Hills, CA: Sage.

Erikson, E. (1968). *Identity youth and crisis.* New York: Norton.

Falvo, D., & Tippy, P. (1988). Communicating information to patients: Patient satisfaction and adherence as associated with resident skill. *Journal of Family Practice, 26,* 643.

Farrand, L. L., & Cox, C. L. (1993). Determinants of positive health behaviors in middle childhood. *Nursing Research, 42,* 208–213.

Finney, J. W., Friman, P. C., Rapoff, M. A., & Christopherson, E. R. (1985). Improving compliance with antibiotic regimens for otitis media. *American Journal of Diseases of Children, 139,* 89–95.

Fishbein, M., & Ajzen, I. (1975). *Belief, attitude, intention and behavior.* Reading, MA: Addison-Wesley.

Friman, P. C., Finney, J. W., Rapoff, M. A., & Christopherson, E. R. (1985). Improving pediatric appointment keeping with reminders and reduced response requirement. *Journal of Applied Behavioral Analysis, 18,* 315–321.

Gillmore, M. R., Catalano, R. F., Morrison, D. M., Wells, B., Iritani, E. A., & Hawkins, J. D. (1990). Racial differences in acceptability and availability of drugs and early initiation of substance use. *American Journal of Drug and Alcohol Abuse, 16,* 185–206.

Ginsburg, H., & Opper, S. (1979). *Piaget's theory of intellectual development.* Englewood Cliffs, NJ: Prentice-Hall.

Glik, D. C., Greaves, P. E., Kronenfeld, J. J., & Jackson, K. L. (1993). Safety hazards in households with young children. *Journal of Pediatric Psychology, 18,* 115–131.

Glynn, T. J. (1981). From family to peer: A review of transitions of influence among drug-using youth. *Journal of Youth and Adolescence, 10,* 363–383.

Gochman, D. S. (1971). Some correlates of children's health beliefs and potential health behavior. *Journal of Health and Social Behavior, 12,* 148–154.

Gochman, D. S., & Saucier, J. (1982). Perceived vulnerability in children and adolescents. *Health Education, 9,* 142–155.

Gordis, L., Markowitz, M., & Lilienfeld, A. M. (1969). Why patients don't follow medical advice: A study of children on long-term antistreptococcal prophylaxis. *Journal of Pediatrics, 75,* 957–968.

Greenberger, E. (1984). Defining psychosocial maturity in adolescence. In P. Karoly & J. Steffen (Eds.), *Adolescent behavior disorders: Foundations and contemporary concerns* (pp. 54–81). Lexington, MA: Heath.

Gustafson-Larson, A. M., & Terry, R. D. (1992). Weight-related behaviors and concerns of fourth-grade children. *Journal of the American Dietetic Association, 92,* 818–822.

Hackworth, S. R., & McMahon, R. J. (1991). Factors mediating children's health care attitudes. *Journal of Pediatric Psychology, 16,* 69–85.

Haight, W. L., Black, J. E., & DiMatteo, M. R. (1985). Young children's understanding of the social roles of physician and patient. *Journal of Pediatric Psychology, 10,* 31–43.

Hansen, W. B., Graham, J. W., Sobel, J. L., Shelton, D. R., Flay, B. R., & Johnson, C. A. (1987). The consistency of peer and parent influences on tobacco, alcohol, and marijuana use among young adolescents. *Journal of Behavioral Medicine, 10,* 559-579.

Hansen, W. B., Johnson, C. A., & Flay, B. R. (1988). Affective and social influences on approaches to the prevention of multiple substance abuse among seventh grade students: Results form Project SMART. *Preventive Medicine, 17,* 135-154.

Hawkins, J. D., Catalano, R. F., & Miller, J. L. (1992). Risk and protective factors for alcohol and other drug problems in adolescence and early adulthood: Implications for substance abuse prevention. *Psychological Bulletin, 112,* 64-105.

Haynes, R. B., Taylor, D. W., & Sackett, D. L. (1979). *Compliance in health care.* Baltimore: Johns Hopkins University Press.

Hofman, A., & Walter, H. J. (1989). The association between physical fitness and cardiovascular disease risk factors in children in a five-year follow-up study. *International Journal of Epidemiology, 18,* 830-835.

Howland, J., Sargent, J., Weitzman, M., Mangione, T., Ebert, R., Mauceri, M., & Bond, M. (1989). Barriers to bicycle helmet use among children. *American Journal of Diseases in Children, 143,* 741-744.

Hunt, L. M., Jordan, B., Irwin, S., & Browner, C. H. (1989). Compliance and the patient's perspective: Controlling symptoms in everyday life. *Culture and Medicine in Psychiatry, 13,* 315.

Iannotti, R. J., & Bush, P. J. (1992a). The development of autonomy in children's health behavior. In E. J. Susman, L. V. Feagans, & W. Ray (Eds.), *Emotion, cognition, health, and development in children and adolescents: A two-way street* (pp. 53-74). Hillsdale, NJ: Erlbaum.

Iannotti, R. J., & Bush, P. J. (1992b). Perceived or actual friends' use of alcohol, cigarettes, marijuana and cocaine: Which has the most influence? *Journal of Youth and Adolescence, 21,* 833-847.

Iannotti, R. J., & Bush, P. J. (1992c). Towards a developmental theory of compliance. In N. Krasnagor, L. Epstein, S. Johnson, & S. Yaffe (Eds.), *Developmental aspects of health compliance behavior* (pp. 59-76). Hillsdale, NJ: Erlbaum.

Iannotti, R. J., O'Brien, R. W., Cowen, E., & Wilson, K. (1990). *Understanding and response to minor injury and illness among pre-adolescents.* Poster presented to the Conference on Human Development, Richmond, VA.

Inhelder, B., & Piaget, J. (1964). *The early growth of logic in the child* [translated by E. A. Lunzer & D. Papert]. London: Routledge & Kegan Paul.

Jeffrey, D. B., McLellarn, R. W., & Fox, D. T. (1982). The development of children's eating habits: The role of television commercials. *Health Education Quarterly, 9,* 174-189.

Jessor, R., & Jessor, S. L. (1977). *Problem behavior and psychosocial development—A longitudinal study of youth.* New York: Academic Press.

Johnson, S. R., Schonfeld, D. J., Siegel, D., Krasnovsky, F. M., Boyce, J. C., Saliba, P. A., Boyce, W. T., & Perrin, W. C. (1994). What do minority elementary students understand about the causes of acquired immunodeficiency syndrome, colds, and obesity? *Developmental and Behavioral Pediatrics, 15,* 239-247.

Kandel, D. B. (1986). Processes of peer influence in adolescence. In R. Silberstein (Ed.), *Development as action in context, problem behavior, and normal youth development* (pp. 87-113). New York: Springer.

Kandel, D. B., & Lesser, D. S. (1972). *Youth in two worlds.* San Francisco: Jossey-Bass.

Kaplan, R. M., & Simon, H. J. (1990). Compliance in medical care: Reconsideration of self-predictions. *Annals of Behavioral Medicine, 12,* 67-71.

Keane, M., O'Brien, R. W., Connell, D. C., & Close, N. C. (1996). *A descriptive study of the Head Start health component.* Final report prepared for the Administration on Children, Youth and Families. Washington, DC.

Kimmel, S. R., & Nagel, R. W. (1990). Bicycle safety knowledge and behavior in school age children. *Journal of Family Practice, 30,* 677-680.

Koocher, G. P. (1981). Children's conceptions of death. In R. Bibace & M. E. Walsh (Eds.), *New Directions in Child Development: Children's Conceptions of Health, Illness and Bodily Function, 14,* 85-100.

Korsch, B. M., & Negrete, V. F. (1972). Doctor-patient communication. *Scientific American, 227,* 66.

Korsch, B. M., Gozzi, E. K., & Francis, V. (1968). Gaps in doctor-patient communications: Doctor-patient interaction and patient satisfaction. *Pediatrics, 42,* 855.

Levitt, M. Z., Selman, R. L., & Richmond, J. B. (1991). The physiological foundations of early adolescents' high risk behavior: Implications for research and practice. *Journal of Research on Adolescence, 1,* 349-378.

Lewis, C. E., & Lewis, M. A. (1982a). Determinants of children's health-related beliefs and behavior. *Family and Community Health, 44,* 85-97.

Lewis, C. E., & Lewis, M. A. (1982b). Children's health-related decision making. *Health Education Quarterly, 9,* 129-141, 225-237.

Lewis, C. E., & Lewis, M. A. (1983). Improving the health of children: Must the children be involved? *Annual Review of Public Health, 4,* 259-283.

Lewis, C. E., & Lewis, M. A. (1984). Peer pressure and risk-taking behaviors in children. *American Journal of Public Health, 74,* 580-584.

Lewis, C. E., Lewis, M. A., Lorimer, A., & Palmer, B. (1977). Child-initiated care: The use of school nursing services in an "adult-free" system. *Pediatrics, 60,* 499-507.

Maiman, L. A., & Becker, M. H. (1974). The health belief model: Origins and correlations in psychological theory. *Health Education Monographs, 2,* 336-353.

McCarthy, D. (1974). Communication between children and doctors. *Developmental Medicine and Child Neurology, 16*, 279.

Mitchell, J. M., O'Brien, R. W., Semansky, R. M., & Iannotti, R. J. (1995). Sources of AIDS information for parents and children. *Medical Care, 33*, 423–431.

Moore, L. L., Lombardi, D. A., White, M. J., Campbell, J. L., Oliveria, S. A., & Ellison, R. C. (1991). Influence of parents' physical activity levels on activity levels of young children. *Journal of Pediatrics, 118*, 215–219.

National Council on Patient Information and Education. (1989). *Children and America's other drug problem: Guidelines for improving prescription medicine use among children and teenagers.* Washington, DC.

Needle, R., McCubbin, H., Wilson, M., Reineck, R., Lazar, A., & Mederer, H. (1986). Interpersonal influences in adolescent drug use: The role of the older siblings, parents, and peers. *International Journal of Addictions, 21*, 739–766.

Newcomb, M. D., & Bentler, P. M. (1986). Substance use and ethnicity: Differential impact of peer and adult models. *Journal of Psychology, 120*, 83–95.

NIDA Notes. (1992). A comparison of drug use among 8th, 10th, and 12th graders from NIDA's high school senior survey. May/June, p. 19.

Obeidallah, D., Turner, P. T., Iannotti, R. J., O'Brien, R. W., Haynie, D., & Galper, D. (1993). Investigating children's knowledge and understanding of AIDS. *Journal of School Health, 63*, 125.

O'Brien, R. W., & Bush, P. J. (1993). Helping children learn how to use medicines, *Office Nurse, 6*, 14–19.

O'Brien, R. W., Bush, P. J., & Parcel, G. S. (1989). Stability in a measure of children's health locus of control. *Journal of School Health, 59*, 161–164.

O'Brien, R. W., & Iannotti, R. J. (1993). Differences in mother's and children's perceptions of urban, black children's life stress. *Journal of Youth and Adolescence, 22*(5), 543–557.

O'Brien, R. W., Smith, S., Bush, P. J., & Peleg, E. (1990). Obesity, self-esteem, and health locus of control in black youths during transition to adolescence. *American Journal of Health Promotion, 5*, 133–139.

Pantell, R. H., & Lewis, C. C. (1986). Physician communication with pediatric patients: A theoretical and empirical analysis. *Advances in Developmental Behavioral Pediatrics, 7*, 65–119.

Pantell, R. H., Stewart, T. J., Dias, J. K., Wells, P., & Ross, W. (1982). Physician communication with children and parents. *Pediatrics, 70*, 396.

Parcel, G. S., & Baranowski, T. (1981). Social learning theory and health education. *Health Education, 123*, 14–18.

Parcel, G. S., & Meyer, M. P. (1978). Development of an instrument to measure children's health locus of control. *Health Education Monographs, 6*, 149–159.

Parke, R. D., & Tinsley, B. J. (1987). Family interaction in infancy. In J. D. Osofsky (Ed.), *Handbook of infant development*, 2nd ed. (pp. 579–641). New York: Wiley.

Perlman, N., & Abramovitch, R. (1987). Visit to the pediatrician: Children's concerns. *Journal of Pediatrics, 110*, 988–990.

Perrin, E. C., & Gerrity, S. (1981). There's a demon in your belly. *Pediatrics, 67*, 841–849.

Perry, C. L., & Kelder, S. H. (1992). Models for effective prevention. *Journal of Adolescent Health, 13*, 355–363.

Perry, C. L., & Murray, D. M. (1985). The prevention of adolescent drug abuse: Implications from etiological, developmental, behavioral and environmental models. *Journal of Primary Prevention, 6*, 31–52.

Peterson, C., & Stunkard, A. J. (1989). Personal control and health promotion. *Social Science and Medicine, 28*, 819–828.

Peterson, L., Farmer, J., & Kashani, J. H. (1990). Parental injury prevention endeavors: A function of health beliefs? *Health Psychology, 9*, 177–191.

Pratt, L. (1973). Child learning methods and children's health behavior. *Journal of Health and Social Behavior, 14*, 61–69.

Rapoff, M. A., & Christopherson, E. R. (1982). Improving compliance in pediatric practice. *Pediatric Clinics of North America, 29*, 339–357.

Rapoff, M. A., Purviance, M. R., & Lindsley, M. D. (1988). Educational and behavioral strategies for improving medication compliance in juvenile rheumatoid arthritis. *Archives of Physical Medicine and Rehabilitation, 69*, 439–441.

Remy, R., & Power, T. G. (1995). *Maternal socialization strategies and children's health locus of control beliefs.* Paper presented to the Society for Research in Child Development, Indianapolis.

Rogers, K. D., & Reese, G. (1965). Health studies—presumably normal high school students: III. Health room visits. *American Journal of Diseases of Children, 109*, 28–42.

Sallis, J. F., Alcaraz, J. E., McKenzie, T. L., Hovell, M. F., Kolody, B., & Nader, P. R. (1993). Parental behavior in relation to physical activity and fitness in 9-year-old children. *American Journal of Diseases in Children, 146*, 1383–1388.

Sallis, J. F., & Nader, P. R. (1988). Family determinants of health behavior. In D. S. Gochman (Ed.), *Health behavior: Emerging research perspectives* (pp. 107–124). New York: Plenum Press.

Sanz, E. J., Bush, P. J., & Garcia, M. (1996). Medicines at home: The contents of medicine cabinets in eight countries. In P. J. Bush, D. J. Trakas, E. J. Sanz, R. Wirsing, T. Vaskilampi, & A. Prout (Eds.), *Children, medicines and culture* (pp. 77–104). Binghamton, NY: Haworth.

Schonfeld, D. F., Johnson, S. R., Perrin, E. C., O'Hare, L. L., & Cicchetti, D. V. (1993). Understanding of acquired immunodeficiency syndrome by elementary school children—a developmental survey. *Pediatrics, 92*, 389–395.

Shear, C. L., Freedman, D. S., & Burke, G. L. (1988). Secular trends of obesity in early life: The Bogulosa Heart Study. *American Journal of Public Health, 78*, 75–77.

Shute, R., Pierre, R., & Lubell, E. (1981). Smoking awareness and practices of urban preschool and first grade children. *Journal of School Health, 5,* 347-351.

Simons-Morton, B. G., Parcel, G. S., O'Hara, N. M., Blair, S. N., & Pate, R. R. (1988). Health related physical fitness in childhood: Status and recommendations. *Annual Review of Public Health, 9,* 403-425.

Simons-Morton, B. G., Taylor, W. C., Snider, S. A., & Huang, I. W. (1993). The physical activity of fifth-grade students during physical education classes. *American Journal of Public Health, 83,* 262-264.

Smith, S. A., Zuckerman, A. E., & Bush, P. J. (1990). *Autonomy in children's food intake: Implications for dietary intervention in cardiovascular disease (CVD) risk reduction.* Paper presented at the annual meeting of the Society for Behavioral Medicine, Chicago.

Taggart, V. S., Zuckerman, A. E., Sly, R. M., Steinmueller, C., Newman, G., O'Brien, R. W., Schneider, S., & Bellanti, J. A. (1991). Evaluation of an asthma education program for hospitalized innercity children. *Patient Education and Counseling, 17,* 35-47.

Tebbi, C. K. (1992). Treatment compliance in childhood and adolescence. *Cancer, 71,* 3441-3449.

Thompson, B., Butcher, A., & Berenson, G. (1987). Children's beliefs about sources of health: A reliability and validity study. *Measurement and Evaluation in Counseling and Development, 20,* 80-88.

Tinsley, B. J. (1992). Multiple influences on the acquisition and socialization of children's health attitudes and behavior: An integrative review. *Child Development, 63,* 1043-1069.

Van Arsdell, W. R., Roghmann, K. J., & Nader, P. R. (1972). Visits to an elementary school nurse. *Journal of School Health, 42,* 142-147.

Vaughn, G. F. (1957). Children in hospital. *Lancet, 1,* 1117.

Walsh, M. E., & Bibace, R. (1991). Children's conceptions of AIDS: A developmental analysis. *Journal of Pediatric Psychology, 16,* 273-285.

Weinfurt, K. P., & Bush, P. J. (1996). Contradictory subject response in longitudinal research. *Journal of Studies on Alcohol, 57,* 273-282.

Williams, R. (1989). Illness visualization and therapeutic adherence. *Journal of Family Practice, 28,* 185-192.

Williams, R. L., Maiman, L. A., Broadbent, D. N., Kotok, D., Lawrence, R. A., Longfield, L. A., Mangold, A. H., Mayer, S. J., Powell, K. R., Sayre, J. W., & Webb, S. (1986). Educational strategies to improve compliance with an antibiotic regimen. *American Journal of Diseases of Children, 140,* 216-220.

Wolf, A. M., Gortmaker, S. L., Cheung, L., Gray, H. M., Herzog, D. B., & Colditz, G. A. (1993). Activity, inactivity, and obesity: Racial, ethnic, and age differences among schoolgirls. *American Journal of Public Health, 83,* 1625-1627.

Zuckerman, A. E., Olevsky-Peleg, E., Bush, P. J., Horowitz, C., Davidson, F., Brown, D., & Walter, H. (1989). Cardiovascular risk factors among black schoolchildren: Comparisons among four Know Your Body studies. *Preventive Medicine, 18,* 113-132.

4

Health Behavior in Adolescents

Julia Muennich Cowell and Beth A. Marks

DEVELOPMENTAL PERSPECTIVE

Adolescents appear to be among the healthiest group of Americans by traditional measures, such as mortality rates (OTA, 1991a). Unfortunately, despite their apparent good health status, adolescents are the only age group in the United States that has not experienced an improvement in health status over the past 30 years (Blum, 1987). Estimates show that 1 in 5 adolescents aged 10–18 suffers from at least one serious health problem (OTA, 1991a). The leading causes of death among adolescents differ from those of other age groups in that unlike older and younger Americans, adolescents are more likely to die of unintentional injuries, suicide, and homicide. Consequently, the use of traditional measures of health may not be an adequate reflection of adolescent health.

Definitions of health and of perceptions of health are essential to the understanding of health promotion. Perceptions about health and health promotion have changed as society has

Julia Muennich Cowell and Beth A. Marks • Department of Public Health, Mental Health, and Administrative Nursing, University of Illinois at Chicago, Chicago, Illinois 60612-7350.

Handbook of Health Behavior Research III: Demography, Development, and Diversity, edited by David S. Gochman. Plenum Press, New York, 1997.

evolved (Millstein, Nightengale, Peterson, Mortimer, & Hamburg, 1993). Health promotion models have been expanded to include psychosocial and environmental aspects of health instead of being limited to the biological model. In the context of a broadened view of health, a definition of adolescent health in particular involves more than the presence or absence of physical disease and disability, since morbidity and mortality of adolescents are associated with biopsychosocial and environmental factors (OTA, 1991a; Imai & Schydlower, 1994). Thus, the core of major health concerns for adolescents is not only physical disease, but also their health behaviors, such as their engagement in risk-taking behaviors related to violence, mental health, substance abuse, sexually transmitted disease, and unintended pregnancy (Imai, 1989; Blum, 1991).

Adolescence is a period in human development that is characterized by change and transitions. Consequently, adolescence should be the focus of efforts to promote healthful behaviors that are specific for individuals who are in a state of change and transition (Brooks-Gunn & Warren, 1989). Basic to efforts in health promotion in adolescence is an understanding of adolescence itself. An understanding of the developmental perspective of adolescent health behavior poses questions about the relationship of genetic and environmental processes across the period of late childhood to older adolescence, roughly age 8 to age 18 (*Health Promotion for Older Children and Adolescents*, 1993). The relative contribution of heredity and environment to adolescent behavior remains unclear and highly debated. Heuristically, the environment provides for external inputs to the human system.

Contributing to the controversial nature of the debate about relative influence of heredity and environment is the complexity of the period in terms of specific transitions. The developmental view of adolescence as a period of transitions can be discussed on the basis of specifically biological, cognitive, emotional, and social transitions.

Biological Transitions

The primary biological change in adolescence is puberty. Puberty consists of two basic developments, adrenarche or the development of the adrenal glands, and gonadarche, the development of the gonads and secondary sex characteristics. These changes occur rapidly and pervasively. Although the specific effects of hormones on behavior are not clearly understood, researchers have found significant relationships between increased levels of testosterone and sexual motivation and aggressiveness in boys and androgen and estrogen levels and initiation of sexual activity in girls (Smith, Udry, & Morris, 1985; Udry, 1988).

Cognitive Transitions

During the period of older childhood and adolescence, there are significant changes in cognition. The quantity of information that can be processed increases with age, as do the knowledge base and the ability to apply what one knows in static settings (Keating, 1990). Adolescents demonstrate an ability to think more abstractly than young children and can view information in relative rather than in absolute terms. Interestingly, older children and adolescents have demonstrated a lack of ability to apply their complex cognitive skills to practical problem solving in dynamic, stressful situations—exactly the type of situations in which health decisions related to substance use and sexual behavior are often made. Further inhibiting the application of complex skills is the egocentric nature of adolescence. Researchers have found that these cognitive constructs often contribute to the sense of invulnerability (Pesce & Harding, 1986). The nature of these cognitive processes in adolescence underscores the importance of encouraging adolescents to rehearse decision making on the basis of relevant content.

Emotional Transitions

Researchers have hypothesized several views of emotion in late childhood and adolescence. One view suggests that emotions are a component of temperament (Buss & Plomin, 1984). Thus, emotions are central to controlling arousal tendencies. The control of arousal tendencies may contribute to protective health behavior as well as risk behavior. For example, one's gentler emotions may mediate anger and consequently protect against cardiovascular disease; conversely, such emotions may give way to greater anger and support aggressive behavior.

Social Transitions

Family continues to be an important influence on youth throughout the adolescent period, despite a wealth of research demonstrating the changes in family during adolescence (Coates, 1987; Cochran & Riley, 1988). The familial transitions that have been identified as significant are the increasing independence given to adolescents, family relocations, parental separation or divorce, loss of siblings, and natural disasters (Amato & Keith, 1991; Simmons & Blyth, 1987).

Peer-group transitions also occur in adolescence. During early adolescence, same-sex friends are preferred, with male friendships being more intense than female friendships (Tietjen, 1982). Social skill is defined differently for boys and girls, with number of friends more important for boys and intensity of friendships more important for girls (Bryant, 1985). Friendships with peers increase among adolescents as contact with adults diminishes. The continued support of adults would be helpful, however, in the adaptation to mature roles (Feiring & Lewis, 1991). The importance of both peer and family role models in supporting a health-promoting lifestyle is underscored.

School transitions occur for most American youth, with the transitions to middle school or junior high school and then to high school being the norm. Studies have demonstrated that transitions to junior high and high school are often associated with decreased academic achievement for girls (Blyth, Simmons, & Carlton-Ford, 1983; Crockett, Petersen, Graber, Schulenberg, & Ebata, 1989). In addition to decreased academic achievement, girls have been found to have lower self-esteem (Wigfield, Eccles, MacIver, Reuman, & Midgley, 1991) and increased psychological symptoms (Hirsch & Rapkin, 1987) after school transitions. Multiple school transitions can produce a cumulative effect, particularly for girls (Simmons & Blyth, 1987).

Future research needs to be directed toward healthy development rather than the typical problem-focused approach, which has resulted in a paucity of theoretical models based on positive human development for conducting research on adolescent health behaviors (Millstein et al., 1993). Furthermore, health promotion programming is enhanced if it is designed to take into account the uniqueness of adolescents in the context of their biological, cognitive, emotional, and social transitions.

CONCEPTUALLY DERIVED DETERMINANTS OF ADOLESCENT HEALTH BEHAVIOR

Examination of the determinants of adolescent health behavior requires a review of the conceptual approaches utilized to research adolescent health behavior. There are a variety of theoretical approaches for studying determinants of health behaviors among adolescents. Researchers have now reached a general consensus, however, regarding the major variables that mediate adolescent health behaviors. These variables may be viewed in two domains, external and internal.

External Variables

Access to Health Care

Health care providers, such as physicians, nurses, psychologists, and social workers, are important mentors in health promotion for many adolescents. Because of the importance of health care providers in giving cues to adolescents, access to health care is a major consideration for many American adolescents (Kaplan, 1990; Wood, Hayward, Corey, Freeman, & Shapiro, 1990). Adolescents' access to needed health care, in particular early intervention services, may be difficult as a result of numerous barriers (Dougherty et al., 1992). Although some of the barriers, such as lack of health insurance coverage, geographic unavailability of health services, and legal barriers, are universal to Americans of all ages, additional issues uniquely affect adolescents (Dougherty, 1993). For example, legal requirements for parental consent and notification for services and lack of trained and acceptable providers, along with a lack of information regarding the need for services and the location of services, can be found to specifically affect adolescent health behaviors and health status.

Financial Barriers. In the United States, health insurance is essentially mandatory for access to the health care system due to the high cost of health services (OTA, 1992). This cost presents a significant financial barrier for adolescents without insurance coverage. Despite the inconsistent data concerning the rate at which the proportion of uninsured adolescents has increased, in general studies do reflect a growing number of adolescents who do not have insurance coverage.

Estimates from the National Health Interview Survey demonstrated that 1 in 7 individuals (15%, or 4.7 million) aged 10–18 did not have any form of health insurance coverage in 1989 (Newacheck, McManus, & Gephart, 1992). Additionally, regional variations exist among adolescents with insurance coverage. Reports document that more than 1 of every 5 adolescents are uninsured in southern and western states, while fewer than 1 in 10 adolescents have no coverage in northeastern and midwestern states (OTA, 1991c). These differences have been attributed to income-specific rates of Medicaid and rates of private health insurance coverage (*Business & Health*, 1990; OTA, 1991c). Lower Medicaid income eligibility requirements in the South and lower percentages of private insurance coverage in the West have been associated with the higher numbers of uninsured adolescents in southern and western states, respectively (OTA, 1991c).

Among the 85% of adolescents who had insurance coverage in 1989, 73% were privately insured, 10% had public insurance, and 2% reportedly were both privately and publicly insured (Newacheck et al., 1992). Many of these adolescents with health insurance coverage are underinsured and are experiencing decreased coverage under private insurance. Additionally, coverage under public programs has not increased substantially (Newacheck et al., 1992).

Determinants of health insurance coverage. The most significant determinant of health insurance coverage for both adolescents and individuals in all other age groups is family income (OTA, 1991c). Studies have shown that financial causes, such as the cost of insurance, are the most often cited reasons for lack of insurance coverage (Newacheck et al, 1992). The study by Newacheck and McManus (1989) reported that poverty and family income were associated with insurance coverage and the type of coverage. Data show that 1 in 3 poor adolescents (below 100% of the federal poverty level) do not have access to Medicaid (OTA, 1991c).

Researchers report that financial barriers to regular source of care were more likely for poor, near-poor, or nonwhite children (Newacheck & McManus, 1989; Wood, Hayward, Corey, Freeman, & Shapiro, 1990). A 1990 study demonstrated that a higher proportion of blacks (16%) and Hispanics (28%) compared to whites (11%) were uninsured (Wood et al., 1990). Black adolescents have been reported as being more likely to be uninsured and covered by public programs than white adolescents (Newacheck & McManus, 1989). Lieu, Newacheck, and McManus (1993) reported in their study that black and Hispanic adolescents were at greater risk than white adolescents for health needs and access problems. Despite the apparent racial disparities, when family income is taken into account, the correlation between race and lack of health insurance coverage almost disappears (Newacheck & McManus, 1989; OTA, 1991c).

Several other factors predict insurance coverage. One powerful factor that influences health insurance coverage for adolescents is parental education level (Newacheck & McManus, 1989). For example, adolescents of parents with less than nine years of formal education have been found to be 11 times more likely to be uninsured than adolescents whose parents have completed some postbaccalaureate training (Newacheck & McManus, 1989). Type of parental employment has also been associated with adolescent coverage (OTA, 1991c). In middle- and upper-middle-income families, adolescents whose parents are self-employed are more likely to be uninsured. Finally, adolescents are more likely to have private health insurance coverage if they live in intact families than if they live in single-parent homes (Newacheck & McManus, 1989).

Barriers to access for adolescents with insurance coverage. While uninsured adolescents face substantial barriers in obtaining health care, even adolescents with insurance face barriers due to limitations in coverage from both Medicaid and private health insurance. Private insurance and managed care systems, such as health maintenance organizations (HMOs), lead to barriers to access for adolescents due to the structuring of health insurance benefits. For example, access limitations may occur in many of the services that are most applicable to adolescent health care needs, such as mental health services, substance abuse treatment services, prenatal care, orthodontia, contraceptive services, abortion services, and preventive screening procedures and services (OTA, 1991c). Preventive services typically are covered by HMOs, and even then HMOs may limit access by requiring long waits for appointments (Dougherty, 1993).

Insurance coverage by private health insurance is oriented toward physician-directed care rather than care by nonphysician providers (OTA, 1991c). Although nonphysician health care providers, such as nurses, psychologists, and clinical social workers, are licensed to practice in an expanded role, direct reimbursement is often problematic. Because these nonphysician providers are often key providers in adolescent health care settings, such as school-based clinics, inability to obtain direct reimbursement for services has an impact on the availability of such services for adolescents and on the long-term viability of these services.

The exact number of adolescents enrolled in HMOs is unknown. National trends, however, demonstrate increasing numbers of families enrolling in HMOs. The impact of HMOs compared to fee-for-service on access to and quality of care currently remains under study. Although many studies have found little differences between fee-for-service and HMOs, a 1994 study found that HMO enrollees were diagnosed at significantly earlier stages for four cancer sites (female breast, colon, cervix, and melanoma) for which effective screening services were available (Riley, Potosky, Lubitz, & Brown, 1994). Although no research is yet available showing similar effects of early, preventive care in the unique health concerns of adolescents, one could hypothesize that adolescents might receive early health promotion cues for health behaviors that have been related to substance use, sexual behavior, nutrition, and physical activity. Surveys have demonstrated that managed care programs are more widely used in the East and West, while fee-for-service is more predominant in the South and the Midwest (*Business & Health*, 1990). Thus, health promotion opportunities may vary by region, and adoles-

cents in regions with lower HMO enrollments may not have health promotion cues provided to them if they are covered by fee-for-service enrollment programs.

Medicaid has been shown to be effective in reducing barriers to access to needed services (Newacheck, 1989b). Approximately 4 million adolescents are covered by Medicaid (OTA, 1991c). Unfortunately, adolescents insured by Medicaid face unique barriers in obtaining health care. Although Medicaid benefits appear to be quite extensive, many of the services needed by adolescents are optional and vary state to state. Because each state designs and manages its own Medicaid program, eligibility criteria, types of services offered, utilization limits, and provider payment policies vary across the states (OTA, 1991c). Despite the variability in benefit packages between the states, federal guidelines do mandate a core group of services that must be offered. For example, mandatory services include inpatient hospital services, physician services, and early and periodic screening, diagnosis, and treatment (EPSDT), while optional services may offer case management, dental services, home health services, prescription drugs, and psychology services.

Another major barrier for adolescents with Medicaid coverage is finding a provider who will see Medicaid patients. A growing number of physicians are restricting or limiting the number of Medicaid-eligible youths in their practices (Newacheck et al., 1992). Yudkowsky, Cartland, and Flint (1990) reported that approximately half of all pediatricians restricted their Medicaid practice in 1989. Low provider reimbursement, unpredictable payments, and administrative burdens have been cited as resulting in decreasing physician participation. With fewer available physicians, adolescents may experience difficulty in obtaining health care, and continuity of care may be impeded for adolescents with Medicaid coverage (American College of Physicians, 1990).

Adolescents with unique coverage characteristics. The financial barriers for adolescents in general are a major factor in accessing health care services. Financial barriers to health care services present an even greater concern, however, for adolescents with disabilities (McManus, Newacheck, & Greaney, 1990; Newacheck, 1989a). Adolescents from economically disadvantaged families and from rural areas, along with racial- and ethnic-minority adolescents, have additional issues concerning access to health care services.

Results from the 1984 National Health Interview Survey (NHIS), which collected data from a nationally representative sample of 15,181 randomly selected adolescents aged 10–18, demonstrated that approximately 6% of adolescents, or about 2 million nationwide, suffered from some degree of chronic health problem (Newacheck, 1989b). A chronic health problem was defined as a limitation in the amount of school, work, or extracurricular activities that the adolescent could engage in due to illness or impairment.

Adolescents with disabling conditions reportedly used 3 times as many physician services and 9 times as many hospital days as their non-disabled peers in 1984 (Newacheck, 1989a). Similarly, Cowell (1988) found that children with special needs consumed 48% of school nursing primary care services but constituted only 10% of the school enrollment. Despite the reported greater need for health care services among adolescents with disabilities, the NHIS data showed that 14% of adolescents with a disability had no health insurance, which translated into approximately 270,000 adolescents with disabilities who have no insurance protection for health care bills (Newacheck, 1989a). The lack of health insurance or the inadequacy of such health coverage as the adolescent has may result in a significant burden on family savings and ultimately present a substantial barrier in obtaining needed health care services (Newacheck, 1989a).

Adolescents from economically disadvantaged families also face increased risks for health problems and increased utilization of ambulatory and hospital services due to barriers to access to other forms of health care. In families with income below the poverty level, adolescents have been shown to be significantly less likely to re-

port excellent health (Newacheck & McManus, 1989). Research has also demonstrated that adolescents from poor families were 47% more likely to suffer from a chronic disabling condition than their peers whose families were above the poverty level (Newacheck, 1989b). Although poor adolescents have more health problems, they have been shown to be 35% more likely to have waited 2 or more years between physician contacts.

For adolescents residing in nonmetropolitan areas, there are also additional barriers to access to health care services (McManus, Newacheck, & Weader, 1989). Rural adolescents are more likely to be poor and to try to solve problems on their own, rather than seek help; they also have more problems gaining physical access to health care, due to lack of available health and mental health care providers, along with transportation problems (OTA, 1991a). According to McManus, Newacheck, and Weader (1989), approximately one third (or 10.8 million) of all adolescents resided in nonmetropolitan areas in 1984. About 50% of these adolescents lived in the South and 25% in the Midwest. This concentration of adolescents is in contrast to the metropolitan adolescent population, which is spread fairly evenly throughout the four regions (McManus, Newacheck, & Weader, 1989). Accordingly, despite the similarities in the health status of metropolitan and nonmetropolitan adolescents, the patterns of utilization of health services and of health insurance coverage differed substantially among these two groups of adolescents. The nonmetropolitan adolescents made fewer physician visits and were more likely to delay seeking physician care than adolescents living in metropolitan areas. Also, adolescents in nonmetropolitan areas were 39% more likely to be hospitalized and 30% more likely to have no form of insurance coverage than adolescents living in a metropolitan area. Additionally, although nonmetropolitan adolescents had higher rates of poverty, they were 20% less likely to have public health insurance coverage, a lack that is probably related to the high concentration of nonmetropolitan youths in the South, where Medicaid is less generous (McManus, Newacheck, & Weader, 1989).

Racial- and ethnic-minority adolescents face barriers to health care similar to those faced by adolescents who are economically disadvantaged, in that they are more likely to be poor and uninsured (OTA, 1991a). Reports state that about 50% of black, Hispanic, and American Indian adolescents and 32% of Asian-American adolescents are living below 150% of the federal poverty level. The disparity in the occurrence of health problems in racial- and ethnic-minority adolescents is partly attributable to their poverty status. The pervasive discrimination against persons of different races and ethnicity, however, may compound the health care access barriers for minority adolescents (OTA, 1991a).

Legal Barriers. The legal requirement to provide informed consent for medical services and payment of services is a major barrier. This requirement often gives rise to conflict between adolescents and their parents and may hinder the delivery of health services for adolescents. Concerns about confidentiality in revealing sensitive issues relating to their health is a significant factor that may lead some adolescents to suppress relevant information or delay or avoid seeking health services (Council on Scientific Affairs, 1993). Their failure to fully disclose all the pertinent information thwarts identification of health problems and provision of appropriate health care. Furthermore, delaying or failing to obtain care may result in a more serious problem or long-term complications.

According to OTA (1991a), the parental consent and notification requirements are based on two major assumptions. The first is that adolescents as minors are unable to make health care decisions. The second rationale is embedded in the belief that parental consent and notification requirements will encourage family autonomy and support parental authority over their minor adolescents. Family autonomy and parental authority are postulated to maintain the family structure and ensure that the parents play a role in educating their children about health care decisions (Cartoof & Klerman, 1986; OTA, 1991c).

Currently, there is a paucity of data regarding adolescents' participation in health care decision making. Research suggests, however, that adolescents of ages 14 and older may have the capacity for informed consent (OTA, 1991a). Additionally, a small number of studies have examined the impact of mandatory parental consent on adolescents' use of reproductive health service. In particular, these studies have focused on the decision to terminate pregnancy (Council on Scientific Affairs, 1993). Studies have demonstrated that mandatory notification laws have caused adolescents to put off seeking health services, which has increased health risks rather than promoted parental participation in adolescents' health decisions (Blum, Resnick, & Stark, 1987; Cartoof & Klerman, 1986; Council on Scientific Affairs, 1993; Yates & Pliner, 1988).

Provider Barriers. The scarcity of providers appropriately trained to address the particular needs faced by adolescents may result in health care that is inappropriate for or unacceptable to adolescents. Available evidence suggests that the contemporary mainstream primary health care system is not meeting the needs defined by adolescents (OTA, 1991a). A 1990 study demonstrated that 10% of the sample had no regular source of care, and 18% identified emergency rooms, community clinics, or hospital outpatient departments as their usual site of medical care (Wood et al., 1990). Furthermore, adolescents utilize the private office-based primary care physician services less than any other age group (OTA, 1991a). A 1985 survey showed that United States citizens of all ages made an average of 2.74 visits to private office-based physicians, whereas adolescents of ages 10–18 made an average of 1.6 visits (OTA, 1991a). The 1990 study by Wood et al. (1990) showed that use of emergency rooms, community clinics, or hospital outpatient departments was more common among poor and nonwhite children and children with Medicaid insurance. Another disturbing finding is that despite the increasingly recognized importance of anticipatory guidance among adolescents, pediatricians have been found to spend very little time on anticipatory guidance during office visits (OTA, 1991a).

Several nonfinancial and nonlegal reasons for the low use of primary care physician services have been hypothesized. Among such reasons are the lack of availability and the unwillingness of physicians to treat adolescents (OTA, 1991a). Furthermore, physicians and other health care providers, because of the biomedical focus of their training, often lack the competence to identify and treat the health problems of adolescents (Graves, Bridge, & Nyhuis, 1987; Kaplan, 1990).

Anecdotally, school nurses have suggested additional reasons for the low use of primary care physician services. The reasons include inconsistencies between adolescents' perceived health needs or problems and the traditional problem-oriented care provided by physicians and other health care providers. Adolescents may also disagree with health care providers about what should be discussed during health care visits. Problems and concerns identified by adolescents tend to be related to adolescent life-adjustment issues such as self-image, separation from parents, and future orientation (Giblin & Poland, 1985). Additionally, a study examining the health needs and perceptions of 158 inner city adolescent males found that the major areas of concern were school, drugs, sex, parents, and family (Frank, 1990). Frank (1990) also found that the health questions identified as being the most frequently asked by the adolescent males were how far to go with sex, care of acne, treatments for depression, and fears about their personal safety. In an anecdotal review, Bailey (1992) found that a small number of adolescent females asked for personal counseling, specifically for an opportunity to just talk. Giblin and Poland (1985) observed that older adolescents were more likely to report problems with substance abuse, sexuality, and interpersonal relationships. Furthermore, females expressed greater needs relating to sexuality, emotional problems, appearance, and interpersonal relationships.

Adolescents who seek and gain access to traditional primary health care are likely to be met by health care providers who have not had specialized training in adolescent health and to receive services that may not be appropriate to their developmental and experiential levels (OTA, 1991a). Although health care providers acknowledge that special skills and knowledge are necessary to treat adolescents, limited available data suggest that the number of health care providers with the interest, willingness, and special skills to treat adolescents is small (OTA, 1991a; Society for Adolescent Medicine, 1992). Table 1 summarizes barriers to health care services that adolescents may encounter.

Social and Environmental Influences

Conventional wisdom has recognized only since the early 1990s that contemporary adolescents' health and behavior are influenced by social and environmental factors, such as family members, peers, schools, and communities (Dougherty, 1993). Although systematic evidence is scarce concerning the relationship between health status and behavior and social and environmental influences, researchers suggest that adolescents who do well seem to have strong and developmentally appropriate social support (Dougherty, 1993). Appropriate social supports ideally come from the adolescent's family; if the family is not available, however, another adult can provide social support for the adolescent (Dougherty et al., 1992).

Parents can serve as positive or negative behavioral role models to their adolescent children (OTA, 1991b). Additionally, in the positive sense, parents can affect the health of adolescents by providing them emotional support and encouragement and promoting their autonomy. Parents can also be early screeners of health care needs and can play a significant role in connecting adolescents to appropriate and beneficial services (OTA, 1991b). Furthermore, caring adults can promote healthy peer interactions, which can prevent unhealthy behaviors among adolescents (Dougherty et al., 1992).

Table 1. Barriers Encountered by Adolescents Gaining Access to Health Services[a]

Barrier	Estimated proportion and number of adolescents affected
Low income (poor to near-poor)	More than 1 in 4 United States adolescents overall (8.3 million); 2 in 4 black, Hispanic, American Indian, and Alaska Native adolescents; 1 in 3 Asian adolescents.
Lack of health insurance	1 in 7 adolescents (4.6 million).
Lack of Medicaid among poor adolescents	1 in 3 poor adolescents (1.76 million).
Limitations on coverage	Depends on health care need.
Requirements for parental consent to notification	Unknown. Common law requires parental consent to health services for minor (age 18 in all but three states), but there are many exceptions that vary by state and service. Role as a barrier depends on the level of conflict between adolescents and their parents.
Lack of parental availability to accompany adolescent for health services	The parents of 60% of adolescents work full-time.
Lack of information about need for and availability of services	Unknown, but can be assumed to be large based on what is known about the availability of selected services for suicide prevention and treatment for sexually transmitted diseases.
Scarcity of appropriately trained providers	Unknown, but can be assumed to be large because in several studies most providers report not feeling appropriately trained.
Geogrpahic factors	May particularly affect the one third of adolescents who live in rural (nonmetropolitan) communities.
Cultural factors	Unknown, but considered important.

[a]From Dougherty et al. (1992). Reprinted with permission of the American School Health Association, Kent, Ohio.

In contrast to the positive role that parents can play in the health of adolescents, parents who abuse substances and are violent may negatively affect adolescent health and health behaviors. For example, adolescents who smoke are more likely to report that their parents smoke (Haeffle, 1994). Furthermore, parents who convey inaccurate messages may have a detrimental affect on adolescent health.

Parents must be available to adolescents if they are to be positive influences in their lives (OTA, 1991a). In some cases, however, parents may not be available, or able, to provide useful information about health care needs and services. Additionally, parents may not have the time to accompany their adolescent child to health care services and provide support and feedback at the time that services are being rendered. Approximately two thirds of adolescents aged 10–17 live in households where both parents (or a single parent) work full time (OTA, 1991a); anecdotal evidence suggests that other family members do not assume parental roles.

Environmental influences, such as schools, also have an influence on adolescent health and health behaviors. On-site school-linked health centers have been cited as being effective in reducing school absenteeism, alcohol consumption, smoking, sexual activity, and pregnancy in schools with these services available to adolescents (OTA, 1991a). As primary reasons for using school-linked health centers in their schools, adolescents reported that they felt they could trust the service because it was part of the school, because the health center was conveniently located, and because they perceived the staff as caring and responsive to their needs (OTA, 1991a). Additionally, many school-based programs are designed to incorporate positive peer support in designing health promotion programs. On-site school-linked health centers appear to respond to the limitations of the traditional health care system in meeting the needs of adolescents. Many public and private schools, however, have limited health and health education services, along with physical education. Moreover, financial constraints on schools usually limit services that relate to health and health promotion. Consequently, loss of school support for promoting health in adolescents will have a detrimental effect on their health status and health behaviors.

Internal Variables

In addition to external resources of access to health care and social influences for health promotion, personal factors play an important role in determining health behavior. Internal variables to be discussed are cognitive appraisal, and intentions and self-efficacy, along with behavioral skills. The contribution of external variables combined with that of internal variables enhances the predictive power of explanatory health behavior models.

Cognitive Appraisal

Cognitive appraisal is the process of intellectually evaluating and deciding on available options to engage in a particular behavior. Adolescents' use of cognitive appraisal is influenced by their knowledge and beliefs about particular health behaviors. Facts regarding health services, health behaviors, and health risks are important building blocks for behavior, but may not be sufficient to initiate or sustain behavior. Adolescent beliefs about health and health behavior combine with knowledge to produce more powerful influences on health behavior. For example, knowledge of reproduction and contraception has been found to be a significant determinant of contraception use in adolescents (OTA, 1991b).

Lack of Knowledge Regarding Available Health Services. The lack of information about health behaviors, health risks, when health services are appropriate, and where the services are located presents another barrier for the adolescent population (Dougherty et al., 1992). Currently, the knowledge level of adolescents regarding the need for and the availability of health

services is limited (Dougherty, 1993). One national survey reported, however, that most of the adolescents were either unaware or did not believe that they could obtain confidential treatment for sexually transmitted diseases (STDs) (OTA, 1991a). As a result of their lack of knowledge of confidential treatment for STDs, teenagers are unlikely to seek and receive needed services. Although data are sparse, a few reports suggest that adolescents lack necessary information regarding a complicated, fragmented health care system that is frequently difficult even for sophisticated adults to negotiate (Dougherty, 1993).

Beliefs about Health and Well-Being on the Part of Adolescents. Over the past two decades, researchers have determined that the meaning of health to children changes as they grow older. Early work in health perceptions actually defined perceptions of illness (Burbach & Peterson, 1986; Gochman, 1970; Kalnins & Love, 1982). Much of the research on the meaning of health among older children and adolescents has focused on the cognitive aspects rather than on the emotional, cultural, or gender aspects of health. In more recent research, efforts to examine the meaning of health have focused not on the absence of illness, but on a positive, dynamic state. Although much of the research directed to a positive paradigm of health has been cross-sectional (age-specific), it has clarified themes that are functional in nature. Thus, children define health as being able to do what they want to do, having energy, and being in good condition (Hester, 1984; Millstein & Irwin, 1987; Natapoff, 1978). Older children and adolescents identify health and illness as conditions that can exist together (Millstein & Irwin, 1987; Natapoff, 1989). The concept that health and illness can coexist suggests that youth can adopt health-promoting behaviors despite acute or chronic illness. For example, youths with epilepsy can conceive of themselves as healthy persons with epilepsy, with the same lifestyle needs in activity and nutrition as youths without epilepsy.

Data are limited regarding adolescents' beliefs concerning health and well-being and how they present with problems to health care providers. A study by Natapoff and Essoka (1989) examining handicapped and able-bodied adolescents' and children's ideas of health found that younger adolescents (aged 12–14) in both groups were more likely to define the meaning of health as physical fitness than were the younger children (aged 6–11). Also, adolescents (27%) defined health as not being sick more frequently than did younger children (8%), aged 6–7. Natapoff and Essoka found that despite the different life experiences, both handicapped and able-bodied children defined health in similar ways, in that both groups viewed themselves as being healthy.

Studies have found that females were more frequent users of health services than males (Bailey, 1992; Kornfalt & Ejlertsson, 1981). Koppleman (1989) proposed that students needing academic or general support may utilize health services to obtain this support by reporting general health complaints. Bailey (1994) has suggested that social support, counseling, and education on specific health issues may be beneficial interventions for adolescent females. While Koppleman's and Bailey's recommendations provide useful direction in school health services, further study is warranted to examine the influence of menstruation-related factors on the gender difference in health services utilization.

A study by Fox (1991) found that older and more intellectually capable adolescents had a lower tendency to seek medical care. Additionally, Fox's study found that mothers and their adolescent children shared a common factor structure in their tendency to seek medical care, which suggests that adolescent children and their mothers share "adult" understandings of illness, or "adult" definitions of appropriate illness behavior for common symptoms, or both. Moreover, adolescents' understanding of illness and their illness behavior based on that understanding are most likely to be structured by their level of cognitive development (Fox, 1991).

Intentions and Self-Efficacy

The theory of reasoned action was designed to explain behavior and self-efficacy as a result of intention (Ajzen & Fishbein, 1980). The importance of examining intention prior to actual behavior in adolescents is observed in the number of behaviors that result in major health concerns for this population. For example, in cigarette smoking, the *intention* to try cigarette smoking, which is not a behavior, probably precedes an adolescent's experimentation with smoking (American Cancer Society, 1992). Intentions have been found to predict a variety of corresponding action tendencies that are major issues in the lives of adolescents, e.g., having an abortion and smoking marijuana (Ajzen, 1988). Furthermore, the intentions related to the behaviors of having an abortion and smoking were highly compatible with the behaviors in terms of target, action, context, and time elements. Although important, intention alone restricts the explanation of adolescent health behavior. Other factors, such as skill and competency, have enhanced the predictive power of intention.

Skill in a specific health behavior is the cornerstone of the social learning theory of Bandura (1986). Skill can be developed by practicing behavior, from modeling or experiencing others' behavior, from persuasion, and from physical ability (Bandura, 1977). Perceived self-efficacy (or competency) is a determinant of performance that has been reported to operate independently of skill (Bandura, 1986). In adolescents, cultivation of self-efficacy may occur through family sources, peers, and schools. Thus, self-efficacy is qualitatively enhanced through social interactions and quantitatively augmented as adolescents become more self-efficacious.

Research has been designed to test the predictive power of self-efficacy, behavioral skill, and behavioral intention. Outcomes of studies combining these constructs have been mixed in adolescent behavioral research. Intention has been found to be a powerful predictor to have sexual intercourse, to have multiple sexual partners, and to use condoms (Walter et al., 1993). Further, behavioral skill was a variable strongly associated with sexual behavioral intention.

Still other studies have identified intention for behavior as an outcome (Nguyen, Sauçier, & Pica, 1994). The theory of reasoned action and social learning theory have been combined to explain behavioral intention to limit sexual partners. Basen-Engquist and Parcel (1994) found that information provided by parents, peers, school, and media did not have a positive effect on 9th-grade adolescent male's intentions to use condoms. Self-efficacy, norms, and attitudes explained 36% of the variance of intention to limit sexual partners (Basen-Engquist & Parcel, 1994). Similarly, self-efficacy theory framed a study of the intent of older adolescent (average age 17.8 years) male and female high school students to use condoms (Joffe & Radius, 1993). Male students' condom use was predicted by their skill in talking to partners about using condoms and in enjoying sex and by their past condom use. For female students, past use of condoms and ability to enjoy sex were the significant predictors of condom use.

Intervention studies have targeted perceived self-efficacy and behavioral intentions in sexual risk-reduction research. Skill-building interventions had a more positive effect on minority females' intention to use condoms than did information sessions alone (Jemmott, Jemmott, Spears, Hewitt, & Cruz-Collins, 1992). College-age students were surveyed to assess contraceptive use and contraceptive self-efficacy (Heinrich, 1993). Contraceptive self-efficacy was the most powerful predictor of contraceptive use.

Competing findings have demonstrated that research does not show a conclusive positive relationship between self-efficacy and risk-reduction behavior. For example, inner city junior high school students' perceived self-efficacy was not significantly related to consistent condom use (DiClemente et al., 1992). Still other research has demonstrated that stronger perceptions of self-efficacy, along with stronger peer affiliation, were significantly related to higher levels of STD (Sha-

fer & Boyer, 1991). These competing findings probably provide evidence of the effects of developmental transitions (biological, cognitive, social, and emotional) on the constructs embedded in theories that address behavioral intention and behavioral skill. Continued research is needed to clarify the conceptual structures relating to behavioral intention and behavioral skill among adolescents.

METHODOLOGICAL ISSUES

Because of constraints on time and money and the greater ease of collecting data, much of the research on determinants of adolescent health behaviors has relied on descriptive research rather than experimental or quasi-experimental designs. Consequently, results of the studies must be interpreted with a great degree of caution. Another issue is that such research is weighted toward behaviors that adolescents have already adopted. Generally, these adopted behaviors are the risky ones (Baldwin, 1991). Additionally, although researchers discuss the need to examine adolescents' positive health behaviors (Kulbok & Baldwin, 1992), the current literature is focused on these negative behaviors. One disadvantage of this approach can be observed in the preponderance of AIDS research focused on high-risk populations, which are largely minorities. The ability to generalize from studies focused on problem behaviors among high-risk adolescents is limited. Thus, research must be broadened to include not only the groups at high risk for the problem behavior, but also the general adolescent population. The focus also needs to shift from the problem-behavior orientation to an examination of a range of health behaviors utilized by individuals.

Design Issues

Reports by parents or self-reports by adolescents are limited in terms of recall by the respondents and may be inaccurate because the respondent may be unaware of relevant information, have forgotten information, or be unwilling to report certain types of information, such as potentially embarrassing or stigmatic health issues, such as sexual intercourse and attempted suicide (Newacheck & McManus, 1989). Additionally, the perceived social stigma or support for the particular behavior and the perceived confidentiality of responses may also result in under- or overreporting of the behavior in question (Kolbe, Kann, & Collins, 1993).

Reports by parents or self-reports by adolescents can be obtained by several methods, such as face-to-face interviews, telephone surveys, and mail questionnaires. Face-to-face interviews with an adolescent in the presence of an adult may result in the adolescent's responses being biased. Moreover, face-to-face interviews with proxies, such as the adolescent's parent, may be biased in that the parent may be unaware of the adolescent's health care usage patterns and health behaviors and under- or overestimate health status. Additionally, both the adolescent and the parent may minimize health problems that are sensitive in nature, e.g., the presence of mental illnesses.

Questionnaires may bias the respondents' responses in many ways. For example, words may have different meanings to the person writing the question and the person answering the question. Some words may have strong emotional content, which can strongly influence the response to the question. Reading levels maybe inappropriate for the adolescents. Response categories in closed-ended questions may also have an unintended effect on the respondent's answers. For example, use of Likert scales ranging from "never" to "always" for response categories has been found to be more reliable with adolescents than requests for the specific number of times they used a safety belt during a given recall period (Streff & Wagenaar, 1989).

The time frame of the behavior is another consideration that must be accounted for in the questionnaire. The 30-day recall period may be most effective in providing current measures of the behavior. Additionally, is the behavior contin-uous throughout the year or is there only a seasonal exposure period? For example, motorcycle and bicycle riding are seasonal activities; therefore, using a 12-month period for recall may enhance the responses when measuring the frequency of adolescents' helmet use in these activities (Waxweiler, Harel, & O'Carroll, 1993).

Another consideration in surveying health behaviors in adolescents concerns the maintenance of anonymity. Research has demonstrated that adolescents may have more confidence in anonymity and therefore be more likely to respond to school-based surveys than non-school-based surveys, since they may associate the former with common school practice and feel that they are responding as a part of a group with their peers (Kolbe et al., 1993).

Sampling Issues

The use of probability sampling in adolescent health behavior research is difficult to attain, as is the case in much of the research studying human populations. As a result, a majority of the studies on adolescent health behaviors have utilized nonprobability sampling, or convenience sampling, which compromises the ability to generalize beyond the population being studied. Another major concern in adolescent health behavior research involves sample size for minority populations. Measuring health behaviors in minorities is problematic due to the relatively small numbers of minorities and their low response rates. To counterbalance the low numbers of minorities, researchers need to oversample, which may be difficult, in addition to being costly.

Defining Outcomes

Each outcome variable in adolescent research may have unique methodological issues that must be considered. One methodological issue is the need to have consistent measures of behaviors across studies to compare results. For example, questions to measure tobacco use may address experimentation, such as whether an individual has ever tried smoking a cigarette, even one or two puffs (Marcus, Giovino, Pierce, & Harel, 1993). Definitions need to be uniform in terms of the initiation of smoking and current usage. Questions may address age when first whole cigarette was smoked, current pattern of smoking, frequency of smoking during the month, intensity of smoking on days of smoking, age when regular smoking began, and use of smokeless tobacco.

Data Analysis Issues

Analyzing adolescent health behavior data highlights several issues. One question is whether or not the analysis is appropriate for the question and sample. Specifically, does the study utilize appropriate analytical models to respond to research questions that describe, show relationships, explain, and predict? Are sample sizes powerful enough to draw suggested conclusions? Are the samples representative, and what statistical strategies need to be employed? The power of randomization enhances any study. For example, in one study of cardiovascular risk related to physical activity and nutrition behavior among 350 youths from randomly chosen classrooms, efforts were made to compare nonrespondents with respondents. Teachers were asked to rate nonrespondents' obesity, perceived activity, and selected demographics. No significant differences were identified between the nonrespondents and the respondents (Cowell & Montgomery, 1993). Thus, the use of randomization in classroom selection minimized selection bias and enhanced the representativeness of the sample.

Sample decay is a perpetual problem in much of the research with adolescents. Researchers usually handle sample decay by statistical manipulation or by deleting cases with missing data points. Thus, the results must be interpreted with caution, because there is uncertainty as to whether or not the cases with missing data points are the same as the cases that have complete data on all of the variables being examined.

CLINICALLY DERIVED DETERMINANTS OF ADOLESCENT HEALTH BEHAVIOR

Cardiovascular Health Behaviors

Though cardiovascular disease (CVD) is not apparent in adolescence, the precursors to CVD that do appear in adolescents are poor nutrition and inactivity. The long-term consequences resulting from nutritional imbalance that may exist during adolescence can be observed in several chronic diseases that affect the lives of many adults. For example, coronary heart disease, atherosclerosis, cancer, stroke, and diabetes account for much of the morbidity and mortality among adults in the United States (Stamler, 1987).

Nutrition

Available literature, based on food frequencies recommended in the food pyramid as a criteria for nutritional adequacy, provide evidence that the dietary patterns acquired during youth have been associated with the development of obesity, unhealthy weight-loss practices, and eating disorders (National Cholesterol Education Program, 1990). Furthermore, the adverse effects of obesity on psychological and physical health have been well documented. Obesity in adolescents has been correlated with low self-image and self-concept, along with less acceptance by peers, depression, and potentially poor academic performance.

Undernutrition may be a more frequent occurrence among today's adolescents as a result of society's perception of thinness as the ideal for beauty (Trowbridge & Collins, 1993). In the pursuit of thinness, adolescent girls now more frequently practice dangerous weight-control strategies, such as eating low-calorie and unbalanced diets, using diet pills, laxatives, and diuretics, and inducing vomiting (Feldman, McGrath, & O'Shaughessy, 1986).

Results from the National School-Based 1991 Youth Risk Behavior Survey found that 12.9% of all of the students surveyed in grades 9–12 had eaten five or more servings of fruits and vegetables a day (Kann et al., 1993). White students were significantly more likely to have consumed more fruits and vegetables than black or Hispanic students, while more male students than female students had eaten five or more servings of fruits and vegetables. Other researchers have found that youth consume less than the recommended daily allowance of fruits (1.6 servings per day) and vegetables (0.75 servings per day) (Montgomery & Cowell, 1994). In the 1991 Youth Risk Behavior Survey, 64% of all students restricted their dietary intake to no more than two servings of foods high in fat content (Kann et al., 1993f). Females were significantly more likely than males to eat less than two servings of foods high in fat content. This trend was also noted in Hispanic students, who also restricted their intake of foods high in fat content. Intake of foods high in fat content reportedly did not vary significantly by grade. In contrast to the Youth Risk Behavior Survey (Kann et al., 1993), local and regional studies of young adolescents have demonstrated a reversing of the food pyramid, with fat servings per day (3.4 servings of fatty foods) surpassing fruits, vegetables, and protein (Montgomery & Cowell, 1994).

Determinants of Dietary Behavior. Little research has addressed the consumption patterns of adolescents. Traditionally, family nutritional behavior and school meal programming have been viewed as important external variables to consider in explaining adolescent consumption patterns. Cowell and Montgomery (in review) found that fathers' education, age of mothers, and health motivation of children were significant predictors of 13% of the variance in nutrition behavior of 350 African-American, Hispanic, and white older children. Children with older mothers, as well as children who had behaviors consistent with their health goals, had more balanced meals using the food pyramid as a criterion. Interestingly, race and ethnicity were not statistically significant predictors of nutrition behaviors. Although the economic diversity was extreme among sample families with annual income ranging from less than $10,000 to more than $1,000,000, children's consumption patterns were very similar. Paradoxically, children who were given a great deal of freedom in making food choices had families in which parents articulated great concern about their own dietary intake.

Physical Activity

While methods of measurement vary across studies, research has consistently demonstrated an association between physical activity behavior and the incidence of major causes of disability and death. For example, level of physical activity has been linked with hypertension (Paffenberger, Wing, Hyde, & Jung, 1983), diabetes mellitus (Richter & Schneider, 1981), and osteoporosis (Alois, 1978). Studies have also suggested that habitual vigorous physical activity is associated with decreasing the overall risk for coronary heart disease (CHD) (Siscovick, Weiss, Fletcher, & Lasky, 1984). Although adolescents have few chronic diseases that can be prevented by physical activity, research suggests that regular physical activity in adolescents is associated with the maintenance of good mental health and self-esteem (Ross & Hayes, 1988).

Obesity is a CHD risk factor related to amount of physical activity and is a health problem of epidemic proportions (Pender, 1987). Researchers have found increasing rates of obesity among youths (Cowell, Montgomery, & Talashek, 1989, 1992). Although obesity is becoming more prevalent in our society, researchers have shown that obesity is a risk factor for CHD that can be prevented or managed by regular physical exercise within the general population of adults and children (Sallis, Patterson, Buono, & Nader, 1985).

The 1991 Youth Risk Behavior Survey found that 48.9% of students in grades 9–12 were enrolled in physical education (PE) classes and 41.5% attended PE class daily (Kann et al., 1993). Enrollment in PE significantly decreased, however, from 75.8% in 9th grade to 27.4% in 12th grade. Daily PE attendance also showed a similar pattern. White adolescents were the least likely to be enrolled in PE classes (45.5%); black adolescents were significantly more likely than whites to be enrolled (60.7%). Males were significantly more likely (56.5%) to exercise more than 30 minutes per class than females (40.7%).

Kann et al. (1993) found that the type of physical activity also varied by grade level. Moderate physical activity decreased from 49.3% among adolescents in the 9th grade to 32.4% in the 12th grade. Furthermore, black teenagers were more likely to report moderate physical activity than white teenagers. Stretching exercises also decreased from the lower grades to the higher grades.

Determinants of Physical Activity Behavior

Major determinants of adolescent physical activity include parental physical activity, parental involvement, peer activity level, perceived competence, and perceived benefits (Brustad, 1993; Ferguson, Yesalis, Pomrehn, & Kirkpatrick, 1989; Sallis et al., 1993). Children nominated by school nurses as physically fit and active demonstrated higher levels of intrinsic motivation as measured by the Health Self Determinism Index-Child (Cox, Cowell, Marion, & Miller, 1990). In the design of previously cited studies, existing fitness levels were not conceptualized as predictors of physical activity. Cowell and Montgomery (1993) found that children's existing fitness levels were predictive of physical activity. A concern arises from Cowell and Montgomery's data in that school- and community-based programs attract athletic youths, so that adolescents who are not athletic or not fit often do not participate in physical activity programs. As a result of this concern, previous fitness levels should be assessed so that youths who are not fit or athletic are included in programs promoting physical activity.

Sexual Behaviors

A 1991 survey of adolescent behaviors reported that 54.1% of all students in grades 9–12 had engaged in sexual intercourse (Kann et al., 1993). The number of adolescents engaging in premarital sexual activity between the ages of 15 and 19 has reportedly been increasing since 1970 (OTA, 1991b).

Early adolescent sexual activity is associated with several health consequences, such as pregnancy, abortion, parenthood, and STDs. Adolescent females engaging in early sexual activity not only are at risk for unintended pregnancy, but also are at greater risk, as are adolescent males, of acquiring STDs, along with the side effects associated with STDs (OTA, 1991b).

In 1988, approximately 1 million adolescents in the United States became pregnant (OTA, 1991b). Although the birth rate among adolescents declined during the period of 1970–1985, for unknown reasons the birth rate began to increase in 1985 and in 1988 reached its highest level in 10 years. Among pregnant adolescents, about one half of the pregnancies are carried to term. Abortions among adolescents have increased substantially since Roe v. Wade in 1973. The primary reason cited for the disparity between adolescent pregnancy and birth rates is abortion (OTA, 1991b). Researchers have speculated that the differences between pregnancy rate and birth rate might be even greater if poor women had greater access to abortion services in the United States.

Pregnant adolescents are at high risk for many negative health outcomes, such as excessive weight gain during pregnancy, toxemia, anemia, nutritional deficiencies, prolonged or abrupt labors, cephalopelvic disproportion, and maternal mortality (OTA, 1991b). Although research has found, in general, that the physical health risks associated with abortions among adolescent females do not appear to be much greater than those for older women undergoing abortions, there is a paucity of data concerning the long-term consequences of abortions among adolescents (OTA, 1991b). Some studies have suggested that adolescent females may experience more negative emotional reactions than women over the age of 19 because of less social support

(Major, Mueller, & Hildebrandt, 1985); a 1989 study found, however, that adolescents were no more likely to experience psychological problems 2 years after their abortions than were adolescents who carried their pregnancies to term (Zabin, Hirsch, & Emerson, 1989).

Parenthood presents several social and economic consequences for adolescents. For example, teenage females have been found to complete less schooling and to be less likely to receive a high school degree or attend college than their peers who delay parenthood until their 20s (OTA, 1991b). Also, studies have demonstrated that adolescent females typically have lower-status jobs and lower incomes than their counterparts. Another finding is that adolescent mothers report multiple stresses in their lives, such as family conflicts, unstable relationships with the child's father, loneliness, isolation, and depression (OTA, 1991b).

The percentage of sexually active females ages 15–19 using contraceptive methods was higher in 1988 (78.8%) than in 1982 (71%) (Forrest & Singh, 1990). Despite the increased usage of birth control methods, adolescent pregnancy rates are reportedly higher in the United States than in many other developed nations (OTA, 1991b). Although other countries have similar rates of adolescent sexual activity, the higher rates of pregnancy in the United States have been attributed to several factors, such as attitudes denying teenage sexual behavior and the difficulty experienced by adolescents in obtaining contraceptives.

Determinants of Sexual Activity Behavior

Several factors are associated with adolescents' initiating sexual activity prior to marriage, including individual characteristics, familial factors, and social and environmental factors.

Individual Factors. Individual characteristics associated with the initiation of sexual activity among adolescents include physical maturation, age, race, socioeconomic status, academic achievement, intelligence, dating behavior, and degree of religious devotion (OTA, 1991b). Older adolescents are more likely to have had sexual intercourse, and black males and females on average become sexually active about 2 years before white males and females. Additionally, adolescents with higher levels of academic success and educational and life goals are less likely to engage in sexual intercourse at an early age and, when they are sexually active, are more likely to use contraceptives consistently. Dating in early adolescence has also been observed to be predictive of sexual intercourse among younger adolescents (Santelli & Beilenson, 1992). Adolescents who are sexually active at an early age have been found to be involved in other behaviors that move them toward independence and perceived adulthood, such as smoking, drinking, and drug use (Zabin, 1984; Zabin, Hardy, Smith, & Hirsch, 1986).

Family Factors. The factor that has been most strongly associated with an adolescent female's decision to initiate sexual activity prior to marriage is her mother's sexual and fertility experience (OTA, 1991b). Researchers state that the earlier the mother's first sexual experience and childbearing, the more likely it is that the adolescent daughter will engage in sexual activity at an earlier age. Studies have found that adolescent females growing up in fatherless homes are more likely to initiate early sexual activity than adolescents in two-parent homes.

Social and Environmental Factors. Several social and environmental factors have been linked with adolescent sexual activity behavior. Research has suggested that adolescent sexual behavior is influenced more by the teenagers' perception of their peers' sexual activity and attitudes toward sexual behavior (OTA, 1991b). Additionally, research has demonstrated that the influence of peer pressure among adolescents varies by gender and age. Younger white adolescent females have been observed to be the most susceptible to peer pressure (Lewis & Lewis, 1984). The direct relationship of the media to adolescent sexual activity behavior is not known; however, community groups and families have expressed concern abut the influence of the media (e.g., television, music, advertisements).

Determinants of Contraceptive Use

The use of contraception among adolescents also has specific determinants, in addition to the factors associated with the initiation of sexual activity. For example, older adolescents are more likely than younger adolescents to use more effective methods of contraceptives (OTA, 1991b). Also, the older a female adolescent is at her first sexual interaction, the more likely she is to use contraception (OTA, 1991b). In males, age at first intercourse has little association with contraceptive use. Other determinants of contraceptive use include the stability of the relationship. Adolescents involved in steady relationships have been observed to use contraception more frequently than those who are not committed to the relationship. Studies have found that adolescent females with clear academic aspirations and good school performance are more likely to use contraception (OTA, 1991b).

Race has also been found to be a determinant of contraceptive use in general and of the type of contraceptive used. Black adolescent females are reportedly less likely to use contraceptives than white adolescents (OTA, 1991b). This finding has been contradicted in black adolescents whose parents had high educational levels. Black females have also been found to more commonly use a prescription method of contraception, such as a diaphragm and the pill, than their white counterparts (OTA, 1991b).

Use of prescription methods of contraception could be explained in several ways. Researchers have hypothesized that prescription use may be related to a learned helplessness that is more prevalent among the poor. Another explanation is that internally motivated youths may initiate over-the-counter contraceptive methods more readily than externally motivated youths. Conversely, poor youths may have greater access

to free or low-cost care, whereas more affluent youths may not have access to acceptable (confidential and sensitive) family planning services and therefore have to rely on over-the-counter contraceptive methods.

Substance Use

Several factors are associated with the use and abuse of psychoactive substances by adolescents. These factors include physical health, mental health, educational, and employment-related consequences. Additionally, the use of drugs by adolescents may result in sexual activity and pregnancy consequences and in delinquency among adolescents (OTA, 1991b).

The use of alcohol contributes to a significant number of adolescent accidents and consequent physical injuries (OTA, 1991b). Mental health concerns are additional consequences of drug use by adolescents. Although research is limited, illicit drug use has been implicated in the greater likelihood that adolescents using drugs may seek professional mental health services (Kandel, Davies, Karus, & Yanagychi, 1986). Newcomb and Bentler (1989) found that cocaine use decreased social supports and increased loneliness, suicidal thinking, and psychotic behavior. Alcohol by itself, however, reduced loneliness, increased social support, and enhanced the drinkers' feelings about themselves (Kline, Canter, & Robin, 1987). Researchers have also reported that use of marijuana and other illicit drugs in adolescence has been correlated with job instability (Kandel et al., 1986). Also, cigarette smoking among males and marijuana smoking among females has been associated with higher rates of unemployment. Finally, cigarette smoking among teens has been associated with early sexual experimentation (Zabin, 1984).

The exact number of adolescents using addicting substances is difficult to ascertain. Results from the National School-Based 1991 Youth Risk Behavior Survey found that 70.1% of all of the students surveyed in grades 9–12 had tried cigarette smoking, and 21.2% had smoked at one time at least one cigarette per day for 30 days (Kann et al., 1993). The average age at first use was 12.6 years, and older adolescents had been found to be more likely to use psychoactive drugs than younger adolescents (OTA, 1991b). The 1991 Youth Risk Behavior Survey found that 81.6% of all of the students surveyed in grades 9–12 had consumed alcohol during their lifetime, and 50.8% had consumed alcohol during the 30 days prior to the survey (Kann et al., 1993). Among all of the adolescents, use of marijuana during their lifetime was reported by 31.3% of the respondents of the 1991 Youth Risk Behavior Survey. The most regularly used psychoactive drugs by adolescents in the United States are cigarettes and alcohol (one third of self-report survey data from adolescents reported 5 or more drinks on at least one occasion in the previous 2 weeks) (OTA, 1991b). Accordingly, use of illicit drugs has declined considerably among adolescents.

Determinants of Substance Use

Individual Factors. An examination of the determinants of adolescent cigarette smoking in the 1991 Youth Risk Behavior Survey found that white students were significantly more likely to have smoked cigarettes more regularly, currently, and frequently than black and Hispanic students (Kann et al., 1993). Hispanic students, however, were more likely to have smoked cigarettes more regularly, currently, and frequently than black students. In the 1991 Youth Risk Behavior Survey, 9th-grade students were less likely to have smoked ever, regularly, currently, or frequently than 11th-grade students.

Additional personal characteristics that influence adolescent substance use include personality traits, attitudes and beliefs, and interpersonal and peer resistance skills (OTA, 1991b). Factors associated with adolescent alcohol use include poor social skills and positive expectancies for alcohol use (Kline et al., 1987). Baumrind (1991) found that adolescent attributes associated with substance use consist of low cognitive competence, concern for peer approval, and lack

of concern for adult approval. Adolescents who have had prior academic difficulties or who have lost a large number of friends during school transitions have been observed to be at greater risk for adaptational problems and thus may begin using substances.

Family Factors. Adolescents of substance-abusing parents have been reported to be at greater risk to use psychoactive drugs (OTA, 1991b). Several reasons have been postulated for the higher risk of psychoactive drug use among adolescents of substance-abusing parents. Some research has suggested that substance-abusing parents may lack parenting and family management skills, which may result in poor home and school behaviors by the adolescent (OTA, 1991b). Consequently, the adolescent may become more vulnerable to use substances for the purpose of self-medicating. In addition, adolescents of substance-abusing parents are often directly exposed to psychoactive substances and may even be encouraged or permitted to use them.

Baumrind (1991) found that certain family types may affect adolescents using substances. These family types included authoritative families, democratic homes, and directive families. Authoritative (*not* authoritarian) families, i.e., families with confident structures who also demonstrated some nontraditional beliefs, fostered a high level of competence among their adolescent children and reported a low level of drug use. Democratic families fostered similar competence among their children, although these children reported heavy marijuana use. Families who provided more directive environments and had high value for control of children had children who avoided drug use but were less competent.

Social and Environmental Factors. The use of psychoactive drugs by peers has been demonstrated as the most consistent predictor of adolescent substance use (Miller & Slap, 1989). Miller and Slap (1989) found in reviewing the literature that three variables were consistent and strongly related to adolescent smoking behavior: parental smoking, peer smoking, and sibling smoking. Variables that were not strong and consistently associated with smoking behavior by adolescents consisted of knowledge of and attitudes about smoking, demographic factors, school activities, and psychological factors. A study by Robinson et al. (1987) demonstrated that adolescents' perceptions of friends' use of marijuana accounted for 41% of the total variance among 10th-graders' use of various drugs. Factors associated with adolescent alcohol use include the adolescents' ratings of high levels of family disengagement and poor family communication, the adolescents' ratings of peer approval of alcohol use, and parental approval of alcohol use (Kline et al., 1987).

Schools have been found to exert direct and indirect influences on patterns of drug and alcohol use (OTA, 1991b). Reportedly, school can be important in the development of self-concept by the adolescent. Two school transition periods place adolescents at high risk for substance use and abuse—that from elementary to junior high school or middle school and that from junior high school or middle school to high school. Each of these transitions moves the teen to a less protected and personal school environment. Adolescents may also have different levels of exposure to and acceptability of psychoactive substances in the school environments.

COMPARISON OF METHODOLOGICAL ISSUES ACROSS PROBLEMS

Much of the extant research on adolescent health behavior has been limited to the examination of one or two high-risk behaviors. Although this research provides valuable insight into the particular behaviors being studied, it yields little information regarding the multiple and interrelated risk behaviors that adolescents may practice (Kolbe et al., 1993). Researchers have identified a clustering of factors predicting adolescent risk-taking behaviors, including gateway drug use to harder drug use. For example, among

students in grades 5–12, cigarette smoking was found to be a "powerful" predictor for the use of alcohol and other drugs (Torabi, Baily, & Majd-Jabbari, 1993). Initiation of risky behaviors at younger ages is associated with exposure to more frequent risks, adoption of more types of risky activities, and more severe social or health outcomes (Klein et al., 1993; Wierson, Long, & Forehand, 1993).

MATURATION

Researchers often do not include the maturation variables as important correlates to other predictive variables (Brooks-Gunn, Petersen, & Eichorn, 1985). These studies typically compare youths across a number of developmental transitions; consequently, the effects of maturation are not taken into account. Despite the disparate findings across studies designed to identify the predictors of health and risk behaviors, the prevalence of health and health behavior problems is high. The Youth Risk Behavior Survey clarified the prevalence of risk among respondents. Although the sample may have underrepresented some groups, the risk behaviors are pervasive. The importance of developmentally sensitive designs as well as designs that draw on crucial external and internal variables is underscored by this review.

SUMMARY

This chapter has described adolescent health behavior in the context of internal and external factors that affect health behaviors. Researchers and clinicians need to be cognizant of barriers to health care, including financial, legal, and provider barriers, that prevent adolescents from accessing appropriate health care services. Appropriate health care services would provide not only health care but also mentoring for healthy behaviors and lifestyles. Additionally, the importance of family interaction and school support in accessing health care services and the development of health behaviors is underscored. Last, internal variables, such as cognitive appraisal and intentions and self-efficacy, are significant factors that can affect adolescent health behaviors.

The conceptual factors that have been reviewed highlight the complexity of adolescent health care needs that are unique to this population. Unlike other population groups, adolescents are for the most part healthy. The majority of their specific health problems arise from behaviors that contribute to negative health status outcomes, rather than the chronic or infectious conditions that are more prevalent in other groups. Clinicians and researchers are therefore directed toward considering the multiple issues that can affect adolescent health care needs.

REFERENCES

Ajzen, L. (1988). *Personality and behavior*. Chicago: Dorsey.

Ajzen, L., & Fishbein, M. (1980). *Understanding attitudes and predicting social behavior*. Englewood Cliffs, NJ: Prentice-Hall.

Alois, J. R. (1978). Skeletal mass and body composition in marathon runners. *Metabolism, 12*, 1783–1796.

Amato, P. R., & Keith, B. (1991). Consequences of parental divorce for the well-being of children: A meta analysis. *Psychological Bulletin, 110*, 26–46.

American Cancer Society. (1992). *Cancer facts and figures—1992*. Atlanta, GA: ACS.

American College of Physicians. (1990). Position paper: Access to health care. *Annals of Internal Medicine, 112*(9), 641–661.

Bailey, K. S. (1992). *School health services utilization*. Unpublished evaluation study. Bradley-Bourbonnais Community High School, Bradley, IL.

Bailey, K. S. (1994). *Female adolescent social support interventions and implications: An integrative review*. Unpublished master's research project. University of Illinois at Chicago.

Baldwin, W. (1991). Perspectives in research on adolescents. *Bulletin of the New York Academy of Medicine, 67*, 548–554.

Bandura, A. (1977). Self-efficacy: Toward a unifying theory of behavioral change. *Psychological Review, 84*(2), 191–215.

Bandura, A. (1986). *Social foundations of thought and action: A social cognitive theory*. New York: Prentice-Hall.

Basen-Engquist, K., & Parcel, G. S. (1994). Attitudes, norms, and self-efficacy: A model of adolescents' HIV-related sexual risk behavior. *Health Education Quarterly, 19*, 263–277.

Baumrind, D. (1991). The influence of parenting styles on adolescent competence and substance abuse. *Journal of Early Adolescence, 11*(1), 56–94.

Blum, R. (1987). Contemporary threats to adolescent health in the United States. *Journal of the American Medical Association, 257*, 3390–3395.

Blum, R. W. (1991). Global trends in adolescent health. *Journal of the American Medical Association, 265*, 2711–2719.

Blum, R. W., Resnick, M. D., & Stark, T. A. (1987). The impact of parental notification law on adolescent abortion decision-making. *American Journal of Public Health, 77*, 619–620.

Blyth, D. A., Simmons, R. G., & Carlton-Ford, S. (1983). The adjustment of early adolescents to school transitions. *Journal of Early Adolescence, 3*, 105–120.

Bradburn, N. M., & Sudman, S. (1991). The current status of questionnaire research. In P. P. Biemer, R. M. Groves, L. E. Lyberg, N. A. Mathiowetz, & S. Sudman (Eds.), *Measurement errors in surveys* (pp. 30–40). New York: Viking Press.

Brooks-Gunn, J., Petersen, A. C., & Eichorn, E. (Eds.). (1985). Time of maturation and psychosocial functioning in adolescence. Parts I and II. *Journal of Youth and Adolescence, 14*(3 and 4 [special issues]).

Brooks-Gunn, J., & Warren, M. P. (1989). Biological and social contributions to negative affect in young adolescent girls. *Child Development, 60*, 40–55.

Brustad, R. J. (1993). Children's perspectives on exercise and physical activity: Measurement issues and concerns. *Journal of School Health, 61*, 228–230.

Bryant, R. K. (1985). The neighborhood walk: Sources of support in middle childhood. *Monographs of the Society for Research in Child Development, 50* (3 Serial No. 210).

Burbach, D. J., & Peterson, L. (1986). Children's concepts of physical illness: A review and critique of the cognitive-developmental literature. *Health Psychology, 5*, 307–325.

Business & Health. (1990). The 1990 national executive poll on health care costs and benefits. *Business & Health, 8*(4), 25–38.

Buss, A. H., & Plomin, R. (1984). *Temperament: Early developing personality traits*. Hillsdale, NJ: Erlbaum.

Cartoof, V. G., & Klerman, L. V. (1986). Parental consent for abortion: Impact of the Massachusetts law. *American Journal of Public Health, 76*, 397–440.

Coates, D. L. (1987). Gender differences in the structure and support characteristics of black adolescents' social networks. *Sex Roles, 17*, 667–687.

Cochran, M., & Riley, D. (1988). Mother reports of children's personal networks: Antecedents, concomitants, and consequences. In S. Salzinger, J. S. Antrobus, & M. Hammer (Eds.), *Social networks of children, adolescents, and college students* (pp. 113–147). Hillsdale, NJ: Erlbaum.

Council on Scientific Affairs, American Medical Association. (1993). Confidential health services for adolescents. *Journal of the American Medical Association*, *269*, 1420–1424.

Cowell, J. M. (1988). Health service utilization and special education: Development of a school nurse activity tool. *Journal of School Health*, *58*, 355–359.

Cowell, J. M., & Montgomery, A. C. (1993). *Patterns of physical activity among school aged children*. Research paper presented at the American Public Health Association Annual Meeting, San Francisco.

Cowell, J. M., & Montgomery, A. C. (in review). Determinants of physical activity among school aged children and consumption patterns.

Cowell, J. M., Montgomery, A. C., & Talashek, M. L. (1989). School aged cardiovascular risk: A school community partnership. *Public Health Nursing*, *6*, 67–73.

Cowell, J. M., Montgomery, A. C., & Talashek, M. L. (1992). Cardiovascular risk stability: From grade school to high school. *Pediatric Health Care*, *6*, 349–354.

Cox, C. L., Cowell, J. M., Marion, L. N., & Miller, E. H. (1990). The health self-determinism index for children. *Research in Nursing and Health*, *13*, 237–246.

Crockett, L. J., Petersen, A. C., Graber, J. A., Schulenberg, J. E., & Ebata, A. (1989). School transitions and adjustment during early adolescence. *Journal of Early Adolescence*, *9*, 181–210.

DiClemente, R. J., Durbin, M., Siegel, D., Krasnovsky, F., Lazarus, N., & Comacho, T. (1992). Determinants of condom use among junior high school students in a minority, inner-city school district. *Pediatrics*, *89*, 197–202.

Dougherty, D. M. (1993). Adolescent health: Reflections on a report to the U.S. Congress. *American Psychologist*, *48*(2), 193–201.

Dougherty, D. M., Eden, J., Kemp, K. B., Metcalf, K., Rowe, K., Ruby, G., Strobel, P., & Solarz, A. (1992). Adolescent health: A report to the U.S. Congress. *Journal of School Health*, *62*(5), 167–174.

Feiring, C., & Lewis, M. (1991). The transition from middle childhood to early adolescence: Sex differences in the social network and perceived competence. *Sex Roles*, *24*(7/8), 489–509.

Feldman, W., McGrath, P., & O'Shaughessy, M. (1986). Adolescents' pursuit of thinness. *American Journal of Disability and Children*, *140*, 294.

Ferguson, K. J., Yesalis, C. E., Pomrehn, P. R., & Kirkpatrick, M. B. (1989). Attitudes, knowledge and beliefs as predictors of exercise intent and behavior in school children. *Journal of School Health*, *59*, 112–115.

Forrest, J. D., & Singh, S. (1990). The sexual and reproductive behavior of American women, 1982–1988. *Family Planning Perspectives*, *22*, 206–214.

Fox, J. W. (1991). Mothers' influence on their adolescents' tendency to seek medical care. *Journal of Adolescent Health*, *12*, 116–123.

Frank, B. S. (1990). *Health needs and perceptions of adolescent males*. Unpublished master's research project. University of Illinois at Chicago.

Giblin, P., & Poland, M. (1985). Health needs of high school students in Detroit. *Journal of School Health*, *55*, 407–410.

Gochman, D. (1970). Children's perceptions of vulnerability to illness and accidents. *Public Health Reports*, *85*, 69–73.

Graves, C. E., Bridge, M. D., & Nyhuis, A. W. (1987). Residents' perception of their skill levels in the clinical management of adolescent health problems. *Journal of Adolescent Health Care*, *8*, 413–418.

Haeffle, J. (1994). *Beliefs, pleasures, external and internal attributions and social reinforcements of smoking among adolescents reporting current smoking, intermittent smoking and non-smoking*. Unpublished master's research project. University of Illinois at Chicago.

Health Promotion for Older Children and Adolescents. (1993). A report of the National Institute of Nursing Research. Bethesda, MD: U.S. Department of Health and Human Services.

Heinrich, L. B. (1993). Contraceptive self-efficacy in college women. *Journal of Adolescent Health*, *14*, 269–276.

Hester, N. O. (1984). Child's health self concept scale: Its development and psychometric properties. *Advances in Nursing Science*, *7*(1), 45–55.

Hirsch, B. J., & Rapkin, B. D. (1987). The transition to junior high school: A longitudinal study of self-esteem, psychological symptomatology, school life and social support. *Child Development*, *58*, 1235–1243.

Imai, W. K. (1989). Special problems in adolescent health care. *Quality Assurance and Utilization Review*, *4*, 115–120.

Imai, W. K., & Schydlower, M. (1994). Adolescent health needs and access to care in the Army medical system. *Texas Medicine*, *90*(3), 62–66.

Jemmott, J. B., Jemmott, L. W., Spears, H., Hewitt, N., & Cruz-Collins, M. (1992). Self-efficacy, hedonistic expectancies, and condom-use intentions among inner-city black adolescent women: A social cognitive approach to AIDS risk behavior. *Journal of Adolescent Health*, *13*, 512–519.

Joffe, A., & Radius, S. M (1993). Self-efficacy and intent to use condoms among entering college freshman. *Journal of Adolescent Health*, *14*, 262–268.

Kalnins, I., & Love, R. (1982). Children's concepts of health and illness and implications for health education: An overview. *Health Education Quarterly*, *9*, 8–19.

Kandel, D. B., Davies, M., Karus, D., & Yanagychi, K. (1986). The consequences in young adulthood of adolescent drug involvement. *Archives of General Psychiatry*, *43*, 746–754.

Kann, L., Warren, W., Collins, J. L., Ross, J., Collins, B., & Kolbe, L. J. (1993). Results from the National School-Based 1991 Youth Risk Behavior Survey and progress toward achieving related health objectives for the nation. *Public Health Reports*, *108* (Suppl 1), 47–55.

Kaplan, R. M. (1990). Behavior as the central outcome in health care. *American Psychologist, 45*, 1211–1220.

Keating, D. P. (1990). Adolescent thinking. In S. S. Feldman & G. R. Elliott (Eds.), *At the threshold: The developing adolescent* (pp. 54–58). Cambridge, MA: Harvard University Press.

Klein, J. D., Brown, J. D., Childers, K. W., Oliveri, J., Porter, C., & Dykers, C. (1993). Adolescents' risky behavior and mass media use. *Pediatrics, 92*, 24–31.

Kline, R. B., Canter, W. A., & Robin, A. (1987). Parameters of teenage alcohol use: A path analytic conceptual model. *Journal of Consulting and Clinical Psychology, 55*, 521–528.

Kolbe, L. J., Kann, L., & Collins, J. L. (1993). Overview of the youth risk behavior surveillance system. *Public Health Reports, 108*(Suppl 1), 2–10.

Koppleman, D. (1989). *Student utilization of the high school service*. Unpublished master's research project. University of Illinois at Chicago.

Kornfalt, R., & Ejlertsson, G. (1981). Total consumption of health services by school children in a primary health care district in southern Sweden. *Scandinavian Journal of Social Medicine, 9*, 63–73.

Kulbok, P., & Baldwin, J. (1992). Preventive health behavior to health promotion: Advancing a positive construct of health. *Advances in Nursing Science, 14*(4), 50–64.

Lewis, C. E., & Lewis, M. A. (1984). Peer pressure and risk-taking behaviors in children. *American Journal of Public Health, 74*, 580–584.

Lieu, T. A., Newacheck, P. W., & McManus, M. A. (1993). Race, ethnicity, and access to ambulatory care among US adolescents. *American Journal of Public Health, 83*, 960–965.

Major, B., Mueller, P., & Hildebrandt, K. (1985). Attributions, expectations, and coping with abortion. *Journal of Personality and Social Psychology, 48*, 585–599.

Marcus, S. E., Giovino, G. A., Pierce, J. P., & Harel, Y. (1993). Measuring tobacco use among adolescents. *Public Health Reports, 108*(Suppl 1), 20–24.

McManus, M. A., Newacheck, P. W., & Greaney, A. M. (1990). Young adults with special health care needs: Prevalence, severity, and access to health services. *Pediatrics, 86*, 1990.

McManus, M. A., Newacheck, P. W., & Weader, R. A. (1989). Metropolitan and nonmetropolitan adolescents: Difference in demographic and health characteristics. *Journal of Rural Health, 6*, 39–51.

Miller, S. K., & Slap, G. B. (1989). Adolescent smoking: A review of prevalence and prevention. *Journal of Adolescent Health Care, 10*, 129–135.

Millstein, S. G., & Irwin, C. E., Jr. (1987). Concepts of health and illness: Different constructs or variations on a theme? *Health Psychology, 1*, 512–524.

Millstein, S. G., Nightengale, E. O., Peterson, A. C., Mortimer, A. M., & Hamburg, D. A. (1993). Promoting the healthy development of adolescents. *Journal of the American Medical Association, 269*, 1413–1415.

Montgomery, A. C., & Cowell, J. M. (1994). *School aged children's nutrition behavior in three diverse communities: Differences and similarities*. Research paper presented at the American Public Health Association Annual Meeting, Washington, DC.

Natapoff, J. (1978). Children's views of health: A developmental study. *American Journal of Public Health, 68*, 995–1000.

Natapoff, J. N., & Essoka, G. C. (1989). Handicapped and able-bodied children's ideas of health. *Journal of School Health, 59*, 436–440.

National Cholesterol Education Program. (1990). Report of the Expert Panel on Population Strategies for Blood Cholesterol Reduction. DHHS Publication No. (NIH) 90-3047. Washington, DC: U.S. Government Printing Office.

Newacheck, P. W. (1989a). Adolescents with special health needs: Prevalence, severity, and access to health services. *Pediatrics, 84*, 872–881.

Newacheck, P. W. (1989b). Improving access to health services for adolescents from economically disadvantaged families. *Pediatrics, 84*, 1056–1063.

Newacheck, P. W., & McManus, M. (1989). Health insurance status of adolescents in the United States. *Pediatrics, 84*, 699–708.

Newacheck, P. W., McManus, M., & Gephart, J. (1992). Health insurance coverage of adolescents: A current profile and assessment of trends. *Pediatrics, 90*, 589–596.

Newcomb, M. D., & Bentler, P. M. (1989). Substance use and abuse among children and teenagers. *American Psychologist, 44*, 242–248.

Nguyen, M. N., Sauçier, J. F., & Pica, L. A. (1994). Influence of attitudes on the intention to use condoms in Quebec sexually active male adolescents. *Journal of Adolescent Health, 15*, 269–274.

OTA (Office of Technology Assessment)/U.S. Congress. (1991a). *Adolescent health — Volume I: Summary and policy options* OTA-H-464. Washington, DC: U.S. Government Printing Office.

OTA (Office of Technology Assessment)/U.S. Congress. (1991b). *Adolescent health — Volume II: Summary and policy options* OTA-H-465. Washington, DC: U.S. Government Printing Office.

OTA (Office of Technology Assessment)/U.S. Congress. (1991c). *Adolescent health — Volume III: Summary and policy options*. OTA-H-466. Washington, DC: U.S. Government Printing Office.

OTA (Office of Technology Assessment)/U.S. Congress. (1992). *Does health insurance make a difference?* OTA-H-BP-99. Washington, DC: U.S. Government Printing Office.

Paffenberger, R. S., Wing, A. L., Hyde, R. T., & Jung, D. L. (1983). Physical activity and incidence of hypertension in college alumni. *American Journal of Epidemiology, 117*, 245–256.

Pender, N. J. (1987). *Health promotion in nursing practice* (5th ed.). Norwalk, CT: Appleton & Lange.

Pesce, R. C., & Harding, C. G. (1986). Imaginary audience behavior and its relationship to operational thought and social experience. *Journal of Early Adolescence, 6*(1), 83–94.

Powers, S. I., Hauser, S. T., & Kilner, L. (1989). Adolescent mental health. *American Psychologist, 44,* 200–208.

Richter, E. A., & Schneider, S. H. (1981). Diabetes and exercise. *American Journal of Medicine, 70,* 201–209.

Riley, G. F., Potosky, A. L., Lubitz, J. D., & Brown, M. L. (1994). Stage of cancer diagnosis for Medicare, HMO and fee-for-service enrollees. *American Journal of Public Health, 84,* 1598–1604.

Robinson, T. N., Killen, J. D., Taylor, C. B., Telch, M. J., Bryson, S. W., Saylor, K. E., Maron, D. J., Maccoby, N., & Farquhar, J. W. (1987). Perspectives on adolescent substance use: A defined population study. *Journal of the American Medical Association, 258,* 2072–2076.

Rogoff, B. (1990). *Apprenticeship in thinking: Cognitive development in social context.* New York: Oxford Press.

Ross, C. E., & Hayes, D. (1988). Exercise and psychological well-being in the community. *American Journal of Epidemiology, 127,* 762–771.

Sallis, J. F., Patterson, T. L., Buono, M. J., & Nader, P. R. (1985). Relation of cardiovascular fitness and physical activity to cardiovascular disease risk factors in children and adults. *American Journal of Epidemiology, 127,* 933–941.

Sallis, J. F., Simons-Morton, B. S., Stone, E. J., Corbin, C. B., Epstein, L. H., Faucette, N., Ianotti, R. J., Killen, J. D., Klesges, R. C., Petray, C. K., et al. (1992). Determinants of physical activity and interventions in youth. *Medicine and Science in Sports and Exercise, 24,* 248–257.

Santelli, J. S., & Beilenson, P. (1992). Risk factors for adolescent sexual behavior, fertility, and sexually transmitted diseases. *Journal of School Health, 62,* 271–279.

Shafer, M. A., & Boyer, C. B. (1991). Psychosocial and behavioral factors associated with risk of sexually transmitted diseases, including human immunodeficiency virus infection, among urban high school students. *Journal of Pediatrics, 119,* 826–833.

Simmons, R. G., & Blyth, D. A. (1987). *Moving into adolescence: The impact of pubertal change and school context.* Hawthorne, NY: Aldine de Gruyter.

Siscovick, D. S., Weiss, N. S., Fletcher, R. H., & Lasky, T. (1984). The incidence of primary cardiac arrest during vigorous exercise. *New England Journal of Medicine, 311,* 874–877.

Smith, E. A., Udry, J. R., & Morris, N. M. (1985). Pubertal development and friends: A biosocial explanation of adolescent sexual behavior. *Journal of Health and Social Behavior, 26,* 183–192.

Society for Adolescent Medicine. (1992). Access to health care for adolescents: A position paper of the Society for Adolescent Medicine. *Journal of Adolescent Health Care, 13,* 162–170.

Stamler, J. (1987). Epidemiology, established major risk factors, and the primary prevention of coronary heart disease.

In W. W. Parmley & K. Chatterjee (Eds.), *Cardiology, 2* (pp. 1–41). Philadelphia: J. B. Lippincott.

Streff, F. M., & Wagenaar, A. C. (1989). Are there really shortcuts? Estimating seat belt use with self-report measures. *Accident Analysis Prevention, 21,* 509–516.

Tietjen, A. M. (1982). The ecology of children's social networks in Sweden. *International Journal of Behavioral Development, 5,* 111–130.

Torabi, M. R., Baily, W. J., & Majd-Jabbari, M. (1993). Cigarette smoking as a predictor of alcohol and other drug use by children and adolescents: Evidence of the "gateway drug effect." *Journal of School Health, 63,* 302–305.

Trowbridge, F., & Collins, B. (1993). Measuring dietary behaviors among adolescents. *Public Health Reports, 108* (Suppl. 1), 37–41.

Udry, J. R. (1988). Biological predispositions and social control in adolescent sexual behavior. *American Sociological Review, 53,* 709–722.

Walter, H. J., Vaughan, R. D., Gladis, M. M., Ragin, D. F., Kasen, S., & Cohall, A. T. (1993).Factors associated with AIDS-related behavioral intentions among high school students in an AIDS epicenter. *Health Education Quarterly, 20*(3), 409–420.

Waxweiler, R. J., Harel, Y., & O'Carroll, P. W. (1993). Measuring adolescent behaviors related to unintentional injuries. *Public Health Reports, 108*(Suppl 1), 11–14.

Wierson, M., Long, P., & Forehand, R. (1993). Toward a new understanding of early menarche: The role of environmental stress in pubertal timing. *Adolescence, 28*(112), 913–924.

Wigfield, A., Eccles, J. S., MacIver, D., Reuman, D. A., & Midgley, C. (1991). Transitions during early adolescence: Changes in children's domain-specific self-perceptions and general self-esteem across the transition to junior high school. *Developmental Psychology, 27*(4), 552–565.

Wood, D. L., Hayward, R. A., Corey, C. R., Freeman, H. E., & Shapiro, M. F. (1990). Access to medical care for children and adolescents in the United States. *Pediatrics, 86,* 666–673.

Yates, S., & Pliner, A. J. (1988). Judging maturity in the courts: The Massachusetts consent statute. *American Journal of Public Health, 78,* 646–649.

Yudkowsky, B. K., Cartland, J. D. C., & Flint, S. S. (1990). Pediatrician participation in Medicaid: 1978 to 1989. *Pediatrics, 85,* 567–577.

Zabin, L. S. (1984). The association between smoking and sexual behavior among teens in US contraceptive clinics. *American Journal of Public Health, 74,* 261–263.

Zabin, L. S., Hardy, J. B., Smith, E. A., & Hirsch, M. B. (1986). Substance use and its relation to sexual activity among inner-city adolescents. *Journal of Adolescent Health Care, 7,* 320–331.

Zabin, L. S., Hirsch, M. B., & Emerson, M. R. (1989). When urban adolescents choose abortion: Effects on education, psychological status and subsequent pregnancy. *Family Planning Perspectives, 21*(6), 248–255.

5

Health Behavior in the Elderly

William Rakowski

INTRODUCTION

The primary objective of this chapter is to suggest ideas that may be helpful for integrating the literatures of behavioral and psychosocial epidemiology, in the broader context of the study of health-related behaviors in older adulthood. The chapter is organized into four sections. The first section discusses the importance of understanding the health-related behaviors of older persons. The section reviews studies from the domain of behavioral epidemiology, which link lifestyle habits with the outcomes of mortality and morbidity. The topic of patterns among, and correlates of, health behaviors is also discussed.

The second section addresses the question of whether the health-related behaviors of older persons are amenable to intervention. This section summarizes an area of applied research that is rapidly growing. Results suggest that programs to promote behavioral change do show positive impacts.

The third section introduces research from psychosocial epidemiology. Specifically, the section reviews literature on the predictive associations between variables such as self-rated health and social network, on one hand, and subsequent health status outcomes, on the other. Psychosocial variables themselves are often not explicitly behavioral, yet their associations with health outcomes beg the question of intermediate steps in the causal chain to health status.

Finally, the fourth section offers an integration of behavioral and psychosocial epidemiology, in a somewhat broader framework than that in which either area has usually been studied. As such, the fourth section is somewhat more speculative than the first three. It is expected, however, that the ideas presented are sufficiently grounded in research to be of assistance.

There is *no* attempt made in this chapter to review in detail the literatures on adherence to treatment regimens, on actions taken in response to symptoms, or on medication taking by older persons. This choice was made deliberately, simply because research on the health-, illness-, and symptom-related behaviors of older persons has grown dramatically over the past 15 years, and it was not possible to review all of these domains in the space available. The starting points for this chapter were the literatures on behavioral and

William Rakowski • Department of Community Health and Center for Gerontology and Health Care Research, Brown University, Providence, Rhode Island 02912.

Handbook of Health Behavior Research III: Demography, Development, and Diversity, edited by David S. Gochman. Plenum Press, New York, 1997.

psychosocial epidemiology, and the ideas sug- gested for integration are therefore directed at models appropriate for surveys of the general population. The framework outlined in the fourth section includes, however, a role for symptom- and illness-related actions. This role is important as one of the possible causal links in what so far is an unspecified chain between baseline assess- ments of older persons and longer-term health outcomes.

THE IMPORTANCE OF HEALTH BEHAVIORS AMONG OLDER PERSONS

The period since 1985 has seen a growing awareness in society of the presence of older persons. Certainly, the sheer numbers of persons over age 60 command attention. Another feature that is gradually but steadily being recognized, however, is the vitality shown by many persons in their 70s, 80s, and even older. The active and robust older adult, who once was touted as "unique" even as late as the 1970s, has been joined by more and more age peers. One of the most important developments of older adult- hood has been the realistic *potential* to retain relatively good health and functional status at least through one's 70s.

The key word is, in fact, "potential." Signifi- cant illnesses and the need for supportive care inevitably occur. Nevertheless, the findings from several longitudinal, epidemiological studies of lifestyle practices of older persons have played a major role in stimulating the optimism that exists in gerontology for the potential of health promo- tion programs.

Results from Behavioral Epidemiology

Comprehensive and useful summaries of be- havioral epidemiological research (e.g., Kaplan & Haan, 1989; Kaplan & Strawbridge, 1994) show that some health-related behaviors can make a substantial difference in the morbidity and mor- tality experience of older persons. Physical activ-

ity and smoking are of particular importance, though there is still reason to examine other behaviors. Not all behaviors have received the epidemiological attention that has been given to smoking and physical activity. For example, pre- venting burns and scalds and promoting oral care have not figured prominently in population-level, outcome-oriented epidemiology, even though they are important areas of health protection. This inattention may be due to a traditional em- phasis on "hard" end points such as mortality, and also to a natural tendency of epidemiology to focus on leading causes of death such as lung cancer, heart disease, breast cancer, and stroke. As behavioral epidemiology adopts newer out- come variables that are based on morbidity and functional health, and as linkages to utilization and medical claims databases become more pos- sible, one can expect more behaviors to be used in research.

Nor is the evidence for health benefits clear in all instances—at least on a general population level including those persons who are not at high risk or actively symptomatic. For example, some epidemiological evidence for cholesterol indi- rectly suggests that dietary factors would be im- portant for cholesterol management and there- fore for heart disease. There has been debate, however, regarding the benefits of cholesterol control in the general population of older per- sons, as opposed to control in those at clearly high risk (Berg & Cassells, 1990, chapt. 10). More- over, the specific dietary practices that would comprise cholesterol control have not been ex- amined as predictor variables for older persons in the same manner as have those for smoking and physical activity.

Health Behaviors across Age Groups

One can ask how well—or how badly— older persons compare to other adult age groups in the performance of certain health-related prac- tices. This question is interesting from the stand- point of knowing about age-group differences at a purely descriptive level, but the question can also be moot. That is, little comfort can be taken if the age groups have similar behavior prevalence rates, but the desired health practice is still reported at a low percentage across all ages. In other words, age-group comparisons can be useful to identify substantial gaps and to suggest areas of intervention to address obvious crises, but the comparison is only one part of the larger picture.

Table 1 summarizes data from the 1990 National Health Interview Survey of Disease Prevention and Health Promotion (NHIS-DPHP). This table is based on information from a federal publication (Piani & Schoenborn, 1993), as well as additional tabulations made by this writer. There were over 8000 persons aged 65 and over in the sample, as well as over 10,000 persons aged 45–64 and another 13,500 persons aged 30–44.

Table 1 is instructive because it indicates the difficulty of finding general, descriptive-level trends either across behaviors for older adults, specifically, or among age groups. The table suggests that older persons are at a disadvantage in regard to vigorous activity and recent visits for dental care and, for women, clinical breast exam and Pap testing. On the other hand, older persons are more favorable in the categories of smoking and drinking (perhaps due to a survival effect). All age groups appear to have room to improve in regard to talking with their physician

Table 1. Performance by Adults Aged 30 and Older of Selected Health-Related Behaviors and on Status Suggestive of Behavioral Practices[a]

| Health-related behavior | Adults manifesting the behavior (%) | | | | | |
| | Women | | | Men | | |
	30–44	45–64	65+	30–44	45–64	65+
Above desirable body weight 20% or more	24.7	34.2	28.2	32.0	37.8	26.3
Medical visit in the past 2 years	91.8	90.8	92.3	77.4	82.5	90.4
Blood pressure check in past year	89.9	90.0	91.7	80.6	85.8	90.9
Ever had blood cholesterol checked	53.2	69.4	70.5	48.2	65.9	71.4
Exercises or plays sports regularly	40.1	34.6	29.1	44.3	35.6	36.9
Vigorous leisure activity[b]	25.0	19.5	12.5	36.4	29.3	26.1
Walked for exercise in past 2 weeks	49.7	49.4	44.3	38.9	44.5	51.6
Currently Smokes Cigarettes	25.8	24.8	11.5	33.6	29.3	14.6
If smokes, ≥25 per day	19.6	21.8	12.0	31.0	39.0	26.8
If smokes, knows CHD risk greater	94.0	87.9	77.9	90.0	84.1	73.5
Two or more drinks/day, past 2 weeks	1.6	2.0	1.7	9.7	9.8	8.5
If drinks, drove when should not have	8.0	2.7	2.0	17.0	9.7	3.7
Seen dentist in past 12 months	74.0	64.9	50.2	62.9	60.5	48.7
Has one or more working smoke detectors	82.4	78.3	73.5	81.7	77.4	77.5
Wears seatbelts all/most of time	73.8	72.0	72.2	64.2	63.5	67.3
Daily/sometimes eats breakfast	73.9	80.2	92.8	71.2	77.8	93.0
Often/sometimes discusses food with doctor	31.6	35.7	36.5	22.5	31.3	30.2
Sleeps 7–8 hours per night	68.0	66.0	59.9	65.9	66.4	61.8
For women only						
Pap test in past 2 years	85.3	73.1	57.5	—	—	—
Clinical breast exam in past 2 years	85.6	79.1	70.3	—	—	—
Breast self-exam ≥12×/year	43.6	47.1	45.4	—	—	—

[a]This table was compiled from information in a federal report (Piani & Schoenborn, 1993), as well as by additional tabulations on the data conducted by this author.
[b]Based on a report of specific activities that involve an average of 3 or more kilocalories per kilogram per day. The entry for exercise/sports is based on a single, general self-report item.

about foods, a behavioral area in which at least 60% of all age groups, and of both sexes, do not report even "sometimes" talking with their doctor. For any clinically based indicator, however, high rates of performance also depend on consistent efforts by health care providers.

Other analyses of the 1990 NHIS-DPHP have found that mammography rates were also lower for women aged 65–75 than for younger women (Rakowski, Rimer, & Bryant, 1993). In addition, influenza vaccinations may be underutilized in the older population. Nichol, Margolis, Wuorenma, and Von Sternberg (1994) examined rates in three successive cohorts of persons aged 65 or more in a Minneapolis–St. Paul health maintenance organization. Annual immunization rates were 45%, 58%, and 55% for the years 1991–1993. Being immunized was associated with lower rates of hospitalization, reduction in all-cause mortality, and cost savings.

Research on the personal health behaviors of older persons must still resolve questions in regard to the types of behaviors that are included in surveys and in regard to constructing general profiles that represent "healthful" lifestyles. For example, summaries of older person's health behavior have not considered suicide or self-injurious actions; the literatures on health promotion/ health education and on suicide have been separate. Yet suicide and attempted suicide are realities.

Suicide, living wills, and advance directives pose an interesting circumstance for behavioral epidemiology. Samples in longitudinal research are often divided simply into "Alive" versus "Deceased" at the outcome assessment. Incorporating indicators of self-injurious actions or advance directives into surveys will inevitably bring the academic behavioral epidemiology of aging into contact with the ethical examination of situations in which self-termination may be justified and therefore not be a legitimate "negative" outcome indicator. In fact, there may come a point at which researchers, ethicists, and others debate whether mortality is necessarily an a priori "negative" outcome. Perhaps functional status will be a less debatable criterion. As a whole, a broad range of outcome variables can be considered when examining the potential benefits of health behaviors in later life (Rakowski, 1994).

Correlates of Health-Related Behaviors

Another question is whether a set of predictor or independent variables seem to be consistent indicators of which groups of older persons do (or do not) report favorable health behaviors. Another way of asking this question is whether favorable (or unfavorable) health behaviors cluster strongly in certain subgroups of the older population. The answer to this question is important. A consistent set of correlates across multiple behaviors would suggest that interventions targeted at well-defined subpopulations (e.g., older men who are living alone in rural areas) could produce change in several health behaviors.

The picture here continues to be murky. Some studies have examined the consistency of the correlates of several health behaviors in a single sample of older persons (Jensen, Counte, & Glandon, 1992; Rakowski, Julius, Hickey, & Halter, 1987; Stoller & Pollow, 1994). All of these reports have concluded that each health behavior studied tended to have its own set of correlates; there was not extensive overlap. Another observation has been that even multivariate equations have not yielded extremely high percentages of explained variance (e.g., Stoller & Pollow, 1994). This finding also casts doubt on the existence of a single group of correlates.

An even more important task is to identify the correlates of behavior *change* in longitudinal studies, rather than to look only for the correlates of health practices in cross-sectional data. Currently, there is only limited information on the predictors of change in older adults' health behavior. For example, Kaplan and Haan (1989) reported on the association of changes in health practices with subsequent survival among middle-aged and older persons. Salive et al. (1992) identified predictors of smoking cessation. Interestingly, the incidence of illness between interviews was associated with quitting. It will be important to study whether the benefits of the behavior change outweigh the effects of the incident condition. Illness-related versus volitional change may be an important covariate for longitudinal models.

It also seems not to be the case in general population surveys that two or three consistent, large clusters of health behaviors are found when techniques such as components analysis are applied to the data. For example, Sobal, Revicki, and DeForge (1992) analyzed interrelationships among health practices in the 1979 National Survey of Personal Health Practices and Consequences, which was a survey of 3025 men and women aged 20–64. They found ten clusters of health practices for men and ten for women, which still accounted for only about one third of the variance. Sobal et al. (1992) concluded that relationships among behaviors were weak, except for these very specific clusters. As in other studies (see Appendix A of their article), there was no evidence for a general health behavior factor that spanned several different types of activities (e.g., exercise, beverage use, smoking, use of health services, home safety).

Despite the absence of broad clusters of behaviors, some behavioral relationships do seem to exist, such as the association between smoking and heavier drinking, a tendency for persons who smoke to have somewhat less favorable health habits in other areas, and for a link between the receipt of Pap tests and mammograms. The Alameda health practices index has also been an effective marker for persons at risk of long-term morbidity and mortality (Camacho, Strawbridge, Cohen, & Kaplan, 1993).

Methodological and measurement issues may contribute to not finding clusters of health practices (Rakowski, 1992). It may also be expecting too much, however, to find well-defined clusters of health practices in general surveys of older persons. The list of professionally defined "desirable" practices is continually expanding, the expansion being usually more rapid than the diffusion of the practice into the general population. In addition, most surveys have used a diverse list of health practices, with no clear conceptual reason either that there *should* be consistency of performing them as a group or that the practices should have similar correlates. Even among four dependent measures chosen to be specifically related to cardiovascular disease, there was little evidence for consistent correlates among adults aged 18–64 (Rakowski, Lefebvre, Assaf, Lasater, & Carleton, 1990).

One can derive, however, some general observations concerning the correlates of older adults' health practices. Perhaps the most prevalent tendency, when there is a gender difference in the data, is for women to report more health promoting behaviors than men (e.g., Hibbard, 1988; Jensen et al., 1992; Lubben, Weiler, & Chi, 1989; Rakowski et al., 1987; Stoller & Pollow, 1994). Men do tend to report more vigorous physical activity. Other than a gender difference, it is probably safest to say that better health practices are reported by older persons with better socioeconomic resources, with more social support, and with a more positive psychological outlook—such as an internal locus of control. Basically, "those who have" more when they enter old age also seem to be "those who get" more in the way of favorable health practices and the benefits of those practices. The examination of ethnic differences is still at an early stage, but among ethnic elderly who survive to old age, it is possible that at least some behaviors will actually have a better profile than among the non-Hispanic white population (Lubben et al., 1989). One of the interesting challenges for health behavior research will be to determine whether behavioral and social factors help to account for the mortality and functional health crossovers that have been observed between older African-Americans and whites (D. O. Clark, Maddox, & Steinhauser, 1993; Guralnik, Land, Blazer, Fillenbaum, & Branch, 1993).

Information Seeking

One area in which a consistent behavioral cluster has been found is information seeking. An information-seeking factor has been found in three separate survey samples, two of which were older adults (Rakowski et al., 1987; Rakowski, Assaf, et al., 1990; Rakowski, Rice, & McHorney, 1992). One of these studies was longitudinal and found that the construct was replicated over time (Rakowski et al., 1992). The number of items has varied among surveys, but the primary ones include reading articles about health, listening to programs in the media, talking with friends, and doing general body self-exams. Also studied have been reading food package labels, preparing in advance for medical visits, and asking questions of various health care providers.

The information-seeking variable has been associated with performance of several other behavioral practices. For example, a greater tendency toward information seeking has been related to engaging in physical activity, having emergency numbers by the telephone, having a stocked first aid kit, checking medication expiration dates, using a seat belt more consistently, asking to sit in the nonsmoking section, and conducting breast self-examination (Rakowski et al., 1992). Stoller and Pollow (1994) also used these information-seeking items and found associations with several health practices. One key feature of information seeking is its definition as a generic *process* that underlies behavior change, rather than as the performance of specific behaviors such as number of cigarettes smoked, days of exercise per week, regularity of wearing seatbelts, or intake of particular food groups.

An implication of this definition is that each one of a group of persons can be comparably high on information seeking, but can select different health behaviors to follow at a given point in his or her life. This characteristic makes it empirically possible to find a process-type factor, even if there is no evidence for strong factors when analysis is based on the performance of specific health behaviors.

The existence among older persons of a general behavioral process such as information seeking is not especially surprising in light of other literature (e.g., Bagley-Burnett, 1988). The transtheoretical model of behavior, known more generically as the stages of change model (Prochaska, DiClemente, & Norcross, 1992), also employs a construct labeled "Consciousness-Raising" as one of the key mechanisms by which people change health-related practices. Originally developed for smoking cessation, consciousness raising is one of the fundamental activities by which persons move from not being ready to initiate a behavior to finally initiating it. The definitions of consciousness raising and information seeking are similar. This chapter will return to information seeking in the section that offers an integration of behavioral epidemiology and psychosocial epidemiology with health status outcomes.

HEALTH BEHAVIOR INTERVENTIONS WITH OLDER PERSONS

Behavioral epidemiological data are important, as are data on the correlates of older adults' health practices, but they are still descriptive. Self-selection or contextual forces may explain why some persons show more favorable health behavior in a cross-sectional survey. People who do not report the desired practices may face greater challenges in adopting them. There is no assurance that lifestyle or behavior changes can be accomplished or that changes in behavior will lead to positive outcomes. The results of experimental/control-designed behavioral interventions are therefore important.

Range of Diseases and Conditions

Interventions with older persons have addressed several different health problems and outcomes, including arthritis (e.g., Lorig & Holman, 1993); urinary incontinence, both in women (e.g., Wells, Brink, Diokno, Wolfe, & Gillis, 1991) and in men (Burgio, Stutzman, & Engel, 1989); diabetes, often with an emphasis on dietary management (e.g., Glasgow et al., 1992); falls and injury prevention (e.g., Stevens et al., 1991/1992; Tinetti et al., 1994); heart disease (e.g., N. M. Clark et al., 1992); smoking cessation (e.g., Rimer et al., 1994); colon cancer (e.g., Atwood et al., 1992; Weinrich, Weinrich, Stromberg, Boyd, &

Weiss, 1993); screening mammography (e.g., Rimer et al., 1992); mild hypertension and blood pressure control (e.g., Applegate et al., 1992); stroke education (e.g., Glanz, Marger, & Meehan, 1986); assertiveness training (Franzke, 1987); low impact aerobics and exercise training (Hopkins, Murrah, Hoeger, & Rhodes, 1990; Topp, Mikesky, Wigglesworth, Holt, & Edwards, 1993). Other interventions have had the objective of promoting general wellness and functioning, rather than addressing a specific illness (e.g., Benson et al., 1989; Fries, Bloch, Harrington, Richardson, & Beck, 1993; Fries, Harrington, Edwards, Kent, & Richardson, 1994; Nelson et al., 1984; Vickery, Golaszewski, Wright, & Kalmer, 1988).

Demonstration of Effectiveness

Interventions with older persons have used a wide range of behavior and outcome variables to assess program impact. Some projects have had a limited dependent variable. For example, Weinrich et al. (1993) simply employed the return of a completed occult stool test within about 6 days as their measure of effectiveness.

Other reports have used a wider range of dependent measures. For example, Emery and Blumenthal (1990) had between 15 and 20 indicators of perceived change in several psychosocial domains as a part of their project that included exercise and yoga groups.

Nelson et al. (1984) examined knowledge, self-care skills, lifestyle change, health service use, health status, and quality of life. Glasgow et al. (1992) used several measures specifically relevant to diabetes control (e.g., fasting blood glucose, glycosylated hemoglobin), but also assessed diabetes-related self-efficacy, problem solving, diabetes-related quality of life, and general mood state.

For the most part, effects on at least some outcomes have been positive. Positive effects have not always been found, however, nor should unqualified success on all dependent variables be expected. For example, Wells et al. (1991) studied pelvic muscle exercise versus a 4-week medica-

tion protocol to deal with urinary incontinence. In this study, 6 months of exercise resulted in greater pelvic muscle strength, but the two groups did not differ on other outcomes (self-reported urine control and wetting, urine control when told to cough). Similarly, Nelson et al. (1984) found that their general self-care intervention produced positive effects on skills, confidence, and lifestyle change, but no effects on physician visits, hospital stays, or quality of life. Topp et al. (1993) investigated the effect of dynamic resistance strength training on gait velocity and balance. The comparison group was a contact-only control. The exercise group demonstrated greater strength of knee extensors and flexors after the 12-week program, but showed no improvement on the gait and balance measures. Laboratory-based studies of exercise training routinely show effects on physiological and mood variables, but not on measures of cognition. Finally, Glasgow et al. (1992) found improvements for caloric intake and fat intake, using a comprehensive package targeting diet and exercise. No evidence was found for impact on fiber intake or on exercise.

Mixed findings such as these require explanation, and the authors in the studies cited have attempted to supply it. One consideration can be the diversity of outcomes that are employed. Since it is important to document the impact of intervention as accurately as possible, a broad set of potential outcomes can be of use in investigating the limits of program effectiveness. At the same time, it is equally important to avoid falling into the trap of believing that "more is better" in regard to the number of outcomes to include. The possible impacts of self-care interventions must not be oversold or overpromised.

A second issue has to do with the apparent degree to which causal pathways have been specified *before* the intervention. Benson et al. (1989) provided an a priori classification of their outcomes into expected "direct" and "indirect" effects of the intervention. Their study showed a greater impact on direct effects (i.e., those outcomes with an immediate causal linkage to the intervention) than on indirect outcomes (i.e., those outcomes that were further removed along a causal pathway). This type of prior specification of hierarchy of outcomes is a very helpful addition to the literature.

Length of Follow-up

The duration of program effectiveness beyond immediate, short-term change can be used to argue for the potential of behavioral interventions. Several interventions have looked at outcomes over 3–6 months, while other interventions have used longer periods. Fries et al. (1993) employed a 2-year follow-up. The falls-prevention intervention conducted by Stevens et al. (1991/1992) used a 2-year period, as did the smoking cessation study of Rimer et al. (1994). The arthritis interventions by Lorig and colleagues covered between 20 months and 4 years of follow-up (Lorig & Holman, 1993).

Long follow-up periods (e.g., 2 years or more) are not a prerequisite for judging that an intervention was successful. The decay of an effect between 6 months and 1 year does not necessarily detract from the value of the intervention. Duration of program impact must be evaluated relative to participants' exposure to the intervention.

Types of Comparison/Control Groups

Some studies with older persons have used "usual care" or a no-contact control (e.g., N. M. Clark et al., 1992; Stevens et al., 1991/1992); other projects have used a delayed-intervention, "wait-list" control in order to examine whether effects would be replicated (e.g., Emery & Blumenthal, 1990; Fries et al., 1993).

Still other studies have used comparison groups involving exposure to health-related materials and activities or to an accepted medical regimen in relation to a clinical illness. Rimer et al. (1992) used low-cost mammography plus posters and materials in retirement communities. Nelson et al. (1984) used a lecture/demonstration on foot care and hypertension versus a multiple session general self-care intervention. Topp et al. (1993) used a two-session driver education course as the control for their dynamic resistance training intervention. Wells et al. (1991) employed a standard drug treatment as the comparison group for their pelvic muscle intervention training. Weinrich et al. (1993) used an existing American Cancer Society package on colorectal cancer for their comparison group. Rimer et al. (1994) contrasted three groups in a test of smoking cessation: Clearing the Air, Clear Horizons, or Clear Horizons and two counselor calls.

Because many interventions have employed "usual care" or no-contact controls, a possible impression is that studies with older persons are not examining a very diverse range of behavior change techniques or methodologies. To the extent that the development of an area of intervention is judged by having existing "gold standards" that can serve as the control/comparison groups whose performance should be matched or exceeded, behavior change interventions for older persons, in most areas, have been at early phases of development. Interventions are rapidly becoming more detailed, however, and reflect increasing methodological and technical sophistication.

Methodological Issues

Behavior change with older persons is clearly possible, despite some caveats concerning the biases of some intervention study samples. Perhaps most generally, the participating older persons have somehow been "connected" to traditional recruitment sources such as hospitals and physician offices; senior centers and nutrition sites; residential complexes; older adult organizations such as AARP; newspapers, television, and radio; retiree groups; and health fairs. They may have had to be interested enough to make the effort to respond to advertisements in the media asking for volunteers.

In addition, as a general rule, persons with less than a high school education have not been a prominent part of intervention study samples, though there are exceptions (e.g., Haber, 1986;

Nelson et al., 1984; Morisky, Levine, Green, & Smith, 1982; Weinrich et al., 1993). This general sample pattern is probably a function of the tendency for interventions to focus on older persons who were routinely connected to health care and social organizations, as well as those who were willing to reply to solicitations in the media asking for volunteers.

As might be expected, educational level is closely related to the representation of persons of color in the intervention studies. Again, there are exceptions (e.g., Franzke, 1987; Haber, 1986; Morisky et al., 1982; Weinrich et al., 1993). Positive outcomes were found in many of these programs. As with education, literature indicates that carefully done projects do have the potential to benefit the behavioral skills and health knowledge of older persons from racial- and ethnic-minority groups.

Behavior change interventions may be one area in which it is important to try to oversample men. Some projects do not report on gender composition, but when both sexes are included, the percentage of men is often as low as 20% and also often not above 35%. Although the percentage may mirror rates in the population, their absolute numbers in the project may not be sufficient for detailed analyses.

Low percentages of any particular group are not an especially serious problem if there are large overall samples that were chosen in a way to minimize bias. Many intervention studies with older persons, however, do not have large numbers of participants. Several projects of those reviewed had total samples under 200, and many of those even numbered under 150 or 100. With these small samples, it is extremely difficult to do detailed between-group comparisons along almost any dimension.

PSYCHOSOCIAL EPIDEMIOLOGY AND OLDER PERSONS

A great deal of attention is being given to variables that are often grouped together as the "psychosocial" influences on the health status of middle-aged and older persons. The types of variables that are studied in psychosocial epidemiology include one's social support, participation in community organizations, perceptions of one's health, religiosity, attribution of health problems to "old age", and personal traits such as life satisfaction, locus of control, and depression. Psychosocial epidemiology is therefore complementary to the behavioral epidemiological studies that look at the influence of lifestyle health habits. Sociodemographic factors such as income and education might also be studied under this rubric, but this chapter will not deal with demographic correlates of health.

Findings from Psychosocial Epidemiology

The reader may wish to consult several very good reviews of psychosocial epidemiology (e.g., Berg & Cassells, 1990, chapt. 14; Berkman, Oxman, & Seeman, 1992; House, Landis, & Umberson, 1988; Kahn, 1994). Most of these reviews have concentrated on social network and sociodemographic variables, which have had a longer tradition of epidemiological study than have self-rated health or other personal psychological traits.

A pattern of findings is emerging from this research. It now seems well established that persons with less favorable self-assessments of their health (e.g., ratings as fair, poor, or "bad") tend to have higher mortality than persons who report "excellent" health (e.g., Idler, Kasl, & Lemke, 1990; Kaplan & Camacho, 1983; Mossey & Shapiro, 1982; Rakowski, Fleishman, Mor, & Bryant, 1993; Schoenfeld, Malmrose, Blazer, Gold, & Seeman, 1994; Wolinsky & Johnson, 1992), although there are exceptions (Idler & Angel, 1990). Even a person self-reporting "good" or average health may have an elevated risk. Bivariate associations are reduced when health status and other key demographic factors are introduced as covariates, but self-ratings still are predictive.

In addition, older persons with fewer involvements in groups and organizations, including religious settings, tend to have higher mortality than those who report participating in such activities (e.g., Berkman et al., 1992; Bryant & Rakowski, 1992; House et al., 1988; Kaplan, Strawbridge, Camacho, & Cohen, 1993; Seeman, Kaplan, Knudsen, Cohen, & Guralnik, 1987; Steinbach, 1992; Zuckerman, Kasl, & Ostfeld, 1984). Social network variables have presented more challenges for assessment than self-ratings of health. This difference may well be a function of the greater attention directed at differentiating dimensions of the social context of aging than at the domain of self-ratings of health.

Other self-ratings may also be important for older persons. Rakowski and Hickey (1992) found that attributing difficulties with activities of daily living to old age rather than to a specific illness was associated with a higher risk of mortality. A subsequent analysis (Rakowski, Wilcox, & Clark, 1994) found that attributing difficulty with instrumental activities of daily living to old age was associated with greater functional difficulty at follow-up. Boult, Kane, Louis, Boult, and McCaffrey (1994) reported that an external locus of control over future health was associated with higher 4-year mortality. Additionally, two studies by Grand, Grosclaude, Bocquet, Pous, and Albarede (1988, 1990) reported feelings of usefulness and future planning to be associated with decreased morbidity and mortality.

The predictive importance of certain psychosocial variables in the general population of older persons is still being studied. For example, an independent predictive effect for marital status at a baseline assessment has not yet been established, although *changes* in marital status can be very important. Also, the importance of marital status may be greater for men than for women.

The independent effect of contact with family members, as opposed to contact with friends and involvement in out-of-home activities, is also still being determined. One of the potential confounds with family contact is that health problems can lead to greater contacts and closer residential proximity, so that frequent contact and proximity can be due both to the volitional aspects of social interaction and to health problems. Finally, the significance of personal traits such as life satisfaction and depression is still unknown. Some studies find an association with mortality; others do not.

Methodological Issues

There are several reasons for the impressive results for self-rated health and social context variables from this research. First, these have been studies of general populations, in contrast to studies of patients who presented themselves in clinics for clearly medical problems, or who were recruited to study coping after disruptive events such as stroke, widowhood, or hip fracture. Second, the follow-up periods of these studies have ranged from 2 through almost 20 years. The fact that predictive associations have been found at these extremes suggests that relatively strong processes are operating. Third, studies have used statistical methods to control for other factors that can influence morbidity and mortality, such as age, gender, baseline medical conditions, living arrangements, education, and income. Moreover, the effects for psychosocial variables are often as strong as those for well-known epidemiological risk factors such as age, sex, and medical conditions. Finally, but by no means least, self-rated health and social context variables are often measured in very basic ways, such as on yes/no, high/medium/low, or similarly brief dichotomous or simple categorical scales. Even these basic measures have been predictive of health outcomes. There are methodological issues, however, that future studies should consider.

Number of Follow-up Assessments. Psychosocial and behavioral epidemiology analyses have often been restricted to situations in which a single baseline assessment is used to predict a subsequent outcome. This is a basic design, baseline → outcome, limited to only two points of data collection. Researchers know, however, that even if the survey is "longitudinal," a single baseline assessment is simply a snapshot of the individual's status, which cannot capture an individual's *consistency* over time. It will therefore be important to have multiwave studies in which the stability or change of psychosocial variables can be used as an "extended baseline" predictor of health outcomes.

Measuring Variables. The methodologies for assessing self-rated health have probably been more straightforward than those for assessing social networks. Self-rated health has usually been assessed with single questions. One version is represented by an item such as that in the National Health Interview Survey ("Would you say your health in general is excellent, very good, good, fair, or poor?"). A second version is self-assessment relative to age peers (e.g., "For your age would you say, in general, your health is excellent, good, fair, poor, or bad?" [Mossey & Shapiro, 1982]). Until recently, a single self-rated health item was used in analyses. The Longitudinal Study of Aging included both versions, and Rakowski, Fleishman, et al. (1993) reported that both were predictive of mortality when used simultaneously in an equation. However, a larger construct of self-rated health, based on five self-rating items and supported by LISREL analysis, did not appear to perform any better than the two individual questions.

There is therefore reason to investigate broader definitions of self-rated health, at the same exercising caution in presuming that all self-ratings will be predictive of health outcomes. When self-ratings of health are expanded, and the diversity of content is also broadened, assessment of subjective health may become as diverse as measurement of social networks.

Self-assessment questions also raise the issue of persons who manifest a preference not to respond either by refusing to answer or by simply saying that they "don't know" how to rate their status. An analysis suggests that nonresponse to self-assessments can also be meaningful (Rakow-ski, Mor, & Hiris, 1994). The mortality rate among persons who did not answer a question on perceived control over future health was higher than that among persons who reported that they had a great deal of control and comparable to that among persons who said that they had little if any control.

Social network measures have been more diverse than health self-assessment measures, probably because the social environment and social interaction have so many potential dimensions (e.g., contact with family versus friends, settings in which contacts can occur, subjective versus objective social contact, satisfaction with contact, in-home versus out-of-home). An interesting analysis of the diversity of social network measures that can be constructed from a single database might be performed on several articles that have used the Longitudinal Study of Aging (e.g., Boult et al., 1994; Rakowski & Wilcox, 1994; Rakowski, Fleishman, et al., 1993; Steinbach, 1992; Wolinsky & Johnson, 1992).

Robustness against Covariates. As indicated, one of the themes in psychosocial epidemiology has been an effort to account for the predictive effects of such variables by including as comprehensive a set of covariates as possible. For example, the report by Idler and Angel (1990) was innovative in the study of self-rated health because the NHANES-I Follow-Up Study, rather than relying only on self-reported measures of illness, contained medical diagnoses that could be used as health status covariates. These objective values did not eliminate the association between self-rated health and mortality. Instead, the bivariate association was diminished when other sociodemographic and other covariates were added.

The issue of covariates is important but difficult to resolve. Age and sex must be included, as well as race and indicators of baseline health status. There is no standard in the epidemiological literature, however, for the list of covariates that "should" be included to provide a fair test of the predictive power of a psychosocial variable for older persons. The practice so far has been to test psychosocial variables against as many competing causes and covariates as possible. The impression is that efforts to date have been as much to try and explain away psychosocial variables as to explore the question of why such variables might have an effect. Skepticism is a reasonable first step, especially for variables that have no clearly evident, immediate causal link to health outcomes. At this point, however, the salience of such variables appears to have been demonstrated, and a new set of research questions must be posed. One possible future emphasis is discussed next.

A Question for Intervention

Although the research results of psychosocial epidemiology are impressive, they lead to a very important question in regard to their application to health promotion/disease prevention interventions: whether psychosocial epidemiology, at a population level, is a purely academic area with little if any practical relevance in applied settings. Psychosocial variables such as self-rated health and social participation do not seem to be areas that easily lend themselves as targets of population-level intervention for general public policy.

The reasons they do not can be ethical, legal, or even practical. For example, in the arena of social contacts, minimum levels of religiosity and church attendance cannot be required by law, even if they predict mortality. In the same way, it is not possible to mandate that people be involved in community organizations, that they do volunteer work, or that they regularly go out of their homes and make social contact with others. The absence of a clear chain of causation between social network variables and health status outcomes also makes intervention problematic, regardless of the epidemiological data, because the intermediate mechanisms and objectives are difficult to specify. Some findings have suggested an association between stressors and immunological responsiveness in an elderly sample (Es-

terling, Kiecolt-Glaser, Bodnar, & Glaser, 1994). Seeman, Berkman, Blazer, and Rowe (1994) have reported that some measures of social ties were associated with indicators of neuroendocrine function, particularly for men. The existence of such associations strengthens the social epidemiological data.

The situation with regard to subjective assessments of health is equally unresolved. It is unclear how to go about countering an individual's self-assessments of poor health status; the challenge is even greater in the presence of health problems. An individual's basis for the assessment of risk may also be a barrier to intervention. Persons who want to change lifestyle habits often define activities such as smoking, lack of exercise, a poor diet, and being very overweight as "problems." Effects can be felt directly on areas such as stamina and speed. The popular media also reinforce the message that certain lifestyles create high risk.

It is not yet clear that persons whose self-rated health is less than "excellent" or "very good," or older persons with little social participation, label these statuses as health-related *problems* to as great a degree as poor lifestyle behaviors are considered to be problems. In fact, many persons would say that they voluntarily choose the level of social contact that they have. They may also assert that they have always been a little pessimistic about their health or that "only fair" health is the best they can expect at their age. Of course, some persons with high-risk behavioral practices also deny their situation, but it still seems more difficult for laypersons (and health care professionals) to deny the potential harmfulness of a concrete behavior than that of an attitude.

Existing data tell us that something very important takes place in the psychology and immediate social environment of older persons that affects their health. Unless practical and ethical ways are found to intervene with psychosocial variables, however, these highly important data cannot be used to benefit the health of older persons.

A Possible Resolution of the Question. One approach to the difficult issue of applying the data may lie in discerning what psychosocial variables denote on a level that is more general than the individual measures that have been used in individual studies. It may be helpful to reflect on a person's phenomenology and ask, "What is the *personal experience* and significance of having social connections and of having a positive view of one's health?" Speculating about the answer is a subjective process and therefore entails a certain degree of risk. Without some risk taking, however, it will be difficult for psychosocial epidemiology to advance beyond being largely an academic pursuit.

Taken as a whole, the data on psychosocial epidemiology seem to point to the importance of having an internal motivation and self-perceived reasons for being actively involved in life on a day-to-day basis. In everyday language, such motivation might be stated as simply as the individuals "having a reason to get out of bed in the morning." Psychosocial variables contribute heavily to this motivation.

A somewhat qualitative proposal like this may seem to be too simple for an issue as complex as trying to understand the nonmedical, psychosocial influences on mortality and morbidity. This suggested role for psychosocial variables, however, may also influence the way in which the results of most epidemiological research and statistical analyses with these indicators are considered for application in interventions. A focus on the broader motivational implications of psychosocial factors may even promote different approaches to the manner in which predictor variables are defined in future studies.

In the standard tradition of empirical research, each predictor variable in domains such as self-rated health or social participation is defined by a specific set of questions. The questions used for measuring the variable are the same for everyone in the study. Statistical analyses determine whether enough persons have the same direction of relationship between responses to those questions and an outcome variable to allow the inference of a significant (non-chance) association.

There is, however, a very important assumption implicit in these analyses: that the underlying concept represented by a specific variable in an analysis (e.g., perceived control over health, contact with family members) is subjectively meaningful for a large percentage of the target population. This judgment is a substantial one to make. The psychosocial epidemiology of aging, like epidemiology more generally, places a high priority on finding population-level, general associations. There is an emphasis on finding "independent" or "main effects" of the predictor, controlling for possible confounders.

In other terminology, this approach could be called "nomothetic," which implies an emphasis on looking for variance shared in common among a large segment of the population. This nomothetic assumption is certainly reasonable in research involving biological or medical variables as there is a plausible physiological or biological rationale for most persons to experience a similar effect. For example, blood pressure beyond a certain threshold greatly increases risk of a stroke, smoking causes lung cancer, and glaucoma leads to blindness regardless of gender, race, or income status. The nomothetic assumption may not be as reasonable, however, when dealing with psychosocial variables. Individuals are extremely diverse in regard to their family environments in childhood and adolescence, schools attended, economic status, marital and child-rearing experiences, work histories, and peer-group influences. By middle- and older-adulthood, substantial differences among persons can be expected. The diversity that results from the different paths that persons travel over the first 40–70 years of their lives cannot be dismissed. Even if persons have the same status on a psychosocial variable when surveyed in later life (e.g., attending church regularly, being involved in community groups), the roads to reaching that status are many and varied—a circumstance sometimes referred to as "overdetermination."

There may be little reason to assume that any

one psychosocial variable, measured at baseline, *should* have a consistent association with subsequent health status. From this perspective, it is impressive that population-level, epidemiological research has found *any* consistent associations between any one psychosocial variable and outcomes or morbidity or mortality. To have found such associations, using the nomothetic assumption implicit in the main-effects analytical model, suggests the extremely strong influence of these perceptual and social factors.

The proposition being offered for consideration is *not* that individuals' life courses are random and unpredictable; rather, it is a simple caution. Although any *one* psychosocial variable may not be important for everyone, *at least one* psychosocial variable (and perhaps more) will be important for virtually everyone. This type of individualized approach to defining a variable is sometimes called *idiographic*. Presumably, that particular one or those select few psychosocial variables, which are chosen to be especially meaningful to the individual, will provide the basic motivation to get out of bed on a day-to-day basis, to remain involved in life, and to plan for the future.

One proposal of this chapter, therefore, is that the effectiveness of psychosocial variables for behavioral intervention will be realized most fully when the results from epidemiological, nomothetically based research are tempered (not necessarily replaced) by an idiographic perspective when applied to intervention. An idiographic strategy recognizes that although the importance of "psychosocial variables" for long-term health status lies in keeping persons integrated in daily life, this maintenance of integration will not occur in the same way for everyone. The *domain* of variables may be more crucial than any specific variable. Flexibility in designing intervention strategies also helps obviate attempts to regulate or manipulate psychosocial variables in contexts in which such regulation is unethical or illegal.

An idiographic definition is still consistent with the traditional way of defining a "reinforc-

ing" variable, in this case relative to the dependent variables of mortality and morbidity. The key to defining a reinforcer is to observe its effects. There is no requirement that the same thing be a reinforcer for everyone; it is the *principle* of reinforcement that is important. The same may be true for the salience of psychosocial variables. This approach to psychosocial epidemiology is not a traditional one, so the methodology for assessing idiographic risk factors is not yet established. If such studies are attempted, it is important that the methodologies be standardized, so that replication across samples can occur.

AN INTEGRATION OF BEHAVIORAL AND PSYCHOSOCIAL EPIDEMIOLOGY

As suggested at the outset of this chapter, the behavioral epidemiology and the psychosocial epidemiology of aging face a challenge in common: The findings pertinent to each type of variable need to be placed in more comprehensive causal frameworks. The plural framework*s* is deliberate, since there may not be a single model. For example, gender differences in the salience of social network variables may prompt separate models for women and men. One of the frontiers of the behavioral epidemiology of aging lies in a closer integration with technologies of health education, health psychology, behavioral medicine, and medical sociology to change lifestyle practices that seem to have the best potential for improving the quality of life in old age. Descriptive epidemiology is only one step in the process.

For behavioral epidemiology, a key question is what factors promote the *adoption* of healthful behaviors by older persons or *sustain* performance by the elderly who are currently practicing them. These are especially important issues, complicated by the greater incidence and prevalence of chronic health problems in older adulthood. At the risk of oversimplification, one may say that older persons can be caught in an unbalanced situation. On one hand, changing behavior almost always requires the investment of physical, psychological, and even material resources. Researchers and educators formally operationalize such phenomenological experiences by constructs such as perceived self-efficacy, resisting temptation to relapse, and researching one's routine to identify barriers and facilitators. On the other hand, chronic illnesses and impairments in functional health can serve as drains on energy and resources. Anyone who has tried to break the proverbial "bad habit" or adopt a more healthful lifestyle knows the commitment of time and energy that is needed. From a subjective standpoint, when the basic instrumental activities of daily living are difficult enough, where does the motivation come from to initiate new health practices or to adapt those currently in one's repertoire?

For psychosocial epidemiology, a next key step is to find more proximate mechanisms by which these variables affect mortality and morbidity. Investigating the possibility of operationalizing psychosocial variables in a more idiographic fashion may be helpful. It may also be helpful to study psychosocial variables in subgroups of the older population defined by selected sets of variables. For example, the MacArthur Studies of Successful Aging are examining a robust sample of older adults (Schoenfeld et al., 1994; Seeman et al., 1994).

It may be possible to combine psychosocial variables into composite indicators rather than treat them all individually. Rakowski and Wilcox (1994) integrated self-rated health and social network variables into a single index. Multivariate adjusted odds ratios of between 4.20 and 5.00 were found with mortality over a 4-year follow-up period, when comparing persons with poor self-rated health and few social contacts with older persons who reported positive self-rated health and relatively more contacts. Such strategies can help to refine understanding of the conditions under which psychosocial variables are most important, but they will not necessarily

identify the mechanisms that produce the effect on health status.

A Proposed Framework

The integration proposed here is to investigate causal frameworks in which the variables of psychosocial epidemiology are placed as antecedents of personal health practices. One such generic diagram is offered in Figure 1. Variables would include self-rated health, social participation, social support, the attribution of health problems to aging, and future planning. Their salience comes as sources of motivation for behavior change and positive coping with life events. Status on these psychosocial variables could be assessed idiographically as well as nomothetically. The figure is not presented in the detail needed for a statistical investigation, but it does imply that by controlling for baseline status on psychosocial and behavioral variables, it will be possible to identify predictors of *change* in health-related behaviors.

An integration like that represented in Figure 1 is being proposed because stability and change between a baseline interview and an assessment of longer-term outcomes are the key mechanisms that should be studied. Prohaska and Glasser (1994) have addressed the antecedent role that symptom experience may play in health behavior change. The figure is also proposed for use in epidemiological surveys, in which interest is in aggregate outcomes such as all-cause morbidity and mortality, with general population samples. These suggestions may or may not be appropriate for the investigation of specific behaviors (e.g., physical activity, seat belt use, annual medical checkups) or for research done with high-risk subgroups of the older population.

Health Behavior in Figure 1.   Personal health behaviors are conceptualized in Figure 1 as falling into three broad categories. One is preventive behaviors of the type usually studied in

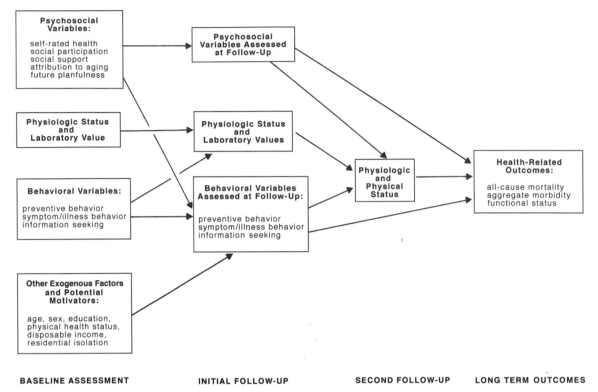

Figure 1. Diagram depicting a possible integration of variables from psychosocial and behavioral epidemiology.

population survey behavioral epidemiology, including physical activity, smoking, alcohol use, regular medical checkups, use of seat belts, and home safety/accident prevention. Prevention-related knowledge could also be included, on the premise that knowledge is necessary but not sufficient for sustained changes in health behavior.

A second category is symptom- and illness-related behaviors. It is important to include both the individual's response to acute conditions and exacerbations of existing chronic problems, as well as the individual's self-care on a day-to-day basis. There are, however, some assessment issues that should be considered. In regard to illness-related behaviors, the *promptness* of response should be addressed, as well as the *appropriateness* of any self-care that is undertaken. It is difficult to study delay in response to symptoms

because individual differences can exist at the level of "appraisal delay" — the process of recognizing that a symptom exists in the first place (Safer, Tharps, Jackson, & Leventhal, 1979). Delay can therefore exist in the period of symptom labeling, which is usually invisible to the outside observer, rather than in the timing of a response after a symptom has been labeled as serious.

In aging research, emphasis has been on studying the observable action; in the process of maintaining one's health, however, the non-occurrence of an event (such as not reacting to a symptom) can be equally important. For example, older adults who believe that their health problems are caused by old age may report acting on a "serious" symptom in the same way as those older persons who do not attribute the problems to aging. Did they act as promptly, however, and did they label the symptom as being serious in the same time frame? In regard to the appropriateness of symptom-related actions, Stoller, Forster, Pollow, and Tisdale (1993) recently reported in their sample that most actions were not harmful, but a small percentage of symptoms had at least one action that was considered problematic by a panel of medical persons.

A related point applies to both preventive and illness-related actions: Surveys might begin to inquire about individuals' tendency *not* to take advantage of opportunities to follow a health-promoting action. The ability to resist tempting contextual and interpersonal situations for unfavorable health practices is sometimes studied, more so, to date, with younger populations than with older persons. The opposite side of the coin, however, is the purposeful avoidance of acting healthfully. The ability to study "nonevents" has been discussed elsewhere as a methodological issue in older adult health behavior research (Rakowski, 1992).

The third category of personal health behaviors is more generic processes, such as the information-seeking construct already discussed. This category seems necessary because a clear, unambiguous course of action rarely exists, even if the ultimate behavioral goal can be specified with reasonable precision. For example, mammography and Pap testing can be beneficial even well into older age, but women are told to talk with their physicians about the best personal schedule to follow, in order to assess risk and benefits in their particular case. Similarly, older adults are encouraged to be physically active, but are also told to consult with their doctors before starting any program of activity. There may also be several options for finding an effective way to reach dietary goals of fat and fiber intake. Even the seemingly straightforward challenge to "stop smoking" can be implemented by several means.

Simply trying to keep up with the incessant flow of health information in the media requires that an individual be willing to implement some generic skills of information seeking, organization, and evaluation. By nature, information seeking is a proactive concept, and any further refinement for measuring the variable might be expanded to assess a tendency to actively avoid such activity. In research that has the luxury of multiple points of assessment, generic behavioral processes could be placed at an intermediate point, between the psychosocial variables and the more specific preventive and illness behaviors. The reasoning here is that the motivational benefits of psychosocial factors operate first on decision-making processes, which are then used to select from several possible courses of action.

Other Pathways and Priorities among Variables. Figure 1 does not presume that a link between psychosocial and behavioral variables is the sole mechanism for effecting longer-term good health status. Some social network variables may directly influence physiological processes (e.g., Esterling et al., 1994; Seeman et al., 1994). In addition, existing behavioral practices at baseline, such as smoking and sedentary lifestyle, may have already affected the individual's potential for improvement in physiological parameters and health benefits even after lifestyle changes are made.

There may also be priorities among the psychosocial variables themselves. There is some evidence that social network factors and self-ratings of health are related. For example, Krause and Borawski-Clark (1994) found evidence that social support contributes to feelings of self-esteem and control under specific situations. Multiwave panel studies may expand the psychosocial domain to investigate whether changes in a given social network variable (perhaps a variable that defines change idiographically) promote changes in self-ratings, which in turn lead to changes in health-related behaviors.

Presumably, behavioral variables also operate through some intermediate steps before influencing long-term health status. One of these steps can be the direct improvement or hampering of physical status and biological processes. This effect can also come from delay of action or failure to act, such as not acting promptly on symptoms of diabetes that then progress to cause some organic damage before treatment is initiated. The possible causal change of "psychosocial change → impact on behavior → physical change" seems to place a priority on conducting longitudinal studies that have at least three assessments before the determination of final status on the dependent variables occurs. The time between survey waves would depend on the time believed necessary for the causal chain to be implemented. Finally, the impact of behavior change can come from greater susceptibility to sudden events such as falls and accidents or as the result of not being prepared for emergencies.

Methodological Issues

Overall, therefore, the premise of Figure 1 is that status on psychosocial variables serves as a motivator for initiating new preventive behaviors, for acting promptly on possible symptoms of illness, and for adapting one's current lifestyle habits to remain as healthful as possible in the face of newly emerging chronic conditions. Generic behavioral processes, such as information seeking, represent a broadly based readiness to evaluate one's situation and explore options for change.

Epidemiological studies of older adults' health practices would continue to include the traditional types of lifestyle and health care utilization questions often used in surveys such as the 1990 National Health Interview Survey of Health Promotion and Disease Prevention, as well as a range of items to assess self-rated health, social connectedness, and other key psychosocial variables. The surveys, however, would also include questions on response to symptoms, lifestyle adjustments to newly emerged chronic problems, and information seeking. No existing national or regional survey contains this diversity of information. The case can now be made that surveys should do so.

At the same time, requesting this scope of information can place a large recall burden on the participant. Moreover, some of the interven-

ing or mediating processes may be too subtle to be captured in a period between resurveys that is sometimes 2–4 years. The fact that psychosocial and behavioral variables have been associated with health status outcomes at even 2–4 years of follow-up implies the desirability of having shorter intervals between resurveys. A six-month period would be good in order to minimize the risk of recall error regarding response to major symptom episodes—unless labor-intensive symptom/behavior diary methodologies were used (e.g., Stoller et al., 1993). Even a 1-year resurvey period would be a major advance over data that have been available so far. It is important to remember that the objective is not only to assess the relationship among these predictor variables at baseline, but also to allow an examination of *change* in antecedents and change in behavior across at least one resurvey before the final assessment of outcome status.

REFERENCES

Applegate, W. B., Miller, S. T., Elam, J. T., Cushman, W. C., Derwi, D. E., Brewer, A., & Graney, M. J. (1992). Nonpharmacologic intervention to reduce blood pressure in older patients with mild hypertension. *Archives of Internal Medicine, 152,* 1162–1166.

Atwood, J. R., Aickin, M., Giordano, L., Benedict, J., Bell, M., Rittenbauch, C., Rees-McGee, S., Sheehan, E., Buller, M., Ho, E. E., Meyskens, F. L., Jr., & Alberts, D. (1992). The effectiveness of adherence intervention in a colon cancer prevention field trial. *Preventive Medicine, 21,* 637–653.

Bagley-Burnett, C. (1988). Measuring information-seeking behaviors. In M. Frank-Stromberg (Ed.), *Instruments for clinical nursing research* (pp. 151–169). Norwalk, CT: Appleton & Lange.

Benson, L., Nelson, E. C., Napps, S. E., Roberts, E., Kane-Williams, E., & Salisbury, Z. T. (1989). Evaluation of the Staying Healthy After Fifty education program: Impact on course participants. *Health Education Quarterly, 16,* 485–508.

Berg, R. L., & Cassells, J. S. (Eds.). (1990). *The second fifty years: Promoting health and preventing disability.* Washington, DC: National Academy Press.

Berkman, L. F., Oxman, T. E., & Seeman, T. E. (1992). Social networks and social support among the elderly: Assessment issues. In R. B. Wallace & R. F. Woolson (Eds.), *The epidemiologic study of the elderly* (pp. 196–212). New York: Oxford University Press.

Boult, C., Kane, R. L., Louis, T. A., Boult, L., & McCaffrey, D. (1994). Chronic conditions that lead to functional limitation in the elderly. *Journal of Gerontology: Medical Sciences, 49,* M28–M36.

Bryant, S., & Rakowski, W. (1992). Predictors of mortality among elderly African-Americans. *Research on Aging, 14,* 50–67.

Burgio, K. L., Stutzman, R. E., & Engel, B. T. (1989). Behavioral training for post-prostatectomy urinary incontinence. *Journal of Urology, 141,* 303–306.

Camacho, T. C., Strawbridge, W. J., Cohen, R. D., & Kaplan, G. A. (1993). Functional ability in the oldest old: Cumulative impact of risk factors from the preceding two decades. *Journal of Aging and Health, 5,* 439–454.

Clark, D. O., Maddox, G. L., & Steinhauser, K. (1993). Race, aging, and functional health. *Journal of Aging and Health, 5,* 536–553.

Clark, N. M., Janz, N. K., Becker, M. H., Schork, M. A., Wheeler, J., Liang, J., Dodge, J. A., Keteyian, S., Rhoads, K. L., & Santinga, J. T. (1992). Impact of self-management education on the functional health status of older adults with heart disease. *Gerontologist, 32* 438–443.

Emery, C. F., & Blumenthal, J. A. (1990). Perceived change among participants in an exercise program for older adults. *Gerontologist, 30,* 516–521.

Esterling, B. A., Kiecolt-Glaser, J. K., Bodnar, J. C., & Glaser, R. (1994). Chronic stress, social support, and persistent alterations in the natural killer cell response to cytokines in older adults. *Health Psychology, 13,* 291–298.

Franzke, A. W. (1987). The effects of assertiveness training on older adults. *Gerontologist, 27,* 13–16.

Fries, J. F., Bloch, D. A., Harrington, H., Richardson, N., & Beck, R. (1993). Two-year results of a randomized controlled trial of a health promotion program in a retiree population: The Bank of America Study. *American Journal of Medicine, 94,* 455–462.

Fries, J. F., Harrington, H., Edwards, R., Kent, L. A., & Richardson, N. (1994). Randomized controlled trial of cost reductions from a health education program: the California Public Employees' Retirement System (PERS) Study. *American Journal of Health Promotion, 8,* 216–223.

Glanz, K., Marger, S. M., & Meehan, E. F. (1986). Evaluation of a peer educator stroke education program for the elderly. *Health Education Research, Theory and Practice, 1,* 121–130.

Glasgow, R. E., Toobert, D. J., Hampson, S. E., Brown, J. E., Lewinsohn, P. M., & Donnelly, J. (1992). Improving self-care among older patients with Type II diabetes: The "Sixty Something…" Study. *Patient Education and Counseling, 19,* 61–74.

Grand, A., Grosclaude, P., Bocquet, H., Pous, J., & Albarede, J. L. (1988). Predictive value of life events, psychosocial factors and self-rated health on disability in an elderly rural

French population. *Social Science and Medicine, 27,* 1377–1342.

Grand, A., Grosclaude, P., Bocquet, H., Pous, J., & Albarede, J. L. (1990). Disability, psychosocial factors and mortality among the elderly in a rural French population. *Journal of Clinical Epidemiology, 43,* 773–782.

Guralnik, J. M., Land, K. C., Blazer, D., Fillenbaum, G. G., & Branch, L. G. (1993). Educational status and active life expectancy among older blacks and whites. *New England Journal of Medicine, 329,* 110–116.

Haber, D. (1986). Health promotion to reduce blood pressure level among older blacks. *Gerontologist, 26,* 119–121.

Hibbard, J. H. (1988). Age, social ties and health behaviors: An exploratory study. *Health Education Research, Theory and Practice, 3,* 131–139.

Hopkins, D. R., Murrah, B., Hoeger, W. W. K., & Rhodes, R. C. (1990). Effect of low-impact aerobic dance on the functional fitness of elderly women. *Gerontologist, 30,* 189–192.

House, J. S., Landis, K. R., & Umberson, D. (1988). Social relationships and health. *Science, 241*(July 29), 540–549.

Idler, E. L., & Angel, R. J. (1990). Self-rated health and mortality in the NHANES-I Epidemiologic Follow-up Study. *American Journal of Public Health, 80,* 446–452.

Idler, E. L., Kasl, S. V., & Lemke, J. H. (1990). Self-evaluated health and mortality among the elderly in New Haven, Connecticut, and Iowa and Washington Counties, Iowa, 1982–1986. *American Journal of Epidemiology, 131,* 91–103.

Jensen, J., Counte, M. A., & Glandon, G. L. (1992). Elderly health beliefs, attitudes, and maintenance. *Preventive Medicine, 21,* 483–497.

Kahn, R. L. (1994). Social supports: Content, causes and consequences. In R. P. Abeles, H. C. Gift, & M. G. Ory (Eds.), *Aging and quality of life* (pp. 163–184). New York: Springer.

Kaplan, G. A., & Camacho, T. (1983). Perceived health and mortality: A nine-year follow-up of the Human Population Laboratory cohort. *American Journal of Epidemiology, 117,* 292–304.

Kaplan, G. A., & Haan, M. N. (1989). Is there a role for prevention among the elderly? Epidemiological evidence from the Alameda County Study. In M. G. Ory & K. Bond (Eds.), *Aging and health care: Social science and policy perspectives* (pp. 27–51). London: Routledge.

Kaplan G. A., & Strawbridge, W. J. (1994). Behavioral and social factors in healthy aging. In R. P. Abeles, H. C. Gift, & M. G. Ory (Eds.), *Aging and quality of life* (pp. 57–78). New York: Springer.

Kaplan, G. A., Strawbridge, W. J., Camacho, T., & Cohen, R. D. (1993). Factors associated with changes in physical functioning in the elderly: A six-year prospective study. *Journal of Aging and Health, 5,* 140–153.

Krause, N., & Borawski-Clark, E. (1994). Clarifying the functions of social support in later life. *Journal of Aging and Health, 16,* 251–279.

Lorig, K., & Holman, H. (1993). Arthritis self-management studies: A twelve-year review. *Health Education Quarterly, 20,* 17–28.

Lubben, J. E., Weiler, P. G., & Chi, I. (1989). Gender and ethnic differences in the health practices of the elderly poor. *Journal of Clinical Epidemiology, 42,* 725–733.

Morisky, D. E., Levine, D. M., Green, L. W., & Smith, C. R. (1982). Health education program effects on the management of hypertension in the elderly. *Archives of Internal Medicine, 142,* 1835–1838.

Mossey, J. M., & Shapiro, E. (1982). Self-rated health: A predictor of mortality among the elderly. *American Journal of Public Health, 72,* 800–808.

Nelson, E. C., McHugo, G., Schnurr, P., Devito, C., Roberts, E., Simmons, J., & Zubkoff, W. (1984). Medical self-care education for elders: A controlled trial to evaluate impact. *American Journal of Public Health, 74,* 1357–1362.

Nichol, K. L., Margolis, K. L., Wuorenma, J., & Von Sternberg, T. (1994). The efficacy and cost effectiveness of vaccination against influenza among elderly persons living in the community. *New England Journal of Medicine, 331,* 778–784.

Piani, A., & Schoenborn, C. (1993). Health promotion and disease prevention: United States, 1990. National Center for Health Statistics. *Vital and Health Statistics, 10,* N. 185 (April).

Prochaska, J. O., DiClemente, C. C., & Norcross, J. C. (1992). In search of how people change: Applications to addictive behaviors. *American Psychologist, 47,* 1102–1114.

Prohaska, T. R., & Glasser, M. (1994). Older adult health behavior change in response to symptom experience. *Advances in Medical Sociology, 4,* 141–161.

Rakowski, W. (1992). Disease prevention and health promotion with older adults: Perspectives on health behavior research and community intervention. In M. G. Ory, R. P. Abeles, & P. D. Lipman (Eds.), *Aging, behavior, and health* (pp. 239–275). Newbury Park, CA: Sage.

Rakowski, W. (1994). The definition and measurement of prevention, preventive health care, and health promotion. *Generations, 18*(1), 18–23.

Rakowski, W., Assaf, A. R., LeFebvre, R. C., Lasater, T. M., Niknian, M., & Carleton, R. A. (1990). Information-seeking about health in a community sample of adults: Correlates and associations with other health-related practices. *Health Education Quarterly, 17,* 379–393.

Rakowski, W., Fleishman, J., Mor, V., & Bryant, S. (1993). Self-assessments of health and mortality among older persons: Do questions other than global self-rated health predict mortality? *Research on Aging, 15,* 92–116.

Rakowski, W., & Hickey, T. (1992). Mortality and the attribution of health problems to aging among older adults. *American Journal of Public Health, 82,* 1139–1141.

Rakowski, W., Julius, M., Hickey, T., & Halter, J. B. (1987). Correlates of preventive behavior in late life. *Research on Aging, 9,* 331–355.

Rakowski, W., Lefebvre, R. C., Assaf, A. R., Lasater, T. M., &

Carleton, R. D. (1990). Health practice correlates in three adult groups: Results from two community surveys. *Public Health Reports, 105,* 481–491.

Rakowski, W., Mor, V., & Hiris, J. (1994). An investigation of non-response to self-assessments of health by older persons: Associations with mortality. *Journal of Aging and Health, 6,* 469–488.

Rakowski, W., Rice, C., & McHorney, C. A. (1992). Information-seeking about health among older adults: An examination of measurement and structural properties. *Behavior, Health, and Aging, 2,* 181–198.

Rakowski, W., Rimer, B. K., & Bryant, S. A. (1993). Integrating behavior and intention regarding mammography by respondents in the 1990 National Health Interview Survey of Health Promotion and Disease Prevention. *Public Health Reports, 108,* 605–624.

Rakowski, W., & Wilcox, V. L. (1994). Integrating self-rated health and social involvement for the examination of mortality among older persons. *Omega, 29,* 95–111.

Rakowski, W., Wilcox, V. L., & Clark, M. (1994). *Attributing functional problems to old age and subsequent functional status.* Poster presented at the 47th Annual Meeting of the Gerontological Society of America; Atlanta, November.

Rimer, B. K., Orleans, C. T., Fleisher, L., Cristinzio, S., Resch, N., Telepchak, J., & Keintz, M. K. (1994). Does tailoring matter? The impact of a tailored guide on ratings and short-term smoking-related outcomes of older smokers. *Health Education Research, Theory and Practice, 9,* 69–84.

Rimer, B. K., Resch, N., King, E., Ross, E., Lerman, C., Boyce, A., Kessler, H., & Engstrom, P. F. (1992). Multistrategy health education program to increase mammography use among women ages 65 and older. *Public Health Reports, 107,* 369–380.

Safer, M. A., Tharps, Q. J., Jackson, T. C., & Leventhal, H. (1979). Determinants of three stages of delay in seeking care at a medical clinic. *Medical Care, 17,* 11–29.

Salive, M. E., Coroni-Huntley, J., LaCroix, A. Z., Ostfeld, A. M., Wallace, R. B., & Hennekens, C. H. (1992). Predictors of smoking cessation and relapse in older adults. *American Journal of Public Health, 82,* 1268–1271.

Schoenfeld, D. E., Malmrose, L. C., Blazer, D. G., Gold, D. T., & Seeman, T. E. (1994). Self-rated health and mortality in the high-functioning elderly—A closer look at healthy individuals: MacArthur Field Study of Successful Aging. *Journal of Gerontology: Medical Sciences, 49,* M109–M115.

Seeman, T. E., Berkman, L. F., Blazer, D., & Rowe, J. W. (1994). Social ties and support and neuroendocrine function: The MacArthur Studies of Successful Aging. *Annals of Behavioral Medicine, 16,* 95–106.

Seeman, T. E., Kaplan, G. A., Knudsen, L., Cohen, R., & Guralnik, J. (1987). Social network ties and mortality among the elderly in the Alameda County Study. *American Journal of Epidemiology, 126,* 713–723.

Sobal, J., Revicki, D., & DeForge, B. R. (1992). Patterns of interrelationships among health-promoting behaviors. *American Journal of Preventive Medicine, 8,* 351–359.

Steinbach, U. (1992). Social networks, institutionalization, and mortality among elderly people in the United States. *Journal of Gerontology: Social Sciences, 47,* S183–S190.

Stevens, V. J., Hornbrook, M. C., Wingfield, D. J., Hollis, J. F., Greenlick, M. R., & Ory, M. G. (1991/1992). Design and implementation of a falls prevention intervention for community-dwelling older persons. *Behavior, Health, and Aging, 2,* 57–73.

Stoller, E., Forster, L., Pollow, R., & Tisdale, W. (1993). Lay evaluation of symptoms by older people: An assessment of potential risk. *Health Education Quarterly, 20,* 505–522.

Stoller, E. P., & Pollow, R. (1994). Factors affecting the frequency of health enhancing behaviors by the elderly. *Public Health Reports, 109,* 377–389.

Tinetti, M. E., Baker, D. I., McAvay, G., Claus, E. B., Garrett, P., Gottschalk, M., Koch, M. L., Trainor, K., & Horowitz, R. I. (1994). A multifactorial intervention to reduce the risk of falling among elderly people living in the community. *New England Journal of Medicine, 331,* 821–827.

Topp, R., Mikesky, A., Wigglesworth, J., Holt, W., & Edwards, J. E. (1993). The effect of a 12-week dynamic resistance strength training program on gait velocity and balance of older adults. *Gerontologist, 33,* 501–506.

Vickery, D. M., Golaszewski, T. J., Wright, E. C., & Kalmer, H. (1988). The effect of self-care interventions on the use of medical service within a Medicare population. *Medical Care, 26,* 580–588.

Weinrich, S. P., Weinrich, M. C., Stromberg, M. F., Boyd, M. D., & Weiss, H. L. (1993). Using elderly educators to increase colorectal cancer screening. *Gerontologist, 33,* 491–496.

Wells, T. J., Brink, C. A., Diokno, A. C., Wolfe, R., & Gillis, G. L. (1991). Pelvic muscle exercise for stress urinary incontinence in elderly women. *Journal of the American Geriatrics Society, 39,* 785–791.

Wolinsky, F. D., & Johnson, R. J. (1992). Perceived health status and mortality among older men and women. *Journal of Gerontology: Social Sciences, 47,* S304–S312.

Zuckerman, D. M., Kasl, S. V., & Ostfeld, A. M. (1994). Psychosocial predictors of mortality among the elderly poor: The role of religion, well-being, and social contacts. *American Journal of Epidemiology, 119,* 410–423.

III

HEALTH BEHAVIOR IN POPULATIONS "AT RISK"

As a complement to the discussion in Part II of a range of health behaviors in the general population across the life span, Part III considers health behavior in populations whose health is at greater risk than that of the general population. Typically, one thinks of racially and ethnically distinguishable minority populations—the oppressed minorities (e.g., Longres, 1995, Chapt. 4) as those most appropriate for consideration in such a discussion. Indeed, there is appreciable evidence (e.g., Cockerham, 1995; Kurtz & Chalfant, 1991) linking race and oppressed ethnicity to mortality and morbidity rates. African-Americans, Hispanic-Americans, and Native Americans, for example, have poorer mortality rates and, for many conditions, poorer morbidity rates than white Americans.

HEALTH BEHAVIORS ACROSS POPULATIONS: RACIAL AND ETHNIC COMPARISONS

Although there is some evidence of differences in selected health behaviors in these different racial and ethnic populations, there is little in the way of systematic, rigorous comparisons.

Berkanovic and Telesky (1985) noted few differences in reporting of illness and complex interactions between ethnicity, health status, perceived seriousness, and social networks in predictions of sick role behavior in Mexican-American, black American and white American samples. On the other hand, Escarce, Epstein, Colby, and Schwartz (1993) noted some racial differences in use of medical services by the African-American and white American elderly covered by Medicare. Black elderly persons were less likely, for example, to receive coronary angiography, coronary angioplasty, or coronary bypass surgery, or a full range of ophthalmological services. Escarce et al. recognize, however, that use of service for these populations is less a health behavior than a treatment decision, and they address institutional barriers that impede use of a fuller range of services by elderly black persons.

Guttmacher and Ellinson (1971), in a frequently cited study, observed how ethnicity is a determinant of beliefs about what behaviors comprise mental illness. Puerto Ricans, Irish, Italian, African-Americans, and Jews in New York City were observed to have consistently different thresholds for tolerance of deviance and for use of the illness metaphor as a way of accounting for deviant behavior.

HEALTH BEHAVIOR WITHIN POPULATIONS

Racial and Ethnic Descriptive Studies. Using the Suchman (1965/1972) model, Farge (1978) reported on an investigation of group structure and health beliefs in a Mexican-American population. Farge proposed a model of Chicano health care based on findings that within the Chicano community, strong family commitments and ties did not necessarily mean that a family member would hold traditional, skeptical beliefs about medicine. Increased knowledge about health and illness was not linked to lesser skepticism, but was linked to increased dependence on lay persons during illness.

More recent and more complete analyses of health behaviors of Hispanic-Americans were provided as part of a large-scale Hispanic Health and Nutrition Examination Survey (HHANES) conducted during the 1980s by the National Center for Health Statistics (e.g., Delgado, Johnson, Roy, & Treviño, 1990). Among the concerns of this study were the data showing that Mexican-Americans had lower levels of health service use than some other Hispanic groups such as Puerto Ricans and Cuban-Americans (Higgenbotham, Treviño, & Ray, 1990). One explanation for this difference was their presumed use of *curanderos*, *sobadores*, herbalists, spiritualists, and other alternative healers. Yet such use was found to be relatively low in the Mexican-American subgroup of this study and was related to perceptions of health status, to satisfaction with care given my medical practitioners, and to the level of commitment to a Mexican cultural orientation. Use of *curanderos* and alternative healers thus cannot account for the lower use of health services by Mexican-Americans. Instead, system barriers are thought to impede use of services (Estrada, Treviño, & Ray, 1990).

Alcohol consumption in Mexican-American women, but not in men, was found to be partially predicted by their degree of acculturation into the larger society interacting with age and social class (Markides, Krause, & Mendes de Leon, 1988; Markides, Ray, Stroup-Benham, & Treviño, 1990). Alcohol consumption in Mexican-Americans was not found to be related to the stresses of acculturation. Neither was acculturation found to be a consistent predictor of preventive behaviors in elderly Hispanic women (Marks et al., 1987) or of a range of preventive, risk, and utilization behaviors in Hispanic-Americans in general (Marks, Garcia, & Solis, 1990; Solis, Marks, Garcia, & Shelton, 1990).

Problems inhere in defining ethnic and racial populations. They are heterogeneous and culturally diverse. For example, Hispanic-Americans include persons of Mexican, Philipine, Cuban, Puerto Rican, and Central American backgrounds (e.g., Gomez, 1987), and African-Americans include persons of Bahamian, Jamaican, Cuban, Haitian, and Puerto Rican backgrounds (e.g., Scott, 1974), those with deep cultural roots in the American South, and those whose families have long lived in other areas of the United States. This diversity creates difficulties in generalizing about health behavior in terms of ethnicity or race. Zimmerman et al. (1994) analyzed the issue of who is "Hispanic" and the implications of self-identification in making this determination, raising questions about the number of generations that should appropriately be included under this rubric. Scott showed distinctively different cultural patterns of beliefs about illness and treatment in her several different African-American samples.

In the first examination of African-American care seeking for acute chest pain in which comparisons of lower and middle socioeconomic status (SES) were made, Ell et al. (1994) observed that delay periods in decisions to seek care are determined by factors similar to those that determine delay in the white population, particularly perceptions of severity of symptoms and use of lay networks. The African-American sample, however, took longer to reach care (including both decision time and travel time) than comparable white samples, reflecting the importance of structural access to care—in this instance, the location of the hospital.

In an analysis of hypertension risks in the African-American community, James (1994) documented the role of what he termed "John Henryism," or the overinvestment in active coping with a socially and economically oppressive environment, as a behavioral risk factor. Data support the John Henry hypothesis, which predicts that such hyperactive persistence in active copying under difficult conditions is a stronger risk factor for African-Americans with lower SES than it is for those with higher SES.

Little research has been done on health behavior in Native American populations. One of the few studies is Hsu and Williams' work (1991) showing that low-income Native Americans were less likely to perceive the risks of ingesting dangerous household items than were other low-income families. In contrast, patterns of hospital use by residents of a Navajo reservation did not differ from patterns in non–Native American comparison populations and were determined primarily by structural factors such as access and location (Davis & Kunitz, 1978).

Racially and ethnically distinctive minority populations such as those just identified are not a primary focus of Part III. Instead, populations were selected whose health behavior has generally been ignored by researchers but is finally receiving attention. There are a large number of such "populations," e.g., inner-city domiciled persons who are not defined as living in poverty (e.g., Hobfoll, Jackson, Lavin, Britton, & Shepherd, 1993, 1994), persons living in rural areas, home health attendants (e.g., Weitzman & Berry, 1992), children with hyperactivity diagnoses (Farmer & Peterson, 1995), and rodeo riders (Bushy, 1990). The selection for discussion from among such populations was aimed at calling attention to those groups about which a corpus of research is emerging, but whose health risk is related either to their being hidden or otherwise "invisible," to economics, to characteristics of the illness itself, or to combinations of these.

Hidden Populations. The first three chapters deal with "hidden" populations whose identity is determined largely—but not solely—by sexual preference. In Chapter 6, Kauth and Prejean provide an analysis of care seeking and risk behaviors in gay men and relates these behaviors to lifestyle components in the gay population.

In Chapter 7, VanScoy emphasizes the barriers to lesbian care seeking and treatment inherent in a patriarchal male-dominated health care system. VanScoy further emphasizes the role of social and community support and of alternatives to the biomedical model in lesbian responses to illness.

In Chapter 8, Thomason and Campos discuss decisions to participate in HIV screening and adhering to treatment in persons living with HIV/AIDS, a population made up largely of gay men and persons who use drugs intravenously.

Economic Risks. Populations put at risk by economic factors include persons in developing countries, homeless persons, and persons living in economic deprivation. In Chapter 9, Coreil discusses transitions in economic development and how these transitions are related to changes in health practices in developing countries, including adoption of oral rehydration therapies, immunizations, weaning, and use of family planning methods.

In Chapter 10, J. D. Wright and Joyner integrate the literatures on health behaviors in the homeless and persons living in poverty, pointing out differences between the two—as well as between them and domiciled and nonpoverty populations—in risk behaviors, lifestyle behaviors, care seeking, and adherence to treatment.

Illness-Linked Risks. Populations whose very identity itself implies a health risk include those living with chronic conditions. In Chapter 11, Gallagher and Stratton examine health behaviors, particularly responses to illness and illness management, in persons living with chronic illnesses. For many of these persons, the illness becomes part of their own identity.

In Chapter 12, Hawley provides extensive discussion of adherence to regimens as well as of perceptions of health status in persons with chronic and severe mental illness. For many of these people, the total engulfment by the illness becomes a barrier both to their adherence and to health professionals' perceiving their somatic health needs.

A final population is one whose risk depends on its role relationships to illness, i.e., to another person who is an identified patient. In Chapter 13, on the health behavior of caregivers, L. K. Wright emphasizes the behavioral component of caregiving and suggests that for this population, mobilization of social support should be considered as a critical health behavior.

REFERENCES

Berkanovic, E., & Telesky, C. (1985). Mexican-American, black-American and white-American differences in reporting illnesses, disability and physician visits for illnesses. *Social Science and Medicine, 20,* 567-577.

Bushy, A. (1990). Understanding health practices and health care needs of western US rodeo participants: An ethnographic approach. *Family and Community Health, 13*(1), 44-54.

Cockerham, W. C. (1995). *Medical sociology* (6th ed.). Englewood Cliffs, NJ: Simon & Schuster.

Davis, S., & Kunitz, S. J. (1978). Hospitalization utilization and elective surgery on the Navajo Indian reservation. *Social Science and Medicine, 12B,* 263-272.

Delgado, J. L., Johnson, C. L., Roy, I., & Treviño, F. M. (1990). I. Hispanic health and nutrition examination survey: Methodological considerations. *American Journal of Public Health, 80* (Suppl.), 6-10.

Ell, K., Haywood, J., Sobel, E., deGuzman, M., Blumfield, D., & Ning, J.-P. (1994). Acute chest pain in African Americans: Factors in the delay in seeking emergency care. *American Journal of Public Health, 84,* 965-970.

Escarce, J. J., Epstein, K. R., Colby, D. C., & Schwartz, J. S. (1993). Racial differences in the elderly's use of medical procedures and diagnostic tests. *American Journal of Public Health, 83,* 948-954.

Estrada, A. L., Treviño, F. M., & Ray, L. A. (1990). IV. Health care utilization barriers among Mexican Americans: Evidence from HHANES 1982-84. *American Journal of Public Health, 80* (Suppl.), 27-31.

Farge, E. J. (1978). Medical orientation among a Mexican-American population: An old and a new model reviewed. *Social Science and Medicine, 12,* 277-282.

Farmer, J. E., & Peterson, L. (1995). Injury risk factors in children with attention deficit hyperactivity disorder. *Health Psychology, 14,* 325-332.

Gomez, E. A. (1987). Hispanic Americans: Ethnic shared values and traditional treatments. *American Journal of Social Psychiatry, 7*(4), 215-219.

Guttmacher, S., & Elinson, J. (1971). Ethno-religious variation in perceptions of illness: The use of illness as an explanation for deviant behavior. *Social Science and Medicine, 5,* 117-125.

Higginbotham, J. C., Treviño, F. M., & Ray, L. A. (1990). V. Utilization of curanderos by Mexican Americans: Prevalence and predictors findings from HHANES 1982-84. *American Journal of Public Health, 80* (Suppl.) 32-35.

Hobfoll, S. E., Jackson, A. P., Lavin, J., Britton, P. J., & Shepherd, J. B. (1993). Safer sex knowledge, behavior, and attitudes of inner-city women. *Health Psychology, 12,* 481-488.

Hobfoll, S. E., Jackson, A. P., Lavin, J., Britton, P. J., & Shepherd, J. B. (1994). Reducing inner-city women's AIDS risk activities: A study of single, pregnant women. *Health Psychology, 13,* 397-403.

Hsu, J. S. J., & Williams, S. D. (1991). Injury prevention awareness in an urban Native American population. *American Journal of Public Health, 81,* 1466-1468.

James, S. A. (1994). John Henryism and the health of African-Americans. *Culture, Medicine and Psychiatry, 18*(2), 163-182.

Kurtz, R. A., & Chalfant, H. P. (1991). *The sociology of medicine and illness* (2nd ed.). Needham Heights, MA: Allyn and Bacon.

Longres, J. F. (1995). *Human behavior in the social environment* (2nd ed.), Itasca, IL: Peacock.

Markides, K. S., Krause, N., & Mendes de Leon, C. F. (1988). Acculturation and alcohol consumption among Mexican Americans: A three-generation study. *American Journal of Public Health, 78,* 1178-1181.

Markides, K. S., Ray, L. A., Stroup-Benham, C. A., & Treviño, F. (1990). VII. Acculturation and alcohol consumption in the Mexican American population in the southwestern United States. *American Journal of Public Health, 90* (Suppl.), 42-46.

Marks, G., Garcia, M., & Solis, J. M. (1990). III. Health risk behaviors of Hispanics in the United States: Findings from HHANES 1982-84. *American Journal of Public Health, 80* (Suppl.), 20-26.

Marks, G., Solis, J., Richardson, J. L., Collins, L. M., Birba, L., & Hisserich, J. C. (1987). Health behavior of elderly Hispanic women: Does cultural assimilation make a difference? *American Journal of Public Health, 77,* 1315-1319.

Scott, C. S. (1974). Health and healing practices among five ethnic groups in Miami, Florida. *Public Health Reports, 89,* 524-532.

Solis, J. M., Marks, G., Garcia, M., & Shelton, D. (1990). II. Acculturation, access to care, and use of preventive services by Hispanics: Findings from HHANES 1982-84. *American Journal of Public Health, 80* (Suppl.), 11-19.

Suchman, E. A. (1965/1972). Social patterns of illness and medical care. In E. G. Jaco (Ed.), *Patients, physicians and illness: A sourcebook in behavioral science and health* (2nd ed.), (pp. 262–279). New York: Free Press. (Reprinted from *Journal of Health and Human Behavior*, 1965, *6*, 2–16.)

Weitzman, B. C., & Berry, C. A. (1992). Health status and health care utilization among New York City home attendants: An illustration of the needs of working poor, immigrant women. *Women and Health*, *19*(2/3), 87–105.

Zimmerman, R. S., Vega, W. A., Gil, A. G., Warheit, G. J., Apospori, E., & Biafora, F. (1994). Who is Hispanic? Definitions and their consequences. *American Journal of Public Health*, *84*, 1985–1987.

6

Health Behavior in Gay Men

Michael R. Kauth and Joseph Prejean

This chapter presents health behavior issues related to acceptance of a gay self-identity, as well as medical, psychological, and substance-use issues specific to gay men. By way of clarification, the term *gay men*, as used herein, refers to nonheterosexual males. The word *gay* without a gender qualifier refers to both nonheterosexual men and nonheterosexual women. While "gay" is a relatively new term, it is less a term of derision than other words once in popular usage, such as "invert," "homosexual," "faggot," and "queer." In discussion of the pathologizing of homosexuality, however, the term *homosexual* is used for semantic and historical accuracy. The term *heterosexual* connotes different-sex eroticism and the presumption of normative sexual behavior; as a "normative" term, it does not suffer from the same limitations as "homosexual."

_____

Michael R. Kauth • Psychology Service, Veterans Affairs Medical Center, New Orleans, Louisiana 70146.   **Joseph Prejean** • Department of Psychology, Louisiana State University, Baton Rouge, Louisana 70803.

Handbook of Health Behavior Research III: Demography, Development, and Diversity, edited by David S. Gochman. Plenum Press, New York, 1997.

THE MEDICALIZATION OF HOMOSEXUALITY: AN OVERVIEW

For many people, *homosexuality* and *health* have little to do with each other. During the past 100 years, same-sex attraction has been viewed as counter to good health and normal development (Halperin, 1990). Within Western culture, heterosexual attraction and behavior are regarded as normal, typical, moral, and healthy, while nonheterosexual feelings and behavior are held to be perverted, rare, destructive, and diseased (Hopkins, 1992). Those who deviate from society's standards of sexuality are pressured to conform and are punished, sometimes violently, if they do not (Center for Population Options, 1992).

In the eyes of contemporary heterosexist society, people with same-sex feelings are not just expressing an alternative way of loving; they are glorifying their disease. Even beyond derogating homosexual behavior, heterosexist culture holds that the gay individual *is* the disease (Foucault, 1978/1990; Katz, 1995). This social context presents unique difficulties for people with same sex feelings in developing a positive nonheterosexual identity and disclosing that identity.

From Vice to Disease

In the United States during the early to mid-19th century, erotic behavior was defined in terms of "true love" or "false love" (Katz, 1995). True love was a pure, spiritual feeling, that did not necessarily include coitus, and certainly not before marriage. False love was earthy, licentious, hedonistic, wasteful, and nonreproductive. Gender was not a defining factor, and nonreproductive different-sex acts as well as same-sex acts were seen as vice.

In the late 19th century, the medical and psychiatric establishment exercised its power to name and invented a norm of sexual behavior (called *heterosexuality* by 1892) by describing "deviant" sexual acts *and persons* (Foucault, 1978/1990; Greenberg, 1988; Halperin, 1990; Katz, 1995). Individuals who engaged in nonnormative acts were defined by that behavior (e.g., homosexuals, transvestites, fetishists, transsexuals, and masturbators) and were assumed to possess certain personality traits (DeCecco, 1990). The focus of sexuality moved from acts to the actor.

In 1869, the term *homosexual* was employed publicly for the first time in a leaflet written and distributed by Kertbeny (Feuray & Herzer, 1990). At that time, the word referred to male–male attraction and to men who enjoyed receptive anal intercourse with men. By the end of the 19th century, the medical community viewed homosexual men as possessing a contrary or inverted (female) sexual attraction (cf., Ellis, 1936; Kiernan, 1892 [cited in Katz, 1995]; Krafft-Ebing, 1893). Homosexuals were thought to have a congenital defect (although environmental stimuli could facilitate such development) and were distinguished by their youthful appearance, broad hips and rounded shoulders, sparse body hair, artistic inclinations, nervousness, frequent masturbation, and inability to whistle (Ellis, 1936). Homosexuality was a disease with little hope of a cure, although several remedies were attempted. Common treatments of the day included surgical and chemical castration, forced heterosexual activity and marriage, hypnosis, counterconditioning, and psychoanalysis (cf. Ellis, 1936; Krafft-Ebing, 1893).

Interestingly, the history of psychoanalysis parallels the medicalization of homosexuality (Lewes, 1988). Sigmund Freud, the father of psychoanalysis, transformed the biological defect of homosexuality into a psychic one (Freud, 1905/1953). The "problem" was seen by his view to be that gay men were fixated at an early psychosexual developmental stage that inhibited their individuation and separation from the mother. Freud not only sexualized identity and social relationships but also asserted that everyone had same-sex feelings, some of which were "latent." Suddenly, this "disorder" was seen to be part of everyone. Homosexuality thus became more pervasive, less easy to discern, and more intractable. Yet Freud later decided that homosexuals did not need psychoanalytic treatment for their same-sex feelings, unless they were also neurotic, and refused to treat them (Greenberg, 1988). Freud's followers disagreed and further pathologized homosexuality, hypothesizing that same-sex feelings were caused by a phobic response to members of the opposite sex (Rado, 1962) or by an absent or hostile father and a domineering mother (Bieber et al., 1962). Whatever the origin of homosexuality, homosexuals were doomed to a life of misery and loneliness, unless they were helped to become heterosexuals.

Beginning in the 1940s, behaviorists or learning theorists, boasting of their nonjudgmentalism and neutrality concerning homosexuality, proposed that same-sex erotic behavior was a consequence of an inappropriate sexual reinforcement history (cf., Barlow & Agras, 1973; Feldman & MacCulloch, 1971; Murphy, 1992). Homosexuality and heterosexuality were viewed as learned behaviors, and people with same-sex feelings had merely learned the wrong one. Through the early 1970s, behaviorists focused their efforts on changing same-sex behavior through aversive conditioning techniques such as electroconvulsive shock and emetics and differential reinforcement (e.g., heterosocial skills training and forced different-sex erotic activity [Murphy, 1992]). Treatment, still no more effective, had changed little since the turn of the century.

In "Sickness" and in Health

Labeling and stigmatizing people with same-sex feelings created the *homosexual* and the gay community (Adam, 1987). Disenfranchised individuals—diagnosed as mentally ill and considered diseased—congregated in large urban settings and eventually refused to be victimized. In one of the more dramatic moments, angry gay citizens in New York City, joined by some empathic straights, flexed their muscle in unison during three days of riots in 1969 (Adam, 1987). At the 1970 American Psychiatric Association (APA) conference, gays demanded that their stories be heard and that psychiatrists take responsibility for diagnosing a group of people as ill. As a result of the efforts of gay activists, the APA removed homosexuality from its list of psychiatric disorders in 1973 (see Bayer, 1981). The American Psychological Association and the National Association of Social Workers took similar action.

Of course, eliminating a diagnostic label did nothing to educate or end prejudicial attitudes or behaviors. Many mental health professionals opposed the removal of homosexuality as a mental disorder (see Bayer, 1981), and some still view it as a pathology (Cameron et al., 1986; Socarides, 1978). The majority of Americans also hold negative beliefs about homosexuality (Gallup Organization, 1992).

Gay men may accept society's stereotype of them as diseased and devalued and then act in ways that are consistent with that belief (cf. Allport, 1954). While some gay men incorporate same-sex attraction into their identity without or with only minimal psychological conflict, others, for a time at least, hate themselves, abuse substances, lead a "double" life, deny their gay relationships, engage in risky sexual activities, and fail to care for their general health (Cass, 1984a,b; Gonsiorek & Rudolph, 1991; Malyon, 1985). Acceptance of a gay identity has been found to be related to greater self-esteem, to disclosure to nongay others, and to ties to the gay community (McDonald, 1982; Paul, Weinrich, Gonsiorek, & Hotvedt, 1982). Although greater self-acceptance reduces the risk of destructive behaviors, positive health behaviors do not necessarily develop in their place. Only since the 1980s has a health-consciousness trend emerged in the gay community (Pronger, 1991).

Other Factors That Mediate Health in Gay Men

In terms of psychological adjustment and health behavior, there are few noted differences between heterosexual and gay men (Gonsiorek & Rudolph, 1991). There appear to be more differences among men in general than there are between heterosexual and gay men. Factors such as developmental phase, ethnicity, race, education, religion, socioeconomic status, and availability of health insurance play a larger role in individual health behavior and attitudes than does gender choice of sexual partner.

Research on homosexuality, however, is in its infancy. Most studies have reported on "pathologies" (e.g., substance abuse and suicide) associated with gay men, without appropriate comparison groups, and few studies have examined general health behaviors. The remainder of this chapter will present published findings on health behavior in gay men.

PHYSICAL AND MEDICAL ISSUES

According to Owen (1985), gay men face specific medical problems that are not as frequently seen in the general population and are largely related to differences in sexual behavior. Practices such as anal intercourse, oral–anal contact, and manual–anal contact, while not unheard of in the heterosexual community, are more common among gay men (Friedman & Downey, 1994). Gay men are also more likely than heterosexual men to become sexually active at a younger age and to have had a greater number of lifetime sexual partners (Judson, 1977; Rotheram-Borus & Gwadz, 1993). These behavioral differences contribute to the higher prevalence of sexually transmitted diseases (STDs) and other sex-related medical problems experienced by gay men (Friedman & Downey, 1994; Paroski, 1987). It should be noted, however, that a higher prevalence of STDs and sex-related problems does not suggest that all gay men experience these complaints.

Owen (1985) noted four categories of medical problems more common among gay men than among heterosexual men: (1) classic venereal diseases, such as gonorrhea, syphilis, herpes simplex, and venereal warts; (2) enteric diseases, including amebiasis, hepatitis, and cytomegalovirus (CMV) infections; (3) traumatic complications of sexual intercourse, such as fecal incontinence, hemorrhoids, or anal fissures; and (4) acquired disorders of cellular immunity, such as those caused by human immunodeficiency virus (HIV).

HIV and AIDS in Gay Men

Perhaps because it was first identified in gay men, and was in fact first called "gay-related immune deficiency" (GRID), acquired immunodeficiency syndrome (AIDS) is associated with homosexuality in the minds of the general population (Shilts, 1987). While the vast majority of AIDS cases have affected gay men, prevention efforts have reduced the number of new cases of HIV infection among gay men from 73% in 1985 to 53% in 1994 (Centers for Disease Control and Prevention [CDC] 1986, 1994). HIV prevention efforts were undertaken by and for the gay community mostly because of the failure of medical and federal authorities to initiate HIV risk reduction campaigns that targeted gay men (Shilts, 1987).

Despite exhaustive HIV education and prevention efforts by the gay community, and some success, a significant proportion of gay men do not practice safer sex consistently. Kelly et al.

(1991) found that among gay men who used condoms regularly, 45% had had a lapse in safer sex practices during the prior 6 months. Subjects reported that the primary reasons for lapses of safer sex behavior were affection for or wanting to please a partner, as well as the spontaneity of sexual activity.

Even consistent condom users, however, do not always feel safe from HIV. Forstein (1984) described a group of people called the "worried well" who are HIV-seronegative but fear infection because of past behaviors. For the worried well, countless deaths of friends and lovers and the association of sex with death create a climate of fear, guilt, and doom that reduces sexual desire and evokes anger, anxiety, depression, hypochondriacal and somatic concerns, and negative feelings about being gay (Harowski, 1988). Given the effect of stress on immune functioning (Antoni, LaPerriere, Schneiderman, & Fletcher, 1991; Baum & Temoshok, 1990), it is not unreasonable to predict that the chronic stress of living with the AIDS epidemic places gay men at increased risk of common illnesses or psychological disorders, although to date there is only limited support for this hypothesis (Martin & Dean, 1993).

Relationship with Physicians and the Medical Establishment

Physicians who assume that all of their patients are heterosexual fail to consider conditions that are more prevalent among gays, avoid discussing gay issues, and use heterosexist language (Owen, 1985). Unfortunately, many gay people do not feel comfortable revealing their sexual orientation to their physicians (Dardick & Grady, 1980), and many physicians are not comfortable hearing it (Douglas, Kalman, & Kalman, 1985; Prichard et al., 1988). Gay men are reluctant to disclose their sexuality to their physicians for fear of humiliation, discrimination, termination, or being "outed" (Savin-Williams, 1994). Kass, Faden, Fox, and Dudley (1992) found that 2% of 852 HIV-seronegative gay men surveyed reported being refused treatment by a physician because of their sexual orientation. Since many gay men choose not to disclose their sexual orientation, this figure probably underrepresents those who are discriminated against because they are gay.

A variety of health care professionals have reported holding prejudicial feelings about gay people, including physicians (Douglas et al., 1985; Prichard et al., 1988), nurses (Douglas et al. 1985), social workers (DeCrescenzo, 1983), and medical students (Kelly, St. Lawrence, Smith, Hood, & Cook, 1987b). In fact, Kelly et al. (1987a,b) found that the majority of 157 physicians and 119 medical students surveyed reported having less sympathy and more blame for gay patients and patients with AIDS than for heterosexual patients with another illness. While negative attitudes of medical students can be altered though education and contact with gay men (McGrory, McDowell, & Muskin, 1990), few medical schools include the topic of homosexuality in their curricula (Townsend, Wallick, & Cambre, 1993).

In sum, the relationship between gay men and health care is largely unexplored. Little is known about how gay men choose a health care provider, under what circumstances a gay patient discloses his sexual orientation to a heterosexual physician, the value of having a gay physician, or gay patients' compliance with medical advice and treatment. It can at least be said, however, that HIV-seropositive gay men appear frustrated with the rigid, dictatorial medical establishment, are able to develop underground medical networks, and are willing to try non-Western medical alternatives (Shilts, 1987).

Health Promotion Behaviors

Recently, gay men have focused greater attention on exercise and health. Popular gay magazines such as *The Advocate*, *OUT*, *genre*, and *10 Percent*, as well as prominent men's fashion magazines such as *Gentlemen's Quarterly* and sports and casual wear catalogs such as *International Male*, feature attractive, healthy-looking, athletic models for their gay readers. In addition,

the public "coming out" of several gay athletes— Greg Louganis, Martina Navratilova, Bob and Rod Jackson-Paris, Billie Jean King, and Bruce Hayes— has effected or echoed a fitness revolution in the gay subculture that parallels the exercise trend in the general population. Playing organized sports or working out at a gym has become a popular way to develop a healthy-looking body and to meet people. When the first Gay Games were held in San Francisco in 1982, fewer than 1800 athletes participated ("Score Card #2," 1994). By 1994, when the fourth Gay Games were held, 15,000 gay people participated.

Without doubt, there are varied reasons for the national fitness trend. Athletics and physical fitness are traditionally viewed as signs of good health and strength. It is possible that gay men (and perhaps the general population) adopted exercise as a reaction to the physical appearance of AIDS: gaunt, frail, pale, and sickly (Pronger, 1991). Looking like the picture of health is one way of countering the feeling of vulnerability to HIV infection. On the other hand, the gay exercise trend could also represent a reclamation of mythic masculinity (Pronger, 1991). The new muscled look challenges the stereotype of the weak, effeminate gay man and the association of homosexuality with disease.

EMOTIONAL AND PSYCHOLOGICAL ISSUES

The sickness model of homosexuality that was prevalent until the mid-1970s held that persistent same-sex feelings alone were indicative of psychological disturbance (Gonsiorek, 1991). It was thus quite remarkable when Hooker (1956) demonstrated in 1956 that clinicians could not distinguish between responses by well-adjusted gay men and heterosexual men on projective tests.

Most gay men appear to cope adaptively with the chronic stressors they experience throughout their lifetime and become healthy functioning adults (Savin-Williams, 1990). While gay men encounter strong oppressive forces at every level of society, there is no evidence that gay men display, overall, greater psychopathology than heterosexual men (Gonsiorek, 1991) or that heterosexism is the sole cause of stress for gay men (Erwin, 1993). Under certain circumstances, however, such as coming out, some gay men appear to be more vulnerable to psychological stress (Newman & Muzzonigro, 1993; Strommen, 1989; Walters & Simoni, 1993).

In a sample of 84 highly functional gay men, subjects revealed few current symptoms of distress, but reported a high prevalence of lifetime emotional disorders (Williams, Rabkin, Remien, Gorman, & Ehrhardt, 1991). What could account for this phenomenon? Walters and Simoni (1993) found that self-esteem scores among 35 adult gay men were lowest for those in the early self-recognition stage of identity development and in a later stage where social integration is the goal, and that these scores were highest for gay men in the final self-acceptance stage of development. Several theorists and observers (Cass, 1984a,b; Garnets, Herek, & Levy, 1992; Gonsiorek & Rudolph, 1991) have noted that for many gay individuals in the initial stage of coming out, recognition of same-sex feelings creates considerable strain between public and private personas, contributing to feelings of inauthenticity, alienation, devaluation, depression, self-destruction, and the fear of discovery. The private–public identity conflict is more evident in the case of a young gay male coming out in an ethnic family that espouses traditional, gender-rigid values. The family may perceive the gay youth as antiethnic and as rejecting the family, while the young gay man feels alienated from both the ethnic and the gay culture (Icard, 1985–1986; Newman & Muzzonigro, 1993).

Other authors (Colcher, 1982; Sadava & Thompson, 1986; Siever, 1994) have reported that gay men struggling with their homosexuality are at increased risk of substance abuse, eating disorders, and engaging in frequent risky sexual activity. Paroski (1987) found that in a sample of 89 gay youths, of ages 14–17, 96% reported using

sex to gain self-validation and information about homosexuality. Furthermore, the majority of a larger sample of 136 mostly Hispanic and African-American gay and bisexual adolescents seeking support services from a gay-related agency in New York City reported having more sexual partners and encounters than the national average for (heterosexuals in) their age group (Rotheram-Borus et al, 1994). In this study, 44% of gay adolescents had 11 or more lifetime sexual partners, and 52% of those surveyed never or only sometimes used condoms with male partners.

Depression and Suicide

Gay men experience a higher incidence of lifetime mood disorders than heterosexual men. Williams et al. (1991) noted that one third of their sample of gay men reported having experienced at least one episode of major depression, compared to 3% of men for all age groups (in studies in which sexual orientation was not assessed). Few gay men evidenced current symptoms of depression, and psychological functioning was high. In a smaller sample of 31 HIV-seronegative gay men, 61% of subjects reported symptoms of lifetime major depression, but only 6% had any current mood-related symptoms (Rosenberger et al. 1993). Again, psychological functioning was high.

Hays, Turner, and Coates (1992) hypothesized that social support acts as a buffer against depression and, in a study of 508 gay men made up of persons with varying HIV serostatus, found that men who were more satisfied with the level of social support they received were significantly less likely to report symptoms of depression 1 year later. However, when social support was used to predict mental health among a sample of 520 gay men with varying HIV serostatues, social support accounted for only 3% of the variance (Lackner et al., 1993). The authors suggested that personality factors and level of social skills play a greater role in fending off depression than does social support alone.

Chronic and severe emotional distress can

contribute to suicidal ideation and behavior. While there has been much speculation about the association between suicide and homosexuality (e.g., Hendin, 1982), the prevalence of suicide attempts or completions among gay men is by no means clear because of the difficulties of determining an individual's sexual identity or motivation or establishing the number of gay people in the population. Even so, it is estimated that gay men and women are 2–7 times more likely than heterosexuals to attempt suicide (Saunders & Valente, 1987). Furthermore, gay people account for 30% of completed suicides, with the majority of attempts being made during youth (Gibson, 1989).

Suicide attempts are highest among the young and minorities, both of which are groups with the fewest personal resources and least social support (Remafedi, 1987). According to the Task Force on Youth Suicide (Gibson, 1989), suicide is the *leading* cause of death among gay, lesbian, bisexual, and transsexual young people in the United States. In a review of the literature on suicide and homosexuality, Savin-Williams (1994) noted that between 20% and 40% of gay youths had made past suicide attempts, most often following significant family problems, first sexual experiences, or recognition of their homosexuality. Interestingly, suicide attempts were not related to running away from home, depression, hopelessness, suicidal ideation, discrimination, loss of friendship, or violence. Hunter (1990) speculates, however, that some homicides among ethnic minority groups that view suicide as shameful may mask actual suicides. Minority youths may use violence as a means of provoking the police or others to kill them because being gunned down carries less stigma than committing suicide.

Remafedi (1987) linked the probability of suicidal behavior to an early recognition of homosexuality. Men who recognized their same-sex feelings early in life experienced more gay-related stressors such as coming out to parents, being discovered by family, and being ridiculed. Saunders and Valente (1987) found that suicide attempts by gay men were often associated with disrupted social relationships, chronic disease and aging, heavy alcohol or drug consumption, and past suicide attempts. Bell and Weinberg (1978) reported, however, that more than one half of initial suicide attempts by gay men in their sample were related to conflicts over sexual identity and rejection from others. Of the 686 gay men and 337 heterosexual men interviewed by the authors, 20% of gay men compared to fewer than 4% of heterosexual men had made past suicide attempts. It is unclear whether suicidal behavior increases in old age for gay men as it does in the general population (Hendin, 1982).

Reminiscent of the Durkheim (1897/1951) social–integration regulation theory of suicide, Saunders and Valente (1987) concluded that men who have accepted their homosexuality and are involved in the gay community are at less risk of suicide than men who are at odds with their same-sex feelings and who have inadequate social support. The authors suggested that low self-acceptance and poor social integration have a greater influence on suicidal behavior than sexual orientation. In a study that produced results consistent with this conclusion, Rich, Fowler, and Blenkush (1986) interviewed the families, friends, and employers of a small sample of 13 gay men and 106 heterosexual men between the ages of 21 and 42 who had committed suicide, inferring sexual orientation and presumptive stressors leading to suicide from these interviews. Their study revealed few differences between the two groups in stressors *presumed* to have contributed to the suicide.

Harassment and Violence

Typically, men identify as gay earlier than women and tend to frequent public gay-related areas, which may account in part for the higher incidence of antigay harassment and physical violence directed at them (Berrill, 1992). For young gay men, victimization is most likely to occur at school and at home, although antigay harassment by one's own family may be more personally threatening and damaging. Boxer, Cook, and Herdt (1991) reported that about 10% of gay youths who disclosed their sexual orientation to their fathers were kicked out of the house. Reviewing 500 case histories of mostly Hispanic and African-American gay and bisexual adolescents (79% males, mean age 17.1 years) who sought services at a gay-identified agency in New York City, Hunter (1990) found that 40% of the youths had experienced violent physical assaults, with 61% of this gay-related violence occurring in the home. Chronic stress from verbal and physical abuse by same-age peers and family members contributes to school-related difficulties such as difficulty concentrating, poor grades, tardiness, absenteeism, and fighting (Savin-Williams, 1994). Other problems resulting from antigay harassment at school and at home include running away, social isolation, conduct and legal problems, substance abuse, prostitution, and suicidal behavior.

The picture changes little for gay college students. In the review by D'Augelli (1992) of antigay violence on college campuses, 55–72% of gay men and lesbians sampled had experienced verbal or physical harassment, with the incidence of physical threats of violence reaching 25% in several studies. A separate review by Berrill (1992) reported that between 16% and 26% of gay college students at four major universities (Yale, Rutgers, Pennsylvania State, and Oberlin) had been threatened with physical violence, and 14–25% had been chased or followed. One third to two thirds of gay students on three of the campuses reported fearing for their safety. In a study of 160 gay college students, men who were less open about their sexual orientation had greater worry about harassment, and students who most feared physical abuse obtained lower life satisfaction scores (D'Augelli, 1991). Some 70–80% of gay male and lesbian college students gave harassment or the fear of it as the reason for remaining closeted (D'Augelli, 1992).

Among adult men and women, a 1984 National Gay and Lesbian Task Force (NGLTF, 1984) study of 1420 gay men and 654 lesbians across eight major cities in the United States (Atlanta, Boston, Dallas, Denver, Los Angeles, New York, St. Louis, and Seattle) found that 94% of those sampled had experienced some form of antigay harassment, and 44% had been threatened with physical violence. More than two thirds of men and women who had received threats of violence and almost half of those who had been physically attacked had experienced multiple assaults. In summarizing data from 24 studies between 1977 and 1991, Berrill (1992) observed that the median proportion of gay people who reported being verbally harassed was 80% (range: 58–91%), and the proportion of those who were threatened by violence was 44% (range: 24–48%). Overall, one third of gay people sampled had been chased, and 17% were assaulted. Finally, the number of antigay or gay-related homicides reported to the NGLTF (1990) fluctuated between 1985 and 1989, but increased during those years from 20 to 62, respectively. In 1986, 80 antigay murders were reported to the NGLTF. These figures, however, are thought to greatly underestimate the number of actual antigay homicides, which are often remarkable in their brutality (Berrill, 1992).

Antigay violence appears to be on the rise. Between 1985 and 1989, the number of antigay assaults reported to the NGLTF more than tripled, from 2042 to 7031, a trend that was mirrored by other studies during the same period (Berrill, 1992). One longitudinal study of several hundred gay men in New York City found that the proportion of men who reported having experienced antigay violence increased from 9% in 1985 to 14% in 1990 (Dean, Wu, & Martin, 1992).

Victims of traumatic assaults can experience a range of symptoms that include sleep disturbances, recurrent nightmares or intrusive thoughts about the event, fear of another assault, chronic headaches, diarrhea, crying spells, depression, social withdrawal, agitation and restlessness, hypervigilance, intense anger, increased use of alcohol and drugs, and deterioration of personal relationships (Garnets et al., 1992). Severe or multiple traumatization can lead to profound life disruption and a diagnosis of posttraumatic stress disorder (American Psychiatric Association, 1994). Janoff-Bulman (1992) purported that being traumatized interferes with basic assumptions that one is safe and secure, people are trustworthy, and the world is an orderly and meaningful place. Victims who blame the trauma(s) on their own character traits ("There is something about me which prompted the attack") rather than on situational factors ("I was in a bad neighborhood") report feelings of low self-worth, depression, and helplessness (Janoff-Bulman, 1982).

In the victim's mind, antigay harassment can "causally link" being gay with the assault, producing a heightened sense of vulnerability and reinforcing negative beliefs about homosexuality (Garnets et al., 1992). Furthermore, gay men who disclose their victimization are sometimes viewed by others as weak, inferior, incompetent, foolish, or even deserving of the event. Victims of antigay violence in rural areas experience considerable stigma and have more difficulty finding support than urban gays (D'Augelli & Hart, 1987), while closeted gay men, fearing discovery, have few if any social resources to cope with being victimized.

Runaways and the Homeless

In his review, Savin-Williams (1994) concluded that 30–40% of homeless street youths are gay, lesbian, or bisexual and that one quarter of them are HIV-infected. He warned that if homeless youths fail to find support services within 1–2 weeks of their arrival on the streets, they face an increased risk of substance abuse, pregnancy, criminal activity, HIV infection, or prostitution. In one sample of 620 homeless adolescents, 75% of those sampled were involved in prostitution (Yates, MacKenzie, Pennbridge, & Swofford, 1991).

Aging

There are few studies of older gay men or their relationships. Aging gay men are a neglected community who are susceptible to ageist

stereotypes about older men, isolation, loss of significant relationships, illness, legal and inheritance concerns, and feelings of "accelerated aging" in a society that (over)values youth and beauty (Friend, 1988). If in good health, however, older gay men may be better equipped to handle aging than heterosexual men. Quam and Whitford (1992) postulated that coming out tempers adjustment to the aging process because gay men tend to perceive social roles as flexible. Furthermore, older men who are out have developed a degree of competency in crisis management and have created a supportive network of friends (Quam & Whitford, 1992).

In a sample of 41 gay men who were over age 50, 44% were "very accepting" of growing old, although greater acceptance of aging was related to current good health (Friend, 1988). What is more, 63% of men sampled lived alone and, for 29%, loneliness was a problem. Older gay men reported fearing rejection by adult children and grandchildren or health professionals because of their sexual orientation. A study of another sample of 27 healthy older gay men (mean age: 66) from the San Francisco Bay area found that high life satisfaction scores, low self-criticism, and few psychosomatic complaints were associated with being *very* satisfied with being gay and with early same-sex sexual experimentation (before age 15) (Adelman, 1991). Men in the sample who were less satisfied with their lives tended to blame their disappointment on being gay.

Seeking of Emotional Help

Bell and Weinberg (1978) reported that 50–58% of adult gay men sampled ($N = 686$) had sought professional help for emotional distress compared with 13–30% of heterosexual men ($N = 337$). Typical presenting complaints among gay men in psychotherapy are (1) coming-out issues such as challenging negative beliefs about homosexuality and establishing a positive self-identity, (2) conflict in or loss of significant relationships, and (3) sexual-performance anxiety and inhibited sexual desire (George & Behrendt, 1988;

Woodman, 1989). A sample of 50 gay men entering psychotherapy most frequently cited relationship issues—communication and sexual problems—as their reasons for seeking treatment (Modrcin & Wyers, 1990). As well as psychotherapy, community-based support groups that provide a forum for debunking cultural stereotypes and nurturing a positive gay identity are particularly important to young gay people in the initial stages of coming out (Gibson, 1989).

Fear of being humiliated or identified as gay prevents some gay men from obtaining help from traditional mental health sources such as psychiatrists, psychologists, social workers, and clergy (Paroski, 1987). Unfortunately, a portion of gay men who disclose their sexual orientation to a psychotherapist are not supported and are sometimes encouraged to change their feelings (Gibson, 1989). In other cases, gay men do not disclose their sexual orientation unless asked, and psychotherapists who assume that all of their patients are heterosexual are unlikely to ask (Gibson, 1989). Counselors who hold negative attitudes about homosexuality communicate their discomfort in various ways to gay clients, although perhaps unintentionally (Hayes & Gelso, 1993). Psychotherapists who cannot be supportive of gay clients should refer them elsewhere.

While it may be presumed that gay men would prefer gay male psychotherapists, when 128 gay men in psychotherapy were asked whether having a gay male psychotherapist was important, only half agreed (Modrcin & Wyers, 1990). Good psychotherapy skills and a knowledge of gay issues appear to be more essential psychotherapist characteristics than being gay.

Summary

It is unclear from the literature what factors contribute to good adjustment and a sense of fulfillment among gay men. The bulk of psychosocial research has focused on problems experienced by gay men and has failed to examine how most gay people cope adaptively.

ALCOHOL AND SUBSTANCE USE

From convenience samples, it is estimated that one third of gay men in metropolitan areas abuse alcohol (Smith, 1982). Zehner and Lewis (1983) asserted that alcoholism is 2–3 times more prevalent in the gay community than in the general population. Ostrow et al. (1990) described "near universal" use of alcohol in their cohort of 3916 gay men from the Multicenter AIDS Cohort Study. The prevalence of illicit substance use mirrors this trend. Rotheram-Borus et al. (1994) reported high usage of several classes of drugs such as marijuana, cocaine/crack, and hallucinogens among their sample of gay adolescents from New York City. Saghir and Robins (1973) found use of illegal substances to be higher and more frequent among gay men than among heterosexual men. Few studies, however, employed age-matched heterosexual comparison groups or explored the possibility that gay men may be more likely than heterosexual men to report substance abuse and seek treatment.

Researchers have hypothesized that gay men turn to alcohol and drugs to cope with anxiety, loneliness, social isolation, societal disregard of gays, and internalized homophobia (Colcher, 1982; Kus, 1987; Sadava & Thompson, 1986). Possibly the same defenses that enable gay men to survive in an essentially hostile world (e.g., masking, denial, humor, and sedation) also contribute to the development and maintenance of alcoholism (Finnegan & Cook, 1984). On one hand, being secretive or attempting to pass as heterosexual decreases the likelihood of meeting other gay men and increases feelings of loneliness and depression; on the other hand, gay bars have typically been the places where gay men go to meet other gay people. Being in a drinking establishment increases the chances of alcohol use, and the anxiolytic effects of alcohol and drugs reward their use by reducing social anxiety and lowering inhibitions (Isrealstam & Lambert, 1984). Additionally, disinhibition spills over into the bedroom when alcohol and drugs (e.g., amyl nitrate or "poppers") are employed to lessen the sense of guilt or shame associated with sexual behavior and facilitate or enhance the performance of certain sexual acts practiced by some gay men, such as anal intercourse (Goode & Troiden, 1979; Mayer, 1983).

With disinhibition comes the loss of control, often in a situation in which reduced self-control can have life-threatening consequences. Several researchers have reported that recreational drug use among their samples was associated with having more than one sexual partner and engaging in high HIV-sexual-risk behavior (Ostrow et al., 1990; Rotheram-Borus et al., 1994; Siegel, Mesagno, Chen, & Christ, 1989). These findings have serious implications for HIV prevention and for substance abuse treatment of gay men. The relationship of drugs and alcohol to unsafe sexual practices, however, may not be a causal one and is complicated by other factors such as anxiety reduction and thrill seeking (Leigh & Stall, 1993; Siegel et al., 1989).

Treatment Issues

Most reports about drug and alcohol treatment approaches for gay men have come from clinical lore rather than from scientific comparison of treatment modalities. Discussions of counseling issues regarding the gay substance abuser have focused on the similarities between gay and heterosexual consumers. With both gay and nongay clients, the counselor is initially directive in helping the recovering individual to structure leisure time, minimize loneliness, and avoid friends who continue to use substances, all of which may trigger relapse (Colcher, 1982). Involvement with supportive organizations is central to all recovery programs.

After helping the client to achieve sobriety, the addictions counselor then examines issues related to the client's abuse. Issues that are unique to the gay substance abuser include (1) his particular experiences as a gay man (e.g., coming out and adjustment), (2) particular features of the gay

subculture (e.g., the focus on drinking and bars), (3) diversity within the subculture, and (4) cultural attitudes that differ from the mainstream (Smith, 1982). Colcher (1982) pointed out that the recovering gay alcoholic or substance abuser can participate in gay social activities that include drinking, if he does so with sober peers. It is also essential, however, that he participate in non-alcohol-oriented gay activities to maintain sobriety.

Smith (1982) suggested taking a "bifocal view" of treatment of the gay alcoholic, viewing the problem simultaneously as unconnected to sexual orientation and highly related to it. Smith (1982) maintains that while the goals for treatment—sobriety and social support—are the same for gay and nongay clients, being gay can play a large role in the etiology and maintenance of alcoholism. The same can be said of the abuse of other substances. Both in treatment and on the outside, stigma against homosexuality and perceptions of intolerance of the gay substance abuser inhibit recovery (Colcher, 1982).

Again, counselors who intend to work with gay substance abusers should assess their ability to treat gay people, and, if they feel they cannot, refer them. They should also be familiar with resources in the community, such as gay Alcoholics Anonymous groups and non-alcohol-related gay organizations and activities.

METHODOLOGICAL CONCERNS AND FUTURE RESEARCH DIRECTIONS

Many methodological problems in research on homosexuality limit the generalizability of most studies. First, samples are not representative of gay men. Nearly all data cited in this chapter come from convenience samples, or small samples, or both, of bar patrons, community center members, social and support group attendants, personal friends, and receivers of gay-related health services. Consequently, data are confounded with degree of comfort with a gay identity, connectedness to the (white) gay community, health risk activities (e.g., drinking), and motivation to participate in a study about homosexuality (Berrill, 1992). Participants from special-interest activities (e.g., activist groups, AIDS support groups, or therapy clients) tend to overrepresent or underrepresent features of gay subgroups (see Harry, 1986). Several studies also have, for convenience, combined bisexual men with self-identified gay individuals on the basis of behavioral similarities. These two groups, however, vary considerably on psychological variables and are not similar at all. Most gay studies tend to include predominantly white, urban, highly educated, middle-income, "out," male subjects. It is unknown whether these samples reveal anything about ethnic, less educated, rural, or closeted gay men and lesbians. Future research with gay people should strive for larger and less urban samples, more ethnic minorities and women, and comparison groups of matched heterosexuals.

Methodology for hard-to-reach populations of uncertain demographic composition and prevalence, like gay men, must be more creative than that for sampling conventional, well-defined groups, (e.g., Herek & Berrill, 1992). "Snowballing," a common current survey strategy, employs social networking to tap into hidden communities. Another strategy is to survey from as many different sources as possible, including non-gay-identified agencies or services utilized by marginalized individuals, in order to increase the heterogeneity of the sample. Uncontrolled dissemination of questionnaires through reprints in newspapers, however, prevents accurate estimation of sample characteristics. Tracking the number of questionnaires distributed allows for calculation of response rates, and data about survey nonresponders provides important information concerning potential sampling bias.

Research on gay men has been limited by the questions asked. Many studies reviewed for this chapter examined gay men only in relationship to AIDS or with the purpose of describing the problems they experience. Future research should

investigate aging and generational differences among gay men, the prevention of substance abuse and suicide, and factors that predict a positive gay identity. Other neglected areas of concern to gay men's lives include health promotion, quality of life, and coping with the chronic stress of living in a heterosexist culture. Cross-cultural studies of people with same-sex attraction will be particularly important in discerning how culture influences health behavior for Western gay men. At present, in brief, there appears to be more unknown than known about gay men.

REFERENCES

Adam, B. D. (1987). *The rise of the gay and lesbian movement*. Boston: Twayne Publishers.

Adelman, M. (1991). Stigma, gay lifestyles, and adjustment to aging: A study of later-life gay men and lesbians. *Journal of Homosexuality*, 20(3-4), 7-32.

Allport, G. (1954). *The nature of prejudice*. New York: Addison-Wesley.

American Psychiatric Association. (1994). *Diagnostic and statistical manual of mental disorders* (4th ed.). Washington DC: Author.

Antoni, M. H., LaPerriere, A., Schneiderman, N., & Fletcher, M. A. (1991). Stress and immunity in individuals at risk for AIDS. *Stress Medicine*, 7, 35-44.

Barlow, D. H., & Agras, W. S. (1973). Fading to increase heterosexual responsiveness in homosexuals. *Journal of Applied Behavior Analysis*, 6, 355-366.

Baum, A., & Temoshok, L. (1990). *Psychological Perspectives on AIDS*. Hillsdale, NJ: Erlbaum.

Bayer, R. (1981). *Homosexuality and American psychiatry: The politics of diagnosis*. Princeton, NJ: Princeton University Press.

Bell, A., & Weinberg, M. (1978). *Homosexualities: A study of diversity among men and women*. New York: Simon and Schuster.

Berrill, K. T. (1992). Anti-gay violence and victimization in the United States: An overview. In G. M. Herek & K. T. Berrill (Eds.), *Hate crimes: Confronting violence against lesbians and gay men* (pp. 19-45). Newbury Park, CA: Sage.

Bieber, I., Dain, H. J., Dince, P. R., Drellich, M. G., Grand, H. G., Gundlach, R. H., Kremer, M. W., Rifkin, A. H., Wilber, C. B., & Bieber, T. B. (1962). *Homosexuality: A psychoanalytic study*. New York: Basic Books.

Boxer, A. M., Cook, J. A., & Herdt, G. (1991). Double jeopardy: Identity transitions and parent-child relations among gay and lesbian youth. In K. Pillemer & K. McCartney (Eds.),

Parent-child relations throughout life (pp. 59–92). Hillsdale, NJ: Erlbaum.

Cameron, P., Proctor, K., Coburn, W., Jr., Forde, N., Larson, H., & Cameron, K. (1986). Child molestation and homosexuality. *Psychological Reports, 58*, 327–337.

Cass, V. C. (1984a). Homosexual identity: A concept in need of definition. *Journal of Homosexuality, 9*, 105–126.

Cass, V. C. (1984b). Homosexual identity formation: Testing a theoretical model. *Journal of Sex Research, 9*, 143–167.

Center for Population Options. (1992). *Lesbian, gay and bisexual youth: At risk and underserved.* Washington, DC: Author.

Centers for Disease Control. (1986). *Acquired immunodeficiency syndrome (AIDS) weekly surveillance report— United States.* Washington, DC: Author.

Centers for Disease Control and Prevention. (1994). *HIV/ AIDS surveillance report, 6*(2), 1–39.

Colcher, R. W. (1982). Counseling the homosexual alcoholic. *Journal of Homosexuality, 7*, 43–52.

Dardick, L. & Grady, K. E. (1980). Openness between gay persons and health professionals. *Annals of Internal Medicine, 93*, 115–119.

D'Augelli, A. R. (1991). Gay men in college: Identity processes and adaptations. *Journal of College Student Development, 32*, 140–146.

D'Augelli, A. R. (1992). Lesbian and gay male undergraduates' experiences of harassment and fear on campus. *Journal of Interpersonal Violence, 7*, 383–395.

D'Augelli, A. R., & Hart, M. M. (1987). Gay women, men, and families in rural settings: Toward the development of helping communities. *American Journal of Community Psychology, 15*(1), 79–93.

Dean, L., Wu, S., & Martin, J. L. (1992). Trends in violence and discrimination against gay men in New York City: 1984 to 1990. In G. M. Herek and K. T. Berrill (Eds.), *Hate crimes: Confronting violence against lesbians and gay men* (pp. 46–64). Newbury Park, CA: Sage.

DeCecco, J. P. (1990). Confusing the actor with the act: Muddled notions about homosexuality. *Archives of Sexual Behavior, 19*(4), 409–412.

DeCrescenzo, T. A. (1983). Homophobia: A study of the attitudes of mental health professionals toward homosexuality. *Journal of Social Work and Human Sexuality 2*, 115–136.

Douglas, C. J., Kalman, C. M., & Kalman, T. P. (1985). Homophobia among physicians and nurses: An empirical study. *Hospital and Community Psychiatry, 36*, 1309–1311.

Durkheim, E. (1897/1951). *Suicide.* New York: Free Press.

Ellis, H. (1936). *Studies in the psychology of sex.* New York: Random House.

Erwin, K. (1993). Interpreting the evidence: Competing paradigms and the emergence of lesbian and gay suicide as a "social fact." *International Journal of Health Services, 23*(3) 437–453.

Feldman, M. P., & MacCulloch, M. J. (1971). *Homosexual behavior: Therapy and assessment.* Oxford: Pergamon Press.

Feuray, J. C., & Herzer, M. (1990). Homosexual studies and politics in the nineteenth century: Karl Maria Kertbeny [translated by Glen W. Peppel]. *Journal of Homosexuality, 19*(1), 23–47.

Finnegan, D. G., & Cook, D. (1984). Special issues affecting the treatment of male and lesbian alcoholics. *Alcoholism Treatment Quarterly, 1*, 85–98.

Forstein, M. (1984). AIDS anxiety in the "worried well." In S. Nichols & D. Ostrow (Eds.), *Psychiatric implications of acquired immune deficiency syndrome* (pp 50–60). Washington, DC: Monograph Series of the American Psychiatric Press.

Foucault, M. (1978/1990). *The history of sexuality: Vol. I. An introduction* [translated by Robert Hurley]. New York: Vintage Books.

Freud, S. (1905/1953). Three essays on the theory of sexuality. In J. Strachey (Ed.), *The standard edition of the complete psychological works of Sigmund Freud: Vol. 7* (pp. 123–246). London: Hogarth.

Friedman, R. C., & Downey, J. I. (1994). Homosexuality. *New England Journal of Medicine, 331*, 923–930.

Friend, R. A. (1988). The individual and social psychology of aging: Clinical implications for lesbian and gay men. In E. Coleman (Ed.), *Psychotherapy with homosexual men and women: Integrated identity approaches for clinical practice* (pp. 307–331). New York: Haworth Press.

Gallup Organization. (1992, June). *Nationally representative telephone poll of 1002 noninstitutionalized adult Americans.*

Garnets, L., Herek, G. M., & Levy, B. (1992). Violence and victimization of lesbians and gay men: Mental health consequences. In G. M. Herek & K. T. Berrill (Eds.), *Hate crimes: Confronting violence against lesbians and gay men* (pp. 207–226). Newbury Park, CA: Sage.

George, K. D., & Behrendt, A. E. (1988). Therapy for male couples experiencing relationship problems and sexual problems. In E. Coleman (Ed.), *Psychotherapy with homosexual men and women: Integrated identity approaches for clinical practice* (pp. 77–88). New York: Haworth Press.

Gibson, P. (1989). Gay male and lesbian youth suicide. In *Report of the secretary's task force on youth suicide: Vol. III: Prevention and interventions in youth suicide.* DHHS Publication No. (ADM)89-1623. Washington, DC: U.S. Government Printing Office.

Gonsiorek, J. C. (1991). The empirical basis for the demise of the illness model of homosexuality. In J. C. Gonsiorek & J. D. Weinrich (Eds.), *Homosexuality: Research implications for public policy* (pp. 115–136). Newbury Park, CA: Sage.

Gonsiorek, J. C., & Rudolph, J. R. (1991). Homosexual identity: Coming out and other developmental events. In J. C.

Gonsiorek & J. D. Weinrich (Eds.), *Homosexuality: Research implications for public policy* (pp. 161–176). Newbury Park, CA: Sage.

Goode, E., & Troiden, R. R. (1979). Amyl nitrite use among homosexual men. *American Journal of Psychiatry, 136,* 1067–1069.

Greenberg, D. F. (1988). *The construction of homosexuality.* Chicago: University of Chicago Press.

Halperin, D. M. (1990). *One hundred years of homosexuality and other essays on Greek love.* New York: Routledge.

Harowski, K. J. (1988). The worried well: Maximizing coping in the face of AIDS. In E. Coleman (Ed.), *Psychotherapy with homosexual men and women: Integrated identity approaches for clinical practice* (pp. 299–306). New York: Haworth Press.

Harry, J. (1986). Sampling gay men. *Journal of Sex Research, 22,* 21–34.

Hayes, J. A., & Gelso, C. J. (1993). Male counselors' discomfort with gay and HIV-infected clients. *Journal of Consulting and Clinical Psychology, 40*(1), 86–93.

Hays, R. B., Turner, H., & Coates, T. J. (1992). Social support, AIDS-related symptoms, and depression among gay men. *Journal of Consulting and Clinical Psychology, 60*(3), 463–469.

Hendin, H. (1982). *Suicide in America.* New York: W. W. Norton.

Herek, G. M., & Berrill, K. T. (1992). Documenting the victimization of lesbians and gay men: Methodological issues. In G.P. Herek and K. T. Berrill (Eds.), *Hate crimes: Confronting violence against lesbians and gay men* (pp. 270–286). Newbury Park, CA: Sage.

Hooker, E. (1956). The adjustment of the male overt homosexual. In H. M. Ruittenbeck (Ed.), *The problem of homosexuality in modern America* (pp. 141–161). New York: Dutton.

Hopkins, P. D. (1992). Gender treachery: Homophobia, masculinity, and threatened identities. In L. May & R. Strikwerda (Eds.), *Rethinking masculinity* (pp. 111–131). Boston Way, MD: Littlefield Adams.

Hunter, J. (1990). Violence against lesbian and gay male youths. *Journal of Interpersonal Violence, 5*(3), 295–300.

Icard, L. (1985–1986, Fall–Winter). Black gay men and conflicting social identities: Sexual orientation versus racial identity. *Social Work, 4*(1–2), 83–93.

Isrealstam, S., & Lambert, S. (1984). Gay bars. *Journal of Drug Issues, 14,*637–653.

Janoff-Bulman, R. (1982). Esteem and control bases of blame: "Adaptive" strategies for victims versus observers. *Journal of Personality, 50,* 180–192.

Janoff-Bulman, R. (1992). *Shattered assumptions: Towards a new psychology of trauma.* New York: Free Press.

Judson, F. N. (1977). Sexually transmitted disease in gay men. *Sexually Transmitted Diseases, 4,* 76–78.

Kass, N. E., Faden, R. R., Fox, R., & Dudley, J. (1992). Homosexual and bisexual men's perceptions of discrimination in health services. *American Journal of Public Health, 82,* 1277–1279.

Katz, J. N. (1995). *The invention of heterosexuality.* New York: Dutton.

Kelly, J. T., Kalichman, S. C., Kauth, M. R., Kilgore, H.G., Hood, H. V., Campos, P. E., Rao, S. M., Brasfield, T. L., & St. Lawrence, J. S. (1991). Situational factors associated with AIDS risk behavior lapses and coping strategies used by gay men who successfully avoid lapses. *American Journal of Public Health, 81,* 1335–1338.

Kelly, J. A., St. Lawrence, J. S., Smith, S., Jr., Hood, H. V., & Cook, D.J. (1987a). Medical students' attitudes toward AIDS and homosexual patients. *Journal of Medical Education, 62,* 549–556.

Kelly, J. A., St. Lawrence, J. S., Smith, S., Jr., Hood, H. V., & Cook, D. J. (1987b). Stigmatization of AIDS patients by physicians. *American Journal of Public Health, 77*(7), 789–791.

Kiernan, J. G. (1892, May). Responsibility in sexual perversion. *Chicago Medical Recorder, 3,* 185–210.

Krafft-Ebing, R. v. (1893). *Psychopathia sexualis, with especial reference to contrary sexual instinct: A medico-legal study* [translated by Gilbert Chaddock]. Philadelphia: F. A. Davis.

Kus, R. J. (1987). Alcoholics Anonymous and gay American men. In E. Coleman (Ed.), *Psychotherapy with homosexual men and women: Integrated identity approaches for clinical practice* (pp. 253–276). New York: Haworth Press.

Lackner, J. B., Joseph, J. G., Ostrow, D. G., Kessler, R. C., Eshleman, S., Wortman, C. B., O'Brien, K., Phair, J. P., & Chmiel, J. (1993). A longitudinal study of psychological distress in a cohort of gay men: Effects of social support and coping strategies. *Journal of Nervous and Mental Disease, 181,* 4–12.

Leigh, B. C., & Stall, R. (1993). Substance use and risky sexual behavior for exposure to HIV: Issues in methodology, interpretation, and prevention. *American Psychologist, 48,* 1035–1045.

Lewes, K. (1988). *The psychoanalytic theory of male homosexuality.* New York: Simon and Schuster.

Malyon, A. K. (1985). Psychotherapeutic implications of internalized homophobia in gay men. In J. C. Gonsiorek (Ed.), *A guide to psychotherapy with gay and lesbian clients* (pp. 59–69). New York: Harrington Park Press.

Martin, J. L., & Dean, L. (1993). Effects of AIDS-related bereavement and HIV-related illness on psychological distress among gay men: A 7-year longitudinal study, 1985–1991. *Journal of Consulting and Clinical Psychology, 61*(1), 94–103.

Mayer, K. H. (1983). Medical consequences of the inhalation of volatile nitrites. In D. G. Ostrow, T. A. Sandholzer, & Y. M. Felman (Eds.), *Sexually transmitted diseases in homosexual men: diagnosis, treatment and research* (pp. 237–242). New York: Plenum Press.

139

McDonald, G. J. (1982). Individual differences in the coming out process for gay men. *Journal of Homosexuality, 8,* 47–60.

McGrory, B. J., McDowell, D. M., & Muskin, P. R. (1990). Medical students' attitudes toward AIDS, homosexuals, and intravenous drug-abusing patients: A re-evaluation in New York City. *Psychosomatics, 31,* 426–433.

Modrcin, M. J., & Wyers, N. L. (1990). Lesbian and gay couples: Where they turn when help is needed. *Journal of Gay & Lesbian Psychotherapy, 1*(3), 89–104.

Murphy, T. F. (1992). Redirecting sexual orientation: Techniques and justifications. *Journal of Sex Research, 29*(4), 501–523.

National Gay and Lesbian Task Force. (1984). *Anti-gay/lesbian victimization: A study by the National Gay Task Force in cooperation with gay and lesbian organizations in eight U.S. cities.* Washington, DC: Author.

National Gay and Lesbian Task Force. (1990). *Anti-gay violence, victimization and defamation in 1989.* Washington, DC: Author.

Newman, B. S., & Muzzonigro, P. G. (1993). The effects of traditional family values on the coming out process of gay male adolescents. *Adolescence, 28*(109), 213–226.

Ostrow, D. G., VanRaden, M. J., Fox, R., Kingsley, L.A., Dudley, J., Kaslow, R. A., & the Multicenter AIDS Cohort Study (MACS) (1990). Recreational drug use and sexual behavior change in a cohort of homosexual men. *AIDS, 4,* 759–765.

Owen, W. F. (1985). Medical problems of the homosexual adolescent. *Journal of Adolescent Health Care, 6,* 278–285.

Paroski, P. A. (1987). Health care delivery and the concerns of gay and lesbian adolescents. *Journal of Adolescent Health Care, 8,* 188–192.

Paul, W., Weinrich, J. D., Gonsiorek, J., & Hotvedt, M. (1982). *Homosexuality: Social, psychological, and biological issues.* Beverly Hills, CA: Sage.

Prichard, J. G., Dial, L. K., Holloway, R. L., Mosley, M., Bale, R. M., & Kaplowitz, H. J. (1988). Attitudes of family medicine residents toward homosexuality. *Journal of Family Practice, 27,* 637–639.

Pronger, B. (1991). *The arena of masculinity: Sports, homosexuality, and the meaning of sex.* New York: St. Martin's Press.

Quam, J. K., & Whitford, G. S. (1992). Adaptation of age-related expectations of older gay and lesbian adults. *Gerontologist, 32*(3), 367–374.

Rado, S. (1962). *Psychoanalysis of behavior II.* New York: Grune & Stratton.

Remafedi, G. (1987). Male homosexuality: The adolescent's perspective. *Pediatrics, 79,* 326–330.

Rich, C. L., Fowler, R. C., & Blenkush, M. (1986). San Diego suicide study: Comparison of gay to straight males. *Suicide and Life Threatening Behavior, 16*(4), 448–457.

Rosenberger, P. H., Bornstein, R. A., Nasrallah, H. A., Para, M. F., Whitaker, C. C., Fass, R. J., & Rice, R. R. (1993).

Psychopathology in human immunodeficiency virus infection: Lifetime and current assessment. *Comprehensive Psychiatry, 34*(3), 150–158.

Rotheram-Borus, M. J., & Gwadz, M. (1993). Sexuality among youths at high risk. *Child and Adolescent Psychiatric Clinics of North America, 2,* 415–431.

Rotheram-Borus, M. J., Rosario, M., Meyer-Bahlburg, H. F. L., Koopman, C., Dopkins, S. C., & Davies, M. (1994). Sexual and substance use acts of gay and bisexual male adolescents in New York City. *Journal of Sex Research, 31*(1), 47–57.

Sadava, S. W. & Thompson, M. M. (1986). Loneliness, social drinking, and vulnerability to alcohol problems. *Canadian Journal of Behavioral Science, 8,* 133–139.

Saghir, M. T., & Robins, E. (1973). *Male and female homosexuality: A comprehensive investigation.* Baltimore, MD: Williams & Wilkins.

Saunders, J. M., & Valente, S. M. (1987). Suicide risk among gay men and lesbians: A review. *Death Studies, 11,* 1–23.

Savin-Williams, R. C. (1990). *Gay and lesbian youth: Expressions of identity.* Washington, DC: Hemisphere.

Savin-Williams, R. C. (1994). Verbal and physical abuse as stressors in the lives of lesbian, gay male, and bisexual youths: Associations with school problems, running away, substance abuse, prostitution, and suicide. *Journal of Consulting and Clinical Psychology, 62*(2), 261–269.

"Score card #2." (1994, June). *OUT,* No. 13, 103.

Shilts, R. (1987). *And the band played on: Politics, people, and the AIDS epidemic.* New York: St. Martin's Press.

Siegel, K., Mesagno, F. P., Chen, J. Y., & Christ, G. (1989). Factors distinguishing homosexual males practicing risky and safer sex. *Social Science Medicine, 28,* 561–569.

Siever, M. D. (1994). Sexual orientation and gender as factors in sociocultural acquired vulnerability to body dissatisfaction and eating disorders. *Journal of Consulting and Clinical Psychology, 62*(2) 252–260.

Smith, T. M. (1982). Specific approaches and techniques in the treatment of gay male alcohol abusers. *Journal of Homosexuality, 7,* 53–69.

Socarides, C. W. (1978). *Homosexuality.* New York: Jason Aronson.

Strommen, E. F. (1989). "You're a what?": Family member reactions to the disclosure of homosexuality. *Journal of Homosexuality, 18*(1/2), 37–58.

Townsend, M. H., Wallick, M. M., & Cambre, K. M. (1993). Gay and lesbian issues in residency training at U.S. psychiatry programs. *Academic Psychiatry, 17,* 67–72.

Walters, K. L., & Simoni, J. M. (1993). Lesbian and gay male group identity attitudes and self-esteem: Implications for counseling. *Journal of Counseling Psychology, 40*(1), 94–99.

Williams, J. B. W., Rabkin, J. G., Remien, R. H., Gorman, J. P., & Ehrhardt, A. A. (1991). Multidisciplinary baseline assessment of homosexual men with and without human immunodeficiency virus infection: Standardized clinical assessment of current and lifetime psychopathology. *Archives of General Psychiatry, 48,* 124–130.

Woodman, N. J. (1989). Mental health issues of relevance to lesbian women and gay men. *Journal of Gay & Lesbian Psychotherapy, 1*(1), 53–64.

Yates, G. L., MacKenzie, R. G., Pennbridge, J., & Swofford, A. (1991). A risk profile comparison of homeless youth involved in prostitution and homeless youth not involved. *Journal of Adolescent Health, 12,* 545–548.

Zehner, M. A., & Lewis, J. (1983). Homosexuality and alcoholism: Social and developmental perspectives. *Journal of Social Work and Human Sexuality, 2,* 75–89.

7

Health Behavior in Lesbians

Holly C. VanScoy

INTRODUCTION

There is a considerable body of scholarly research on the health behavior of lesbians in the United States. Most of this research has been undertaken since the mid-1970s; the number of articles and books published from 1984 to 1993 was approximately 5 times greater than the number published in the previous 10-year period (VanScoy, in press). This increase generally parallels the growth in most fields of practice and research, of awareness of two phenomena: (1) that health issues for all groups in the general population are not identical and (2) that neither the treatment of all groups by nor the responses of all groups to the health care system are necessarily comparable.

Lesbians are members of two specific populations—women and homosexuals—whose health behavior has received increased attention in the professional literature over the last decade. Without question, lesbian health research has been strongly influenced by and clearly reflects society's increased interest in and support for schol-

arly inquiry into the activities of females and homosexuals in general. But the most recent research—particularly since 1985—has focused on lesbians as a distinct population, moving well beyond considering them merely as subsets of the female and homosexual populations. These newer works implicitly reject the assumption that lesbian health behavior can be understood simply as an intersection of the attitudes, motivations, needs, or actions of other groups (e.g., Eliason, Donelan, & Randall, 1992). Many researchers make this sharpened focus on lesbians explicit in their work and take care to explain that lesbians have often been overlooked in studies of women's health care, as well as in studies of the homosexual population. Trippet and Bain (1992, p. 145) note that "lesbians perceive themselves differently from the way opposite-sex-oriented women or same-sex-oriented men perceive themselves."

As this chapter will demonstrate, although the health behavior of lesbians has only recently begun to gain recognition and acceptance as unique, a number of themes and issues have already begun to be identified. This emerging research base, in combination with valuable evidence from earlier, less specifically focused inquiries, provides a valuable starting point for understanding and serving the lesbian health care consumer and for framing additional schol-

Holly C. VanScoy • Academic Research Associates, Inc., Grand Rapids, Michigan 49506.

Handbook of Health Behavior Research III: Demography, Development, and Diversity, edited by David S. Gochman. Plenum Press, New York, 1997.

arly inquiries into the health behavior of this population.

LESBIAN PERSPECTIVES ON SELF, ILLNESS, AND HEALTH

The Multiple Constructions of Lesbian Identity

There is no single definition of the word *lesbian*, although many adults—and probably most individuals providing health services—consider the term appropriately applied to a woman who engages or desires to engage in sexual behavior with another female. As Lynch (1993, p. 196) observed, however, "Heterosexual people are not solely defined by their sexual activity; neither should be lesbian women." The term *lesbian identity*, coined by Browning (1984), is a much broader and more comprehensive term and one that takes into account considerably more than the type of sexual relationships in a woman's life.

The importance of understanding the multifaceted influences on the construction of lesbian identity is reflected strongly in most post-1980s research on the health behavior of this population. This emphasis has gradually begun to encourage health care providers to take into account the social, emotional, economic, affectional, political, and medical contexts of this population's identity, rather than to focus solely on overt or explicit sexual activities (Stevens & Hall, 1991). As Lynch (1993, p. 196) noted, the term "lesbian" may accurately be used to refer to the social, emotional, erotic, and political identity of homosexual women.

Within the lesbian population, the most general understanding of the term—and the meaning with which most lesbians most readily agree—is that a *lesbian* is a *woman-identified woman*, or a woman for whom other females play the majority of, if not all, important life roles, including but not limited to friend, confidant, political associate, co-parent, business associate, and spouse

or sexual partner. Lesbians are therefore not dependent upon males in the same ways as or to the same extent that heterosexual females in American society are, and this independence almost always extends well beyond the realm of sexual relationships. A woman, in fact, may identify herself as a lesbian but have no female partner (or spouse); it may even be the case, if she does have a female partner, that their relationship may not include sexual behavior. When lesbian identity is constructed by lesbians themselves, it generally has a much broader meaning than the identity ascribed by nonlesbians, including nonlesbian individuals or groups within the health care system. Moreover, it is likely to be constructed in terms of contexts other than sexual (Lockard, 1985).

Only since the mid-1980s has it become relatively common for research on the health issues, health care needs, and health behaviors of this population to reflect consideration of the importance of understanding lesbians' own construction of their identity (e.g., Dritz, 1985; M. Smith, Heaton, & Siever, 1990) or, as Eliason et al. (1992, p. 133) have termed it, *lesbian epistemology*, or ways of knowing the world.

Stevens and Hall (1988, p. 69) proposed that "for lesbian women, the cultural meanings of illness and wellness are linked to lesbian identity, which is an immutable quality that permeates and differentiates the self." A relatively early work by Ponse (1978) on the social construction of lesbian identity continues to be among the most widely cited in the health literature. More recent research, however, has provided descriptions and elaborations of additional contexts, most of which have a strong emphasis on understanding the developmental character of personal identity formation. These studies include Hollander and Haber's (1992) adaptation of Brofenbrenner's model and Lynch's (1993) refinement of Raymond and Blumfield's (1988) developmental schema. These identity models have generally been used as the underpinning for explorations of self-disclosure as a health behavior with significant implications for the lesbian population. (Exceptions to this use of an identity model include Hepburn and Gutierrez's [1988] more holistic approach to identity development, which is infused throughout their work, *Alive and Well: A Lesbian Health Guide*, and Hetrick and Martin's [1987] model describing adolescent social development in homosexuals.)

The purpose of including various identity models in research studies has at times been discussed openly by authors, most with the same goal in mind. Hollander and Haber (1992), for example, viewed the inclusion of identity contexts in research as an important part of efforts to effect change in the behavior of *health care providers*, suggesting that further education would afford them an ecological base for understanding lesbian lifestyles and would allow them to recognize that "lesbians are multifaceted just like everyone else and not merely women who have sex with other women" (p. 128).

Western Medical Tradition as Patriarchy

In addition to describing lesbian health behavior in terms of identity contexts, a number of works provide insight into this population's perspective on Western (allopathic) medical tradition, particularly the institutional characteristics of this tradition that have been incorporated into the health care system in the United States. As scholarship on lesbians makes evident, the health care behavior of this population must be interpreted within this perspective to be fully understood.

In this respect, research on lesbians' health experiences shows considerable kinship with feminist efforts on the same topic (Pharr, 1988). From a feminist perspective, the health care system in the United States (and other Western democracies) is viewed as a system that has historically been dominated by men and oppressive of women. French (1992, p. 132), in fact, asserted, "The male medical profession *began as a war on women*." Two of the weapons employed by the medical profession in waging this war have been

ignoring and medicalizing women's health concerns. The process of *medicalizing* has meant that the health care system defined female "distinctives" (such as pregnancy, childbirth, menstruation, and menopause) as abnormal, i.e., in need of medical intervention. The process of *ignoring* has meant that valid and common health concerns of women received little or no systematic attention in health care research, education, or practice. Wallick, Cambre, and Townsend (1992), for example, found that the mean amount of time devoted to the topic of homosexuality in a 4-year medical program was about 3½ hours; only a small fraction of this brief period was addressed specifically to lesbian concerns.

A valuable contribution to the process of developing the widest contextual framework for understanding lesbian health behavior was made by Stevens and Hall (1991), who discussed the medical construction of lesbianism as a potent force that, in conjunction with traditional cultural ideologies regarding female and homosexual behavior, created a health care system in which lesbian behavior has been pathologized. Moreover, because of the status and power that health professions—particularly medicine—have had in Western culture, the medical construction of lesbianism has been viewed as having strong influence on a variety of public policies, as well as on the treatment by the health care system. This influence was codified in 1942 when the American Psychiatric Association (APA) declared homosexuality (including lesbianism) to be a medical diagnosis (Gonsiorek & Weinrich, 1991), an action that produced far-reaching implications for lesbians legally, economically, politically, socially, and medically. As a population considered "sick" or "crazy" by virtue of their identity, lesbians became increasingly subjected to the health care system's treatment-oriented efforts to modify (i.e., "cure") their thoughts, feelings, and behaviors—including those that had little or nothing to do with sexual expression or affectional preference.

Reversal of this medicalization of lesbian identity has been and continues to be slow in coming. It was not until 1973, when the APA finally removed homosexuality from the list of mental disorders, that significant modifications in the process began to occur. Even this progress has been halting, at best. In 1974, for instance, the re-incorporation of homosexuality into the list of mental disorders was considered by the APA, garnering the support of 37% of its members—not enough to reverse the decision of the previous year, but enough to provide evidence that even within the enlightened field of psychiatric practice, more than one third of the practitioners had not accepted the premise that homosexuals are inherently normal human beings. Schwanberg (1985, 1990) and others have discussed at length the considerable body of medical research that has been directed toward establishing *lesbianism* itself as a medical disorder (Romm, 1965; Socarides, 1992). Lynch (1993, p. 196) suggested that "allopathic medicine and psychiatry, in particular, have been the main agents for the 'disease' or 'disorder' view" of this population. The more recent medical research base is not without similar works, although current efforts generally seek to provide genetic, hormonal, or psychological explanations for lesbianism (e.g., Bower, 1992; Dancey, 1990).

Stevens (1992) concluded that medical theories throughout the 20th century scapegoated and pathologized lesbians, noting that until the mid-1970s this population was characterized by the medical profession as "sick, dangerous, aggressive, tragically unhappy, deceitful, contagious, and self-destructive" (p. 91). In addition, lesbians were subjected—at times involuntarily—to exploitative medical care designed to cure their lesbianism, including commitment to psychiatric treatment facilities, electroshock treatment, genital mutilation, aversive therapy, psychosurgery, hormonal injection, psychoanalysis, and psychotropic chemotherapy. These treatments continued despite mounting evidence that no scientific research evidence was ever produced to support their effectiveness (Gonsiorek & Weinrich, 1991).

Lesbians' encounters with the health care system have reflected not only the system's diagnosis and treatment of lesbianism as illness, but also its incorporation of the larger society's judgment that lesbianism is a crime and a sin. The impact of this perspective has been evident in health care research as well as health care practice: The only studies about lesbian health concerns for many decades were those focused on diagnosing lesbianism and discovering its "causes" and "cure." This history of medicalizing lesbian identity as well as other concerns of women while ignoring other female health issues is well known to much of the lesbian population today, and this knowledge has a significant impact on their health care behaviors (Stevens, 1992, pp. 91–92).

As O'Donnell, Pollack, Leoffler, and Saunders (1979) noted in *Lesbian Health Matters!*: "It seems unlikely that a sexist and heterosexist power structure would support work that could prove lesbians are healthy human beings." This echoed Chafetz, Sampson, Beck, and West's (1974, p. 714) conclusion that "male-dominated science has not taken women, including lesbians, seriously enough to engage in the necessary research on which the helping professions could adequately base their theory and practice."

It is not uncommon for lesbians to view the United States medical care system as an extension of patriarchal society, a society that devalues women generally and homosexual women specifically (Dworkin & Gutierrez, 1989; Stevens & Hall, 1990). Eliason, et al. (1992, pp. 132–133) discussed the relationship of this perspective to lesbians' health behaviors, suggesting that lesbians are perceived as a major threat to the patriarchy because they are not potential partners for men and do not follow traditional rules for women in contemporary society. Homophobia is generally viewed as the primary response to this threat and has been documented as pervasive in all health care professions—including psychology, medicine, social work, and nursing—where it has been clearly seen to have detrimental effects on lesbians seeking care.

Homophobia and Heterosexism in the Health Care System

A number of studies have documented lesbians' perceptions that the health care system harbors any or all of homophobic, heterosexist, and sexist attitudes, and most have included an interpretation of lesbian health behavior as a reaction to these systemic characteristics. Many of these studies have explored the influences of homophobia, heterosexism, and sexism on lesbians within the health care system as a whole (e.g., Douglas, Kalman, & Kalman, 1985; Gentry, 1992). Others have focused on the impacts of homophobic, heterosexist, and sexist attitudes and behaviors on lesbians requiring or receiving services in specialized fields of professional practice, including mental health and substance abuse (e.g., Browning, Reynolds, & Dworkin, 1991; Hall, 1990, 1993, 1994; Neisen, 1990), sex education and therapy (Ellis, 1985; Nichols, 1989), gynecological–obstetric care (e.g., Conway & Humphries, 1994; Johnson, Smith, & Buenther, 1987; Zeidenstein, 1990), gerontology (e.g., Deevey, 1990; LoBiondo-Wood, 1986), and adolescent health care (e.g., Owen, 1985; Remafedi, 1990).

In such research, *homophobia* is most often defined as "an irrational fear of homosexuality" (Eliason et al., 1992, p. 132); *heterosexism*, as an assumption that heterosexuality or male–female sexual expression is the "superior and only life option" (Lynch, 1993, p. 193); and *sexism*, as a focus primarily or exclusively on male health concerns or services, or on health roles for women (including those of service providers or service recipients or both) that are subordinate to those of men (Elder, Humphreys, & Lakowski, 1988).

When the homophobic, heterosexist, and sexist characteristics of the health care system collide, as it were, with the personal identity issues of the lesbian population, a constellation of behaviors—which may be broadly characterized as the health behaviors of lesbians—have been repeatedly documented by researchers. The consensus of findings is that these behaviors result not so much from different health care needs or concerns in this population as from lesbians' reactions to the homophobic, heterosexist, and sexist characteristics of the health care system. Simply stated, lesbian health behavior has been generally documented to result most directly from the way lesbians have historically been diagnosed and treated (or ignored)—or from the ways they anticipate being treated (or ignored)—in health settings, and not from any inherent health concerns related principally or solely to their lesbian identity (Johnson, Guenther, Laube, & Keettel, 1981; M. Smith et al., 1990).

Lynch (1993, p. 196) found that women who are lesbians did not have any "discreet clinical problems 'caused' by their lesbianism." Their health issues were no different from other women's health issues. They primarily wanted good health care, meaning they wanted to (1) be viewed holistically; (2) receive the correct information about prevention, diagnosis, and treatment for their legitimate health concerns, and (3) receive respectful and sensitive physical examinations and care, including prevention services.

HEALTH ACTIONS OF THE LESBIAN POPULATION

Enough specific actions have been discussed with sufficient detail in the professional literature to provide meaning to a collective term such as *lesbian health action* or *activity*. It is important to recognize, however, that lesbian health actions may vary considerably among individual lesbians and that their actions are strongly influenced not only by their lesbianism, but also by such factors as their age, race, ethnic and/or linguistic background, economic resources, occupational status, experience with (or desire to experience) pregnancy and parenting, and particular health or wellness concern (Cochran & Mays, 1988; Stern, 1993). Lesbians are no more homogeneous than any other population in these respects. As the landmark women's alternative health publication *The New Our Bodies, Ourselves* (Lesbian Revisions Group, 1992, p. 178) explained, they are "numerous in every economic group, social class, and political persuasion"; are employed in every occupational setting, experience physical disabilities and illness just as other women do, may have or plan to have children or be certain they will remain childless and "find this a freeing choice"; have relationships that last a lifetime or are celibate; and may be "married to men and cannot easily leave ... marriages," yet they all "make primary commitments to women."

Some of the research on the health behavior of lesbians is careful to underscore the importance of considering individual lesbians' characteristics and not overgeneralizing the findings of studies with relatively limited samples (usually comprised of women who are young, English-speaking, white, middle-class, well educated, and comfortable identifying themselves as lesbians) to all homosexual women (Greene, 1994; Stevens, 1994). Even when a research effort has included a large sample of lesbians (e.g., Bradford & Ryan, 1988; Michigan Organization for Human Rights [MOHR], 1991), the investigators have cautioned others about the inherent limitations of their findings because so much of the health behavior within many lesbian subcultures has yet to be systematically examined.

On the basis of the evidence provided by the current research base, however, certain health care actions or activities can be viewed as representative of the segments of the lesbian population that have received attention. A recent study by Stevens (1994)—notable, in part, for its inclusion of a multiethnic, socioeconomically diverse sample—formulated a description for certain health activities described as "protective strategies for unsafe environments." These strategic actions include rallying support, screening providers, maintaining vigilance, controlling information, bringing a witness, challenging mistreatment (negotiating, registering complaints, and striking a pose [i.e., assuming an assertive role]), and escaping danger. Hitchcock and Wilson

(1992) described and labeled several other lesbian health activities, many of which overlap with Steven's, including formalizing the lesbian relationship (e.g., securing a durable power of attorney for a partner to make medical decisions), scouting out (which is similar to Stevens's "maintaining vigilance"), screening, and networking. It is likely that future research will explore the prevalence and varied forms of these particular activities within other lesbian cohorts.

Six specific actions, including some of those described by Stevens (1994) and Hitchcock and Wilson (1992), have received the greatest attention in the literature through the mid-1990s and will be discussed in greater detail:

- Avoiding the traditional health care system altogether (with the exception of mental health services).
- Relying on any or all of alternative health care providers, partners, friends, and self for broadly based, holistic health care.
- Delaying health care.
- Not disclosing lesbian identity to health care providers.
- Selecting lesbian or other female providers, when available.
- Seeking and using substance abuse and mental health services, programs, or support groups.

Each of these actions or activities has been documented many times in the professional literature on this population, and although the actions have been described with a variety of terms, there is considerable overlap in the specific behavior manifestations documented. The most cogent of these are summarized below.

Avoiding the Traditional Health Care System

More than a decade ago, the Lyon-Martin Clinic in San Francisco reported that the most significant risk to lesbians' health was their avoidance of routine health care (Peteros & Miller, 1982). The growing research base provides support for the conclusion that a greater percentage of lesbians, in comparison to heterosexual females, avoid seeking health care within the traditional health care system (e.g., Jay & Young, 1979; O'Donnell, 1978). The evidence available suggests that this avoidance may be either the result of a negative personal experience within health care settings, the anticipation of encountering a negative experience (based on the experiences of other lesbians), or both (Beunting, 1992; Stevens & Hall, 1988).

Stevens (1994, p. 218) reported that this population is "commonly subjected to antagonism when they seek care." Rooted in the homophobia, heterosexism, and sexism discussed earlier, the activities of health care providers have been perceived by lesbian research subjects as uncaring, intolerant, ill-informed, hostile, negative, voyeuristic, rough, threatening, insensitive, irrelevant, offensive, derogatory, and demeaning (e.g., Geddes, 1994; Saunders, Tupac, & MacCullough, 1988). In a review of 19 studies on lesbian health care experiences published in the 20-year period from 1970 to 1990, Stevens (1992, p. 109) found that anti-lesbian ideas and sentiments were obvious in the behaviors of providers. Moreover, trends in the research findings remained unchanged over time and were similar in all parts of the country. Subjects generally believed that health care providers knew little about lesbians, but condemned their lifestyle. These women viewed health care providers as hostile and rejecting and feared for their own safety in health care interactions. They were often reluctant to seek care as a result of these attitudes and behaviors.

The finding that lesbians "feared for their safety" suggests a subjective perception of danger that is usually considered antithetical to competent, useful health care, yet this perception has been reported frequently in the literature (e.g., Lucas, 1992; Zeidenstein, 1990). The research by Stevens (1994) detailing 223 health encounters by lesbians provided confirmation of previous findings. This multiethnic, socioeconomically diverse sample of lesbians were in agreement in

their belief that as a general rule, obtaining health care was a dangerous undertaking (p. 220).

In the largest study focused on this population's "failure to seek traditional health care," Trippet and Bain's (1992, p. 148) sample of 503 women—78% of whom identified themselves as lesbian on the research instrument—provided five specific reasons for their avoidance: (1) Low-cost, natural, or alternative care is not provided; (2) holistic care is not provided; (3) little preventive care and education are provided; (4) communication and respect are lacking; and (5) few women-managed clinics are available. Dardick and Grady (1980), Reagan (1981), and others confirmed that anticipation of negative reactions from health care providers was the greatest factor influencing lesbians' avoidance. This conclusion was supported by Stevens and Hall's (1988) finding that 72% of the lesbians surveyed *had* experienced a negative reaction when they disclosed their sexual identity. As within any non-majority population, the experience of one lesbian often has a significant impact on the subsequent activities of other lesbians, who may (accurately) anticipate like experiences in a similar situation. Thus, one woman's negative health care interaction can have a "ripple effect" through a much larger segment of the lesbian community and deter many others from seeking care in that particular setting, from that specific provider, or anywhere within the traditional system. Thus, 84% of Stevens and Hall's sample described a general reluctance to seek health care, not only because of how they had been treated, but also because of what they knew about the treatment of other lesbians.

Hepburn and Gutierrez (1988), writing as two openly lesbian women, acknowledged the difficulty lesbians have in confronting the medical establishment in the person of a professional health care provider. The assumption of heterosexuality and the affectation of superiority were noted to be "too much for most of us" (p. 11). The result, they suggest, is that lesbians are likely to avoid routine health care and seek help only when faced with a specific crisis.

In Robertson's (1992) study of 10 lesbians, "none of the subjects received any routine health care, and some felt yearly examinations were not necessary" (p. 161). E. M. Smith, Johnson, and Guenther (1985) found that 58% of their sample sought gynecological care only when a problem occurred, while Stevens and Hall (1988) reported an even larger percentage (84%) of their sample "reluctant" to seek health care. Bradford and Ryan (1988) reported that for women who did not seek health care, the principal reasons were financial constraints and lesbians' reliance on self-care (largely as a consequence of an earlier negative health care experience).

The contrasting effect of positive health care experiences on lesbian activities has also been documented (Stevens & Hall, 1988). Not surprisingly, lesbians reported that they sought out health care settings in which and providers from whom they knew other members of the lesbian population had received sensitive, accepting, and competent health care. In many communities across the country, an informal "referral network" among lesbians facilitates the connection between individual women in need of health services and providers who have delivered appropriate care to other members of this population (Hitchcock & Wilson, 1992).

Relying on Alternative Providers, Friends, or Self for Care

Numerous studies have examined the types of health care providers used by lesbians who do not access the traditional system (e.g., Johnson & Palermo, 1984; Johnson et al., 1981; Robertson, 1992). In general, at least some use of "alternative" (i.e., other than allopathic) health care providers has been reported by about 35–45% of each sample. Alternative providers specifically named included women's health clinics, chiropractors, homeopathic practitioners, masseuses, body workers, acupuncture and accupressure practitioners, biofeedback specialists, nutritionists, nurse-midwives, yoga and meditation instructors, and herbalists (Hepburn & Gutierrez,

1988; Robertson, 1992; Stevens & Hall, 1988; Trippet & Bain, 1992).

Beunting's (1992) comparison of 27 lesbians to 52 heterosexual women found that the "health lifestyles" of the two groups were significantly different in terms of six characteristics, with lesbians showing higher mean scores on incorporation of alternative diet, meditation/relaxation techniques, and use of recreational drugs. Study results were reported to "contribute to a perception of a more holistic health orientation among the lesbian women in this sample" (p. 170). Trippet and Bain (1992) found that as a result of dissatisfaction with Western medical approaches of medication and surgery, lesbians in their sample "sought alternative health practices that are less invasive and more in tune with the human body and nature" (pp. 148–149). Studies by Johnson, Smith, and Guenther (1987) and E. M. Smith et al. (1985) based on a large sample of lesbians also found that use of alternative health care was positively correlated with women's beliefs that personal disclosure would negatively affect the quality of health care provided within the traditional system.

Another finding of interest has been that a significant number of lesbians provide their own health care. In their 1984 survey of more than 2000 lesbians nationwide, Bradford and Ryan (1988) found that many of their respondents, particularly those between the ages of 40 and 60, were meeting their own health care needs. In this study, 9% of their sample said they cared for their own obstetrical–gynecological needs, and 24% reported that they cared for other health problems (Bradford & Ryan, 1991).

Bradford and Ryan (1991, p. 155) also reported on their sample's heavy reliance on alternative mental health resources, noting that "over 60 percent relied upon non-professional sources, primarily from friends, support groups or peer counselors. Nine percent had consulted psychics and seven percent, religious counselors." Several older works also documented the tendency of lesbians to utilize friends as health care providers (Chafetz et al., 1974; Saunders et al., 1988). More recently, Stevens (1994, p. 221) documented lesbians' reliance on friendship networks as an important aspect of the health action strategy described as *rallying support*. When lesbians rallied support, they offered each other health information, diagnostic suggestions, tangible assistance with activities of daily living, and caregiving. The behavior also included validating one another's strengths and competencies and commiserating about losses and discomforts, as well as helping each other bear the weight of infirmity and entering into legal contracts, when appropriate (e.g., legal or durable power of attorney).

Delaying Health Care

Rather than avoiding the traditional health care system altogether, many lesbians simply delay or postpone their utilization of this system until a health care need constitutes a medical crisis or emergency (e.g., Glascock, 1981; Stevens & Hall, 1988; Zeidenstein, 1990). Again, much of the research suggests that delaying is related to lesbians' perception of a real or potential threat within the health care environment. A participant in Stevens's (1994) research expressed this concern vividly, noting that as a lesbian, she had tried to "stay away" as a method of dealing with "health care providers' assumptions and their homophobia" (p. 220).

Stevens (1992) noted several other characteristics of the health care system that were associated with both delayed help seeking and avoidance, including institutional structures and policies (such as denying partner participation, visitation, or other involvement), locating women's preventive health clinics in obstetric and birth control clinics (where the assumption of females' heterosexuality may be especially strong), ignoring outreach to the lesbian community, and inhibiting lesbian health care providers' disclosure of their own lesbianism (p. 113). Stevens and others (e.g., Bradford & Ryan, 1988; Glascock, 1981) also found that financial barriers prevent lesbians from seeking or securing care when treatment need arises and often result in delayed help seeking.

Not Disclosing Lesbian Identity to Health Care Providers

Without question, the lesbian health behavior discussed most widely in the literature is disclosure (or nondisclosure) of identity to health care providers or within the health care system (e.g., Deevey, 1990; Hall, 1994; Jones et al., 1984). Self-disclosure research gains particular relevance in a population such as lesbians, where an aspect of identity that is potentially problematic for an individual is not readily discernible to others (despite some health care providers' beliefs to the contrary). Unlike race, age, physical or mental ability, linguistic competence, weight, or ethnic origin—all of which may result in a negative response from members of the majority culture—a female's lesbianism cannot be detected by others. She must disclose her identity—or *come out*—to them if they are to know this aspect of her life (Moses, 1978). When a lesbian comes out to a health care provider, however, she generally knows or believes that she may be placing herself in an even more vulnerable situation than she was in as simply a female within a sexist system. Having come out, she will carry the identity of *homosexual* female in a sexist, heterosexist, and homophobic system, with all the stigma associated with this label (e.g., Markowitz, 1991; Sang, 1989).

Stevens (1992) noted that the degree of lesbians' openness about themselves is guided by the contingencies of particular interactions. Depending on the context, members of this population "must imaginatively construct the anticipated responses of others while balancing personal vulnerability and available resources, in an attempt to avoid social rejection, humiliation, restriction or attack" (p. 111). The question may well arise: Why would a woman voluntarily come out as a lesbian under such conditions? The research on self-disclosure provides a number of answers to this query.

Several works confirm that lesbians believe that the quality of their relationship with health providers would be improved if they felt free and safe to disclose their identities and share appropriate details of their social, emotional, and sexual lives (e.g., Johnson et al., 1981; Stevens, 1992). Moreover, many lesbians are aware that there are times when inappropriate care may be provided or necessary care overlooked if the provider assumes they are heterosexual. Nondisclosure in such instances creates circumstances in which they feel medically at risk or unsafe. These reasons for disclosure are often counterbalanced, however, by a host of compelling reasons to remain silent, including the fact that the topic of lesbianism is seldom introduced by health care providers, and this silence is perceived to signal the provider's lack of comfort with this information.

This provider behavior has been explored variously, including research on the belief that physicians can ascertain lesbian identity when it is not specifically disclosed to them. Good (1976) inquired about the process by which a sample of physicians determined whether a patient was a lesbian. Of the 72 subjects in this study who believed that they had ever provided services to at least one lesbian, more than one third claimed they were able to make this judgement using clinical observation. Of these 72 physicians, 9 reported that they asked women directly about their lesbian identity, while 38 noted that patients voluntarily disclosed it. Several studies of lesbians (e.g., E. M. Smith et al., 1985; Zeidenstein, 1991) have reported that most members of the study samples have never been asked directly about their lesbianism in a health care setting. A 1991 study of lesbian health by the Michigan Organization for Human Rights (MOHR) (1991) found that 61% of the 1681 respondents did not feel able to share their homosexuality with health providers.

Good (1976) also reported that more than 50% of the physician subjects—including 6 of the 7 female gynecologists in the sample—thought that they had never treated a lesbian. Commenting on these findings, Robertson (1992) noted that "this would seem unlikely, considering the estimate of female homosexuality by Kinsey is approximately 5%…[and] recent fig-

ures place the lesbian population at a minimum of 10%" (p. 126).

Many scholars, including Cochran and Mays (1988) and Hitchcock and Wilson (1992), have documented the persistence of health care providers' beliefs and activities related to the presumption of heterosexuality for all females over the past 15 years, a period during which—paradoxically—lesbian issues became quite visible in society as a whole. In every study, lesbians consistently reported subjectively experiencing the presumption of heterosexuality in medical history taking; discussions with providers about their sexual activities, need for and use of birth control, and sexually transmitted diseases; questions about marital status and family; and health care providers' tendency to discredit their partners and friends as significant others. The literature review by Stevens (1992) convincingly established that providers' heterosexual assumptions constitute a formidable obstacle to the delivery of effective health services to lesbians within the traditional system. The study found that providers usually assume that their female clients are heterosexuals who have male sexual partners and perform within normative social roles as wives and mothers in traditional family units (p. 110). This overwhelming assumption of heterosexuality undoubtedly has the effect of silencing lesbians who would otherwise be willing to disclose their identity, if they (1) were asked in a fashion that normalized the inquiry process, (2) were confident the information would remain confidential, and (3) believed that the information would be used to ensure the provision of care that did not harm or further stigmatize them.

The term *lesbian invisibility* has been coined and used extensively in the literature to describe one of the pervasive effects of this assumption of heterosexuality in all women (e.g., Deevy, 1990; Robertson 1992). This term has been used not only to describe health care interactions between patients and health providers, but also to indicate that the health care literature (both periodicals and textbooks) on lesbian concerns is relatively sparse considering the magnitude of this population, that inclusion of information on lesbians is virtually non-existent in health care education, and that provision of health care benefits for lesbians is markedly different from the health care benefits of women with male partners. The term *lesbian* is not used as a matter of course and frequently enough in the health care system to make providers comfortable with its use in everyday health care transactions.

Worth noting is the assertion by some researchers that lesbian invisibility is further exacerbated by health care providers' inability to distinquish lesbians' issues, needs, and concerns from those of homosexual males (Eliason & Randall, 1991). Their invisibility as women in a male-oriented society is mirrored to a considerable extent by their invisibility as lesbians in a homosexual subculture in which gay males receive the greatest public (and health care) attention. Although the modern "gay rights" movement has accomplished much in terms of providing visibility to the social, political, and civil rights concerns of all homosexuals, it has, in a sense, further blurred the distinctions between the behaviors and health care needs of lesbians and gay men, a distinction that has important ramifications in the provision of health services. For example, AIDS has often been characterized as a "gay disease," but according to the Centers for Disease Control and Prevention, lesbians with no self-history or partner history of bisexuality, heterosexuality, or intravenous drug use in the last 10 years are the lowest-risk group for contracting AIDS sexually (Chu, Beuhler, Fleming, & Berkleman, 1990; Zeidenstein, 1990). Yet several studies have documented a number of erroneous beliefs held by the public generally and health care providers specifically about the lesbian population and this viral disease (e.g., Gentry, 1992; Robertson, 1992). For instance, Randall (1987) found that 20% of nursing educators believed that lesbians are an important source of AIDS transmission; Douglas et al. (1985) reported that the association of AIDS with the homosexual population as a whole may increase lesbian phobia; and Randall (1987, 1989), Eliason and Randall (1991), and

Eliason et al. (1992) found that between 18% and 28% of the nursing students in their samples believed that lesbians are a high-risk group for HIV infection. Eliason et al. (1992, p. 371) concluded that although most of the subjects had been exposed to factual knowledge that explicitly stated that lesbians are a low-risk group for HIV infection and transmission, these nurses continued to associate lesbians with the disease because HIV, AIDS, and the gay lifestyle are inextricably linked in their minds.

Stevens's (1993) research on nonsexually transmitted HIV infection (via such behaviors as injection drug use, blood transfusion, and artificial insemination) in lesbians is an example of new scholarship that may eventually serve to dispel these misconceptions.

Eliason et al. (1992) provided additional information about lesbian stereotypes that has relevance to discussions of disclosure behaviors. Several major themes or *lesbian stereotypes* emerged from their research on the perceptions of 278 female nursing students. These students believed that (1) lesbians seduce heterosexual women; (2) lesbians have an "aura of masculinity" (i.e., "want to be men"); (3) lesbianism is biologically unnatural, or in violation of moral, ethical or religious principles; (4) lesbians are "rampantly sexual" or "too blatant" about their lifestyles; (5) lesbians are a bad influence on children; and (6) lesbians spread sexually transmitted diseases (pp. 138–140). It is not difficult to predict what type of reflexive actions these stereotypes would provoke in almost any population to which they are systematically applied. Stevens's (1994) notion of lesbian "protective strategies" seems especially relevant in this context—i.e., lesbian nondisclosure can be viewed as one protective response to these stereotypical views.

Although some evidence has suggested that nondisclosure allows lesbians to "maintain a total charade" with health care providers about their identity (Hitchcock & Wilson, 1992, p. 182), nondisclosure has been found to exact a toll in terms of increased stress for the lesbian seeking health services (Franke & Leary, 1992; Gillow & Davis,

1987). For example, some research exploring disclosure patterns in greater detail has found that many lesbians do not feel that the revelation of their identity is wholly, or even partially, under their personal control. These studies document that physicians are not alone in believing in the omniscience of providers: Some lesbians themselves believe providers can discern their lesbianism from their physical appearance, mannerisms, friends or social networks, or marital status and living arrangements (Moses, 1978; Stevens & Hall, 1988). This ability was not generally perceived to have positive consequences by lesbians who subjectively experienced losing control of a closely guarded secret in this fashion.

Hitchcock and Wilson (1992, p. 180) contributed a typology describing four different personal disclosure "stances" used by lesbians: (1) passive disclosure, (2) passive nondisclosure, (3) active disclosure, and (4) active nondisclosure. The two passive stances were found to be the most commonly used strategies. In both, the woman provides clues about her sexual identity, but does not directly either affirm or deny it. Passive disclosure was defined as a lesbian's electing not to deny an assumption of or conjecture as to her identity; passive nondisclosure, as her "posing" as a heterosexual or "passing as straight" by allowing her "heterosexuality" to be assumed. Active disclosure was defined as explicit revelation of her identity by a lesbian; active nondisclosure, as her affirmation of providers' assumptions of heterosexuality.

This work also suggested that the disclosure process is determined by three interacting conditions: personal attributes, health care context, and relevancy of disclosure to a health care need; it concluded, however, that the decision of what disclosure stance to use is also significantly related to the anticipated consequences. Robertson (1992, p. 158) asked, "Does one identify oneself in order to receive adequate care, or to risk potential adverse consequences?"

Apart from Hitchcock and Wilson's (1992) study, little is known at present about the consequences of nondisclosure, apart from those briefly noted earlier (i.e., greater subjective feelings of stress and concern with the potential danger of inappropriate treatment based on the presumption of heterosexuality). Previous research does provide, however, a great deal of information about disclosure consequences, particularly those for active disclosure. It is notable that existing works have recorded most vividly the perceptions of lesbians with negative disclosure experiences, while more positive outcomes have been much more rarely recorded. Describing providers' activities, the 19 studies reviewed by Stevens (1992) documented joking, ostracism, refusal to treat, cool detachment, shock, pity, curiosity, avoidance of physical contact, insults to the patient and her partner or friends, invasions of privacy, rough physical handling, and breaches of confidentiality in the literature from 1970 to 1990 (p. 111). In another study, although Robertson's (1992) sample of 10 lesbians generally reported the reactions of their health providers to their disclosure as "fine," they also revealed that "once they came out to the provider, feelings of being 'exposed,' 'embarrassed,' 'less anonymous,' and of a 'void' in the relationship were common" (p. 160). Two of the women in this sample—constituting 20% of the cohort—detailed immediate negative and inappropriate reactions, and others told of "rushed examinations," being made to feel that their physical problem was psychologically based, and having a health concern discounted because it involved a lesbian partner rather than a "legitimate relationship with a male" (p. 160).

Some research has concluded that providers can make changes in the health care system to communicate that accurately disclosed lesbian identity is as valued, respected, and important as heterosexual identity. Most of the suggested changes involve modifying any or all of the knowledge bases, attitudes, and activities of providers themselves. Gentry (1992, p. 179) noted that "health care providers must confront their own feelings, prejudices and beliefs regarding human sexuality and alternative life styles in order to provide optimal health care...." Eliason

(1993, p. 18) added that "education is the key to providing nonhomophobic, nonheterosexist care." Lynch (1993) provided recommendations of a more concrete nature, including intolerance for the shunning of lesbian patients by other staff, respecting confidentiality, and acknowledging lesbian relationships. Lynch (1993, p. 202) concluded that "we cannot leave it to women who are lesbian...to destigmatize themselves because the stigma is externally placed. If health care providers are unable to work through their homophobia, they should refer their client to a provider who is more accepting and not subject their patient(s) to negative feelings."

Stevens and Hall (1988, 1990) described several specific provider activities perceived by their subjects as encouraging active disclosure, including use of open and inclusive language and approaches, calm and affirming acknowledgment of lesbian identity, provision of positive regard for the lesbian and her partner or friends, and provision of appropriate support. Taken as a whole, the research on disclosure activities confirmed that these activities are used as protective devices, one (of the few) means lesbians believe they have of maintaining control over how they are perceived and treated in health care settings that are perceived (often accurately) as generally hostile to this population's existence and culture (American Academy of Nursing, 1992). When they have little to fear from disclosure of identity, lesbians often disclose their identity, just as they do when they fear the consequences of non-disclosure. Virtually every work cited confirms that most often it is the activities of the health care setting or the provider or both—not those of the lesbian herself—that determine whether a woman will disclose who she is and the full familial, social, cultural, economic, political, and sexual contexts of her health concerns.

Selecting Lesbian or Other Female Health Providers

Several studies have examined the provider preferences of this population. Overwhelmingly,

the results show that when the opportunity is available, lesbians select health providers who are also lesbians. When lesbian providers are not available, they prefer other female providers rather than males (e.g., Paroski, 1987; Trippet & Bain, 1992). This behavior is consistent with Lucas's (1992) findings from a study of the health provider and health service preferences of 178 self-identified lesbians, in which 92% expressed a preference for a lesbian health provider, and females were preferred over males in all provider categories (p. 225). Women in this sample named Pap smear, breast examination, pelvic examination, and well-woman health classes as the services they would prioritize (p. 224); approximately two thirds agreed or strongly agreed that a woman's sexual preference should be asked by the health care provider. About one third of the subjects preferred to have information about their identity recorded in their medical record (p. 226).

Seeking and Using Substance Abuse and Mental Health Services, Programs, or Support Groups

Lesbian health behaviors with respect to mental health and substance abuse have frequently been described in th literature as both quantitatively and qualitatively different from the behaviors of other groups. There is a lengthy history of research reporting that a greater percentage of lesbians than of other women in the United States need, seek, and utilize these mental health and substance abuse services (e.g., Bloomfield, 1993; Fifield, Latham, & Phillips, 1977; Glaus, 1988; McKirnan & Peterson, 1989a,b; Schilit, Clark, & Schallenberger, 1988; VanDenBerg, 1991) although Lucas's (1992) study of 178 self-identified lesbians and Beunting's (1992) survey of 79 lesbians and heterosexual women are two studies that recently reached conclusions somewhat inconsistent with this overall trend.

Although substance abuse needs, services, and behaviors may be broadly construed to be a subset of mental health needs, services, and behavior (i.e., substance abuse disorders have been included within the *Diagnostic and Statistical Manual for Mental Disorders* since its first edition), for purposes of clarity the two will be considered separately in this discussion.

Substance Abuse Needs, Services, and Behaviors

As Hepburn and Gutierrez (1988, p. 186) noted, "Addictions, whatever the specific addicting agent, have an enormous impact on Lesbian individuals and communities." Among the various addicting substances used by this population are tobacco, prescribed medications, alcohol, and illicit drugs such as marijuana, cocaine, hashish, peyote, and other hallucinogenic drugs, crack, heroin, LSD, and Ecstasy. This list is not exhaustive and may be expected to expand whenever new substances are introduced into society as a whole. The lesbian population differs from other populations, not in the *type* of substances used, but in the *overall quantity and quality* of such use.

Except for studies of alcohol, research specifically focused on lesbian patterns of substance use is conspicuously missing from the literature, although studies of substance use for women as a whole undoubtedly have included lesbian subjects. No research was located that analyzed lesbianism as an important or interesting variable in understanding women's use of most other drugs, probably because the assumption of heterosexuality is as strong in this area of health care research as it is in others. The notable exception is in the area of alcohol use, in which studies of lesbians are relatively plentiful.

Hall (1990, p. 89) reported that lesbians have an incidence rate for alcoholism "perhaps three times the general population." This corresponds with findings that approximately 30% of lesbians report drinking problems compared to 10% of the general public (Nardi, 1981; Saghir & Robins, 1973). Hepburn and Gutierrez (1998, p. 193) provided estimates of the extent of alcohol problems in this population that were even higher—noting

that some 30–38% of lesbians experience difficulty in this area. Bradford and Ryan's (1988) national lesbian health survey found that 6% consumed alcohol every day. Only a single study (Bloomfield, 1993) has reported no significant differences in alcohol consumption and drinking patterns between lesbians and heterosexual women.

A variety of explanations have been advanced for the findings of rather dramatic differences between homosexual and heterosexual alcohol consumption patterns, some of which were extrapolated from studies of homosexual samples that included only gay males or a disproportionate number of lesbians. One theory relates alcoholism within the broader homosexual community to the tendency of gay and lesbian people to socialize in gay bars (L. R. Schwartz, 1980). When Lewis, Saghit, and Robins (1982) studied lesbian alcoholism and controlled for bargoing behavior, it was found that this population's rates of heavy drinking and alcoholism still exceed those of heterosexuals. Another theory suggests that an individual's nonacceptance of a homosexual identity may be responsible (Kus, 1990), while other evidence points to membership in a stigmatized group—and the general stress, isolation, and low self-esteem associated with this membership (Israelstrom & Lambert, 1986; Nicoloff & Stiglitz, 1987)—as an important factor promoting substance abuse, which within this frame of reference is frequently termed *self-medication* or an effort to ameliorate psychological discomfort with alcohol ingestion. (The problematic use of alcohol and other substances in the general population has frequently been framed in similar terms.)

Hall (1990) acknowledged the influence of these factors, but suggested that they may be less helpful in understanding lesbians' alcohol use patterns than a holistic approach incorporating the overall community context of lesbian experience. This approach includes consideration of lesbian community dynamics, the lifestyle of "covert" lesbians, the dynamics of lesbian's affectional relationships, and the potential for loss of self (pp. 97–99). Eight conclusions about lesbian alcoholism that utilized this context were derived in terms of three perspectives—developmental, symbolic interactionist, and critical theory. These conclusions included (1) the likelihood that genetic factors have an impact on lesbian alcoholism; (2) the possibility that alcohol use (as well as depression and suicidal behavior) may be related to the intrapsychic and interactional effects of stigmatization; (3) the probability that culture and ethnicity are factors in etiology; (4) the influence of sociocultural differences and inequalities related to sex differences (including the perception of researchers that alcoholism is a "male" disease); (5) the historical stigmatization, oppression, and marginalization of homosexuals in cultures worldwide; (6) the multiple negative attributions for lesbian alcoholics of being female homosexual substance abusers; (7) the influence of one stigma on the process of acquiring another; and (8) the experience of "losing self" through a variety of critical processes (pp. 100–101).

Finnegan and McNally (1987) developed a five-stage model to explicate the relationship between alcoholism and lesbian identity, with an emphasis on the recovery process. Deevey and Wall (1992) reframed and critiqued this model specifically in terms of lesbian experiences, then proposed an alternative model that incorporated more of the social contexts of lesbians' experiences with alcohol to describe the same process. Social shaming of lesbians was highlighted by Deevey and Wall as having a particularly potent influence on the development of alcoholism in this population, as well as on recovery, referred to as "the serenity of lesbian self-affirmation" (p. 207).

Hall (1990, 1992) interviewed 35 lesbians to explore the images of the recovery process in this population, noting that such explorations were important, in part, because of "the recent cultural trend away from substance abuse in lesbian communities" (p. 181). An important health behavior identified in this population was their willingness to recognize alcohol problems and work toward recovery well before members of other populations acknowledged this need. Because lesbians have a generally longer experience, as a group, with the process of recovery from problems of substance addiction, they may be a valuable resource for populations that have just begun to explore recovery options.

Hall's (1994) work included examination of the role of Alcoholics Anonymous (AA) and other Twelve Step programs based on the AA model in the lesbian recovery process. It concluded that this model utilizes a primary image of recovery as conversion. Lesbian images of recovery, on the other hand, focus not only on conversion, but also on physical transition, personal growth, struggle with compulsivity, reclaiming of self, connection/reconnection with other women/lesbians, cyclical/celebratory commemoration, vocational change, and social transition (pp. 185–193). The research concluded that "the uncritical promotion of AA and other Twelve Step groups as the single or even the best model of recovery is inappropriate" (p. 194). This finding reinforced Herman's (1988) conclusion that addiction programs have generally negative impacts on the political vitality of homosexuals.

Hall (1994) used information from the same sample to describe the health care experiences of lesbians recovering from alcohol problems, an aspect that was discussed only very briefly in the earlier work (Hall, 1990, 1992). This publication reported that 91% of the subjects had abused other substances, and significant numbers had difficulties with food, codependency, sex, and money. Other findings were that 46% had been heavy drinkers and there were no light drinkers. Length of abstinence from substance use ranged from 1 to 25 years, with a mean of 6 years. About two thirds of the sample reported having experienced some form of childhood abuse; 46% specifically referred to childhood sexual abuse. About two thirds of the sample had received treatment for their alcohol problems, usually as outpatients. Most of the same barriers within the health care system cited earlier were noted by this sample, including financial constraints and the perception that the treatment was unsafe for lesbians. Additional barriers described by these subjects were lack of child care and limited number of patient "slots," both probably more problematic in substance abuse treatment than in some other forms of health care.

This study also evaluated barriers to recovery related to interactions with health care providers or the health care system. These barriers were discovered to include lack of trust in providers (based on providers' assumptions of heterosexuality, ignorance of lesbianism and lesbian culture, violations of confidentiality, and instructions not to disclose lesbian identity in the treatment setting); absence of conceptual congruence with the provider (i.e., disagreement about how the problem and interventions were constructed); and paradoxical provider persuasive styles (characterized as paternalistic, maternalistic, confrontational, and influential) that, rather than aiding lesbians' recovery from alcoholism, impeded it (pp. 240–243).

Other work has explored substance abuse treatment and recovery issues of this population (e.g., Underhill, 1991). The work of Hellman, Staunton, Lee, Tyton, and Vauchon (1989) based on responses from 36 treatment providers in New York City found that knowledge of appropriate evaluation and treatment methods for homosexuals was limited, most did not discuss their clients' homosexuality (even though they considered it to be important), supervision and training of most providers was substandard or nonexistent, and development of specific treatment programs for this population had little priority in their facilities. Many of the 164 respondents felt that treatment programs would benefit from openly lesbian or gay male staff and that there would be little professional risk for these providers. Respondents also believed that homosexual alcoholics are less likely to seek help and have more problems reaching the recovery stage of maintaining sobriety.

As a whole, the research on substance-abuse-related health behavior in this population suggests that it is consistent with their behavior within the health care system as a whole. The primary difference is that the confluence of familial, social, political, and personal experiences of lesbians has resulted in circumstances that have promoted and sustained problem drinking and other substance abuse at a rate that appears to exceed that of the general population. Although lesbians may be generally more willing than members of other populations to seek help with these substance abuse problems, they encounter all of the same provider behaviors that characterize the health care system when they do, and their attitudinal and behavioral responses to these provider behaviors are consistent with other lesbian health behavior patterns, including avoidance, delay, preference for lesbian or female providers, and experiencing conflicts about self-disclosure needs and consequences in substance abuse treatment settings.

Mental Health Needs, Services, and Behaviors

Although the mental health behavior of lesbians has long received scholarly attention, a significant amount of the early research focused on lesbianism as a mental illness. After 1973, when this diagnostic position was modified by the psychiatric community, research on this population lagged somewhat behind explorations of physical health and substance abuse needs, services, and behaviors for a period; however, this situation began to change with the initiation of the *Journal of Gay and Lesbian Psychotherapy*, a professional publication focused on the mental health needs and services, in 1989. Combined with the encouragement afforded researchers in this field by the *Journal of Homosexuality*, which began publishing in the early 1970s, this new journal touched off a wave of thinking and writing about lesbian (and gay) mental health that shows little sign of abating. Further, as the lesbian and gay rights movement gained greater visibility, lesbian-focused mental health information began to appear in a wide range of professional journals for health providers.

A significant amount of this literature examines aspects of the lesbian–therapist/counselor relationship, with an overarching emphasis on the relational contexts for individual or group therapy (e.g., Modricin & Wyers, 1990; Ussher, 1990, 1991). A few works are focused on developing theoretical models to explicate and improve therapeutic efforts (e.g., Brown, 1989).

The mental health issues highlighted by the National Lesbian Health Care Survey (Bradford & Ryan, 1988) included suicidal ideation (noted by more than 50% of the respondents), suicide attempts (reported by 18%), childhood or adult sexual abuse (cited by 37%), rape or sexual attack (described by 32%), and incest (reported by 19%). About 75% of the sample had participated in mental health counseling at some time in their lives, about half of these for feelings of depression.

Trippet's (1994) study on lesbians' mental health needs and behaviors largely confirms previous findings. The findings were based on a qualitative and qualitative analysis of the responses of 503 women to questions regarding mental health problems for which they would seek help, as well as their recommendations for changes needed in the mental health system. The percentage of respondents personally experiencing each mental health concern was as follows (p. 320): relationship issues, 76.5%; conflict about being in the closet at work and out socially, 66.2%; depression, 66%; conflict over coming out, 60.2%; contemplation of suicide, 38%; conflict over religion, 27.4%; alcohol abuse, 23.7%; drug abuse, 16.7%; attempted suicide, 10.7%; bulimia, 5.6%; anorexia, 2.8%. As is evident, the majority of these issues would require disclosure of lesbian identity to a therapist/counselor for effective resolution; however, the subjects had experienced or anticipated many of the same provider behaviors that create barriers to the delivery of other health services to this population. The systemic changes they recommended included (1) changes in treatment modalities (including less use of medication and greater knowledge on the part of therapists/counselors about

women and lesbians; (2) practical changes (including making therapy more accessible and affordable, and providing insurance coverage for mental health practitioners other than psychologists and psychiatrists; (3) provider attitudinal changes (specifically reduction in homophobia); and (4) changes in the gender distribution of mental health providers, to include more women and openly lesbian therapists/counselors (pp. 321–322). These findings are consistent with those of Bradford and Ryan (1988), Diamond and Wisnack (1978), R. D. Schwartz (1989), and many others who have explored similar issues.

Trippet's (1994) results regarding suicide—considered to be among the most serious mental health issues of this population—are congruent with those of Saunders and Valente (1987), who reported that lesbians attempt suicide 7 times more often than heterosexual women, and with those of Kremer and Rifkin (1969), who found that rates of suicide for adolescent lesbians was 300% higher than rates of comparison groups. Moreover, suicidal ideation and attempts, depression, and alcoholism have been considered to be co-morbid conditions for this population.

Despite research findings suggesting that lesbians as a group have a greater willingness to utilize mental health services, extensive documentation that the mental health needs of this population are serious and pervasive, and a rather extensive base of literature providing therapists with information on appropriate provider behavior, the mental health system has moved no further than the rest of the health care system in the design and delivery of services that adequately address this population's needs. The finding that 60% of the lesbians surveyed nationwide use their partner or other lesbians to meet mental health needs supports this conclusion (Bradford & Ryan, 1988). Rothblum (1994) encouraged further research to determine the relative salience of gender versus sexual orientation in the development and treatment of mental disorders. This work proposed that the experiences of lesbians (and gay men) in society "may place them at increased risk for some mental health problems and may protect them from other mental health problems" (p. 215).

ADDITIONAL RESEARCH WITH IMPLICATIONS FOR LESBIAN HEALTH BEHAVIOR

There has been a great deal of research on other topics that relate to or affect lesbian health behavior. This research includes works on lesbians and gay males as health care students or providers (e.g., Cotton, 1993; Geraci, 1994; Stephany, 1989, 1992, 1993); on lesbian reproductive issues, particularly artificial insemination (e.g., Curtin, 1994; Zeidenstein, 1990); on specific settings in which lesbians may require care, such as hospices (Stephany, 1989); on violence toward lesbians, particularly lesbian battering (e.g., Klinger, 1991; Renzetti, 1992); and on specific illnesses or health concerns for which lesbians may require care or services (e.g., Ball, 1994; White & Levinson, 1993).

METHODOLOGICAL ISSUES IN LESBIAN HEALTH BEHAVIOR RESEARCH

Analysis of the research methodologies employed in studying lesbian health behavior provides additional support for the conclusion that this field of inquiry is in its infancy and that it has not been as rigorously pursued as other topics in health care research. Although there is certainly no shortage of publications on the topic, many of these publications may be considered *research* only in the broadest construction of the term: A great number are reports, not scientific studies.

The specific methodological shortcomings of this research base are relatively easy to enumerate. They include:

- Difficulties in defining the lesbian population (Donovan, 1992).

- Reliance on convenience, snowball, or other nonrandomly selected samples of lesbians, most of whom are young, Caucasian, and middle class, and all of whom are comfortable being out (or self-identified) enough as a lesbian to participate in a survey, interview, or other data-gathering process.
- Generally small sample size compared to size of the population(s) of interest.
- Use of nonstandardized instruments (generally questionnaires or surveys designed for the specific study and having reliability and validity that have either not been established or are not reported).
- Extensive use of survey methodology and descriptive techniques, generally to the exclusion of more rigorous methods.
- Absence of research with randomly assigned interventions or treatments.
- Complete reliance on lesbians' self-reports of their behavior rather than on observational methods.
- Lack of clear definitions of research variables or aspects of interest, many of which (e.g., fear, disclosure, hostility) have ambiguous meanings.
- Overgeneralization of results to the entire population of lesbians based upon nonrepresentative samples.
- Failure to consider and/or report all study limitations or threats to validity as a part of the study's findings or conclusions, especially the impact of social stigma on the participation of members of the population in the research effort and *demand characteristics*.

The level of statistical analysis in these works, while not a weakness per se considering the types of research represented, provides another indication that this research lacks rigor. When quantitative results are provided, the usual statistics employed are descriptive rather than comparative, except in the broadest sense of this term, even when comparisons are made or implied. Percentages are employed frequently to summarize data; when means (statistical averages) are provided, standard deviations usually are not. For example, in studies comparing lesbians and heterosexual women, percentages are often provided for both groups, and the reader is left to make a comparison between the figures. The handful of works using χ^2-square or t-tests to analyze data do not report probability levels or degrees of freedom, and the terms *significant* or *significance* are used to mean "important" and "importance" rather than a statistically based conclusion. Imprecise terms such as *more than* and *less than* are utilized in lieu of providing exact figures.

The greatest strengths of the methodologies employed are in the use and adaptation of qualitative methodologies, particularly in more recent studies that utilize ethnographic, phenomenological techniques to explore lesbian health behaviors within an elaborated theoretical context. The creative use of these methods has generated data that are rich and meaningful, particularly for theory-building and definitional purposes.

This research base contains no meta-analyses and only a single literature review. (This work spanned a 20-year period and analyzed 19 research efforts. The method of selecting this sample of works was not specified.) Although most of these publications utilize many citations, the most evident connections in this body of research exist within the collective output of an individual author, pairs of authors, or relatively small groups of individuals who appear to be consistently pursuing the same or similar topics (e.g., Stevens and Hall; Deevey; Eliason, Donelan, and Randall; Johnson, Geunther, E. M. Smith, Laube, Palermo, and Keetle; Robertson and Schacter; Stephany; and Trippet and Bain). Otherwise, the research as a whole is linear—i.e., the studies follow one another in time, but neither build upon nor are related to one another in any other way—and generally disconnected, lacking any consistent theme or focus, except for works by the same author or authorship groups. In several instances, a single survey was utilized as the basis for more than one publication, often quite similar in content, but published in different professional journals. In short, there is clearly no "research agenda" on lesbian health among professionals who publish.

Considered collectively, these works establish lesbian health behavior as an emerging rather than an established area of research and scholarship. This summary illustrates, however, that existing efforts provide a strong and interesting foundation of descriptive studies upon which to base more rigorous and methodologically elegant research efforts in the future.

REFERENCES

American Academy of Nursing. (1992). Expert panel report: Culturally competent care. *Nursing Outlook, 40,* 277–283.

Ball, S. (1994). A group model for gay and lesbian clients with chronic mental illness. *Social Work, 39*(1), 109–115.

Beuting, J. A. (1992). Health life-styles of lesbian and heterosexual women. *Health Care for Women International, 13*(2), 165–171.

Bloomfield, K. (1993). A comparison of alcohol consumption between lesbians and heterosexual women in an urban population. *Drug and Alcohol Dependency, 33*(3), 257–269.

Bower, B. (1992). Genetic clues to female homosexuality. *Science News, 142,* 117.

Bradford, J., & Ryan, C. (1988). *The national lesbian health care survey.* Washington, DC: National Gay and Lesbian Health Foundation.

Bradford, J., & Ryan, C. (1991). Who we are: Health concerns of middle-aged lesbians. In B. Sang, J. Warshow, & A. Smith (Eds.), *Lesbians at midlife: The creative transition* (pp. 147–163). San Francisco: Spinsters Book Co.

Brown, L. S. (1989). New voices, new visions: Toward a lesbian/gay paradigm for psychology. *Psychology of Women Quarterly, 13,* 445–458.

Browning, C. (1984). Changing theories of lesbianism: Challenging the stereotypes. In T. Darty & S. Potter (Eds.), *Women-identified women.* Palo Alto, CA: Mayfield.

Browning, C., Reynolds, A. L., & Dworkin, S. M. (1991). Affirmative psychotherapy for lesbian women. *Counseling Psychologist, 19,* 177–196.

Chafetz, J., Sampson, P., Beck, P., & West, J. (1974). A study of homosexual women. *Social Work, 19,* 714–723.

Chu, S. Y., Beuhler, J. W., Fleming, P. L., Berkleman, R. L. (1990). Epidemiology of AIDS in lesbians, U.S., 1980–1989. *American Journal of Public Health, 80,* 11, 1380–1381.

Cochran, S. D., & Mays, V. M. (1988) Disclosure of sexual preference to physicians by black lesbian and bisexual women. *Western Journal of Medicine, 149,* 616-619.

Conway, M., & Humphries, E. (1994). Bernard clinic meeting need in lesbian sexual health care. *Nursing Times, 90,* 40-41.

Cotton, P. (1993). Gay, lesbians meet, march, tell Shalala bigotry is health hazard. *Journal of the American Medical Association, 269,* 2611-2612.

Curtin, L. L. (1994). Lesbian, single and geriatric women: To breed or not to breed? *Nursing Management, 25,* 14-16.

Dancey, C. P. (1990). Sexual orientation in women: An investigation of hormonal and personality variables. *Biological Psychology, 30*(3), 251-264.

Dardick, L., & Grady, K. (1980). Openness between gay persons and health professionals. *Annals of Internal Medicine, 93,* 115-119.

Deevy, S. (1990). Older lesbian women: An invisible minority. *Journal of Gerontological Nursing, 16*(5), 35-37.

Deevey, S., & Wall, L. (1992). How do lesbian women develop serenity? *Health Care for Women International, 13,* 199-208.

Diamond, D. W., & Wisnack, S. C. (1978). Alcohol abuse among lesbians: A descriptive study. *Journal of Homosexuality, 4,* 123-142.

Donovan, J. M. (1992). Homosexual, gay, and lesbian: Defining the words and sampling the populations. *Journal of Homosexuality, 24,* 27-47.

Douglas, C. J., Kalman, C., & Kalman, T. P. (1985). Homophobia among physicians and nurses: An empirical study. *Hospital and Community Psychiatry, 36,* 1309-1311.

Dritz, S. (1985). Medical aspects of homosexuality. *New England Journal of Medicine, 302,* 463-464.

Dworkin, S. H., & Gutierrez, F. (1989). Counselors, be aware, clients come in every size, shape, color and sexual orientation. *Journal of Counseling and Development, 68,* 6-10.

Elder, G. E., Humphreys, W. & Lakowski, C. (1988). Sexism in gynecology textbooks: Gender stereotypes and paternalism, 1978 through 1983. *Health Care for Women International, 9,* 1-17.

Eliason, M. (1993). Cultural diversity in nursing care: the lesbian, gay or bisexual client. *Journal of Transcultural Nursing, 5*(1), 14-20.

Eliason, M., Donelan, C., & Randall, C. (1992). Lesbian stereotypes. *Health Care for Women International, 13,* 131-144.

Eliason, M. J., & Randall, C. E. (1991). Lesbian phobia in nursing students. *Western Journal of Nursing Research, 13*(3), 363-374.

Ellis, M. J. (1985). Eliminating our heterosexist approach to sex education: A hope for the future. *Journal of Sex Education and Therapy, 11*(1), 60-65.

Fifield, L., Latham, J. D., & Phillips, C. (1977). *Alcoholism and the gay community: The price of alienation, isolation, and oppression.* Los Angeles: Gay Community Services Center.

Finnegan, D. G., & McNally, E. B. (1987). *Dual identities: Counseling chemically dependent gay men and lesbians.* Center City, MN: Hazelden.

Franke, R., & Leary, M. R. (1992). Disclosure of sexual orientation by lesbians and gay men: A comparison of private and public processes. *Journal of Social and Clinical Psychology, 10,* 262-269.

French, M. (1992). *The war against women.* New York: Summit Books.

Geddes, V. A. (1994). Lesbian expectations and experiences with family doctors: How much does the physician's sex matter to lesbians? *Canadian Family Physician, 40,* 908-912.

Gentry, S. E. (1992). Caring for lesbians in a homophobic society. *Health Care for Women International, 13,* 173-180.

Geraci, A. P. (1994). Earring etiquette in medical schools. *Journal of the American Medical Association, 271,* 716.

Gillow, K., & Davis, L. (1987). Lesbian stress and coping methods. *Psychological Nursing and Mental Health, 25*(9), 28-32.

Glascock, E. (1981). *Access to the traditional health care system by nontraditional women.* Paper presented at the American Public Health Association Annual Meeting, Los Angeles.

Glaus, K. O. (1988). Alcoholism, chemical dependency and the lesbian client. *Women and Therapy, 8,* 131-144.

Gonslorek, J. C., & Weinrich, J. D. (1991). *Homosexuality: Research implications for public policy.* Newbury Park, CA: Sage.

Good, R. (1976). The gynecologist and the lesbian. *Clinical Obstetrics and Gynecology, 19,* 473-481.

Greene, B. (1994). Ethnic minority lesbians and gay men: Mental health treatment issues. *Journal of Consulting and Clinical Psychology, 62*(2), 243-249.

Hall, J. M. (1990). Alcoholism in lesbians: Developmental, symbolic interactionist and critical perspectives. *Health Care for Women International, 11*(1), 89-107.

Hall, J. M. (1992). An exploration of lesbians' images of recovery from alcohol problems. *Health Care for Women International, 13,* 181-198.

Hall, J. M. (1993). Lesbians and alcohol: Patterns and paradoxes in medical notions and lesbians' beliefs. *Journal of Psychoactive Drugs, 25*(2), 109-119.

Hall, J. M. (1994). Lesbians recovering from alcohol problems: An ethnographic study of health care experiences. *Nursing Research, 43*(4), 238-244.

Hellman, R. E., Staunton, M., Lee, J., Tytun, A., & Vauchon, R. (1989). Treatment of homosexual alcoholics in government-funded agencies: Provider training and attitudes. *Hospital and Community Psychiatry, 40*(11), 1163-1168.

Hepburn, C., & Gutierrez, B. (1988). *Alive and well: A lesbian health guide.* Freedom, CA: Crossing Press.

Herman, E. (1988). Getting to serenity: Do addiction programs sap our political vitality? *Outlook, 1*(2), 10-21.

Hetrick, E. S., & Martin, A. D. (1987). Developmental issues and their resolution for gay and lesbian adolescents. *Journal of Homosexuality, 14*(1–2), 25–43.

Hitchcock, J. M., & Wilson, H. S. (1992). Personal risking: Lesbian self-disclosure of sexual orientation to professional health care providers. *Nursing Research, 41*, 178–183.

Hollander, J., & Haber, L. (1992). Ecological transitions: Using Brofenbrenner's model to study sexual identity change. *Health Care for Women International, 13*, 121–129.

Israelstrom, S., & Lambert, S. (1986). Homosexuality and alcoholism: Observations and research after the psychoanalytic era. *International Journal of the Addictions, 21*, 509–537.

Jay, K., & Young, A. (1979). *The gay report* (2nd ed.). New York: Summit.

Johnson, S. R., Guenther, S., Laube, D. W., and Keettel, W. C. (1981). Factors affecting lesbian gynecologic care: A preliminary study. *Journal of Obstetrics and Gynecology, 140*(1), 20–24.

Johnson, S. R., Smith, E. M., & Guenther, S. M. (1987). Comparison of gynecologic health care problems between lesbians and bisexual women: A survey of 2,345 women. *Journal of Reproductive Medicine, 1*, 805–811.

Johnson, S. R., & Palermo, J. L. (1984). Gynecologic care for the lesbian. *Clinical Obstetrics and Gynecology, 27*, 724–730.

Johnson, S. R., Smith, E. M. & Geunther, S. M. (1987). Comparison of gynecologic health care problems between lesbians and bisexual women: A survey of 2,345 women. *Journal of Reproductive Issues, 32*, 805–811.

Jones, E. E., Farina, A., Hastorf, A. H., Markus, H., Miller, D. T., Scott, R. A., & French, R. (1984). *Social stigma: The psychology of marked relationships*. New York: W. H. Freeman.

Klinger, R. (1991). Treatment of a lesbian batterer. In C. Silverstein (Ed.), *Gays, lesbians, and their therapists* (pp. 126–142). New York: W. W. Norton.

Kus, R. J. (1990). *Keys to caring: Assisting your gay and lesbian clients*. Boston: Alyson.

Leaman, T. L. (1987). The lesbian patient: When she is your patient. *Female Patient, 12*(5), 10–14.

Lesbian Revisions Group. (1992). Loving women: Lesbian life and relationships. In The Boston Women's Health Collective (Eds.), *The new our bodies, ourselves* (pp. 177–203). New York: Simon & Schuster.

Lewis, C. E., Saghir, M. T., & Robins, E. (1982). Drinking patterns in homosexual and heterosexual women. *Journal of Clinical Psychiatry, 43*(7), 277–279.

LoBiondo-Wood, G. (1986). Health education for the homosexual female. In V. M. Littlefield (Ed.), *Health education for women: A guide for nurses and other health care professionals*. Norwalk, CT: Appleton.

Lockard, D. (1985). The lesbian community: An anthropological approach. *Journal of Homosexuality, 11*(3-4), 83–95.

Lucas, V. A. (1992). An investigation of the health care preferences of the lesbian population. *Health Care for Women International, 13*, 221–228.

Lynch, M. A. (1993). When the patient is also a lesbian. *AWHONN Clinical Issues Pertaining to Women's Health, 4*(2) 196–202.

Markowitz, L. M. (1991). Homosexuality: Are we still in the dark? *Family Therapy Networker, 15*(1), 26–35.

McKirnan, D. J., & Peterson, P. L. (1989a). Psychosocial and social factors in alcohol and drug abuse: An analysis of a homosexual community. *Addictive Behaviors, 14*, 41–52.

McKirnan, D. J., & Peterson, P. L. (1989b). Alcohol and drug use among homosexual men and women: Epidemiology and population characteristics. *Addictive Behaviors, 14*, 555–563.

Michigan Organization for Human Rights (MOHR). (1991). *Michigan lesbian health survey*. Detroit: MOHR.

Modricin, M. J., & Wyers, N. L. (1990). Lesbian and gay couples: Where they turn when help is needed. *Journal of Gay and Lesbian Psychotherapy, 1*, 89–104.

Morin, S. F., & Rothblum, E. D. (1991). Removing the stigma: Fifteen years of progress. *American Psychologist, 46*, 947–949.

Moses, A. (1978). *Identity management in lesbian women*. New York: Praeger.

Nardi, P. M. (1981). Alcoholism and homosexuality: A theoretical perspective. *Journal of Homosexuality, 7*(4), 9–26.

Neisen, J. P. (1990). Heterosexism: Redefining homophobia for the 1990s. *Journal of Gay and Lesbian Psychotherapy, 1*, 21–23.

Nichols, M. (1989). Sex therapy with lesbians, gay men, and bisexuals. In S. Leiblum & R. C. Rosen (Eds.), *Principles and practice of sex therapy: Update for the '90s* (2nd ed.). (pp. 269–297). New York: Guilford Press.

Nicoloff, L. K., & Stiglitz, E. A. (1987). Lesbian alcoholism: Etiology, treatment, and recovery. In Boston Lesbian Collective (Eds.), *Lesbian psychologies* (pp. 283–293). Urbana: University of Illinois Press.

O'Donnell, M. (1978, May). Lesbian health care: Issues and literature. *Science for the People, 9*.

O'Donnell, M., Pollack, K., Leoffler, V., & Saunders, Z. (1979). *Lesbian health matters!* Santa Cruz, CA: Women's Health Collective.

Owen, W. F. (1985). Medical problems of the homosexual adolescent. *Journal of Adolescent Health Care, 6*(4), 278–285.

Paroski, P. A. (1987) Health care delivery and the concerns of gay and lesbian adolescents. *Journal of Adolescent Health Care, 8*(2), 188–192.

Peteros, K., & Miller, F. (1982). Lesbian health in a straight world. *Second Opinion*, April 4.

Pharr, S. (1988). *Homophobia: A weapon of sexism*. Inverness, CA: Chardon Press.

Platzer, H. (1993). Ethics: Nursing care of gay and lesbian patients. *Nursing Standards, 7*(17), 34–37.

Ponse, B. (1978). *Identities in the lesbian world: The social construction of the self*. Westport, CT: Greenwood.

Randall, C. E. (1987). Lesbian-phobia among BSN educators: A survey. *Cassandra: Radical Nurses Journal*, 6, 23–26.

Randall, C. E. (1989). Lesbian phobia among BSN educators: A survey. *Journal of Nursing Education*, 28, 303–306.

Raymond, D., & Blumfield, W. (1988). *Looking at gay and lesbian life*. New York: Philosophical Library.

Reagan, P. (1981). The interaction of health professionals and their lesbian clients. *Patient Counseling and Health Education*, 3, 21–25.

Remafedi, G. (1990). Fundamental issues in the care of homosexual youth. *Medical Clinicians of North America*, 74(5), 1169–1179.

Renzetti, C. M. (1992). *Violent betrayal: Partner abuse in lesbian relationships*. Newbury Park, CA: Sage.

Robertson, M. M. (1992). Lesbians as an invisible minority in the health services arena. *Health Care for Women International*, 13(2), 155–163.

Romm, M. E. (1965). Sexuality and homosexuality in women. In J. Marmor (Ed.), *Sexual inversion: The multiple roots of homosexuality* (pp. 288–301). New York: Basic Books.

Rothblum, E. D. (1994). "I only read about myself on bathroom walls": The need for research on the mental health of lesbians and gay men. *Journal of Consulting and Clinical Psychology*, 62, 213–217.

Saghir, M. T., & Robins, E. (1973). *Male and female homosexuality*. Baltimore: Williams & Wilkins.

Sang, B. E. (1989). New directions in lesbian research, theory, and education. *Journal of Counseling and Development*, 68, 92–96.

Saunders, J. M., Tupac, J. D., & MacCulloch, B. (1988). *A lesbian profile: A survey of 1000 lesbians*. West Hollywood: Southern California Women for Understanding.

Saunders, J. M., & Valente, S. M. (1987). Suicide risk among gay men and lesbians: A review. *Death Studies*, 11, 1–23.

Schilit, R., Clark, W. M., & Shallenberger, E. A. (1988). Social supports and lesbian alcoholics. *Affilia*, 3(2), 27–40.

Schwanberg, S. L. (1985). Changes in labeling homosexuality in health science literature: A preliminary investigation. *Journal of Homosexuality*, 12(1), 51–73.

Schwanberg, S. L. (1990). Attitudes toward homosexuality in American health care literature, 1983–1987. *Journal of Homosexuality*, 19(3), 117–136.

Schwartz, L. R. (1980). *Alcoholism among lesbians/gay men: A critical problem in critical proportions*. Phoenix, AZ: Do It Now Foundation.

Schwartz, R. D. (1989). When the therapist is gay: Personal and clinical reflections. *Journal of Lesbian and Gay Psychotherapy*, 1, 41–51.

Smith, E. M., Johnson, S. R., and Guenther, S. M. (1985). Health care attitudes and experiences during gynecological care among lesbians and bisexuals. *American Journal of Public Health*, 75(9), 1085–1088.

Smith, M., Heaton, C., & Seiver, D. (1990). Health concerns of lesbians. *Physician Assistant*, 14(1), 81–94.

Socarides, C. W. (1992). Sexual politics and scientific logic: The issue of homosexuality. *Journal of Psychohistory*, 19, 359–380.

Stephany, T. M. (1989). Lesbian hospice nurse. *American Journal of Hospital Care*, 6(5), 13–14.

Stephany, T. M. (1992). Promoting mental health: Lesbian nurse support groups: *Journal of Psychosocial Nursing and Mental Health Services*, 30(8), 2.

Stephany, T. M. (1993). Lesbian hospice patients. *Home Health Nurse*, 11(6), 11–13.

Stern, P. N. (1993). *Lesbian health: What are the issues*. Bristol, PA: Taylor & Francis Group.

Stevens, P. E. (1992). Lesbian health care research: A review of the literature from 1970 to 1990. *Health Care for Women International*, 13, 91–120.

Stevens, P. E. (1993). Lesbians and HIV: Clinical, research, and policy issues. *American Journal of Orthopsychiatry*, 63, 289–294.

Stevens, P. E. (1994). Protective strategies of lesbian clients in health care environments. *Research in Nursing and Health*, 17, 217–229.

Stevens, P. E., & Hall, J. M. (1988). Stigma, health beliefs, and experiences with health care in lesbian women. *Image: Journal of Nursing Scholarship*, 20, 69–73.

Stevens, P. E., & Hall, J. M. (1990). Abusive health care interactions experienced by lesbians: A case of institutional violence in the treatment of women. *Response: To the Victimization of Women and Children*, 13(3), 23–27.

Stevens, P. E., & Hall, J. M. (1991). A critical historical analysis of the medical construction of lesbianism. *International Journal of Health Services*, 21, 291–307.

Trippet, S. E., (1994). Lesbians' mental health concerns. *Health Care for Women International*, 15, 317–323.

Trippet, S. E., & Bain, J. (1992). Reasons American lesbians fail to seek traditional health care. *Health Care for Women International*, 13, 145–153.

Underhill, B. L. (1991). Recovery needs of alcoholics in treatment. In N. VanDenBerg (Ed.), *Feminist perspectives on addictions* (pp. 73–86). New York: Springer.

Ussher, J. M. (1990). Couples therapy with gay clients: Issues facing counselors. *Counseling Psychology Quarterly*, 3, 109–116.

Ussher, J. M. (1991). Family and couples therapy with gay and lesbian clients. *Journal of Family Therapy*, 13, 131–148.

VanDenBerg, N. (Ed.). (1991). *Feminist perspectives on addictions*. New York: Springer.

VanScoy, H. (in press). Lesbian health care research since 1973: Patterns and trends across helping professions.

Wallick, M. M., Cambre, K. M., & Townsend, M. H. (1992). How the topic of homosexuality is taught in U.S. medical schools. *Academic Medicine*, 67(9), 601–603.

White, J., & Levinson, W. (1993). Primary care of lesbian patients. *Journal of General Internal Medicine*, 8, 41–47.

Zeidenstein, L. (1990). Gynecological and childbearing needs of lesbians. *Journal of Nurse-Midwifery*, 35(1), 10–16.

8

Health Behavior in Persons with HIV and AIDS

Bradley T. Thomason and Peter E. Campos

INTRODUCTION

In just over a decade, from the mid-1980s to the mid-1990s, acquired immunodeficiency syndrome (AIDS) has become a universal health problem challenging virtually every branch of the health sciences. For behavioral scientists, the challenge posed by AIDS is accompanied by the frustration of knowing that AIDS is preventable. Unlike previous diseases that devastated communities around the globe, AIDS can be halted at the behavioral level without a vaccine, physician visit, or medical system intervention. Infection with and transmission of the human immunodeficiency virus (HIV), in most cases, can be stopped by responsibly governing one's behavior. Behavioral choices accurately predict susceptibility to HIV exposure. For the millions of individuals infected with

HIV, health behaviors are crucial to one's livelihood and longevity. Certain health behaviors (e.g., coping styles, social support utilization) are known to affect the rate of HIV disease progression and subsequently determine the quality of life for those living with HIV and AIDS (Ostrow, 1990; Thomason, Jones, McClure & Brantley, 1996).

When epidemiological tracking of HIV began in the mid-1980s, gay and bisexual men constituted the highest-risk group for HIV infection, accounting for approximately 75% of documented AIDS cases at that time (Nash & Said, 1992). As knowledge surrounding HIV transmission modes became evident, the gay community responded comprehensively. Aided by health professionals and social scientists, the gay community launched HIV education and prevention campaigns in major cities of the United States. The focus of the campaigns pertained to sexual behavior and lifestyle changes (e.g., condom use, monogamy, sexual communication and negotiation). A decade later, data indicate that prevention programs have been successful and the overall prevalence of AIDS among gay and bisexual men has decreased dramatically (Nash & Said, 1992).

Bradley T. Thomason • Department of Family and Preventive Medicine, Emory University School of Medicine, Atlanta, Georgia 30308.   **Peter E. Campos** • Department of Psychiatry and Behavioral Sciences, Emory University School of Medicine, Atlanta, Georgia 30308.

Handbook of Health Behavior Research III: Demography, Development, and Diversity, edited by David S. Gochman. Plenum Press, New York, 1997.

Recently, however, AIDS has become the leading cause of death for all young adults in the United States, expanding beyond gay groups. Given this harrowing news, it is obvious that prevention efforts have not generalized to all individuals at risk. Infection rates among intravenous (IV) drug users have remained consistently high. Heterosexuals, considered to be a low-risk population at the beginning of the epidemic, have witnessed a steady rise in AIDS cases in recent years. Moreover, a demographic breakdown shows sharp elevations in certain subsections of the United States population. Substantial increases of new AIDS cases have been observed among women, people of color, and the poor (Nash & Said, 1992).

As of December 1994, more than 1 million cases of AIDS had been reported to the World Health Organization (WHO, 1995). In the United States, over 400,000 AIDS cases have been documented by the Centers for Disease Control and Prevention (CDC, 1995). Of the United States adult cases, 97% of individuals were infected via sexual activity or intravenous drug use (IDU). These behaviors facilitate the exchange of body fluids (i.e., blood, blood products, semen, and vaginal fluid) known to carry HIV in high enough portions to infect susceptible hosts upon exposure. Fortunately, effective screening procedures for blood and tissue donors have nearly eliminated the risk of exposure for the recipients of blood products (the remaining 3% of adult United States AIDS cases) (CDC, 1995). Thus, newly infected adults continue to be exposed by two primary modalities, unsafe sexual behavior and IDU. Changing these health risk behaviors is crucial in order to deter the spread of HIV disease and the decimation it brings.

HIV TESTING AND
THE PSYCHOSOCIAL SEQUELAE
OF AN HIV DIAGNOSIS

In 1985, laboratory tests designed to detect HIV antibodies were approved by the Food and Drug Administration (Schochetman & George, 1992). Since that time, widespread availability of testing sites has facilitated expedient delivery of diagnostic information and clinical services to millions infected with HIV. Today, the purposes of HIV testing extend far beyond medical diagnostics and treatment planning. HIV testing has become an avenue for research and surveillance as well as for public policy making and sociopolitical debate (Johnston & Hopkins, 1990; Schochetman & George, 1992). Consequently, the sometimes volatile climate surrounding the HIV testing and notification process strongly affects an individual's behavioral and emotional responses to HIV (Jacobsen, Perry, & Hirsch, 1990; Landau-Stanton & Clements, 1993).

The decision to be tested for HIV typically involves careful deliberation by the individual. In the minds of those seeking HIV testing are myriad notions, some valid and others misconstrued, about the drawbacks and benefits of having their HIV status revealed. Researchers have begun to identify factors that influence a person's decision to seek testing. From available data, the variable emerging most consistently as a primary predictor of a person's decision to test is fear. In studies conducted at the Center for the Biopsychosocial Study of AIDS in Miami, researchers have examined fear associated with HIV testing and notification. Among HIV-positive individuals, clinically significant anxiety was observed throughout each stage of the testing process. Peak anxiety levels and avoidance behaviors occurred during days just prior to and following serostatus notification (Antoni et al., 1990; Ironson et al., 1990). In addition to anxiety, depression and suicidal behavior may constitute part of the emotional sequelae immediately following an HIV diagnosis (Jacobsen, Perry, & Hirsch, 1990; Landau-Stanton & Clements, 1993; Perry, Jacobsberg, & Fishman, 1990). Pre- and posttest counseling aimed at providing the patient with useful information and support can help buffer the affective distress associated with HIV testing.

In an attempt to identify the mechanisms by which fear and dysphoria affect the decision to be tested, researchers have compared individuals who returned to HIV testing sites for serostatus results following phlebotomy appointments versus those who did not. Interestingly, fear seemed to play a significant role in determining the behaviors of both groups. Lyter, Valdiserri, Kingsley, Amoroso, and Rinaldo (1987) examined notification return rates in more than 2000 gay men. Among those who returned for results, gaining serostatus knowledge was viewed as empowering in their attempts to combat AIDS-associated fear. In contrast, those who chose not to return feared that an HIV diagnosis would be too burdensome and believed that they did not have adequate coping resources to deal with seropositivity (Lyter et al., 1987). It appears, therefore, that one's repertoire of coping skills may be an important factor in mediating the impact of fear on notification return rate.

Manifestations of fear associated with HIV testing and notification take many forms. Common fears include anticipation of decompensating health, physical and emotional suffering, and, ultimately, death. Concerns over discrimination and loss of personal resources (e.g., home, job, insurance, financial stability) also are deterrents to being tested. Policies and guidelines to ensure testing anonymity and confidentiality have eliminated many of the barriers to HIV testing. Too often, however, these fears reflect real threats to a seropositive individual's integrity and are enacted by a social milieu motivated by fear as well.

Denial is often the most immediate reaction to an HIV diagnosis. Denial can serve a defensive function by protecting the individual from decompensation and overwhelming levels of anxiety. If denial persists, however, it may manifest as maladaptive coping behaviors and avoidance strategies. Refusal to seek health care temporarily enables individuals to remove themselves from the reality of an HIV diagnosis. Continued risk behaviors, such as needle sharing and unsafe sex, also may reflect an element of denial (Forstein, 1984; Ostrow, 1990).

Pre- and posttest counseling, when done in a supportive environment by qualified health care providers, can enhance the person's ability to cope with the stress of testing and the subsequent emotional sequelae of an HIV diagnosis. Awareness of social support resources afforded by pretest counseling may improve the likelihood of follow-through on notification. Pre- and posttest counseling not only helps maximize rates of returning for results, but also initiates the process of health maintenance and improvement for individuals living with HIV. Knowledge of serostatus, whether HIV-positive or HIV-negative, may in turn lead to healthy behavioral and lifestyle changes. Improving and protecting one's health were viewed as paramount reasons to be tested by HIV-positive persons in studies by McCusker et al. (1988) and Siegel, Brooks, Kern, and Levine (1989). Concern for the health of one's sexual partner is an important consideration as well, and adds to the motivation to be tested (Ostrow et al., 1989).

Delaney and Goldblum (1987), in *Strategies for Survival: A Gay Man's Health Manual for the Age of AIDS*, offer advice to gay men struggling to cope with an HIV diagnosis. These authors outline strategies used by gay men with HIV disease to improve their quality and quantity of life. Decreased substance use, dietary changes, rest and exercise, and stress management constitute a few of the basic health maintenance tactics employed by gay men to cope effectively with HIV and maximize survival time (Delaney & Goldblum, 1987).

Data suggest that of the individuals who meet phlebotomy appointments for HIV testing, only 31–78% return for serostatus notification (McCusker et al., 1988; Ostrow et al., 1989; Valdiserri et al., 1993). Demography and risk category may account for part of the variance in return rates. In a review of more than 550,000 records of publicly funded HIV testing sites in the United States, Valdiserri et al. (1993) reported significant associations with race and age; subjects who were younger and African-American were less likely to return for testing results. Another study found that sexual orientation predicted return for notification. Cahn, Soriano,

Sumay, and Cahn (1993) reported that homosexuals were more likely than heterosexuals to return for their test results. Collectively, these data may reflect social norms yielded by the AIDS epidemic. It is acceptable and encouraged for gay men to be tested for HIV on a routine basis. Until recently, however, HIV-testing behaviors were not promoted among ethnic minority communities or young, sexually active heterosexuals.

Among IV drug users, length of sobriety and treatment history correlate with notification return rates. In their sample of over 1000 IV drug users, Rockwell et al. (1993) reported higher return rates for individuals who had sought methadone treatment consistently and had at least a 6-month history of sobriety prior to HIV testing. The characteristics of the testing site also have bearing on the decision to test. Proximity and familiarity were important features of the testing site to subjects in the study of Rockwell et al. (1993). Although IV drug users often are considered a difficult population to reach, evidence indicates that these individuals will follow through with HIV testing when consideration is given to their specialized treatment needs and health care accessibility is maximized. Although data regarding risk category and demography are sparse, the overall results suggest that tactics routinely used to encourage testing and notification follow-through may not be reaching a large portion of at-risk individuals. Outreach efforts should focus on HIV subpopulations, improving HIV-testing access and acceptability.

STANDARD MEDICAL TREATMENT: ACCEPTANCE AND ADHERENCE

At the mid-1990s, there is pessimism about finding a cure or vaccine for HIV, though great strides in the clinical management of HIV infection have been made since the mid-1980s. Antiretrovirals (e.g., AZT, ddI, and ddC) and protease inhibitors have become standard treatments and are known to slow the progression of HIV disease. Preventive measures, such as prophylaxis

for *Pneumocystis carinii* pneumonia (PCP) (the pneumonia most commonly associated with AIDS), are frequently part of the treatment protocol and help delay the onset of complicating illnesses for persons with HIV. Treatment approaches must be multifaceted in order to best combat the HIV illness spectrum, which is highly unpredictable and complex (Libman & Wiltzburg, 1993). In addition, a high morbidity of psychiatric illness has been documented in the HIV population (Fernandez & Ruiz, 1989). Thus, if treatment strategies are to be successful, they must be comprehensive and address multiple needs of the HIV-positive patient.

For most people with HIV, there is a substantial time lapse between HIV infection and initiation of treatment. Unfortunately, many seropositive individuals seek treatment late in the stages of HIV disease when CD4 cell counts (CD4 is the blood cell that facilitates immune functioning) are substantially lower than the thresholds at which antiretrovirals and PCP prophylaxis routinely would be introduced (Katz, Bindman, Keane, & Chan, 1992). Following treatment initiation, adherence to health care regimens may wax and wane. Maximizing treatment adherence and promoting healthful behaviors among seropositive individuals presents an unremitting challenge to health care providers.

A number of obstacles may hinder HIV-positive persons' access to and acceptance of health care. Fears similar to those associated with HIV testing may impede an individual's decision to seek medical treatment. Patients fear the breaching of confidentiality or disclosure of their seropositivity will result in multiple personal losses. Employment, insurance, housing, and financial assets may be threatened. Disclosure of serostatus often necessitates divulging additional information about one's lifestyle (e.g., sexual orientation, drug use). These revelations can ostracize a person's social support network. Anticipation of these potential losses may deter HIV-positive individuals from obtaining health care (Katz et al., 1992; Landau-Stanton & Clements, 1993).

Despite the thousands of health care professionals who have devoted time and energy to HIV intervention, some health care climates continue to be rejecting and hostile toward persons living with HIV. A few studies have indicated that attitudes and approaches to patient care adopted by the medical community are important predictors of patients' adherence to treatment. Among HIV patients in experimental treatments, respect and sensitivity from medical staff were viewed as highly influential in their decisions to participate in research protocols. Heightened attention to confidentiality issues and expression of appreciation by staff providers enhanced patients' satisfaction with participation in clinical trials (Johnson, 1994). Having a supportive primary care nurse was one of three crucial predictors of adherence in a study by Morse et al. (1991). In a study of dental care among HIV-positive individuals, the potential for rejection by the dental community was one of the primary reasons for not seeking dental care. Sadly, this concern was validated. One third of subjects in the study were denied or given limited treatment after disclosing their HIV statuses to their dentists (Robinson, Zakrzewska, Maini, Williamson, & Croucher, 1994).

The use of antiretrovirals in the treatment of AIDS has met with controversy. Critics state that antiretrovirals have limited efficacy and might cause more harm than benefit. For example, AZT has known bone marrow toxicity and a number of untoward side effects (e.g., anemia, nausea, headache). Awareness of these potential adverse events has attenuated the acceptance of standard pharmacotherapy practices among some individuals with HIV and AIDS. A few researchers have argued that the toxicity of AZT, coupled with continued unhealthy behaviors (e.g., substance abuse), actually facilitates the progression from HIV to AIDS (see Sonnabend, Witkin, & Purtilo, 1984).

Having faith in traditional medicine and the medical community may be a key factor in determining treatment adherence. Belief in the efficacy of standard pharmacological treatment regimens has been shown to affect adherence significantly. Increased adherence to PCP prophylaxis and anti-retroviral medications was associated with the belief that these medications delayed the onset of illness and increased longevity (Besch et al., 1994; Samet et al., 1992). Mossar, Lefevre, Deutsche, Wesch, and Glassroth (1993) conducted a large-scale, well-controlled study on medication adherence, examining a number of psychological and medical parameters, and matching subjects on demographic and risk category variables. Their general conclusion was that having little faith in traditional Western medicine while practicing alternative therapies was predictive of nonadherence to prophylactic treatments in a large cohort of HIV-positive subjects. No strong association between adherence and emotional indices was reported.

In many chronic-illness populations, the degree of family and social support is indicative of treatment adherence (see McDaniel, Hepworth, & Doherty, 1992). Support from families, significant others, health professionals, and social services has been shown to increase adherence to HIV medical treatment (Genser & Schlenger, 1994; Morse et al, 1991). Intervention programs aimed at increasing social support, such as the FRIENDS program at St. Claire's Hospital in New York City, have been successful in promoting both addiction recovery and treatment adherence among HIV-positive persons with substance abuse problems (Bodnar, Sharp, Mayer, & Rips, 1993). In addition, elevating the level of social support may have direct effects on the physical and psychological well-being of HIV-positive individuals by buffering the effects of stress (Thomason et al., 1996).

Despite the many obstacles to treatment, most studies on the HIV population have indicated high levels of treatment adherence. Rates of adherence to medical appointments and pharmacological regimens between and 80% and 90% have been reported (Besch, Collins, Morse, & Simon, 1992; Meisler et al. 1993; Samet et al., 1992). Sociodemographics, health status, and risk category may also be related to adherence. There is evidence that younger, uneducated, and healthier individuals are less adherent to HIV treatment (Besch et al., 1992; Samet et al., 1992). One study found that African-Americans demonstrated less adherence (Besch et al., 1992); other researchers found no association with race (Meisler et al., 1993).

Several studies have suggested that a history of IDU is associated with poor treatment adherence. For those in recovery, however, adherence levels are similar to levels in those without a history of substance abuse (Besch et al., 1992; Bodnar et al., 1993). Homelessness further complicates treatment adherence. Providing comprehensive medical care in a centralized and accessible site mitigates problems with adherence and facilitates treatment of drug addiction (Broers, Morabia, & Hirschel, 1994; Genser & Schlenger, 1994).

ALTERNATIVE MEDICINE

A lack of faith in traditional medical approaches to HIV care may impede adherence to conventional HIV therapies. Vast numbers of persons with HIV and AIDS, however, have become disenchanted with standard medical practice and have turned to alternative forms of therapy. Surveys of alternative therapy practices among the HIV population have indicated that these treatments are quite popular as replacements for standard medical care or as a complement to allopathic medicine. Studies have suggested that anywhere from 31% to 60% of persons with HIV use at least one form of alternative therapy (Anderson, O'Connor, MacGregor, & Schwartz, 1993; Wolffers & de Moree, 1994; Wolfstadter, Montaocean, Heyman, Bihari, & Buhring, 1993). Some researchers have noted that the higher estimates of usage may be more accurate, given that use of alternative therapies may exclude HIV patients from experimental treatment protocols. Fearing exclusion from these services, HIV patients may be impelled not to inform health care providers of their participation in alternative therapies (Anderson et al., 1993).

Many HIV care providers are wary of advocating alternative treatments due to their lack of empirical support for such treatments and uncertainty regarding their dangers and benefits. Recipients of the therapies, however, have attested overwhelmingly to the direct physical, psychological, and spiritual enhancement of alternative medicine (Wolffers & deMoree, 1994). From limited data, there is evidence to suggest that some forms of alternative therapies may delay the onset and progression of HIV disease, boost immune functioning, and help manage symptoms and side effects associated with pharmacotherapy (Gustafson, Cardellina, & Fuller, 1989; Nesetril, 1994). There is some speculation that they may increase survival time (Nesetril, 1994). In contrast, other researchers have described known toxicities of certain homeopathic drugs and their tendency to mimic HIV symptomatology (Gowen, Erksine, McAskill, & Hawkins, 1993). Furthermore, in one case study of an AIDS patient, death from an unconventional treatment (hydrogen peroxide therapy) has been reported (Hirschtick, Dydra, & Peterson, 1994).

Anderson et al. (1993) attempted to identify the most common modalities of alternative treatments and patterns of their usage in a study of nearly 200 HIV-positive subjects. These researchers found immune-enhancing agents such as interferon alpha, Chinese herbs, and cimetidine to be the most popular (used by 83% of subjects). Spiritual healing practices (used by 39%), however, were rated as the most satisfying. Most individuals availed themselves of more than one type of therapy, and studies have identified at least 100 types of alternative therapies being undertaken routinely by persons with HIV and AIDS (Anderson et al., 1993; Laifer, Ruettimann, Langewitz, Maurer, & Kiss, 1992). In addition to those already mentioned, common practices include special diets (e.g., vegetarian, high-protein, high-cereal, macrobiotic); body work, including yoga, massage therapy, and acupuncture; vitamin therapy; osteopathy; New Age methods (e.g., crystal therapy); and visual techniques (imagery and meditation) (Anderson et al., 1993; Barton, Davies, Schroeder, Arthur, & Gazzard, 1994; Hand, 1989; Laifer et al., 1992). Many individuals with HIV are engaged in some form of psychotherapy or support group. Studies have suggested that psychotherapeutic modalities may improve both physical and mental health and increase survival time for individuals with AIDS (Antoni et al., 1991; Thomason et al., 1996). Federally unapproved medications are available via underground networks and are taken frequently by persons with HIV and AIDS (Anderson et al., 1993). There are few rigorous studies and little hard data on the effectiveness of these interventions.

Collectively, traditional medical providers advocate the use of unconventional therapies to varying degrees. Knowing the hesitancy of some providers to support alternative medicine, however, most HIV-positive individuals do not disclose information about their engagement in these forms of therapies. Alternatively, many HIV-positive individuals have begun to identify alternative or holistic practitioners as their primary care providers. Seropositive persons who utilize holistic care providers rate them as more attentive to their health care needs than traditional providers. Alternative practitioners encourage patients to be proactive in their treatment regimens, and in doing so elevate patients' sense of empowerment and self-control (Harrington, 1992; Simms & McCann, 1992).

Most individuals seeking alternative therapies are informed of their availability by peers and HIV-related literature (Gowen et al., 1993; O'Connor, 1991). Engendered by limited access to unapproved therapies and the belief that many health professionals are unapproachable, extensive and sophisticated networks have evolved to meet the unaddressed needs of the AIDS community. Dispensing unapproved and unconventional therapies comprises one of their goals. Disseminating uncensored information and political activism are high on their agendas as well. The success of these groups (e.g., ACT-UP) has done a great deal to heighten AIDS awareness among the lay public, government, and health care community.

Financial burdens are commonplace for persons with AIDS, and the exorbitant cost of health care further complicates their financial stress. Money is often a factor in the decision to seek alternative treatments. The annual cost of standard pharmacotherapy and medical services for an AIDS patient was approximately $40,000 in 1987 (Johnston & Hopkins, 1990). Comparatively, HIV-positive individuals spent an average of $18 per month on alternative treatments in a study by Kassler, Blanc, and Greenblatt (1991). Costs of alternative therapies annually range from $40 to $8000, with a median of $700 (Anderson et al., 1993). As health care costs continue to rise, the large fiscal discrepancy between alternative and traditional medicine provides additional incentive for persons with HIV and AIDS to explore cost-effective, unconventional therapies.

There are no consistent data on what type of person is more likely to choose alternative therapies in managing HIV disease. Anderson et al. (1993) found associations with risk group, duration of illness, and sex; that is, gay men with a longer duration of seropositivity were more likely to engage in alternative treatment practices. Results from other studies have supported the finding that alternative therapies are employed more frequently among gay men relative to other risk groups (O'Connor, 1991), as well as among those in more advanced stages of disease (Greenblatt, Hollander, McMaster, & Henke, 1991).

With regard to sex as a predictor of alternative medicine utilization, results have been inconsistent. Anderson et al. (1993) reported that none of the female subjects in their study used alternative therapies. In stark contrast, Harrington (1992) documented the popularity of such treatment practices among HIV-positive women and noted the lack of efficacy with which standard medical practices address the health problems of women with HIV. All of the women who participated in this study incorporated some form of alternative therapy in their overall treatment regimens (Harrington, 1992).

BEHAVIORAL RISK REDUCTION AND PREVENTION: BASIC ELEMENTS

Behavioral risk reduction remains the only way to stop the rising incidence of HIV infection. Initial prevention efforts were focused on gay men, and effective elements of these programs have been successfully extended to diverse groups. These groups include women, ethnic minorities, young adults and adolescents, and those with severe and persistent mental illness, the highest-risk groups for HIV infection today (CDC, 1995; Nash & Said, 1992; WHO, 1995). As the demography of AIDS changes, prevention programs must be geared toward specific groups in culturally appropriate language and contexts. The basic elements of risk reduction, however, remain the same regardless of any particular subgroup or culture.

In their most generic form, HIV prevention programs are designed to eliminate or reduce the chances of HIV transmission from an infected person to someone else. As noted previously, HIV infection is possible only when direct blood-stream access is afforded to infected blood, blood products, semen, or vaginal fluid; additionally, breast milk carries the virus. Most cases of HIV transmission are due to specific sexual or drug use behaviors. Prevention efforts must focus on risk behaviors and psychosocial cofactors that facilitate risk. These specific behaviors include sexual intercourse without latex protection (e.g., condoms, dental dams), any sexual act that exposes open sores or cuts to infected body fluids, and sharing IDU apparatus. In the early years of the epidemic, gay men were cautioned to decrease their numbers of sexual partners and to avoid other behaviors that were thought to be potentially dangerous (e.g., oral–anal contact, hand–anal contact). The focus of most prevention efforts in the mid-1990s, however, is on the aforementioned specific sexual and drug use risk behaviors.

Psychosocial cofactors that facilitate engagement in high-risk behaviors have been found among all demographic groups, irrespective of an individual's knowledge of AIDS or HIV transmission. These cofactors include specific actions (e.g., alcohol and drug use), negative emotional states (e.g., depression, boredom, anger), dysfunctional cognitions (e.g., "He'll leave if I insist on him using a condom," "She looks healthy, so I

don't have to worry this time"), and social styles (e.g., a couple believing each is the other's only sexual partner). These cofactors make up the context in which risk behaviors occur and negatively influence personal perceptions of risk, self-efficacy, and coercion resistance. In behavioral terms, they are antecedents to risk behavior and must be addressed in prevention programs in order to ascertain behavior change. They are discussed later in this chapter.

Basic to all successful prevention programs is an educational component and a risk-reduction intervention. The vast majority of early AIDS prevention programs focused at the first level; i.e., increasing AIDS knowledge was seen as the goal of the programs. The implication was that behavioral change would result from an increased awareness of AIDS and HIV transmission risk. Evidence from other fields of health and clinical psychology suggested that this approach was oversimplified and risk behavior change could be made only through specifically targeting behaviors, their antecedents, and their consequences. Few programs (e.g., Kelly, St. Lawrence, Hood, & Brasfield, 1989) have offered comprehensive interventions focussing on these variables. The paucity of such programs is due in part to the slow response of fields such as psychology to the AIDS health crisis (see Campos, Brasfield, & Kelly, 1989) despite effective application of behavior change principles to other community health problems.

Education

Education about AIDS, HIV transmission, and the necessity of preventing transmission is an essential and important initial step in prevention programming. This is the educational foundation upon which further decisions about risk engagement, risk perception, and risk behavior change are made. Education is also the primary stage hypothesized in several health promotion models, such as the health belief model (Rosenstock, Strecher, & Becker 1994).

Specific knowledge about AIDS varies among

diverse populations, although most groups studied today tend to exhibit high general levels of knowledge about AIDS (see DiClemente, Forrest, & Mickler, 1990; Kelly et al., 1991). The failure of general education programs to change risk behaviors was also noted, however, in some of these studies (e.g., Bandura, 1994; Becker & Joseph, 1988; DiClemente & Peterson, 1994). Effective prevention of HIV transmission must move beyond educational approaches and include specific interventions to change risk behavior. Sexual and drug use risk behaviors can be divided into the general categories of "high-risk," "moderate-risk," "lowered-risk," and "no-risk," depending on the likelihood of HIV transmission.

In the "high-risk" category are vaginal or anal intercourse without a condom and sharing drug use apparatus. "Moderate-risk" behaviors include using a condom for vaginal or anal intercourse, nonprotected oral sex without orgasm, and boiling or bleaching needles and syringes prior to using them. In the "lowered-risk" category are oral sex with latex protection, nonpenetrative sexual acts, and cleaning drug paraphernalia at least three times before each use. Transmission of HIV by sexual means is not possible if a person abstains from sex, or engages exclusively in masturbation with no contact with open cuts or sores. Likewise, transmission via IDU is not possible if an individual refrains from using IV drugs. These are the only truly "no-risk" practices.

The examples given for "moderate-risk" and "lowered-risk" behaviors may not be widely accepted; i.e., some might argue that any condom use or any attempt to clean needles and syringes automatically constitutes "lowered-risk" practices. Use of a condom during vaginal or anal intercourse carries higher risk of infection than use during oral sex and therefore should be placed in a higher risk category. It could be argued that oral sex should be classified in the same way as anal or vaginal intercourse, although the notion that oral sex poses any risk at all is under debate. Nonetheless, the use of risk categories can be helpful in educating individuals about relative risks of certain practices and in assessing risk when moving from one behavioral category to another.

Effective prevention programs must include information about establishing lower-risk behaviors. One way to decrease high-risk behaviors may be to introduce competing behaviors lower in HIV-transmission risk. For sexual behaviors, such behaviors are termed "safer sex practices." They can include any behaviors that do not involve the exchange of body fluids (e.g., use of condoms) and any sexual acts that are nonpenetrative (e.g., mutual masturbation).

Surveys of sexual behaviors among United States adults have documented that practices termed "safer sex practices" may already be common as "foreplay" in the repertoires of persons with sexual experience (Kelly, 1995). Contrary to the goals of prevention programs, however, the adoption of safer sex practices does not automatically mean the exclusion or replacement of higher-risk behaviors. Instead, safer sex practices might be preludes to higher-risk behaviors. Although the introduction of lowered-risk alternatives is important in prevention programming, all programs must nonetheless focus on decreasing high-risk behaviors specifically.

Changing Risk Behavior

The ultimate goal of all prevention programs must be the cessation, or at least the decrement, of high-risk behaviors. If behavior change technology is applied to HIV prevention, risk-behavior change involves four components: (1) changing antecedents that trigger high- and lower-risk behaviors; (2) changing the specific risk behaviors; (3) changing the consequences of risk behaviors; and (4) preventing relapse into high-risk practices.

Changing the Antecedents of Risk Behavior. Behavioral antecedents are important psychosocial triggers. For HIV-transmission risk, antecedents can include a wide variety of variables. The behaviors in question are circumscribed:

sexual intercourse, with or without latex protection; sharing drug use apparatus; and safer sex behaviors. The possible triggers of each, however, are potentially overwhelming and highly individualistic. The best approach would be to consider what particular antecedents act as triggers under specific circumstances for each individual. It is not always feasible or cost-effective to do so, however, given the epidemic nature of the AIDS health crisis. An alternative approach must be to include attention to potential triggers in all group prevention programs so individuals can assess and change their own antecedents.

Although few investigators specifically address the concept of behavioral antecedents, several prevention approaches acknowledge controlling potential trigger variables in their application. For example, the idea of antecedent control is not explicitly identified in the area of risk perception. Risk perception is an important construct in many prevention models. It usually refers to how well individuals assess the degree to which their own behaviors may be putting them at risk for HIV infection. Risk perception is influenced by several psychosocial factors, including identification with affected groups, personally knowing people living with AIDS, geographic location, demographics, substance use, and prior experience with risk behaviors. Self-efficacy, self-esteem, social skills, culturally normative practices, and peer pressure might also influence one's ability to evaluate personal risk and subsequent engagement in risk behavior (e.g., Bandura, 1994; Kalichman, 1995).

The explicitness of the prevention message will influence risk perception. Risk perception is enhanced when explicit and clear descriptions of sexual and IDU behaviors are incorporated into the strategy. Moreover, language usage is an important consideration when designing a prevention message. For example, asking whether someone "engaged in sexual intercourse" is vague and often misunderstood. One must specifically define *intercourse* in culturally appropriate and lay terminology.

Some risk-perception variables (e.g., belief systems, self-efficacy) may be construed as antecedents to risk behaviors and therefore be amenable to behavioral interventions themselves. These variables may be considered psychosocial cofactors of HIV transmission insofar as negative mood states and beliefs provide a context for establishing and maintaining risk behavior (i.e. low self-efficacy may lead to reduced risk protection [e.g., Bandura, 1994]). Changing antecedents is an effective way of ameliorating target behaviors through their situational and personal triggers. This approach has yet to be systematically applied in AIDS prevention work. Part of the challenge may be defining specific antecedents to specific risk practices; to the knowledge of the authors, such studies have not been reported. Another challenge to dealing with antecedents is the diversity found among cues to action. The accuracy with which antecedents predict behavior varies across individuals, situations, and emotional states. A possible means to help clarify the value of identifying particular antecedents with given behaviors would be a series of single-subject studies, focusing specifically on HIV transmission behaviors.

Changing the Specific Risk Behavior.   Although changing antecedents and consequences of behaviors are themselves risk-change interventions, HIV prevention must include highly specific behavioral training as well. This training involves skill mastery, during which individuals are taught how to use condoms or "clean the works" with bleach. Another cardinal element is behavioral rehearsal, in which individuals practice these new, safer actions beyond the prevention seminar. Prostheses (e.g., "dildos") and various other paraphernalia may be used to illustrate the actions. Several highly innovative programs have been created using only this notion of explicit skill building.

In planning behavior change, the target population must be defined if the program is to be successful. In most programs, the population would be comprised of individuals attending the prevention seminars. Kelly, et al. (1992) focused their "Popular People" program, however, on key members of gay communities rather than on general consumers. Their approach is highly innovative. These investigators conceptualized a change in peer norms regarding acceptable and unacceptable sexual behaviors by intervening with men identified by their community as leaders. These leaders were trained specifically in risk reduction techniques and held private parties where they invited guests to participate in further prevention training. This strategy resulted in positive changes community-wide and had the additional bonus of influencing cultural norms that dictate the expression of behavior. Leaders of the social network were the specific targets of intervention, but the ultimate impact was felt on a global level within the community.

Changing the Consequences of Risk Behavior. As with any behavior change program, it is important to attend to the consequences of behavior. Consequences affect the probability of repetition or nonrepetition of an action and are crucial in predicting behavioral maintenance. HIV risk behaviors are highly pleasurable, while the negative consequences (e.g., HIV infection, immune compromise) are rarely immediate. This remoteness of consequences presents unique challenges to behavioral risk-reduction efforts.

There can be several interpersonal (e.g., relationship), social (e g., peer norms), and personal (e.g., self-esteem) consequences as the result of changing risk behaviors. Consequences that are positively reinforcing might include sustaining a monogamous relationship (interpersonal), acceptance by peers for being "clean" of drugs (social), and feeling empowered by resisting coercion (personal). These rewards help maintain lower-risk alternatives. Conversely, negative consequences of risk behavior can impede further development of safe behaviors, lead to relapse into higher-risk patterns, and create strong resistance to becoming safer. Examples might

include rejection threats from partners (interpersonal), peer resistance to safer norms (social), and feeling rejected if others deride safer practices (personal). These negative events act as punishment for lower risk efforts and may become antecedents to higher-risk practices (Kelly, 1995).

The positive and negative consequences resulting from risk-behavior change often create a double-bind for the individual. For example, teaching clients assertion skills to resist coercive sexual requests may be personally rewarding but simultaneously create a power imbalance in individuals' relationships. As individuals change risk patterns, different peer groups and relationships may need to be formed in order to garner support and reinforce new behavioral norms (Kelly, 1995).

Prevention of Relapse. Finally, effective prevention programs must also attend to the possibility of lapsed behavior, or relapse in general. "Lapses" are defined as temporary, usually one-time, recurrences of high-risk behaviors. "Relapse" is the sustained involvement in high-risk behaviors to preintervention levels or even higher levels. In studies of gay men, several factors were found to influence reengagement in higher-risk practices. Kelly et al. (1991) reported that high-risk lapses were inversely related to situational and personal efficacy variables. In addition, the data suggested that high-risk lapses may be dictated in part by affective states. Interestingly, these authors found a higher degree of relapse associated with positive emotional experiences and cognitions (e.g., "I wanted to please my partner," "It felt better") than with negative emotional experiences (e.g., "I was depressed," "I felt inadequate").

In standard relapse-prevention work, lapses are permissible events. Individuals are instructed not to consider the event an irremediable catastrophe, but instead to use the information to plan against future lapses. With respect to HIV infection, this intervention would be a difficult reconciliation, given that even one lapse into high-risk behavior has potentially devastating consequences. That is, behavioral lapses might lead to infection of HIV-negative individuals or to reinfection with perhaps a more virulent or lethal strain of the virus for seropositive persons.

In classic work by Marlatt and Gordon (1985) with substance abuse, *planned* lapses were found to enhance relapse prevention in certain circumstances. As a result of this paradoxical strategy, treated subjects were able to maintain a sense of control over changed behaviors. Unfortunately, planned lapses into high-risk behaviors might lead to HIV infection or reinfection and are therefore unacceptable, for obvious medical and ethical reasons. Alternatively, given that lapses into high-risk behavior are found in a substantial percentage of individuals who have made significant behavioral changes (e.g., Kelly et al., 1991), a planned program of cognitive behavioral intervention might enhance maintenance of behavioral changes without the need for "planned empowerment."

In summary, the overall approach to preventing HIV transmission through behavioral risk reduction must be comprehensive and multifaceted. Thus far, successful prevention programs have included educational approaches to increase AIDS knowledge, specific interventions to reduce high-risk behaviors and increase lower-risk alternatives, attention to contextual and antecedent conditions (e.g., psychosocial factors influencing risk perception, cultural variables), personal contingencies to reinforce positive changes, and enhancement of relapse prevention. In addition, researchers must search for new prevention elements as the demography of AIDS changes daily and the pandemic continues to grow exponentially.

METHODOLOGICAL CONSIDERATIONS AND FUTURE DIRECTIONS IN HIV HEALTH BEHAVIOR RESEARCH

Halfway through the second decade of the AIDS health crisis, the literature on HIV health behavior remains sparse. At the beginning of the epidemic, social scientists were among the first proactive professionals to address HIV health behavior by planning and implementing AIDS prevention programs in major United States cities (McKusick, Conant, & Coates, 1985). Unfortunately, the initial motivation for applied research on HIV health behavior has lost momentum. Unlike other health concerns, behavioral aspects of HIV have not been popular foci on the research agendas of behavioral medicine scientists (Kelly, 1994). Applying theoretical principles and research strategies from related areas of health psychology may provide a stronger empirical foundation for HIV behavioral research as well as stimulate the interests of potential investigators.

The available data on HIV health behavior are limited not only in number but also in scope. HIV research, in general, has been criticized for selective sampling procedures. The majority of published studies have been conducted on gay men, most of whom are Caucasian, educated, socioeconomically stable, and reside close to AIDS epicenters in large urban areas. Given the dynamic nature of AIDS demography, the generalizability of existing data is stifled. Future investigations must include heterogeneous samples of the HIV population. Health concerns and behaviors of HIV-positive persons often excluded from research endeavors (i.e., women and ethnic minorities of varying socioeconomic status) must be addressed. Additionally, recent data indicate a rise of HIV infection among certain subsections of homosexual men (i.e, rural, young, ethnic minority, and "closeted" homosexual men) (Centers for Disease Control, 1993). Prevention efforts targeting the gay community, must, therefore, be re-examined both theoretically and empirically.

Finally, as research efforts expand, attention should focus on designing methodologically sound investigations. The selection of appropriate outcome variables in HIV behavioral research may need closer scrutiny. Gibson and Young (1994) have pointed out that commonly employed outcome measures, such as condom use, may not be relevant to all interventions or population samples. Kelly (1994) cautioned against overreliance on self-report indices, noting the traditional concerns of social desirability, errors in recall, and response sets when using self-report. More prospective studies with adequate sample sizes and incorporating objective parameters are needed before definite conclusions about HIV behavioral research can be drawn.

CONCLUSION

The AIDS health crisis has had a profound impact on the attitudes and behaviors of millions globally. For those living with HIV, health behaviors may dictate quality of life and survival time. The complexity of HIV disease has challenged traditional Western medicine while providing fertile ground for the proliferation of alternative therapies. "Safe sex" has become a buzz phrase of the '90s, evidencing an increased awareness of preventive health behaviors among both the HIV-affected community and the general population. Unfortunately, this heightened awareness has not been paralleled by a slowing of the epidemic, and the decimation of AIDS has advanced without reprieve. Until a cure is found, changing health behaviors remains paramount in combatting HIV disease.

REFERENCES

Anderson, W., O'Connor, B. B., MacGregor, R. R., & Schwartz, J. S. (1993). Patient use and assessment of conventional and alternative therapies for HIV infection and AIDS. *AIDS, 7,* 561-566.

Antoni, M., August, S., LaPerriere, A., Baggett, H. L., Klimas, N., Ironson, G., Schneiderman, N., & Fletcher, M. A. (1990). Psychological and neuroendocrine measures related to functional immune changes in anticipation of HIV-1 serostatus notification. *Psychosomatic Medicine, 52,* 496-510.

Antoni, M., Baggett, L., Ironson, G., LaPerriere, A., August, S., Klimas, N., Schneiderman, N., & Fletcher, M. A. (1991). Cognitive-behavioral stress management intervention buffers distress responses and immunologic changes following notification of HIV-1 seropositivity. *Journal of Consulting and Clinical Psychology, 59,* 906-915.

Bandura, A., (1994). Social cognitive theory and exercise of control over HIV infections. In R. J. DiClemente & J. L. Peterson (Eds.), *Preventing Aids: Theories and methods of behavioral interventions* (297-317). New York: Plenum Press.

Barton, S. E., Davies, S., Schroeder, K., Arthur, G., & Gazzard, B. G. (1994). Complementary therapies used by people with HIV infection. *AIDS, 8,* 561.

Becker, M. H., & Joseph, J. G. (1988). AIDS and behavioral change to reduce risk: A review. *American Journal of Public Health, 78,* 394-410.

Besch, C. L., Collins, G., Morse, E., & Simon, P. (1992). *Cofactors associated with participant compliance in two CPCRA trials.* Abstract presented at the 8th International Conference on AIDS, Amsterdam.

Besch, C. L., Morse, E. V., Simon, P. M., Bincsik, A., Cefali, P., Connett, J., Child, C., Costanzo, L., Cox, L., & Landry, S. (1994). *Determinants of levels of compliance in patients enrolled in a PCP prophylaxis protocol (Community Programs for Clinical Research on AIDS [CPCRA]): Baseline data.* Abstract presented at the 10th International Conference on AIDS, Yokohama.

Bodnar, S., Sharp, V., Mayer, J., & Rips, J. (1993). *Friendship and the facilitation of medical care among HIV-infected substance abusers.* Abstract presented at the 9th International Conference on AIDS, Berlin.

Broers, B., Morabia, A., & Hirschel, B. (1994). A cohort study of drug users' compliance with zidovudine treatment. *Archives of Internal Medicine, 154,* 1121-1127.

Cahn, R., Soriano, S., Sumay, A., & Cahn, P. (1993). *Desertion during HIV testing process.* Abstract presented at the 9th international conference on AIDS, Berlin.

Campos, P. E., Brasfield, T. L., & Kelly, J. A. (1989). Psychology training related to AIDS: Survey of doctoral graduate programs and predoctoral internship programs. *Professional Psychology: Research and Practice, 20,* 214-220.

Centers for Disease Control. (1993). *HIV/AIDS surveillance.* Atlanta, GA: U.S. Public Health Service.

Centers for Disease Control and Prevention Studies (1995). Statistics from the Centers for Disease Control and Prevention. *AIDS, 9,* 103-105.

Delaney, M., & Goldblum, P. (1987). *Strategies for survival: A gay man's health manual for the age of AIDS.* New York: St. Martin's Press.

DiClemente, R. J., Forrest, K. A., Mickler, S., and Principal Site Investigators (1990). College students' knowledge and attitudes about AIDS and changes in HIV-preventive behaviors. *AIDS Education and Prevention, 2,* 201-212.

DiClemente, R. T., & Peterson, J. L., (1994). Changing HIV/AIDS Risk Behaviors: The role of behavioral intervention. In R. J. DiClemente, & J. L. Peterson (Eds.), *Preventing AIDS: Theories and methods of behavioral interventions.* (pp. 1-4). New York: Plenum Press.

Fernandez, F., & Ruiz, P. (1989). Psychiatric aspects of HIV disease. *Southern Medical Journal, 82,* 999-1004.

Forstein, M. (1984). The psychosocial impact of the acquired immune deficiency syndrome. *Seminars in Oncology, 11,* 77–82.

Genser, S. G., & Schlenger, W. (1994). *Retaining at-risk drug abusers in drug treatment and medical care: Strategies for HIV risk intervention.* Abstract presented at the 10th International Conference on AIDS, Yokohama.

Gibson, D. R., & Young, M. (1994). Importance of appropriate outcome measures in HIV behavioral research. *Journal of Acquired Immune Deficiency Syndromes, 7,* 631–632.

Gowen, S. L., Erskine, D., McAskill, R., & Hawkins, D. (1993). *An assessment of the usage of non-prescribed medication by HIV positive patients.* Abstract presented at the 9th International Conference on AIDS, Berlin.

Greenblatt, R. M., Hollander, H., McMaster, J. R., & Henke, C. J. (1991). Polypharmacy among patients attending an AIDS clinic: Utilization of prescribed, unorthodox, and investigational treatments. *Journal of Acquired Immune Deficiency Syndromes, 4,* 136–143.

Gustafson, K. R., Cardellina, J. H., & Fuller, R. W. (1989). AIDS antiviral sulfolipids from cyanobacteria (blue-green algae). *Journal of the National Cancer Institute, 81,* 1254–1258.

Hand, R. (1989). Alternative therapies used by patients with AIDS. *New England Journal of Medicine, 320,* 672–673.

Harrington, I. (1992). *The use of complementary therapies by HIV+ women.* Abstract presented at the 8th International Conference on AIDS, Amsterdam.

Hirschtick, R. E., Dydra, S. E., & Peterson, L. C. (1994). Death from an unconventional therapy for AIDS. *Annals of Internal Medicine, 120,* 694.

Ironson, G., LaPerriere, A., Antoni, M., O'Hearn, P., Schneiderman, N., Klimas, N., & Fletcher, M.A. (1990). Anticipation and reaction to news of HIV-1 antibody status. *Psychosomatic Medicine, 52,* 247–270.

Jacobsen, P. B., Perry, S. W., & Hirsch, D. A. (1990). Behavioral and psychological responses to HIV antibody testing. *Journal of Consulting and Clinical Psychology, 58,* 31–37.

Johnson, L. M. (1994). *An assessment of satisfaction of clinical research participants in a long term study.* Abstract presented at the 10th International Conference on AIDS, Yokohama.

Johnston, W. B., & Hopkins, K. G. (1990). *The catastrophe ahead: AIDS and the case for a new public policy.* New York: Praeger.

Kalichman, S. C. (1995). *Understanding AIDS: A guide for mental health professionals,* Washington, DC: American Psychological Association.

Kassler, W.J., Blanc, P., & Greenblatt, R. (1991). The use of medicinal herbs by human immunodeficiency virus-infected patients. *Archives of Internal Medicine, 151,* 2281–2288.

Katz, M., Bindman, A., Keane, D., & Chan, A. (1992). CD4 lymphocyte count as an indicator of delay in seeking human immunodeficiency virus-related treatment. *Archives of Internal Medicine, 152,* 1501–1504.

Kelly, J. A. (1994). HIV prevention among gay and bisexual men. In R. J. DiClemente & J. L. Peterson (Eds.), *Preventing AIDS: Theories and methods of behavioral interventions* (pp. 297–317) New York: Plenum Press.

Kelly, J. A. (1995). *Changing HIV Risk Behavior: Practical Strategies.* New York: Guilford Press.

Kelly, J. A., Kalichman, S., Kauth, M., Kilgore, H., Hood, H. V., Campos, P.E., Rao, S. M., Brasfield, T. L., & St. Lawrence, J. S. (1991). Situational factors associated with AIDS risk behavior lapses and coping strategies used by gay men who successfully avoid lapses. *American Journal of Public Health, 81,* 1335–1337.

Kelly, J. A., St. Lawrence, J. S., Hood, H. V., & Brasfield, T. L. (1989). Behavioral intervention to reduce AIDS risk activities. *Journal of Consulting and Clinical Psychology, 57,* 60–67.

Kelly, J. A., St. Lawrence, J. S., Stevenson, L. Y., Hauth, A. C., Kalichman, S. C., Diaz., Y. E., Brasfield, T. S., Koob, J. J., & Morgan, M. G. (1992). Community AIDS/HIV risk reduction: The effects of endorsements by popular people in three cities. *American Journal of Public Health, 82,* 1483–1489.

Laifer, G., Ruettimann, S., Langewitz, W., Maurer, P., & Kiss, A. (1992). *Frequent use of alternative therapies and higher subjective benefit compared to traditional medicine in HIV-infected patients.* Abstract presented at the 8th International Conference on AIDS, Amsterdam.

Landau-Stanton, J., & Clements, C. D. (1993). *AIDS, health, and mental health: A primary sourcebook.* New York: Brunner/Mazel.

Libman, H., & Witzburg, R. A. (1993). *HIV infection: A clinical manual.* Boston Little, Brown.

Lyter, D. W., Valdiserri, R. O., Kingsley, L. A., Amoroso, W. B., & Rinaldo, C. R. (1987). The HIV antibody test: Why gay and bisexual men want or do not want to know their results. *Public Health Reports, 102,* 468–474.

Marlatt, A., & Gordon, J. R. (1985). *Relapse prevention: Maintenance strategies in the treatment of addictive behaviors.* New York: Guilford Press.

McCusker, J., Stoddard, A. M., Mayer, A. H., Zapka, J., Morrison, C., & Saltzman, S. P. (1988). Effects of HIV antibody test knowledge on subsequent sexual behaviors in a cohort of homosexually active men. *American Journal of Public Health, 78,* 462–467.

McDaniel, S. H., Hepworth, J., & Doherty, W.J. (1992). *Medical family therapy: A biopsychosocial approach to families with health problems.* New York: Basic Books.

McKusick, L., Conant, M., & Coates, T. J. (1985). The AIDS epidemic: A model for developing intervention strategies for reducing high risk behavior in gay men. *Sexually Transmitted Disease, 12,* 229–234.

Meisler, A., Ickovics, J., Walesky, M., Fiellin, M., Skowronski, C., & Friedland, G. (1993). *Adherence to clinical trials among women, minorities, and injection drug users.* Abstract presented at the 9th International Conference on AIDS, Berlin.

Morse, E. V., Simon, P. M., Coburn, M., Hyslop, N., Greenspan,

D., & Balson, P. M. (1991). Determinants of subject compliance within an experimental anti-HIV drug protocol. *Social Science & Medicine, 32*, 1161–1167.

Mossar, M., Lefevre, F., Deutsche, J., Wesch, J., & Glassroth, J. (1993). *Factors predicting compliance with prophylactic treatments among HIV positive patients.* Abstract presented at the 9th International Conference on AIDS, Berlin.

Nash, G., & Said, J. (1992). *Pathophysiology of AIDS and HIV infection.* Philadelphia: W. B. Saunders.

Nesetril, F. (1994). *Alternative treatments for HIV infection.* Abstract presented at the 10th International Conference on AIDS, Yokohama.

O'Connor, B. B. (1991). *PWA use and evaluation of alternative therapies in Philadelphia.* Abstract presented at the 7th international conference on AIDS, Florence.

Ostrow, D. G. (Ed.). (1990). *Behavioral aspects of AIDS.* New York: Plenum Press.

Ostrow, D. G., Joseph, J. G., Kessler, R., Soucy, J., Tal, M., Eller, M., Chmiel, J., & Phair, J. P. (1989). Disclosure of HIV antibody status: Behavioral and mental health characteristics. *AIDS Education and Prevention, 1*, 1–11.

Perry, S., Jacobsberg, L., & Fishman, B. (1990). Relationships between CD4 lymphocytes and psychological variables among HIV positive adults. Abstract presented at the Sixth International Conference on AIDS, San Francisco.

Robinson, P., Zakrzewska, J.M., Maini, M., Williamson, D., & Croucher, R. (1994). Dental visiting behaviour and experiences of men with HIV. *British Dental Journal, 176*, 175–179.

Rockwell, R., Bardell, B., Sotheran, J. L., Wenston, J. A., Friedman, S. R., & DesJarlais, D. C. (1993). *Predictors of return by IDUs to an HIV clinic for post-HIV test counseling on the lower east side, NYC.* Abstract presented at the 9th International Conference on AIDS, Berlin.

Rosenstock, I. M., Strecher, V. J., & Becker, M. H. (1994). The health belief model and HIV risk behavior change. In R. J. DiClemente & J. L. Peterson (Eds.), *Preventing AIDS: Theories and methods of behavioral interventions* (pp. 5–24). New York: Plenum Press.

Samet, J. H., Libman, H., Steger, K. A., Dhawan, R. K., Chen, J., Shevitz, A. H., Dewees-Dunk, R., Levenson, S., Kufe, D., & Craven, D. E. (1992). Compliance with zidovudine therapy in patients infected with human immunodeficiency virus, type 1: A cross-sectional study in a municipal hospital clinic. *American Journal of Medicine, 92*, 495–502.

Schochetman, G., & George, J. R. (1992). *AIDS testing: Methodology and management issues.* New York: Springer-Verlag.

Siegel, K., Brooks, C., Kern, R., & Levine, M. (1989). *Gay men's decisions about taking the HIV antibody test.* Abstract presented at the 5th International Conference on AIDS, Montreal.

Simms, M., & McCann, K. E. (1992). *The use of and attitudes to alternative medicine on the part of gay men with AIDS or HIV infection.* Abstract presented at the 8th International Conference on AIDS, Amsterdam.

Sonnabend, J. A., Witkin, S. S., & Purtilo, D. T. (1984). AIDS: An explanation for its occurrence among homosexual men. In P. Ma & D. Armstrong (Eds.), *Acquired immune deficiency syndrome and infections of homosexual men.* New York: York Medical Books.

Thomason, B., Jones, G., McClure, J., & Brantley, P. (1996). Psychosocial co-factors in HIV illness: An empirically-based model. *Psychology and Health, 11*, 385–393.

Valdiserri, R. O., Moore, M., Gerber, A. G., Campbell, C. H, Dillon, B. A., & West, G. R. (1993). A study of clients returning for counseling after HIV testing: Implications for improving rates of return. *Public Health Reports, 108* 12–18.

Wolffers, I., & de Moree, S. (1994). *Alternative treatment as contribution to care of pwHIV/AIDS.* Abstract presented at the 10th International Conference on AIDS, Yokohama.

Wolfstadter, D., Montaocean, K., Heyman, J., Bihari, B., & Buhring, M. (1993). *Survey study on distribution, risks and benefits of alternative treatments in HIV and AIDS.* Abstract presented at the 9th international conference on AIDS, Berlin.

World Health Organization. (1995). Statistics from the World Health Organization. *AIDS, 9*, 409–410.

9

Health Behavior in Developing Countries

Jeannine Coreil

INTRODUCTION

The distinction between developed and developing countries has become increasingly blurred as many less developed countries make important strides in social conditions as well as economic development. While it long has been recognized that the nations of the world do not fall neatly into two categories of "more" and "less" developed, but instead extend across a wide continuum of socioeconomic diversity, only recently have observers noted that health and quality of life indicators can be quite variable within countries traditionally considered underdeveloped (Pillai & Shannon, 1995). Some very poor countries have made remarkable improvements in the health of their populations, while comparatively wealthier nations have not fared so well (Caldwell, 1990). It is common to find a fourfold typol-

ogy by which nations are classified as least developed, less developed, newly industrialized, and developed.

The criteria used to define development have included economic, demographic, social, and political indicators. By World Bank (1993) definitions, the term *developing economies* refers to those that fall within the low to middle range of gross national product (GNP) per capita. Low-income economies are those with a GNP of $635 (U.S.) or less; middle-income economies include those with a GNP above $635 but less than $7911. Low- and middle-income countries are also defined as demographically developing, in the sense that their age distributions are young, compared with those of industrialized nations, owing to their high fertility rate. Composite social–health indicators have been devised to measure quality of life conditions such as the Physical Quality of Life Index (PQLI) and the Index of Suffering (Pillai & Shannon, 1995). In recent decades, the term *Third World* is often used synonymously with *developing countries* in the economic sense; the term as originally used, however, was primarily political in meaning, growing out of the Cold War era when three worlds of development corresponded to demo-

Jeannine Coreil • Department of Community and Family Health, College of Public Health, University of South Florida, Tampa, Florida 33612.

Handbook of Health Behavior Research III: Demography, Development, and Diversity, edited by David S. Gochman. Plenum Press, New York, 1997.

cratic, Communist, and nonaligned nations (Horowitz, 1966). This chapter uses the terms "developing" and "Third World" countries interchangeably.

In discussions related to health, it is helpful to consider the social- and health-related indicators that are often cited in discussions of the health conditions of developing countries. These indicators include urban/rural population distribution, literacy rate, access to clean water, infant and under-5 mortality, maternal mortality, fertility rate, and life expectancy. Table 1 contrasts typical norms for these indices for developing and developed countries. It should be borne in mind that many countries fall somewhere between these two ideal types. While developed countries are highly urbanized and industrialized, developing countries have predominantly agricultural economies supported by rural-dwelling populations with little education. Access to clean water and modern medical services is comparatively low, with infant mortality, child malnutrition, and maternal mortality very high in the less developed areas. Life expectancy is considerably lower and fertility much higher.

Research on health behavior in developing countries differs markedly from its counterpart in developed countries, for several reasons. First, child health and survival is the most important public health problem in the Third World because of the predominance of youth in the population (a product of high fertility) and because mortality in this age group exceeds adult mortality. Second, infectious and parasitic diseases are more prevalent in developing countries than chronic, noncommunicable diseases, and environmental risk factors for these health problems are more important than individual health behavior. Third, while health behavior research in developed countries tends to be organized around particular behaviors (e.g., smoking, exercise, diet, use of seat belts), behavioral research in developing countries is largely centered around biomedically defined diseases and organized efforts to control them (e.g., malaria, AIDS, tuberculosis, diarrhea).Fourth, governments and families in developing countries have fewer resources to invest in lifestyle change, and individuals have less choice of and control over their health-related behavior than is typical in developed countries. Thus, behavioral research on health in developing countries is shaped by the dominant health goal of reducing child mortality from preventable infectious diseases, while in developed countries the emphasis is on reducing adult morbidity from chronic diseases, primarily through lifestyle modification.

**Table 1. Indicators of Health
in Developing and Developed Areas**

Indicator	Developing areas	Developed areas
Health-related demographic rates		
Infant mortality	100	10
Under-5 mortality	175	13
Maternal mortality	500	11
Total fertility	5	2
Life expectancy	53 years	75 years
Population urban	30%	73%
Adults literate (M/F)	53%/33%	97%/90%
Access to clean water	37%	95%
Ratio of expenditures for health/defense	4/33	50/50

DEVELOPMENTAL TRANSITIONS

Developing societies are undergoing complex transitions in the areas of population trends, disease patterns, and health behavior. These processes have been described as, respectively, the demographic, epidemiological, and health transitions. Each will be discussed briefly, to set the stage for a more detailed discussion of health behavior in developing countries.

Demographic Transition. History has shown that as societies undergo the shift from rural agricultural economies to urban industrialized ones, population processes follow a predictable course of change referred to as the *demographic transition.* The pretransition period is characterized by high rates of fertility and mortality, particularly infant and child mortality, producing moderate rates of population growth. During the period of transition, death rates first begin to decrease in response to improvements in living conditions and health care, but there is a lag time during which fertility remains high because the factors that favor large family sizes, such as expectations for high mortality among children, are slow to change. This lag results in elevated population growth rates, which is the situation in which many developing countries find themselves in the latter part of the 20th century and the reason that population growth is sometimes used to define underdevelopment. Over time, fertility decreases in response to falling mortality, producing the low growth rates characteristic of industrialized nations.

Epidemiological Transition. Along with the demographic changes just described, corresponding changes occur in the pattern of diseases that dominate the health profile of a society. The pretransition situation is characterized by high rates of infectious disease, including diarrheal diseases, respiratory infections, and parasitic diseases, which, coupled with poor nutritional status, lead to excess deaths in the younger age groups. As infectious diseases decline, more

children survive to adulthood, life expectancy increases, and chronic diseases that affect the older population become the major health problems of a society, as currently seen in industrialized countries. These processes are referred to as the *epidemiological transition* (Omran, 1971), and most developing countries are currently in the early stages of this transformation.

Table 2 illustrates common health problems experienced by young and older age groups pre- and posttransition. It has become apparent in recent years, however, that population subgroups within a single country may experience very different rates of disease change, creating an "epidemiologic polarization" (Frenck, Bobadilla, Sepulveda, & Cervantes, 1989) between the disadvantaged and wealthier classes. It is also important to consider variation across ethnic groups, time periods, and geographic zones (Phillips, 1991).

Health Transition. The concept of the "health transition" is a more recently defined area of study that seeks to elucidate the cultural, social, and behavioral determinants of health that underlie the epidemiological transition (Caldwell, 1993). Health transition research looks beyond changes in material standard of living and medical services to understand the behavioral and sociocultural factors that influence health conditions in all societies, with most work concentrated in poor countries. Some of the important findings to emerge from this work include the far-reaching effects of maternal education on a variety of health activities and the impact of household organization on health-related behavior. The accumulating body of research on health behavior in developing countries would fall within the health transition rubric, although many such studies are not explicitly identified as health transition research.

METHODOLOGICAL ISSUES

Overreliance on Aggregate Data. The most serious methodological issue of concern to

**Table 2. Illustrative Health Problems
of Children and Adults Pre- and
Postepidemiological Transition**[a]

Pretransition	Posttransition
Children	
Diarrhea	Congenital defects
Acute respiratory infections	Growth failure
Polio, tetanus	Micronutrient deficiency
Undernutrition	Mental development problems
Malaria	Injury
Intestinal helminths	
Adults and elderly	
Tuberculosis	Mental disorders
Malaria	Circulatory disease
AIDS/STDs	AIDS/STDs
Parasitic diseases	Cancers
Injury	Injury
Maternal problems	Chronic pulmonary disease

[a]Reproduced with permission from the *Annual Review of Public Health*,
Volume II. © 1990 by Annual Reviews, Inc.

this chapter is the paucity of available research conducted in developing countries on specific health-related behaviors. The bulk of the literature focuses on epidemiological trends, mortality patterns, availability of services, evaluation of programs, and policy issues such as the relative merits of alternative strategies for improving health. Much of the research relies on aggregate data, vital statistics, broad population indicators, and the like, with little attention to individual-level data, which would allow analysis of the predictors of health behavior. For example, much of the health transition research is based on national statistics comparing different societies on indicators such as life expectancy, infant mortality, education of women, and per capita income. Studies that do focus on individual behavior have been largely concentrated on utilization of health services and, to a lesser extent, on performance of health-promoting actions in the home. Comparatively little research has addressed personal attributes such as beliefs, expectations, motives, values, perceptions, and other cognitive

elements. Studies that have addressed these kinds of factors derive primarily from operational research on externally funded programs aimed at high-profile health problems that affect children and childbearing women. Thus, available research is skewed toward issues important to donor agencies that fund large-scale public health initiatives.

Knowledge, Attitudes, and Practices (KAP) Surveys. Research on individual health behavior in developing countries has been heavily skewed toward the standard KAP survey, which segments behavior into discrete elements such as knowledge of disease risk factors, use/nonuse of a health practice/service, and perceptions of therapeutic efficacy. The KAP survey for decades served as the standard for applied behavioral research in the Third World, providing quantifiable demographic data and behavioral indices amenable to statistical analysis (Hursh-Cesar, 1988). For example, KAP-type variables (e.g., contraceptive prevalence, breast-feeding rate, and use of oral rehydration therapy for diarrhea) are often measured in large-scale surveys such as the Demographic and Health Survey and the World Fertility Survey. The utility of the KAP survey method for understanding health behavior has been criticized on several grounds, including the validity of responses (Schopper, Doussantousse, & Orav, 1993), the limited explanatory power of survey items, and the moderate impact on policy that expensive national surveys have achieved (Davis, 1987).

Qualitative Methods. In contrast to the KAP survey approach, anthropological research on health behavior has traditionally relied on qualitative ethnographic methods and small-sample community studies. Both theoretically oriented and applied research on ethnomedical beliefs and practices have followed this approach. This tradition has stimulated the development of specialized methodologies, variously referred to as "rapid ethnographic assessment," "rapid anthropological procedures," and "focused ethnographic studies," which share a basic grounding in qualitative methods applied to a specific domain of inquiry (Manderson & Aaby, 1992). These methods aim to collect in-depth data on the cultural construction of health problems and identify local patterns of prevention and treatment. Rapid assessment grew out of the need of applied researchers to provide policy-relevant information about how people think and act in a relatively short time frame. In addition, the qualitative data complemented KAP studies by addressing questions such as why people acted as they do and by providing insights into the social context of behavior.

With the popularization of social marketing approaches to behavior change in Third World settings in the past decade, group interview methods, and focus groups in particular, have gained prominence in health behavior research (Coreil, 1995). Like its ethnographic cousin, the "consumer" approach to research seeks to illuminate how people think about a health issue, but it is more explicitly oriented toward uncovering values and motives that underlie behavioral decisions and choices. Identifying barriers and incentives to behavior change is an important process in this endeavor, with the aim of applying the information to program design.

Integration of Qualitative and Quantitative Methods. Contemporary discussions of methodological issues in applied behavioral research reflect a growing consensus that an integration of qualitative and quantitative data provides the most powerful analysis, and multimethod approaches increasingly are viewed as the standard for applied research in developing countries (Yach, 1992). For example, it is common for community-based studies to include a household survey, focus group interviews, key informant interviews, and participant observation as complementary sources of data to address a research problem.

THEORETICAL PERSPECTIVES

Health behavior research in the United States has focused primarily on individual behavior change, drawing on conceptual frameworks from social psychology and health education such as the health belief model, social learning theory, the PRECEDE model, and the transtheoretical model. In contrast, behavioral research on health in developing countries has been much less conceptually oriented. The literature is heavy in empirical studies organized around an essentially biomedical/epidemiological framework of disease-focused studies that seek to identify specific determinants of health practices. Much of the research is purely descriptive, with no stated theoretical underpinnings. Overall, the field is less focused on individual behavior and more oriented toward family and community contexts of behavior. In line with this pattern, anthropological and culture change perspectives have figured importantly in research traditions, and in recent decades economic models have gained increasing prominence.

Health Communication Models. In the 1970s, innovation theory gained popularity as researchers sought to explain why some people adopt healthy behaviors more readily than others and to identify the characteristics of people who try new behaviors early versus late in the culture change process (Valente & Rogers, 1995). This approach was applied to a variety of public health problems including family planning, breast-feeding, dietary change, and, more recently, oral rehydration therapy and condom use. Early anthropological research in this vein tended to conceptualize the issues in terms of determinants of culture change, with traditional cultural patterns often assumed to serve as barriers to successful innovation, or "acculturation," if a culture-contact situation was involved. The outcomes of change studied, however, were usually specific behavioral practices (Paul, 1955).

What was described as directed culture change programs in that era would appropriately fall within the field of applied health communication in the 1990s. Health communication models have continued to evolve over the years, experiencing a burst of development in the 1980s and 1990s as social marketing intervention strategies gained importance (Ling, Franklin, Lindsteadt, & Gearom, 1992). In the 1990s, variants of health communication/innovation/social marketing/behavior change models are found in a wide range of international health projects.

Ecological Models. Much of the anthropological research conducted on health behavior in developing countries uses, either explicitly or implicitly, an ecological conceptual model that situates human behavior within a broadly defined physical, biological, and sociocultural environment (Pelto, Bentley, & Pelto, 1990). Decision making about treatment choices (often involving an array of modern and traditional alternatives) is analyzed in terms of the influence of factors such as climatic and seasonal conditions, subsistence patterns, social organization (including household dynamics), and ethnomedical systems (e.g., illness beliefs and treatment options). Behavior is conceptualized as "adaptive" in the sense of being the best solution to a given set of circumstances, resources, and constraints in a particular situation. The unit of analysis in most ecological studies has been a defined population or community.

Since the 1980s, researchers have developed microlevel ecological models that focus on the household or family as the unit of analysis, an approach sometimes referred to as the "household production of health and nutrition" (Bentley & Pelto, 1991; Berman, Kendall, & Bhattachyara, 1994). For example, the "developmental niche" framework of Harkness and Super (1990) focuses on the domestic context of child care. Derived from studies of children's behavior and development in different cultural contexts, the developmental niche framework builds on recent theoretical advances in anthropology, psychology, and biological ecology and reflects current thinking in developmental systems theory. In this view, the child and the child's environment are viewed as interactive systems, and "the household, as the center of early human life, is seen to be the focal mediator of this relationship, working largely through culturally constructed mechanisms" (Harkness & Super, 1990; p. 218). The developmental niche is conceptualized in terms of three integrated subsystems: the physical and social setting in which the child lives, culturally regulated customs of child care and child rearing, and the psychology of the caretakers. Health-related behavior is analyzed in terms of the influence of these interacting subsystems on care provided to the child.

Still other approaches encompass a much broader sociocultural context of health behavior, such as those that rely heavily on political economic analyses of social inequality and differential access to power and resources as explanations for individual behavior (Turshen, 1989). For example, political economic analyses of AIDS risk behavior have underscored the effects of gender relations and limited employment opportunities that constrain the degree of control women have in sexual relationships (Miles, 1993).

Cultural Construction of Health and Illness. A large number of studies have been conducted on health beliefs and practices and on use of services in different cultural settings of the developing world. Very often, the notion of "cultural differences" is invoked to explain observed patterns of behavior. Sometimes more specific cultural concepts are applied to the problem, such as the notion of explanatory model of illness, folk illness or culture-bound syndrome, indigenous categories of illness, and preferred traditional methods of treatment. What these broad fields of study have in common is an underlying assumption that the ways in which people think about, make sense of, and act on illness are profoundly determined by the shared understandings and interpretations given the raw events of sickness, i.e., how the events are culturally "constructed" to be meaningful.

For example, numerous studies that sought to explain why people choose modern versus traditional medicine for treatment of different episodes of illness have stressed the importance of perceived etiology in determining appropriate treatment. Early work of this nature emphasized a dichotomy between natural, biomedically defined illnesses and supernatural or folk illnesses, with the former perceived to fall within the realm of modern medical treatment and the later within the traditional domain. Later studies described a more complex system integrating multiple kinds of therapies within single illness episodes.

Although a large part of such studies have been conducted by anthropologists, many health and social scientists have implicitly or explicitly invoked a constructivist paradigm to explain health behavior. For example, numerous studies examine local perceived causes of illness as explanatory constructs for understanding behavioral response to illness episodes. Because of the disease focus of international health research, often such studies examine local ethnomedical

models of a single illness category with an implied comparative framework, and a few projects have been designed as multicultural comparative studies of particular illness problems (e.g., Weller, Patcher, Trotter, & Baer, 1993).

Analytical Frameworks for the Study of Child Survival. In the mid-1980s, international attention became increasingly focused on understanding the determinants of child survival as many countries adopted interventions identified as "selective primary health care," an approach aimed at reducing the occurrence of the major diseases that contribute to child mortality (Walsh & Warren, 1979). An influential model that guided the research of many investigations of this nature was Mosley and Chen's "An Analytical Framework for the Study of Child Survival in Developing Countries" (Mosley & Chen, 1984). A key component of the model was a set of proximate determinants that directly influence the risk of morbidity and mortality in children, grouped into five categories: maternal factors, environmental contamination, nutrient deficiency, injury, and personal illness control. The latter category of personal illness control is the component that incorporates health behavioral factors, including both preventive practices (e.g., antenatal care, immunization, malaria prophylaxis) and curative practices (e.g., medical treatment). Cognitive variables such as beliefs about disease causation are grouped with socioeconomic determinants, which are viewed as operating through the proximate determinants to affect child survival.

Operational Research Model. A great deal of international health research, including health behavior studies, is conducted within the context of specific health programs sponsored by local governments, bilateral and international agencies, private foundations, and other organizations. Research components are built into the overall project with very specific, problem-focused aims of providing practical information applicable to the design and evaluation of such programs. Studies of this nature are referred to as "operations research" or "operational research" to reflect their direct links to actual program operations and objectives. The delineation of research questions tends to be based on narrowly defined, pragmatic needs of decision makers and administrators rather than on theoretical models of human behavior (although some concepts and theory might be used selectively in designing the research). Consequently, a large number of health behavior studies follow what can be called the operational research model, which gives primacy to program needs and practical use of findings in selection of methods, analysis, and reporting of information. Operational research begins with this central question: "What do we need to know about the behavior of our target population in order to most effectively achieve the aims of the program?" Subsequent decisions about the who, what, where, and how of collecting data flow directly from this basic question.

More than any other category of behavioral health research in developing countries, operational research tends to be documented in the "gray literature" of project reports, monographs, agency publications, and other nonindexed sources, as opposed to books and peer-reviewed journal articles. Another characteristic of this type of program-specific study is the use of structured data collection guides, which are usually focused on a single health domain or problem (as are programs), and sometimes involve cross-national comparisons. In order to standardize indices for comparison, a number of manuals have been developed to guide the collection of ethnographic data by researchers working in different cultural settings (Herman & Bentley, 1992).

HEALTH BEHAVIOR ACROSS THE LIFE SPAN

Since the kinds of health problems that afflict individuals in all societies are so closely linked to age and life course, this chapter will structure the discussion of health behavior in developing countries from a life-span perspec-

tive. The review will address health issues in three broad categories: infancy and childhood, the reproductive years, and the adult and older age groups. The focus of the discussion is on determinants of health behavior and utilization of modern health services. Related issues of the social and behavioral consequences of disease, the relative merits of alternative intervention programs to prevent or control disease, and the use of traditional and alternative medical services are not systematically addressed.

Infancy and Childhood

A discussion of health behavior in relation to the youngest age group must of necessity focus on the perceptions and actions of the caregivers on whom infants and children depend for their survival. In large measure, this approach boils down to understanding the behavior of mothers, who hold primary responsibility for the care and feeding of their children. Indeed, because international health efforts accord so much emphasis to the well-being of children, the bulk of research on health behavior in developing countries in fact focuses on mothers as the subjects of study. There is a large literature on mothers' knowledge and practices regarding child health issues, including infant feeding, child care, home management of diarrhea, preventive services (immunization, growth monitoring), and therapeutic responses to acute respiratory infections. This body of research seeks to identify the characteristics of mothers and their households that are associated with desirable behavior. As noted earlier, maternal education has been consistently correlated with positive health practices. Other predisposing factors include exposure to health information, positive experiences with the modern health care system, social support (e.g., the availability of substitute caregivers), economic roles and resources, and personality characteristics. Some studies have also given attention to child variables that affect health, such as gender differences in family response to illness and how infant behavior can influence feeding practices.

To illustrate some of these issues, selected

studies will be reviewed in the areas of breast-feeding, immunization, and home management of diarrhea. These interventions are three of the four cornerstone child survival interventions subsumed under the acronym GOBI (growth monitoring, oral rehydration, breast-feeding, and immunization), which have dominated child health programs in developing countries since the early 1980s.

Breast-Feeding. Of the child survival interventions, breast-feeding promotion has the longest history in international health research because recognition of its importance for the developing world predates child survival programs per se. Very often, behavioral studies of breast-feeding have been conducted within the broader context of infant feeding and weaning practices. A review by Brownlee (1990) of behavioral issues in this area highlights several problems that are common in many developing countries. First, there are detrimental feeding practices such as discarding colostrum, giving prelacteal feeds before breast milk comes in, introducing supplemental food too early or too late, preparing breast milk substitutes improperly, and using weaning foods with inadequate nutritional value. Second, infant feeding practices are influenced by sociocultural variables such as social networks, urbanization and social change, women's work patterns, household income, gender biases (e.g., differential feeding of female babies), maternal health and nutrition, and advertising of commercial infant formulas. Third, interventions to promote optimal infant feeding practices must address the problem at the levels of the community, health institutions, national policy, and regulation of the commercial sector.

Although breast-feeding rates have fallen in some developing countries, the most serious problem in most Third World settings is not the total abandonment of breast-feeding, but the premature introduction of supplementary foods and liquids into the infant's diet, leading to suboptimal nutrition and exposure of the infant to infectious agents (WHO, 1981). While the choice of bottle-feeding is strongly correlated with urban residence, exposure to mass media, economic status, and maternal employment, the decision to introduce supplementary foods is attributed to mothers' beliefs about the perceived adequacy of their milk production. The most common reason given by women for introducing other foods is insufficient milk, whether caused by their own inadequate diet, stress, illness, or deviation from behavioral norms (e.g., sexual misconduct). The insufficient-milk explanation probably subsumes a variety of psychosocial mechanisms, including poor understanding of lactation, lack of social support for breast-feeding, and stressful life situations that undermine lactation (Huffman, 1984).

Immunization. In developing countries, routine childhood immunizations are recommended for six preventable diseases: diphtheria, pertussis (whooping cough), tetanus, polio, measles, and tuberculosis. The study of immunization behavior is conceptually significant because it encompasses a constellation of factors germane to understanding the use of preventive health services in general (Coreil, Augustin, Halsey, & Holt, 1994). It requires multiple occasions of seeking care at a health facility in the absence of child illness and involves complex knowledge and costs in the process. Research on the determinants of immunization use has identified both "user" and "service delivery system" variables operating in different settings (Heggenhougen & Clements, 1987; Pillsbury, 1990). On the user side of the equation, studies have pointed to barriers such as maternal time constraints and competing priorities, socioeconomic factors, lack of knowledge, low motivation, fears, and community opinion. On the service delivery end, factors related to accessibility, availability, acceptability, affordability, education, and communication have received attention.

Overall, the immunization literature has stressed the importance of parental knowledge about the kinds and schedule of recommended vaccines and the difficulties families face in seeking care. Many parents have a very sketchy understanding of how vaccines work; some even think they cure the illnesses in question. Others have difficulty getting away from work and family demands on their time. Clinic schedules are often not compatible with the time availability of clients, and the way parents are treated by clinic staff often discourages utilization. Analyses of successful immunization programs have underscored the importance of education, outreach, monitoring, and client-friendly delivery systems in overcoming these obstacles (Sherris, Blackburn, Moore, & Mehta, 1986).

It should be noted that these barriers to immunization use, and the ways found to overcome them in developing countries, are very similar to those relevant for the industrialized world (Orenstein et al., 1990). It appears that the behavioral issues important in preventive health service utilization transcend national differences in economic development. Indeed, the advances made by developing countries in immunization coverage in the 1980s and early 1990s have prodded industrial countries like the United States (which now lags behind many developing countries on immunization coverage) to draw upon the experience of Third World nations and mount comprehensive public health initiatives to improve access to immunization services (Interagency Committee to Improve Access to Immunization Services, 1992).

Management of Diarrhea.   One outcome of the worldwide attention given to control of diarrheal diseases during the 1980s has been the accumulation of a large body of comparative research on local perceptions of digestive disorders and home management of diarrhea, including use of oral rehydration therapy (ORT) and other home-based remedies (Sukkary-Stolba, 1990). Research on the cultural construction of diarrhea has shown that in most settings, there are several named categories of illness that include the symptom of watery stools in their definition, often discriminated into simple and complicated types, and that there may be multiple etiologies for similar illness categories, each variant being perceived to have a unique pathophysiology and appropriate set of treatment guidelines (Coreil &

Mull, 1988). For example, cross-cultural studies of diarrhea have identified etiological beliefs related to hot and cold body states, intestinal worms, teething, diet, indigestion, germs, sorcery, violation of taboos, evil eye, fallen fontanelle, and numerous folk medical conditions. Perceived severity, prognosis, and appropriate care may vary considerably across illness categories. These insights have highlighted the importance of elucidating culturally valid definitions of terms used in investigations of knowledge and behavior related to any illness.

Discussions of the help-seeking process in management of diarrhea have accorded considerable attention to the domestic domain of care, in part because much of the research was aimed at understanding and promoting the use of ORT in the home. In this research, the key role mothers play as therapy managers for sick children was highlighted, including the importance of maternal characteristics and knowledge, gender roles, and economic factors such as maternal time availability (Leslie, 1987). Household variables also received attention in these analyses, such as studies that documented the importance of family structure and resources in therapeutic response patterns. In order to understand how the new therapy could be integrated into traditional practices, researchers identified a range of indigenous treatments for diarrhea, including dietary modifications, herbal remedies, purgatives, massage, ritual practices, and pharmaceutical medicines. Findings from studies of traditional dietary management of diarrhea contributed to the shift in WHO policy emphasis away from home use of ORT as the first response to diarrhea and toward the recommendation of continued usual feeding and giving of locally available fluids (WHO, 1995).

Reproductive Years

Health issues related to reproductive years overwhelmingly concern women, mostly because of the high rates of maternal mortality found in developing areas. While infant mortality is roughly 10 times greater in developing countries compared to developed, maternal mortality is 50 times greater or more. There are a number of factors that account for this high rate, including disadvantaged social and economic status of women in the Third World, their poor nutritional status, maternal depletion from frequent childbearing, and inadequate access to maternity services. Furthermore, unlike most health problems of the developing world, which are largely avoidable through environmental improvements, good nutrition, preventive care, and early detection, maternal mortality can be reduced significantly only through access to technological interventions for complications of pregnancy and childbirth (Freedman & Maine, 1993). Attempts to identify risk factors for the four main complications—hemorrhage, eclampsia, infection, and obstructed labor—have been unsuccessful at providing early detection criteria. Thus, it is the availability of emergency acute care for these problems that makes a difference in whether women die from childbirth, and its lack explains the profound maternal mortality differential between industrial and preindustrial societies.

Family Planning. Although not directly practiced for prevention of maternal deaths, family planning can lower current maternal mortality by 25% (Freedman & Maine, 1993) through birth spacing, prevention of unsafe abortions, and reduction of the severity of the maternal depletion syndrome. In addition to this advantage, family planning, again through birth spacing, promotes improved child health and nutrition and reduces the enormous economic and social costs of high fertility.

Earlier research on family planning focused on the cultural acceptability of different methods of contraception (Polgar & Marshall, 1978). Current discussions are more concerned with the factors that favor the practice of family planning in general (McNicoll, 1992). The prevalence of modern contraceptive use is 32% in the developing world, excluding China (Robey, Rutstein, Morris, & Blackburn, 1992). The demographic factors associated with contraceptive use are ma-

ternal age, number of children, urban residence, and maternal education. As would be expected, older women with more children are more likely to seek to delay having additional children, and women who have more education and live in urban areas are more likely to limit their family size. In countries in which the fertility transition is well advanced (e.g., Sri Lanka and Thailand), however, education has much less impact on family planning use; in these areas, women of all educational levels seek to limit their fertility.

The emphasis on education and other demographic factors in explanations of contraceptive behavior reflects the influence of economic models of fertility change that have dominated this field, particularly in the past two decades. These analyses are guided by the "rational actor" model of human behavior, which assumes that decisions are based on assessments of costs, benefits, opportunities, and constraints, factors largely accounted for by demographic transition processes.

Some researchers have argued, however, that both cultural change and the diffusion of contraceptive technology (i.e., health transition processes) are also important variables in explaining change in contraceptive practice (Pollak & Watkins, 1993). Much attention has been focused on explaining the so-called KAP gap, i.e., the disparity between measures of the number of reproductive-age women who do not desire more children, or who wish to delay childbearing, and the rate of contraceptive practice. Planners use this disparity as an indicator of unmet need for family planning services, and there has been much discussion of the validity of the methods used to calculate this need. To the extent that some unmet need exists, researchers have investigated the reasons for nonuse of modern contraceptives, with their results pointing to behavioral factors such as fears of side effects or health concerns, disapproval of contraceptives by women or their partners, and religious beliefs (Nair & Smith, 1984; Williams, Baumslag, & Jelliffe, 1994).

Use of Maternity Services. In contrast to its low impact on maternal mortality, prenatal care can significantly improve child health outcomes in developing countries, and there are maternal health advantages as well. Assuming that prenatal services are, in fact, available, what are the behavioral determinants of their use? Studies have consistently found an inverse relationship between age and parity, on one hand, and use of formal antenatal care on the other. Given that age and parity are strongly intercorrelated, this finding suggests that older women with greater experience having children are less likely to use services, perhaps because their prior experience increases their confidence. Evidence from the Philippines indicates, however, that it is the presence of other children that restricts high-parity women from seeking care, a behavior that is little affected by age (Leslie & Gupta, 1989). It is probable that other situational factors also interact with maternal age in its influence on service utilization.

There is substantial evidence indicating that education is positively correlated with use of maternal health and nutrition services, for both urban and rural areas of developing countries (Leslie & Gupta, 1989). A later section addresses possible explanations for the relationship between education and mother's health behavior. Related to education, income also has been found to influence use of prenatal health services positively (Timyan, Brechin, Measham, & Ogunleye, 1993). Apart from its obvious importance for expensive services, income level can affect utilization of free services as well because of the opportunity costs associated with the time demands of careseeking, which are particularly acute among poor women. The distribution of income within a family can also affect its availability for health care, and competing demands on women's time have been reported to influence use of prenatal care (Leslie & Gupta, 1989). Moreover, the aggressive promotion of family planning in the Third World has made some women suspicious of all health services; in some areas, for example, women report that they avoid going to clinics for fear of being sterilized.

In the domain of reproductive health behav-ior, childbirth practices in developing countries have been the least responsive to the forces of modernization. If one ranks the different types of maternity care help seeking, curative and emergency care is utilized most often, prenatal care is second, and childbirth services are sought least often (Royston & Ferguson, 1985). For normal, uncomplicated pregnancies, women prefer home deliveries attended by family members or traditional midwives. Roughly 80% of deliveries in the Third World take place at home, but the percentages attended by trained midwives vary greatly across areas. While medical institutions are perceived as providing help with complications, the normal birth process is perceived to be a natural event that is best managed within the context of home, where the attention of loved ones and midwives provides emotional and spiritual support during labor and delivery (Jordan, 1990). Hospitals are avoided because of the stark, unfriendly environment, the frequently dirty wards and beds, and the technologically invasive procedures that typify modern obstetrics. Also, the risk of infection is often greater in crowded hospitals that lack hygiene, supplies, and personnel. Traditional birthing practices allow the parturient woman to maintain greater control over the birth process, such as allowing her to move around in a familiar setting during labor and to deliver the baby in a manner that is preferable to her and protects her privacy (Pillsbury & Brownlee, 1989).

Adult and Older Years

While child and reproductive health has been the dominant focus of public health research and policy in developing countries for many decades, there has been increasing concern about the neglected needs of the growing adult population (Mosley, Jamison, & Henderson, 1990). Adult mortality from chronic diseases is increasingly becoming a serious public health problem in Third World countries, but not because the rates for these diseases are escalating, as is commonly believed. Age-specific mortality from noncommunicable diseases actually is decreasing, but the magnitude of the problem has increased because adults make up a growing proportion of the population (Phillips, Feachem, Murray, Over, & Kjellstrom, 1993). Although tropical diseases and other communicable diseases are a significant cause of morbidity and mortality in developing countries, the leading causes of adult death are cardiovascular diseases, cancer, and unintentional injuries.

AIDS-Related Behavior. Research on AIDS-related behavior has had more of a purely behavioral orientation than research on other health problems in developing countries, primarily because prevention is so strongly dependent on deliberate individual action. Consequently, there has been comparatively greater attention directed at developing theoretical models focused on AIDS-related behavior. For example, the applied behavior change model (W. A. Smith, Helquist, Jimerson, Carovano, & Middlestadt, 1993) and the AIDS risk reduction model (Catania, Kegeles, & Coates, 1990), and other adaptations of behavior change theory, have been applied in studies of AIDS-prevention behavior. While early research focused primarily on the association between predictor variables and HIV risk factors, more recent work addresses the psychosocial and cultural influences on decision-making and outcomes at different stages of the behavior change process. At the same time, others have directed attention to the social structural and political conditions that create so-called "high-risk" groups, such as the economic pressures that force poor, marginal women into formal sex work or multiple sexual partnerships in order to survive (McGrath et al., 1992; Miles, 1993).

Like the research on contraception discussed earlier, behavioral research on AIDS faces all of the challenges posed by research on socially sensitive topics, in this case sexual behavior associated with a highly stigmatized disease. Many of the studies rely on KAP surveys for measures of sexual activity, but there can be problems with the accuracy and validity of reported information (Schopper et al., 1993). In light of such po-

tential problems, anthropological research has figured importantly in the AIDS literature, because of its attention to cultural sensitivity and social context of behavior; even anthropological research, however, cannot be used uncritically (Standing, 1992). Indeed a diversity of methodological approaches have been applied to the study of AIDS-related sexual behavior, including complex mathematical modeling of sexual contacts (Anderson, 1992).

Among the developing areas of the world, Africa is the most severely affected by the AIDS pandemic. Within Africa, women are at greater risk for exposure to the human immunodeficiency virus than men, not so much because of their own behavior as because of the sexual behavior of men. Males report a higher number of female sexual partners, and they tend to have relations with younger women, who form a larger cohort within the population. Consequently, the prevalence of HIV infection is higher among females in this region, and this pattern has implications for maternal–infant transmission (Decosas & Pedneault, 1992). Because women have traditionally been the target group of public health interventions, AIDS prevention programs have likewise aimed safe sex messages at women, but in reality women have little control over the risk behavior of their male partners.

Tropical Diseases and Behavior. A distinctive component of health behavior in developing countries is the importance of individual, household, and community activities related to tropical diseases. Although not the leading causes of adult mortality, tropical diseases such as malaria, yellow fever, filariasis, schistosomiasis, dengue fever, dracunculiasis (guinea worm), onchocerciasis, and trachoma account for a significant amount of morbidity and mortality in developing areas. These infectious and parasitic diseases are closely tied to environmental conditions, including poverty and inadequate water and sanitation, and many of the available control strategies are community-based public health interventions. Large scale public works, however, such as improved water supply and chemical vector control, often require a level of funding and infrastructural development that is beyond the reach of local governments.

In the wake of unsuccessful efforts at environmental control, behavior change has gained increased attention in the control of tropical diseases in recent years. Depending on the disease in question, the specific behavioral control measure often involves a technological aspect (e.g., prophylactic pills for malaria, bednets for dengue fever, water filters for guinea worm) or a hygienic practice (face-washing for trachoma, latrine use for schistosomiasis). Efforts to encourage people to adopt such measures often encounter complex socioeconomic and cultural constraints that hinder the incorporation of recommended behavior change into everyday activities. Intensive health education and community organization efforts are required to support the behavior change (Gordon, 1988).

Studies of the transmission of tropical diseases have identified various human behaviors (e.g., water-, habitation-, and subsistence-related activities) associated with exposure to disease vectors. Not surprisingly, the theoretical models that have guided behavioral research on tropical disease have had a strong ecological orientation, with emphasis on environmental influences and individual adaptive response. In recent years, researchers have integrated household production perspectives with the traditional ecological approach to tropical diseases. For example, Castro and Mokate (1988) analyzed the individual, household, and community determinants of malaria in Colombia, highlighting the importance of variables such as work and water collection patterns that regulate exposure to mosquito bites. Similarly, Coreil, Whiteford, and Salazar (in press) apply a model for studying the household ecology of disease transmission to dengue fever in the Dominican Republic, examining aspects of the biophysical, social, and cultural environments that affect risk behavior, transmission behavior, and risk protection for mosquitos.

In their review of the social patterning of schistosomiasis, Huang and Manderson (1992) identified schistosomiasis as a *behavioral* disease, in which exposure to the snail vector is conditioned by factors such as gender, age, occupation, and religion. While acknowledging the political context of development projects that propagate the vectors, the reviewers note the importance of women's roles, which bring them into greater contact with water than men, and religious proscriptions, which produce the reverse gender effect. Furthermore, knowledge and perceptions of the illness have been found to influence exposure to risk as well as treatment-seeking behavior, an important component of disease control, since chronic sufferers can infect others through water contact.

Cross-cultural studies of malaria have documented the importance of indigenous explanatory models for various fevers, of which malaria is often one type, in local responses to control measures (Oaks, Mitchell, Pearson, & Carpenter, 1991). There are usually multiple perceived causes for malaria-type fever, some of which are perceived to be beyond control of individuals (e.g., hard work, getting cold). Thus, communities often remain skeptical about the possibility of preventing this infection.

RESEARCH ISSUES

While the preceding review has focused on separate health problems across the life stages, it is useful to examine some of the recurrent issues that weave common threads across the disparate domains of investigation. Though by no means an exhaustive discussion, this section will briefly address the issues of maternal education, time allocation, and future directions for health behavior research in developing countries.

Maternal Education

While the education–health behavior link is significant for both mothers and fathers in developing countries, the effects of maternal education are most striking in their impact and scope. Moreover, the effects of maternal education have been shown to be independent of economic factors and access to health services. The preceding review highlighted its influence on behavior promoting child health (immunization, breast-feeding, management of diarrhea) and on reproductive practices (family planning, use of perinatal services). Discussions of possible mechanisms that link maternal education and positive health actions have suggested a variety of pathways of influence (Cleland & van Ginneken, 1988; Caldwell, 1990). First, education is likely to alter a person's worldview such that the more educated are more receptive to new ideas and novel ways of responding to life situations. Education probably enhances one's sense of control over the outside world, fostering confidence in one's ability to seek out resources and manipulate the social environment. Formal schooling undoubtedly imparts important communication and management skills that can be applied in diverse situations. These factors may account for the increased propensity of educated mothers to seek services for themselves and their children. A related argument stresses the empowering role of education for women within their families and communities, leading to more assertive action in favor of health (e.g., allocation of household resources).

Second, there may be direct benefits of education apart from perceptual changes. For example, through school experiences, women may acquire specific knowledge and skills related to hygiene, health, nutrition, and availability of services. Educated mothers may be better able to recognize the signs and symptoms that indicate a health problem needing professional attention. Also, literate persons may receive better treatment by medical personnel, and they may be more able to understand the educational messages imparted by health workers in clinical settings.

Third, it is likely that the effects of education interact with other societal factors to influence health behavior. For example, in settings in which it is normative for females to attend school, the general status of women is probably enhanced such that women's roles favor a more active involvement in public life, including interactions with organized health institutions. Additionally, aspects of the social environment, such as father's behavior and support from other family members, may enable mothers in such settings to provide better care to children.

Cleland and van Ginneken (1988) summarize the potential mechanisms whereby maternal education may influence positive behavior by listing six hypotheses (p. 1364): "Compared to the uneducated, educated mothers may:

- Attach a higher value to the welfare and health of children.
- Have greater decision-making power on health-related and other matters.
- Be less fatalistic about disease and death.
- Be more knowledgeable about disease prevention and cure.
- Be more innovative in the use of remedies.
- Be more likely to adopt new codes of behavior that improve the health of children though they are not perceived as having direct consequences for health."

Although the effects of maternal education on different kinds of health behavior have been fairly well documented, there have been few attempts to elucidate which of these hypotheses account for the observed relationships. Focused studies are needed to illuminate the mediating links in order to guide policy development that goes beyond the obvious need to strengthen educational opportunities for women in developing countries.

Time Allocation

In a manner similar to maternal education, the importance of women's time constraints has emerged as a recurrent determinant of health behavior in Third World settings. Here, the discussion has focused on the effects of competing demands on women's time deriving from multiple role functions in the economic and domestic spheres of family life. Analyses of barriers to use of health services as well as home-based interventions have repeatedly cited the time costs of engaging in the desired action, as reflected in the review presented in this chapter. A number of issues have surfaced in the discussion of maternal time allocation for health, including the opportunity costs of time lost from income-generating activities, the increased time demands of new health technologies introduced through child survival programs, and the relative impact of expanded economic roles (e.g., in agricultural development) that increase women's financial resources but take them away from home for greater lengths of time.

Recognition of the deterrent role that maternal time constraints place on health behavior has led to surprisingly little discussion of ways to ameliorate the situation. When solutions have been addressed, attention has been focused primarily on altering domestic organization in various ways, such as improving child care resources in mothers' absence (Engle, 1989). Although researchers have cited the need for changes in service delivery systems to accommodate maternal time limitations, a responsive call to action at this level is not evident. In fact, comparatively little attention has been directed toward ways that the health establishment, which includes sociomedical researchers, can redefine its mission to respond to the needs of populations being served.

Future Directions

Looking to the future of health behavior research in developing countries, the most important new trends will likely be linked to changes in disease patterns within the growing adult and older populations. Increased attention to behavioral factors in chronic and noncommunicable diseases can be expected over the next few decades.

Men, Risk Behaviors, and Lifestyle.   While women have been the focus of attention in the past because of their pivotal role in child and reproductive health, men soon will have their day as the "target" of research, policy, and planning in the Third World. One area in particular in which males will take center stage is that of personal health behavior or lifestyle patterns. Consider, for example, the problem of tobacco use in developing countries, which shows signs of becoming a public health problem of magnitude equal to or greater than that found in the developed world. While cigarette consumption has declined in most industrial countries, it has shown an alarming rise in the world's poorer countries, where transnational tobacco companies have been intensively marketing their products (Stebbins, 1990). People in the Third World currently consume between one third and over one half of the world's tobacco, a proportion likely to increase if cigarette marketing continues to flourish under the limited restrictions typically imposed in developing countries. Moreover, it is primarily men who are taking up the smoking habit in developing countries, where in general about 50% of males and 5% of females use tobacco (Crofton, 1984). The impact of male smoking on lung cancer rates is already evident in several countries and will surely magnify over succeeding decades. This increase, in turn, will prompt researchers to study the social and behavioral factors that influence cigarette use in these populations.

Unintentional Injuries.   Another repercussion of the ongoing epidemiological transition in developing countries is the rise in unintentional injuries, most notably from motor vehicle accidents and occupational risks, which, like tobacco use, affect males disproportionately (G. S. Smith & Barss, 1991). Death and disability from other injuries such as drowning, poisoning, burns, and falls variably affect age and sex groups and will become increasingly important public health problems as countries modernize. Since few studies of risk behaviors and preventive measures have been conducted on unintentional injuries in Third World settings, a new item will be added to the agenda of behavioral research.

Adherence to Regimens. Implicit in the vast literature on health behavior in developing countries is the underlying premise that the goal of research is to identify the factors that enhance or impede the performance of desirable actions that improve health and prevent disease. Broadly defined, this endeavor can be described as compliance research, although some researchers may object to the use of this value-laden term, which has connotations of authoritarian ideology and medical control. In the broad sense, research on compliance with recommended health actions has been conducted on a wide range of health behavior in developing countries. In the more restricted sense of patient adherence to therapeutic regimens, however, the literature is sparse for the developing world (Homedes & Ugalde, 1994). As Third World societies undergo health transition processes that entail increasing use of modern medical services, there will be a need for empirical research on factors that affect patient response to prescribed medical treatment, the use of pharmaceutical medicines, and the ability to sustain healthful lifestyle changes. Adaptations of traditional approaches to the study of compliance will be needed to ensure that concepts and methods are appropriate for diverse cultural settings, health care systems, and patient characteristics.

Self-Care and Elderly Populations. Given the scarcity of resources for health care in developing countries, particularly since the introduction of economic structural adjustment measures in the late 1980s, there will be greater interest in promoting self-care, another fertile ground for health behavior study. This area will be especially important for the growing elderly populations in Third World areas, where social welfare programs are much less developed than in industrial

countries (Koseki & Reid, 1991). The entire field of research on elderly health behavior in developing countries will undoubtedly develop in coming years as the public health needs of older persons grow in priority on national planning agendas.

Commonalities and Differences. As the Third World is transformed by the various demographic, epidemiological and health processes discussed in this chapter, health professionals can expect to find a convergence of problems and trends in global health behavior. Future studies may increasingly emphasize the commonalities in determinants of health behavior across variously developed countries, in contrast to the differences stressed in this review. Only in that future, however, will researchers see the extent to which the health transition will unfold in predictable ways in the developing world or take uncharted paths and result in heterogeneity of behavior patterns. Whether the transition leads to less differentiation or not, it will be important to study the processes and outcomes in order to profit from the lessons such research will have for understanding health behavior generally.

REFERENCES

Anderson, R. M. (1992). Some aspects of sexual behavior and the potential demographic impact of AIDS in developing countries. *Social Science and Medicine, 34*(2), 271–280.

Bentley, M. E., & Pelto, G. H. (1991). The household production of nutrition: Introduction to special issue, *Social Science and Medicine, 33*(10), 1101–1102.

Berman, P., Kendall, C., & Bhattachyar, K. (1994). The household production of health: Integrating social science perspectives on micro-level health determinants. *Social Science and Medicine, 38*(2), 205–215.

Brownlee, A. (1990). Breastfeeding, weaning and nutrition: The behavioral issues. Behavioral Issues in Child Survival Monograph No. 3. Washington, DC: U.S. Agency for International Development.

Caldwell, J. C. (1990). Cultural and social factors influencing mortality levels in developing countries. *Annals of the*

American Academy of Political and Social Sciences, 510, 44-59.

Caldwell, J. C. (1993). Health transition: The cultural, social and behavioral determinants of health in the third world. *Social Science and Medicine, 36,* 125-135.

Castro, E. B., & Mokate, K. M. (1988). Malaria and its socio-economic meanings: The study of Cunday in Colombia. In A. N. Herrin & P. Rosenfield (Eds.), *Economics, health and tropical diseases* (pp. 159-189). Manila: University of the Philippines, School of Economics.

Cantania, J. A., Kegeles, S. M., & Coates, T. J. (1990). Towards an understanding of risk behavior: An AIDS risk reduction model (ARRM). *Health Education Quarterly, 17*(1), 53-72.

Cleland, J. G., & van Ginneken, J. K. (1988). Maternal education and child survival in developing countries: The search for pathways of influence. *Social Science and Medicine, 27,*(12), 1357-1368.

Coreil, J. (1995). Group interview methods in community health research. *Medical Anthropology,16,* 193-210.

Coreil, J., Augustin, A., Halsey, N., & Holt, E. (1994). Social and psychological costs of preventive child health services in Haiti. *Social Science and Medicine, 38*(2), 231-238.

Coreil, J., & Mull, J. D. (Eds.). (1988). Anthropological studies of diarrheal illness. *Social Science and Medicine* (Special Issue), *27*(1).

Coreil, J., Whiteford, L., & Salazar, D. (in press). The household ecology of disease transmission: Dengue fever in the Dominican Republic. In M. Inhorn & P. Brown (Eds.), *The anthropology of infectious disease.* New York: Gordon & Breach.

Crofton, J. (1984). The gathering smoke clouds: A worldwide challenge. *International Journal of Epidemiology, 13,* 269-270.

Davis, K. (1987). The world's most expensive survey. *Sociological Forum, 2*(4), 829-835.

Decosas, J., & Pedneault, V. (1992). Women and AIDs in Africa: Demographic implications for health promotion. *Health Policy and Planning, 7*(3), 227-233.

Engle, P. (1989). Child care strategies of working and non-working women in rural and urban Guatemala. In J. Leslie & M. Paolisso (Eds.), *Women, work and child welfare in the third world* (pp. 179-200). Boulder, CO: Westview.

Freedman, L. P., & Maine, D. (1993). Women's mortality: A legacy of neglect. In M. Koblinsky, J. Timyan, & J. Gay (Eds.), The health of women: A global perspective (pp. 147-170). Boulder, CO: Westview.

Frenk, J., Bobadilla, J. L., Sepulveda, J., & Cervantes, M. L. (1989). Health transition in middle income countries: New challenges for health care. *Health Policy and Planning, 4*(1), 29-39.

Harkness, S., & Super, D. (1994). The developmental niche: A theoretical framework for analyzing the household production of health. *Social Science and Medicine, 38*(2), 217-226.

Heggenhougen, K., & Clements, J. (1987). Acceptability of childhood immunization. World Health Organization, EPC Publication No. 14.

Herman, E., & Bentley, M. E. (1992). Manuals for ethnographic data collection: Experience and issues. *Social Science and Medicine, 35*(11), 1369-1378.

Homedes, N., & Ugalde, A. (1994). Research on patient compliance in developing countries. *Bulletin of the Pan American Health Organization, 28*(1), 17-33.

Horowitz, I. L. (1966). *Three worlds of development.* New York: Oxford University Press.

Huang, Y., & Manderson, L. (1992). Schistosomiasis and the social patterning of infection. *Acta Tropica, 51,* 175-194.

Huffman, S. L. (1984). Determinants of breastfeeding in developing countries: Overview and policy implications. *Studies in Family Planning, 15*(4), 170-183, 1984.

Hursh-Cesar, G. (1988). UNICEF KAP studies. *Report to Office of Evaluation, Office of Programme Communication, UNICEF.* Washington, DC: Intercultural Communication.

Interagency Committee to Improve Access to Immunization Services. (1992). The public health service action plan to improve access to immunization services. *Public Health Reports, 107*(3), 243-251.

Jordan, B. (1990). Technology and the social distribution of knowledge: Issues for primary health care in developing countries. In J. Coreil & J. D. Mull, (Eds.), *Anthropology and primary health care* (pp. 98-136). Boulder, CO: Westview.

Koseki, L. K., & Reid, S. E. (1991). Elderly self-care education: A low technology primary health care option for developing countries. *Asia-Pacific Journal of Public Health, 5*(4), 322-330.

Leslie, J. (1987). *Time costs and time savings to women of the child survival revolution.* Washington, DC: International Center for Research on Women.

Leslie, J. (1989). Women's time: A factor in the use of child survival technologies? *Health Policy and Planning, 4*(1), 1-16.

Leslie, J., & Gupta, G. R. (1989). *Utilization of formal services for maternal nutrition and health care in the third world.* Washington, DC: International Center for Research on Women.

Ling, J. C., Franklin, B. A. K., Lindsteadt, J. F., & Gearon, S. A. N. (1992). Social marketing: Its place in public health. *Annual Review of Public Health, 13,* 341-362.

Manderson, L., & Aaby, P. (1992). An epidemic in the field? Rapid assessment procedures and health research. *Social Science and Medicine, 35*(7), 839-850.

McGrath, J. W., Schumann, D., Pearson-Marks, J., Rwabukwali, C. B., Mukasa, R., Namande, B., Nakayiwa, S., & Nakyobe, L. (1992). Cultural determinants of sexual risk behavior for AIDS among Baganda women. *Medical Anthropology Quarterly, 6*(2), 153-161.

McNicoll, G. (1992). Changing fertility patterns and policies in the third world. *Annual Review of Sociology, 18,* 85-108.

Miles, L. (1993). Women, AIDS, and power in heterosexual sex: A discourse analysis. *Women's Studies International Forum, 16*(5), 497–511.

Mosley, W. H., & Chen, L. C. (1984). An analytical framework for the study of child survival in developing countries. In W. H. Mosley & L. C. Chen (Eds.), *Child survival: Strategies for research. Population and Development Review, 10* (Suppl.) 25–45.

Mosley, W. H., Jamison, D. T., & Henderson, D. A. (1990). The health sector in developing countries: Problems for the 1990s and beyond. *Annual Review of Public Health, 11,* 335–358.

Nair, N. K., & Smith, L. (1984). Reasons for not using contraceptives: An international comparison. *Studies in Family Planning, 15*(2), 84–92.

Oaks, S. C., Jr., Mitchell, V. S., Pearson, G. W., & Carpenter, C. J. (Eds.). (1991). *Malaria: Obstacles and opportunities.* Washington, DC: National Academy Press.

Omran, A. R. (1971). The epidemiological transition: A theory of the epidemiology of population change. *Milbank Memorial Fund Quarterly, 49,* 509–538.

Orenstein, W. A., Atkinson, W., Mason, D., & Bernier, R. H. (1990). Barriers to vaccinating preschool children. *Journal of Health Care for the Poor and Underserved, 1,* 315–330.

Paul, B. D. (1955). *Health, culture and community: Case studies of public reactions to health programs.* New York: Russell Sage.

Pelto, P. J., Bentley, M. E., & Pelto, G. H. (1990). Applied anthropological research methods: Diarrhea studies as an example. In J. Coreil & J. D. Mull, (Eds.), *Anthropoloy and primary health care* (pp. 253–277). Boulder, CO: Westview.

Phillips, D. R. (1991). Problems and potential of researching epidemiological transition: Examples from Southeast Asia. *Social Science and Medicine, 33*(4), 395–404.

Phillips, M., Feachem, R. G. A., Murray, C. J. L., Over, M., & Kjellstrom, T. (1993). Adult health: A legitimate concern for developing countries. *American Journal of Public Health, 83,* 1527–1530.

Pillai, V. K., & Shannon, L. W. (1995). Introduction: Definition and distribution of developing areas. In V. K. Pillai & L. W. Shannon (Eds.) *Developing areas: A book of readings and research* (pp. 1–13). Oxford: Berg.

Pillsbury, B. (1990). *Immunization: The behavioral issues.* Washington, DC: Agency for International Development.

Pillsbury, B., & Brownlee, A. (1989). *Household and community beliefs and practices that influence maternal health and nutrition.* Washington, DC: International Center for Research on Women.

Polgar, S., & Marshall, J. F. (1978). The search for culturally acceptable fertility regulating methods. In M. H. Logan & E. E. Hunt (Eds.), *Health and the human condition* (pp. 328–340). North Scituiate, MA: Duxbury.

Pollak, R. A., & Watkins, S. C. (1993). Cultural and economic approaches to fertility: Proper marriage or *mésalliance? Population and Development Review, 19*(3), 467–496.

Robey, B., Rutstein, S. O., & Morris, L., with the assistance of Blackburn, R. (1992). *The reproductive revolution: New survey findings. Population Reports,* Series M, No. 11.

Royston, E., & Ferguson, J. (1985). The coverage of maternity care: A critical review of available information. *World Health Statistics Quarterly, 38*(3), 267–273.

Schopper, D., Doussantousse, S., & Orav, J. (1993). Sexual behaviors relevant to HIV transmission in a rural African population: How much can a KAP survey tell us? *Social Science and Medicine, 37*(2), 401–412.

Sherris, J. D., & Blackburn, R., with the assistance of Moore, S. H., & Mehta, S. (1986). *Immunizing the world's children. Population Reports: Issues in World Health,* Series L, No. 5.

Smith, G. S., & Barss, P. (1991). Unintentional injuries in developing countries: The epidemiology of a neglected problem. *Epidemiologic Reviews, 13,* 228–266.

Smith, W. A., Helquist, M. J., Jimerson, A. B., Carovano, K., & Middlestadt, S. E. (1993). *A world against AIDS: Communication for behavior change.* Washington, DC: Academy for Educational Development.

Standing, H. (1992). AIDS: Conceptual and methodological issues in researching sexual behavior in sub-Saharan Africa. *Social Science and Medicine, 34*(5), 475–483.

Stebbins, K. R. (1990). Transnational tobacco companies and health in underdeveloped countries: Recommendations for avoiding a smoking epidemic. *Social Science and Medicine, 30*(2), 277–235.

Sukkary-Stolba, S. (1990). *Oral rehydration therapy: The behavioral issues.* Washington, DC: U.S. Agency for International Development.

Timyan, J., Brechin, S. J. G., Measham, D. M., & Ogunleye, B. (1993). Access to care: More than a problem of distance. In M. Koblinsky, J. Timyan, & J. Gay (Eds), *The health of women: A global perspective* (pp. 217–234). Boulder, CO: Westview.

Turshen, M. (1989). *The politics of public health.* New Brunswick, NJ: Rutgers University Press.

Valente, T. W., & Rogers, E. M. (1995). The origins and development of the diffusion of innovations paradigm as an example of scientific growth. *Science Communication, 16*(3), 238–269.

Walsh, J., & Warren, K. S. (1979). Selective primary health care: An interim strategy for disease control in developing countries. *New England Journal of Medicine, 301,* 967–974.

Weller, S. C., Patcher, L. M., Trotter, R. T., II, & Baer, R. D. (1993). Empacho in four Latino groups: A study of intra- and inter-cultural variation in beliefs. *Medical Anthropology, 15,* 109–136.

Williams, C. D., Baumslag, N., & Jelliffe, D. B. (1994). *Mother and child health: Delivering the services* (3rd ed.). New York: Oxford University Press.

World Bank. (1993). *Investing in health*. New York: Oxford University Press.

World Health Organization. (1981). *Contemporary patterns of breastfeeding: Report on the WHO collaborative study on breastfeeding*. Geneva: WHO.

World Health Organization. (1995). *How research findings have improved diarrhea case management guidelines*. Geneva: WHO.

Yach, D. (1992). The use and value of qualitative methods in health research in developing countries. *Social Science and Medicine, 35*(4), 603–612.

10

Health Behavior among the Homeless and the Poor

James D. Wright and Laurie M. Joyner

INTRODUCTION: HEALTH BEHAVIORS AND HEALTH OUTCOMES

The growing emphasis on health behavior among health researchers and the parallel emphasis on prevention among health practitioners should not be allowed to obscure critically important relationships between health behavior and larger social, cultural, and economic forces. In the language of research methods, behavior is an intervening variable, not an independent one. The complex relationships among behavior, culture, and social structure are all too easily ignored in the rhetoric of public policy debates and in simple-minded thinking about issues that arise in these debates.

It is convenient but frequently wrong to believe that health behaviors arise from the free choices and free wills of the people involved;

James D. Wright • Department of Sociology, Tulane University, New Orleans, Louisiana 70118.   **Laurie M. Joyner** • Department of Sociology, Loyola University, New Orleans, Louisiana 70118.

Handbook of Health Behavior Research III: Demography, Development, and Diversity, edited by David S. Gochman. Plenum Press, New York, 1997.

such thinking leads, for example, to "Just Say No" as a national drug policy. The link between behavior and health outcomes is, of course, an important one, but it is equally important to understand the reasons people behave as they do. Beliefs, values, and customs—in a word, culture—constrain behavior in powerful ways; so too does the larger structure of society, especially the structure of legitimate and illegitimate opportunities. The unwillingness or inability to recognize cultural and structural determinants of behavior can easily turn the analysis of health behavior into unintended "blaming the victim."

Poverty and homelessness, the subject matter of this chapter, are widely recognized risk factors for a range of deleterious health consequences, and both are also strongly correlated with numerous health behaviors that help to produce those consequences. Summarizing a vast literature, poverty and homelessness are not healthy for children and other living things. Poor and homeless people live disproportionately in unsanitary conditions, eat suboptimal diets, are far less likely to have health insurance and therefore utilize health services at lower rates, smoke more cigarettes, consume drugs at elevated rates, live in violence-prone communities, and, more generally, have fewer economic and social resources to invest in their physical well-being.

The purpose of this chapter is to review evidence on selected health behaviors and their linkages to health outcomes among the homeless and the poor. To foreshadow the obvious conclusion, there is practically nothing about being poor or homeless that is good for one's health. People, however, generally do not choose to be homeless or poor; rather, these conditions are thrust upon them by larger social forces. Nor do people always "choose" the behaviors that have come to be associated with poverty and homelessness. Health behavior is important in understanding why poverty and homelessness are so strongly linked to negative health outcomes, but behavior is not the whole story—not by any means.

DEFINITIONS AND CONCEPTUALIZATIONS

Homelessness

There is no generally agreed-upon definition of what constitutes homelessness (Wright, 1989). Many analysts find it useful to distinguish between the *literally homeless* (those who spend their nights either in outdoor locations, in temporary overnight shelters, or in other places not intended for human habitation) and the *marginally housed* (persons with a claim to some minimal housing, but who are at high risk of homelessness) (Rossi, Wright, Fisher, & Willis, 1987). By at least some definitions, the "marginally housed" are nearly isomorphic with the poverty population, and so our focus here is on the literally homeless population. Even this status, however, is not well-defined; indeed, issues of definition and the multiplicity of ways that people become homeless or experience the condition of homelessness complicate all efforts even to count homeless people (Wright & Devine, 1992), much less to examine the correlated health behaviors.

Poverty

In contrast to the case of homelessness, there is an official government definition of poverty used by nearly all analysts and also used in this chapter. The official poverty standard is set by the Bureau of the Census and is derived ultimately from the cost of food, is adjusted annually for inflation, and differs for families and households of varying sizes (Devine & Wright, 1993). In 1992, the official poverty standard for a four-person family was an annual income of $14,355 or less. In the same year, nearly 37 million people, representing about 14% of the population of the United States, lived at or below the federal poverty designation.

It is apparent that there is no sharp line of demarcation between the homeless and the poor, or between the poor and near-poor (the latter being frequently defined as persons and households with incomes between 100% and 150% of the poverty line). Many currently housed poor people will have experienced episodes of homelessness in the recent past or will experience them in the near future. More generally, there is a continuum of housing adequacy and economic well-being, and there is a large population of poor and near-poor people who rise and fall on the continuum largely in response to short-term fluctuations in employment and related factors. In a nontrivial sense, the population "at risk" for homelessness comprises nearly the entire poverty population of the country.

A Note on Sources of Data: Methodological Issues

Nearly without exception, national sample surveys of health and health behavior are derived from samples of households. Thus, institutionalized populations are excluded; so too are persons who do not reside in households, i.e., the homeless. As a result, most of the available data on health behavior among the homeless is derived from special studies done in local facilities that provide services to the homeless (e.g., shelters, soup kitchens, and health care for the homeless clinics). For the most part, these studies are not generalizable in the statistical sense to any known population of homeless persons, and certainly not to the national homeless population. One must, therefore, depend on the consistency of results from multiple studies undertaken in various cities or contexts, rather than on the machinery of statistical inference, to reach plausible conclusions about what is or is not true of the homeless in general.

Unfortunately, much the same is true of poverty. Relatively few of the national health surveys or other health and disease surveillance efforts obtain sufficient data on household composition and income to isolate those persons within the sample who fall below the official poverty standard. In contrast, a measure of race is available in all sources of data; yet, while racial differences in morbidity and mortality are well known (Jepson, Kessler, Portnoy, & Gibbs, 1991) and are now considered a priority in national public health policy, the social-class differences in such matters often *exceed* the racial differences, and by substantial margins (Navarro, 1990). Moreover, racial differences in health status and outcomes are often *explained* by differential rates of poverty or access to health care across racial and ethnic groups.

Race, Poverty, Homelessness, and Health

Poverty rates among African-Americans are roughly 3 times the rates for whites, both in general and for various demographic subgroups (Devine & Wright, 1993); African-Americans and other ethnic minorities are also overrepresented among the nation's homeless population (Burt, 1992). Thus, race and ethnicity interact with both poverty and homelessness in complex relationships that are often difficult to disentangle. In many cases, the only usable indicator of socioeconomic status available in a given data source will be race, and so differences by race figure prominently in the following account. It is therefore important to stress at the outset that while

some of the racial differences in health status, access, or behavior are secondary to correlated differences in income, poverty, education, and related socioeconomic factors, others are due to racial differences in risk factors such as smoking and nutrition, differences in stressful living conditions, cultural differences, and even biological differences in some cases (e.g., sickle cell anemia), and that the data are typically inadequate to differentiate among these effects.

GENERAL HEALTH STATUS OF THE HOMELESS AND THE POOR

It is important to review, if only briefly, some of the health outcomes associated with being homeless and being poor in order to be clear on what the differences in health behaviors are intended to explain.

Physical Morbidity

There is now a large literature on the health status of the homeless (e.g., Brickner, Scharer, Conanan, Savarese, & Scanlan, 1990). This literature shows conclusively that homeless people suffer from practically every ailment of the flesh and spirit at rates far in excess of those in the domiciled population. The only apparent exception to this pattern is for the diseases of old age, specifically cancer and stroke (Wright & Weber, 1987), which occur at lower rates among the homeless mainly because homeless people rarely live long enough to contract these diseases.

Research links physical health outcomes to homelessness in three distinct ways (Institute of Medicine, 1988). First, ill health is frequently a cause of homelessness (Wright & Weber, 1987). Second, the conditions of homelessness indisputably cause a great deal of physical illness (Scharer, Berson, & Brickner, 1990). Third, whatever the pathways of cause and effect, the material conditions of homelessness greatly complicate the delivery of adequate primary health services (Brickner et al., 1990).

There is little doubt that many of the most commonly diagnosed disorders of the homeless result from behavioral and lifestyle factors. A few illustrations will suffice. Excessive rates of alcohol abuse among homeless men are largely although not entirely responsible for the elevated rates of hypertension observed in this population (Wright & Weber, 1987); the high-salt diet provided in most soup kitchens and feeding programs exacerbates the problem (Winick, 1985). Alcohol abuse is strongly implicated in the high rate of gastrointestinal and neurological disorders observed among the homeless.

Perhaps *the* characteristic physical disorder of the homeless is peripheral vascular disease, and in this condition, too, lifestyle factors are strongly implicated (McBride & Mulcare, 1985). Constant forced walking and the tendency to sleep with the legs in a dependent position causes blood and body fluids to pool in the extremities; this pooling in turn requires higher venous pressures in order to return the blood through the circulatory system. Over a sufficient period of time, the venous valves are destroyed, leading to edema, thromboses, cellulitis, and ulceration. Poor hygiene and exposure to the environment will, of course, further increase the possibility and seriousness of these infections.

Exposure to the physical and social environment of the streets increases the incidence of lice and scabies, various exposure disorders, respiratory infections, a wide range of skin ailments, and trauma. In fact, upper respiratory infections, disorders of the skin, and trauma are the most commonly encountered acute diagnoses in every health care setting that serves homeless people. Inadequate hygiene and grossly inadequate treatment histories account for the exceptional rates of dental caries among the homeless. Poor diet causes anemia and a range of other nutritional deficiency disorders, increases susceptibility to infection (Luder, Boey, Buchalter, & Martinez-Weber, 1989), and complicates the management of many chronic medical conditions. Persons denied adequate shelter, in short, not only lose the roof over their heads, but also are exposed to a range of risk factors that are uniquely and strongly destructive of physical health.

What is true of the homeless is more or less true of the poor as well. Setting aside the obvious qualitative differences between homelessness, on one hand, and poverty, on the other, and acknowledging also that the lack of money is not the *only* factor implicated in ill health, it nonetheless remains true that income is probably *the single most important factor* that dictates both health and health behavior in American society today (Battle, 1990).

Perhaps the best-known and most firmly established health correlate of poverty is infant mortality; indeed, "the correlation between poverty and high infant mortality rates is undisputed" (Miller, 1985, p. 35). Infant mortality in the United States has been declining among all socioeconomic groups for decades, but the rate of decline slowed abruptly in the 1980s, mainly among infants of poor mothers (Miller, 1985).

Poverty negatively affects morbidity as well as mortality among children (and adults). Focusing first on children, data from the National Health Interview Survey (NHIS) showed approximately equal prevalences of most acute disorders among poor and nonpoor children, more severe sequelae of those acute disorders among the poor than among the nonpoor, somewhat higher rates of chronic disorders among the poor, and higher hospitalization rates for poor children (Egbuonu & Starfield, 1982, p. 551). Analysis of the Child Health Supplement to the 1981 NHIS (Newacheck & Starfield, 1988) revealed similar results: Poor children were more severely affected by their illnesses (as measured by bed days), were more likely to have multiple illnesses in the 1-year span covered by the study, and utilized fewer physician services.

Poor children in the United States have consistently received insufficient health care despite the widespread availability of Medicaid since 1967 (Gortmaker, 1981). Access to adequate health care is routinely reported to be problematic for the poor in general (Aday, Fleming, & Andersen, 1984) and for poor children in particular (Newacheck & Halfon, 1986). Thus, inadequate access to appropriate care is perhaps the primary mechanism that links poverty to ill health, among both children and adults.

The literature on health consequences of poverty among adults is also vast. Compared to middle-class populations, poor people are often found to have (1) different patterns of health behavior (e.g., see Lewis, Raczynski, Heath, Levinson, & Cutter, 1993), (2) different health beliefs and health practices (Lubben, Weiler, & Chi, 1989), (3) sharply different patterns of health care utilization (Stern, Weissman, & Epstein, 1991), and very different health care outcomes (e.g., see Young, Waller, & Kahana, 1991).

Thus, the poor no less than the homeless also suffer from elevated levels of morbidity and mortality and experience many of the same difficulties accessing and utilizing health care services. Consistent with these findings, the NHIS consistently reports an inverse relationship between income and the number of days spent per person-year under "general activity restrictions" due to acute or chronic conditions (e.g., see National Center for Health Statistics, 1994).

Mental Health

Mental illness is the most heavily researched aspect of the homelessness problem, and the research literature on the topic is therefore quite substantial; a useful overview includes the report of the Federal Task Force on Homelessness and Severe Mental Illness (1992).

Published estimates of the rate of mental illness among the homeless vary from a low of 10% to a high of 90%. The consensus in the field is that approximately a third of homeless adults suffer from nontrivial psychiatric disorders. About the same percentage have been hospitalized for psychiatric reasons at least once. Among the mentally ill homeless (and ignoring for the moment substance abuse disorders), schizophrenia is the most common diagnosis, usually followed by depression (La Gory, Ritchey, & Mullis, 1990).

An association between poverty (or income) and mental health has also been obvious since the advent of community mental health surveys in the 1950s (Gurin, Veroff, & Feld, 1960). The basic result has been replicated literally dozens of times in subsequent literature (e.g., Kessler & Neighbors, [1986] and the references cited therein). The effect of low income on psychological health is apparent in all racial and ethnic categories; poor people of all races and ethnicities report lower levels of mental health than middle-class or affluent people. The exact reason for this effect is less certain; Camasso and Camasso (1986) and others have pointed to higher rates of stressful or undesirable life experiences (e.g., deaths of loved ones, job losses, evictions) and lower levels of social support among the poor as probable contributing factors.

Mortality

Mortality among the homeless has not been extensively researched. One study reports an average age of death for homeless men as being around 51 or 52 years (Wright & Weber, 1987); one study of San Francisco homeless reports an average age at death of 41 years (*Morbidity and Mortality Weekly Report* [*MMWR*], 1991a). It is fairly obvious that mortality among the homeless is astonishingly high. On the basis of this research, one of the "costs of being homeless" in America is roughly 20 years of life expectancy.

The direct effect of poverty on mortality has also not been adequately researched; in this area, as in many others, race is often taken as a proxy. Navarro (1990) pieced together evidence from a variety of sources and concluded that the social-class difference in United States mortality is not only large but increasing. National mortality data can obscure exceptional mortality rates in certain impoverished inner city communities. For example, the age-adjusted mortality rate in Harlem (where 96% of the population is African-American and where more than 40% live below the poverty line) is more than *double* the rate for United States whites and some 50% higher than the overall rate for United States blacks (McCord & Freeman, 1990). Astonishingly, black men in Harlem have a lower chance of surviving to age 65 than men in Bangladesh.

HEALTH BEHAVIORS OF THE HOMELESS AND THE POOR

Perceived Health Status

The effects of poverty and homelessness on health are not lost on poor and homeless people themselves. Ropers and Boyer (1987) investigated the perceived health status of a sample of homeless individuals in Los Angeles. The proportion of homeless reporting themselves to be in "poor" health was 70% greater than the proportion among low-income respondents (family income under $10,000) in the NHIS. Self-reported poor health was higher among homeless respondents with chronic health conditions, among those who had recently seen a physician for an acute health problem, among homeless experiencing chronic depression, and among those with severe alcohol-dependence symptoms (Ropers & Boyer, 1987, p. 673). A large percentage of respondents also stated that their health had deteriorated since the onset of homelessness.

The best and most recent data on perceived health status among the population as a whole are from the 1992 NHIS (National Center for Health Statistics, 1994). These data show significant racial and income differences in self-assessed health status. Compared to whites, African-Americans are less likely to rate their health as excellent, very good, or good, and more likely to rate their health as fair or poor. The percentage of respondents assessing their health as excellent or very good increases regularly as income rises; in the 1992 data, slightly fewer than half the respondents with family incomes under $10,000 reported excellent or very good health, while nearly 80% of those earning $35,000 or more so reported. Likewise, nearly 1 in 4 respondents earning a family income under $10,000 reported

their health as fair or poor compared to only 1 in 25 (4.3%) of those earning incomes of $35,000 or more (National Center for Health Statistics, 1994).

Diet, Nutrition, and Exercise

Diet and exercise are important health behaviors in any population, and in these behaviors too the poor and homeless appear to have significant deficits compared to the rest of the United States population. Unfortunately, the entire topic of hunger, malnutrition, and poverty has become so politicized that the voice of science can barely be heard in the din. Some have claimed that an epidemic of hunger is sweeping across the poverty population of this country, a point of view that is not sustained by serious scientific research (Graham, 1985). Such evidence as there is suggests modest but important dietary deficiencies in some nutrients among poor as opposed to nonpoor persons, not widespread hunger or malnutrition.

The Homeless

Specific studies of dietary intake or nutritional deficiency disorders among homeless persons, whether child or adult, are rare. Winick (1985) has noted that the menu used by the city of New York in its shelters for homeless persons supplies at least one third of the daily requirements for all known nutrients, and is to that extent "sufficient." The shelter and soup kitchen diets, however, are typically high in cholesterol, saturated fats, sugar, salt, and starch, so while they may well offer adequate caloric intake, they are far short of optimal. To our knowledge, no study has yet been published discussing dietary intakes or adequacy for homeless persons who do not avail themselves of shelters and soup kitchens and who eat mainly what they can scavenge from street sources, but it is unlikely in the extreme that such diets are adequate by any criterion.

A few studies have remarked the disproportionate occurrence of nutritional deficiency disorders among homeless children. Wright (1991a) has reported that 2.2% of homeless children who received care during the first year of the National Health Care for the Homeless program were diagnosed with anemias—twice the rate for "normal" children seen in ambulatory pediatric clinics nationwide (see also, Miller & Lin, 1988). An additional 1.6% of the homeless children had nutritional deficiency disorders other than anemia (most of them vitamin deficiency disorders); among children in general, such deficiencies are practically nonexistent (Wright, 1991b). About 2% of the homeless children studied by Miller and Lin were diagnosed with growth problems or anthropomorphic abnormalities possibly secondary to dietary insufficiencies.

In a national probability sample of homeless individuals using shelters and soup kitchens, Burt and Cohen (1989) found that only 29% of single women, 41% of women with children, and 22% of single men reported eating three or more meals on the average day; that homeless people generally do not eat three meals a day is a rather common finding in the literature. Substantial portions in all subgroups of the Burt–Cohen sample reported that they often did not get enough to eat and sometimes went a day or more without food. Lack of money and prohibitively long lines at the feeding outlets are the principal problems in this connection.

Luder et al. (1989) found that diets among their sample of urban homeless and marginally housed single room occupancy residents "deviated substantially from the requirements of the [Recommended Daily Allowance nutritional allocations], placing them at increased risk for nutritional deficiencies" (p. 455). They also found that 92% of their subjects had serum cholesterol levels greater than 200 (milligrams per deciliter), placing them at high risk for coronary heart disease. A large number of participants also had a body mass index above the normal range, which is associated with both hypertension and diabetes. In this sample, 80% reported a chronic medical condition, and a significant proportion had been told to follow special diets, but only

about half of the latter felt that they could realistically comply with these dietary restrictions. Health Care for the Homeless care providers are nearly unanimous in their view that dietary control of diseases such as diabetes and hypertension among a homeless population is practically impossible (see the many entries under "nutrition" in the papers collected in Brickner et al. [1990]).

There appear to be no studies reporting data on patterns of physical exercise among any sample of homeless people.

The Poor

Nowhere is the thinness of the line of demarcation between poor people and homeless people more evident than in studies of soup kitchen users, the majority of whom prove not to be literally homeless, but rather poor people who utilize feeding programs to help "make ends meet." A random sample of soup kitchen clients in New York City found that only 41% were literally homeless (Bowering, Clancy, & Poppendieck, 1991); a similar study of soup kitchens in several New York counties (Rauschenbach, Frongillo, Thompson, Andersen, & Spicer, 1990) found that only 17% of the patrons were actually homeless, although a higher percentage were at risk of homelessness (were temporarily doubled up with friends or had recently experienced some housing instability).

Numerous studies of the housing burdens of the poor have reported that substantial proportions of poor households (on the order of half or more) spend between 60% and 80% of their total monthly income on rent *alone* (Rauschenbach et al., 1990). This expenditure leaves little for other necessities such as food, and indeed survival is possible only if free food can be procured from such sources as soup kitchens and food banks. In an important sense, then, the soup kitchens help *prevent* homelessness among marginal, low-income households; they cut the food bill so that more of the monthly income can be spent on rent.

Many poor people who utilize soup kitchens and other food outlets are also found to participate in government-supported nutrition programs (food stamps in most cases, WIC food allocations in a few) to help stretch incomes around expenses. Numerous studies of families who participate in the food stamp and various other nutrition programs have found that these families continue to request emergency food assistance near the end of the month, suggesting that their food stamps are not an adequate subsidy (Thompson et al., 1988).

A large national "food consumption survey" conducted in the United States in 1977 and 1978 compared average dietary intakes of low-income households receiving food stamps with those of low-income households eligible for but not receiving food stamps (Human Nutrition Information Service, 1982). On the whole, the diets of food stamp recipients were more adequate than those of non-recipients, despite the stereotype that food stamps are often frittered away on non-nutritious "junk" food. In this study, the average diet of poor households in general was deemed "sufficient" in total calories and in 11 specific nutrients; fewer than 40% of the low-income households studied, however, consumed diets meeting the Recommended Daily Allowances (RDAs) for *all* nutrients. RDA-intake deficiencies were particularly widespread for total calories, calcium, magnesium, and vitamin B_6.

These findings have been replicated in a number of more recent surveys investigating the nutritional adequacy of low-income diets (e.g., see Emmons, 1987). In one study of soup kitchen clients, 94% were found to have nutritional deficiencies according to laboratory and anthropometric evidence (Laven & Brown, 1985, p. 875). Emmons (1987) also found that participation in emergency food assistance programs (e.g., soup kitchens, feeding outlets) did not result in higher nutrition scores. The nutritional quality of food offered in these programs clearly requires more attention.

The literature on poverty and nutrition among children is somewhat more developed than the literature on adults. Much of this research is based on inferences from anthropomorphic data

(specifically, age-by-weight-by-height measurements), not on direct nutritional intake surveys or observations. Most studies based on such approaches (e.g., Shah, Kahan, & Krauser, 1987) report disproportionate weight-for-height abnormalities among poor children. There is some literature on nutritional deficiency disorders among poor and nonpoor children. Iron deficiency anemias, for example, are more widespread among poor children than nonpoor children, in both Canada (Shah et al., 1987) and the United States (Singer, 1982). Rickets (resulting from vitamin D deficiency) are also more common in poor than in nonpoor children.

Direct studies of nutritional intakes and ensuing deficiencies are relatively rare. Shah et al. (1987) reported data from the Nutrition Canada Survey showing that mean intakes of all nutrients among children varied directly with family income level, with particularly pronounced differences in the intakes of vitamins A and C, folic acid, and calcium. Shah et al. (1987, p. 486) suggest that "children of low-income families are usually fed lower-quality diets, which consist of more refined carbohydrates and fewer meats, fruits, and vegetables." Similar results are reported by Zee, DeLeon, Robertson, and Chen, (1985). Among 1219 preschoolers from a poverty area of Memphis, Tennessee, between 9% and 18% were observed to have low or deficient levels of vitamins A, C, B_1, and B_2, and hemoglobin and serum iron. Wilton and Irvine (1983) reported relatively small but consistent differences in nearly all nutrients between the daily dietary intakes of low-income and average-income children; as with other studies, the differences in intake of calcium and vitamin C were notably large.

One study in Boston (Meyers, Rubin, Napoleone, & Nichols, 1993) found that children whose families received housing subsidies were less likely than other poor children to experience iron deficiency anemias (19% versus 30%, a very large difference). Presumably, housing subsidies reduce pressure on the monthly food budget, thus allowing a more adequate diet.

The large literature on poverty and nutrition can be summarized as follows (Brown & Allen, 1988, p. 517): (1) Infants of poor mothers die more frequently; they are at greater risk for low birth weight and associated health impairment than middle class children. Many factors are responsible for the difference in infant mortality, but poor maternal nutrition is certainly among them. (2) Poor children are less likely than their better-off peers to be adequately nourished and are more likely to suffer growth deficits. (3) Poor children are at higher risk of nutrition-related illness, including illnesses more commonly associated with extreme malnutrition in various Third World countries. (4) Poor adults are at greater risk of and die younger from nutrition-related diseases than other Americans.

There is no consensual definition of "hunger" in the literature, and the issue is highly politicized. Still, a number of studies have suggested that as many as 20 million Americans suffer from this condition (Brown & Allen, 1988; Physician's Task Force on Hunger in America, 1985), and numerous other studies have documented the growing demand for emergency food relief (e.g., see Cohen, 1990). Whatever the true number of hungry people, it is certain that the poor are overrepresented among them, especially poor women, infants and children, and the elderly—precisely the groups for whom proper nutrition is especially important (Brickner et al., 1990).

There is also a growing literature on physical activity and its socioeconomic correlates, most showing a higher prevalence of sedentary lifestyles among the poor than the nonpoor. Data from the Behavioral Risk Factor Surveillance System show relatively high levels of sedentary living among the lowest-income and lowest-education groups, levels that decline sharply as income and education increase (*MMWR*, 1993, p. 578). Likewise, the 1990 NHIS found that the proportion of persons who exercised regularly increased from 33% among those with incomes less than $10,000 to 52% of those with incomes of $50,000 or more. Consistent with this finding, a study of predominantly poor black residents of public housing in Birmingham reported that "a sedentary life style is common among this low-income minority group" (Lewis et al., 1993, p. 1016).

Access to and Utilization of Health Services

The recent and continuing debate over health care reform has focused national attention on the problems faced by disadvantaged populations in accessing the health care system. A commonly cited statistic in these discussions is that some 37 million Americans lack health insurance, a large fraction of whom are also among the 35–40 million Americans who fall below the poverty line. Lack of access to and underutilization of health services are principal mechanisms that connect homelessness and poverty to poor health outcomes.

The Homeless

Many studies have shown that the homeless have numerous health problems but face profound barriers to accessing health care. Most lack a regular source of medical care, and most are also without health insurance, whether public or private, resulting in costly and inefficient overutilization of inpatient and emergency care services (Robertson & Cousineau, 1986).

Robertson and Cousineau (1986) studied urban homeless adults in Los Angeles and found that fewer than half of those with a chronic medical problem had seen a physician about that problem in the previous year; only 13% had a physician whom they saw regularly. Many said they did not see a doctor because they did not consider their problem sufficiently serious or felt that it could not be treated. About a quarter cited no money or no health insurance as the reason. In these data, 81% reported having no health insurance coverage of any kind; 7% had Medicaid, 4% had Medicare, 5% had private insurance, and 2% had veteran's health benefits. One in five had been hospitalized for a health problem during the previous year. Participants in this study were

3 times more likely than the general urban population to report themselves in fair or poor health, 50% more likely to report a physical health disability, and twice as likely to have been hospitalized in the previous year.

Hilfiker (1989) reported that most homeless individuals could not name a regular source of care, nor did they have health insurance; therefore, when their health degenerated, they frequently turned to the emergency room, an expensive and inefficient alternative. He also reported that most homeless people also received no public assistance and that benefit levels were generally inadequate for those who did. Nationwide, only about 20% of the homeless are covered under Medicaid or other forms of public insurance; even when this coverage is present, patients are often forced into second-rate public systems because private medicine has essentially abandoned the homeless and the poor (Hilfiker, 1989). In the same vein, 79% of homeless soup kitchen users studied by Bowering et al. (1991) did not have health insurance.

The principal barrier to access to health care among the homeless is extreme poverty (Altman et al., 1989), but lack of money and insurance are not the only problems. Wood, Valdez, Hayashi, and Shen (1990) listed the general stresses of a homeless existence, preexisting family problems, and weak support networks as factors that increased the likelihood that homeless families would not seek or obtain access to the health and social service system. Further, amid the daily struggle for survival and the quest to meet even the most basic human needs, health is rarely a high-priority concern (Kerner, Dusenbury, & Mandelblatt, 1993).

The literature suggests three major classes of reasons that homeless people experience difficulties obtaining necessary medical care. First is the health care system itself and the manner in which health care is traditionally delivered. Included in this category would be an inadequate supply of public health facilities, lack of providers for Medicaid patients, geographic factors that limit accessibility, and the forbidding and often unfriendly institutional settings in which care is typically delivered. Second are the many special and unique needs and circumstances of homeless people, their distraction from health concerns by more basic survival issues, and their exceptional rates of morbidity, educational deficits, and high rates of mental illness and substance abuse. The final set of factors inheres in the attitudes of health professionals, who frequently define homeless and indigent persons as unworthy or undesirable clients. This attitude has been called the GOMER problem: Get Out of My Emergency Room (Annas, 1986).

There is also overwhelming evidence from the National Health Care for the Homeless demonstration project (Wright & Weber, 1987) and the larger 109-city Health Care for the Homeless program created by the Stewart B. McKinney Homeless Assistance Act (Vicic, 1991) that all these barriers and others can be overcome. Vicic points out that in the first year of the McKinney program, 231,000 homeless individuals were seen a total of 783,000 times. This result implies, first, that homeless people can indeed be brought into a system of health care if it is designed with their unique circumstances in mind and, second, that some level of continuity of care can be established even among a transient, difficult-to-reach homeless population. The barriers, while formidable, are clearly not insurmountable.

The Poor

Since the poverty of the homeless is the principal barrier to their health care access, it is clear that the differences between homeless people and poor people in access and utilization are matters of degree, not of kind (Elvy, 1985). That access to care is more problematic in the lower socioeconomic strata than among middle-class and more affluent people is a long-standing and widely reported finding (e.g., see Rowland & Salganicoff, 1994).

Aggregate racial differences in physician contacts illustrate the dimensions of the access issue. Whites have more physician contacts per year than blacks (5.5 versus 4.7); this relationship tends to hold across all age and income groups. Likewise, more affluent people have more annual physician contacts than less affluent people, regardless of race. The number of dental visits per year also increases with income; persons with annual incomes above $25,000 have nearly twice as many dental visits per year as their less affluent counterparts (National Center for Health Statistics, 1985).

Insurance status is a, perhaps *the*, key mediating variable between poverty and health care access. More than three quarters of the medically uninsured are poor or near-poor (Weissman & Epstein, 1993). Having no insurance is in turn related to essentially all measures of access: "uninsured persons are more likely than either the privately or the publicly insured to lack a usual source of care" (Weissman & Epstein, 1993, p. 247), are less likely to have a private physician as their usual source of care if they have a usual source of care (and therefore rely more on hospital-based providers), report longer travel times to get to their source of care and longer waiting times once they arrive, are more likely to utilize public hospitals, have fewer ambulatory visits, are more likely to delay or forgo care altogether, are less likely to seek or utilize preventative services, and tend to receive poorer care once they present for treatment (e.g., see Monheit, 1994; Franks, Clancy, Gold, & Nutting, 1993). That all these relationships have been reported in numerous recent studies renders the link between insurance status and access essentially incontrovertible.

Access to health services among the poor is further complicated by fear, isolation, and inability to pay out of pocket (Reuler, Bax, & Sampson, 1986); by lack of supportive social networks (Kroll, Carey, Hagedorn, Fire Dog, & Benavides, 1986); by lack of transportation to care outlets, exposure to violence, and low educational attainments in the poverty population (Rask, Williams, Parker, & McNagny, 1994); and by numerous other factors. Thus, lack of insurance is one but by no means the only barrier.

The tendency for poor, uninsured people to delay or forgo treatment, to eschew preventive services, and to utilize hospital-based providers (mainly emergency room services) when seeking care implies that care is often not sought until health conditions degenerate to emergency status and, moreover, that care is sought in the most expensive and inefficient ways possible. It is therefore possible and even rather likely that a system of universal health coverage would prove cost-beneficial in the long run. Wright and Weber (1987) examined the cost per visit among clients seen in the National Health Care for the Homeless demonstration program and compared those costs to the national costs of emergency room care; on that basis, they concluded that ambulatory clinics for homeless people would "break even" economically if 1 clinical visit in 20 prevented a trip to the ER (see also Stern et al., 1991).

The tendency for poor, uninsured people to receive worse care once they present for treatment (Weissman & Epstein, 1993; Hadley, Steinberg, & Feder, 1991) is an especially disturbing finding that calls attention, once again, to the two-tiered system of health care that exists in this nation: a first tier reserved mostly for the affluent and the insured that offers one of the highest levels of health care available anywhere in the world and a second tier that serves mainly the unaffluent and the uninsured and is characterized by indifferent treatment in second-rate facilities. As the concentration of poverty in the central city neighborhoods worsens, the demands placed on inner city public health care outlets grow increasingly burdensome and the quality of care inexorably suffers.

Compliance Behavior

Another important dimension of health behavior is what is called *compliance behavior*, namely, whether and to what extent patients follow the advice and treatment regimens given to them by health professionals. The conditions for compliance are obvious and well-understood; compliance requires that patients (1) recognize that they have a health problem, (2) believe that the recommended treatment regimen will help to resolve that problem, and (3) possess the personal, social, and financial resources necessary to comply with the regimen (Stephenson, Rowe, Haynes, Macharia, & Leon, 1993).

The Homeless

Numerous barriers to compliance among the homeless have been described in the literature, especially in Brickner et al. (1990), from which the following account is derived. A revealing case is that of homeless diabetics. In a domiciled population, diabetes can be managed more or less adequately by tight dietary control and sometimes multiple daily insulin injections. But what can "tight dietary control" possibly mean to homeless people who eat what is available in the soup kitchens and shelters or what they can scavenge from street sources? Lacking access to a refrigerator or some other means of storage, where are homeless diabetics supposed to keep their insulin? And do we really want to turn vulnerable homeless people loose on the streets with a pocketful of sterile syringes? In these cases, noncompliance stems less from lack of motivation than from the existential conditions of a homeless existence.

Nearly by definition, homeless people lack the commonplace routines of everyday life and therefore have no "routine" into which compliant health behavior can be integrated. Domiciled people easily forget how tightly our notions of time are tied to the routines of family and work. Having neither family nor work, homeless people frequently live disorganized and chaotic lives. "Come back next Thursday" is a sensible request only if the concept of "Thursday" itself has meaning; among many homeless people, and especially among the mentally ill and substance abusive, it does not.

Often, compliance with a treatment regimen means taking daily medication, and in this, too, homeless people confront formidable barriers. With no medicine cabinet in which to store medication, many homeless people carry their medications with them. A few days of walking and sleeping with the vials of pills in their pockets often grinds the pills to a powder. Under the circumstances of homelessness, bottles of medication are also often lost or stolen. Researchers reported that homeless AIDS patients frequently failed to complete antibiotic regimens "because they lost or could not afford to fill their prescriptions" (Torres, Lefkowitz, Kales, & Brickner, 1987, p. 780). Other compliance problems in this population were a greater tendency to leave the hospital against medical advice and to be lost to follow-up.

Maintaining a follow-up schedule (getting to referrals, keeping appointments, and the like) requires access to transportation, which is routinely problematic for the homeless (Elvy, 1985); a daily calendar in which appointment dates and times can be recorded; and sufficient free time to go to doctors' offices or clinics. One might think that "free time" would be the least of a homeless person's worries, but homeless people have less of it than many people realize. Perhaps *the* distinguishing feature of the daily existence of homeless people is that they are required to stand in line for practically everything. In many cities, for example, soup kitchen lines begin to form around 10:00 A.M. for the noon meal; if one is not in line early enough, the food may well be gone. A homeless person with a health follow-up appointment scheduled at, say, 11:00 A.M. may have to choose between keeping the appointment and eating. And there are other lines in which to stand: for the evening meal, for a bed in the shelter, for the clothing outlet, and for other necessities.

The homeless mentally ill and substance abusive face special compliance problems. Both groups can (and often do) have severe memory problems. Both groups have altered perceptions of pain and other somatic states, which can influence their motivation to be compliant. Many medications are strongly contraindicated with alcohol, and so homeless alcoholics frequently must choose between taking their medication and drinking, the latter very much a part and parcel of their daily existence, the former not.

For many homeless people, health care and treatment compliance are luxuries that assume priority only after the more pressing needs of daily existence have been satisfied—the needs to obtain food, find shelter, avoid predators, and the like. Given these far more pressing and immediate needs, it is little wonder that homeless people are frequently noncompliant. One study of referral keeping among homeless women in Seattle reported that "personal stresses and competing priorities, weighed against perceived medical urgency," were the major barriers (Schlosstein, St. Clair, & Connell, 1991, p. 279).

The Poor

Many of the compliance problems faced by the homeless are also faced more generally by the poor: lack of access to necessary transportation, lack of social support, lack of money, subcultural differences in what is considered necessary for good health and in definitions of "good health" itself, complications of child rearing and child care, and diversion by more pressing problems.

Shea, Misra, Ehrlich, Field, and Francis (1992) studied correlates of noncompliance with hypertension treatment in an inner city minority population in New York City. Hypertension is a useful test case because with hypertension, as with many other chronic disorders, compliance with treatment is essential for proper management and also because the disease is often asymptomatic (there is no associated unpleasant somatic state that might represent a motivation to comply with treatment). Younger clients were less compliant than older clients when other factors were controlled; somewhat surprisingly, compliance was not related to insurance status. Dependence on emergency rooms for treatment (to have blood pressures checked and obtain medication prescriptions) and not having a primary care physician were also strongly related to noncompliance. Smokers, problem drinkers, and drug abusers were also less compliant than their opposite numbers.

Several studies of compliance among persons with AIDS and tuberculosis are now available in the literature. Alcohol and drug abuse, poverty, and homelessness are almost always reported as significant barriers (Slutkin, 1986); closely supervised therapy is routinely urged as the only effective means to overcome these barriers. Noncompliance with TB chemotherapy is implicated in recurrent infections in about a third of all cases; patients who received care from private physicians were more compliant with TB drug treatment than clients treated by other health care providers (Kopanoff, Snider, & Johnson, 1988).

It would be remiss not to conclude this discussion with a brief comment about "noncompliance" behavior among health professionals who treat the poor and homeless, since there is often clear evidence of the failure of medical caregivers to comply with standards-of-care guidelines. One study of recurrent TB (Kopanoff et al., 1988) reported that about 20% of the recurrent cases resulted from the fact that patients had *no* chemotherapy prescribed for their previous TB episode; another 20% resulted from inappropriate or inadequate therapy. A chart review for patients being treated in an outpatient sexually transmitted disease (STD) clinic in a public hospital in Los Angeles found that 49 of 176 patients (28%) received care that failed to meet even the *minimum* quality-of-care criteria (Shekelle & Kosecoff, 1992). When physicians judge patients to be "poorly motivated," they are 4 times more likely to relegate these patients to self-care than to so relegate clients who are perceived to be highly motivated (McArtor et al., 1992).

Physician attitudes about indigent and homeless patients apparently underlie these patterns. One study of family practice residents found that a majority believed that "poor patients are more likely than others to miss appointments without canceling (73%), more likely to be late for appointments (51%), and are less knowledgeable about their illnesses (80%)" (Price, Desmond, Snyder, & Kimmel, 1988, p. 615). A majority also felt that poor people are not likely to practice preventive health behaviors or to be compliant with medical regimens, and a substantial minority (41%) believed that poor people simply care less about their health than more affluent people. If physicians *believe* that poor or homeless patients will be noncompliant, and treat such patients on that basis, then such treatment will surely increase the odds that their poor and homeless patients will in fact *be* noncompliant—a classic case of the self-fulfilling prophecy.

Sexuality

As HIV and other sexually transmitted diseases continue to increase in epidemic proportions in the United States, sexuality has come to be recognized as a health behavior of considerable import. The prevalence of syphilis, gonorrhea, HIV disease, and other STDs has increased dramatically among the urban poor in the last decade; homeless people also suffer from these disorders at elevated rates. Another health outcome of sexuality is, of course, pregnancy, whether unwanted or not.

The Homeless

One fairly common but inaccurate stereotype of the homeless is that they are relatively old, generally broken-down and debilitated, and therefore not likely to be sexually active. In fact, the homeless are surprisingly young, with an average age in the middle 30s in most studies (Wright, 1989), and there is both direct and indirect evidence that most of them are sexually active. Direct evidence comes from a sample of homeless black men in Miami (*MMWR*, 1991b). Among the 110 men studied, 31% had had sex with one partner and 39% had had sex with two or more partners within the previous month. Among this 70% who were sexually active, 17% had had sex just once, 49% had done so two to five times, and the remainder had done so six or more times (all, again, within the previous month).

Pregnancy provides direct evidence of sexual activity among homeless women. Nearly a tenth of all women seen in the National Health Care for the Homeless (HCH) program presented with pregnancies (Wright & Weber, 1987, pp. 106–107). Among 16 to 19-year-old homeless women, the figure was 24%, and among 20 to 24-year-olds, 22%. There is evidence, hardly surprising, that homeless women receive inferior prenatal care (Chavkin, Kristal, Seabron, & Guigli, 1987); most care providers consider *all* pregnancies among homeless women as high-risk, especially when other factors (inadequate nutrition, psychiatric illness, substance abuse) are also present, as they frequently are. For these and other reasons, the proportion of low-birth-weight babies and the rate of infant mortality are both elevated among homeless women (Bassuk & Weinreb, 1993; Chavkin et al., 1987).

STDs are among the most common diagnoses in health outlets serving homeless women (Burroughs, Bouma, O'Connor, & Smith, 1990). In the HCH data, STDs were observed in 2.9% of the adult clients (1.9% of the men, 5.4% of the women) (Wright & Weber, 1987). The rate of STD infection among the homeless is about twice that among the ambulatory population in general. Analysis of the rates of STD by age and gender combined showed that these infections are more common among women than men at all ages, and more common among the young than among the old regardless of gender.

There is also evidence that the rate of HIV infection is higher among the homeless than among the general population by a factor of 2–10, depending on study and comparison group (Wright, 1990); in some homeless populations, the rate of HIV seroprevalance is on the order of 5–15% (Raba et al., 1990), an astonishing rate of infection. Certainly, HIV risk behaviors are widespread among the homeless, especially among homeless IV drug abusers (Joseph & Roman-Nay, 1989) and homeless adolescents (Rotheram-Borus & Koopman, 1991).

Little is known about safe sex practices among the homeless, but some data are available for a sample of homeless men in Miami (*MMWR*, 1991b). Among the sexually active men in this sample (78 men who had had sex at least once in the prior month), about 10% were exclusively homosexual, and about half reported having used a condom on one or more occasions in the prior month. Trading drugs for sex or sex for drugs were both relatively common.

The Poor

The reproductive and sexual behaviors of the poor have always seemed perverse when measured against middle-class norms. Summarizing an extensive literature: Poor people become sexually active at earlier ages than middle-class people (Furstenberg, Lincoln, & Menken, 1981), have much higher rates of teen and unwed pregnancies (Devine & Wright, 1993, pp. 132–142), are less likely to use contraception (Upchurch, Farmer, Glasser, & Hook, 1987) or otherwise engage in safe sex practices (Nyamathi, Bennett, Leake, Lewis, & Flaskerud, 1993), contract STDs (Aral & Holmes, 1991) and HIV (Conway et al., 1993) at elevated rates, have much higher rates of infant mortality and other complications of pregnancy (Combs-Orme, Risley-Curtiss, & Taylor, 1993), and probably have more sexual partners (Ford & Norris, 1993). Taken together, the sexual practices of the poor represent an important class of high-risk health behaviors.

Violence

That "violence is a public health issue" has recently become part of the catechism of the public health profession (Koop & Lundberg, 1992; Rosenberg, O'Carroll, & Powell, 1992). Like many other public health issues, this one also has a disproportionate impact on the lower strata of society. The general trend in violence, especially homicide, has been sharply upward over the past several years; poor people in the inner cities are overrepresented among both the perpetrators and the victims of this carnage.

The Homeless

Traumatic injury is among the top three or four presenting conditions in any health care outlet serving predominantly homeless people (Brickner et al., 1990). "Homeless people are at high risk for traumatic injuries for a number of reasons. They are frequently victims of violent crimes such as rape, assault, and robbery" (Institute of Medicine, 1988, p. 44). To illustrate the dimensions of the problem, Kelly (1985) reported that the rate of sexual assault against homeless women exceeds that of United States women in general by a factor of *20*. Other subgroups among the homeless also face higher than average risks of traumatic injury due to intentional violence, among them homeless teens (Wright, 1991c), the homeless mentally ill (French, 1987), and homeless alcoholics and drug addicts (Wright & Weber, 1987).

Homicide is grossly overrepresented among causes of death among homeless people. In any average recent year, about 1% of all deaths in the United States are due to homicide; of the deaths among homeless people investigated in Wright and Weber (1987), 26% were murders. Other studies of mortality among the homeless report similar results (e.g., see *MMWR*, 1991a, p. 879).

Wright, Devine, and Joyner (1993) reported on experiences with violence among a sample of substance-abusive homeless men and women in New Orleans. Respondents in their study were asked how often they had been victimized by robbery, assault, rape, or forcible theft, how many times they had been beaten up, and how many times they had been stabbed with a knife or shot at with a gun. Overall, 91% had experienced one or more of these victimizations (93% of the men, 90% of the women), usually on several occasions. The average woman in the sample had been robbed 3 times in her life, assaulted or beaten up 14 times, raped 5 times, and shot at once; the average male had been shot at twice. Likewise, Gelberg and Linn (1989) reported that 71% of their sample of homeless people in Los Angeles had been victimized by some crime in the previous year.

The pattern of violence against persons who eventually become homeless often begins in childhood (Wright & Devine, 1993). Emotional, sexual, and physical abuse during childhood are common elements in the biographies of homeless people (Burroughs et al., 1990; Susser, Lin, Conover, & Struening, 1991). Homeless women are also frequent victims of family violence; indeed, abusive mates are a leading risk factor for homelessness among women (Browne, 1993).

The exceptional rate of violence against the homeless is a joint function of exposure and vulnerability. The streets (and to a lesser but still significant extent the shelters) are inherently dangerous places, and so exposure to potentially violent situations is widespread. Some homeless people go to truly extraordinary lengths to protect themselves from the inherent dangers (e.g., keeping on the move all night long and sleeping during the day, or sleeping in trees, in dumpsters, or in other concealed places). It is useful to stress that many of the apparently "bizarre" things homeless people do are in fact highly adaptive health behaviors with the purpose of reducing risk of physical harm. Furthermore, many homeless people are of course in poor physical health, or generally debilitated, or mentally impaired, or impaired by alcohol and other drugs, so they are often easy targets. One might think that the homeless are protected to some extent by the fact that they possess practically nothing worth stealing, but Wright and Weber (1987) reported one case in which a homeless alcoholic man was beaten to death for his sack of aluminum cans, worth maybe 3 dollars.

The Poor

Between 1985 and 1990, the age-adjusted aggregate homicide rate increased by 23% and shot up further still in the early years of the 1990s. Homicide is now the leading cause of death for black males of ages 15–34 (Novello, Shosky, & Froehlke, 1992) and is steadily moving up the list in many other age-by-race-by-gender subgroups as well (National Center for Health Statistics, 1993). In several states, death by gunfire has recently overtaken death by automobile accident among causes of premature mortality. Poor inner

city African-Americans are at the forefront of these trends.

Schwarz et al. (1994) reported results from a longitudinal study of injury morbidity in a poor African-American community in Philadelphia (97% black; median income approximately equal to the official federal four-person poverty line). Astonishingly, in the 4-year study period (1987–1990), *half* the residents of the study area sustained one or more injuries that resulted in emergency department treatment (or death). Men of all ages were more likely to experience injury; the distribution of injuries by age shows a marked peak among persons in their 20s. Combining risk factors, "94.3% of men 20 through 29 years old came at least once to an emergency department for an injury" over the 4 years (Schwarz et al., 1994, p. 757). Among young, impoverished, inner city African-American males, in short, the experience is essentially universal.

In the first year of the study (1987), falls accounted for the largest share of all injuries; by the third year, "interpersonal intentional injury" (violence) had moved into first place. The increasing proportion of injuries resulting from gunfire was especially pronounced. Over the entire study period, the estimate is that 41% of all males of ages 20–29 went to an emergency department for treatment of a violence-related injury at least once, a truly stunning number. The study also documents a 179% increase in firearms injuries over the 4 years, a 26% increase in stabbings, and a 41% increase in other injuries secondary to violence. Among all violence-related injuries in the analysis, 8% were inflicted by firearms, 15% by knives, and 24% by other weapons.

Much of the violence that now plagues the inner cities is perpetrated by and against young males (Fingerhut, Ingram, & Feldman, 1992a; *MMWR*, 1990). Some of this youth violence, although certainly not all, is connected to the urban traffic in narcotics, and some is linked to the growing problem of inner city youth gangs. A great deal apparently stems from the growing practice of carrying guns among inner city teens. Sheley and Wright (1993) have reported data on gun ownership and carrying practices among a sample of incarcerated juvenile offenders in inner city areas of five major cities in the United States. Among the incarcerated juveniles, 86% had owned at least one firearm at some time in their young lives; 83% owned a gun at the time they were incarcerated. Of those who had ever owned a gun, two thirds acquired their first firearm by the age of 14. The practice of *carrying* guns was also relatively common; 55% carried a gun "all" or "most of the time" in the year or two before being incarcerated, and 84% carried a gun at least "now and then."

Gun carrying among inner city males reflects family and peer influence in large measure. About 80% of the incarcerated juveniles studied by Sheley and Wright came from families in which at least some of the males owned guns; most significantly, 62% had male family members who carried guns as they went about their daily business, at least from time to time. The practice was even more widespread among peers; 90% of the incarcerated juveniles reported having at least some friends and associates who owned and carried guns.

Gun possession and carrying are not confined just to young, inner city male criminals; these practices have also begun to spill over into the larger inner city high school population (Callahan & Rivara, 1992; Sheley & Wright, 1993). In a parallel sample of male high school students in the same five cities, Sheley and Wright (1993) reported that nearly a third had owned at least one gun in their lives, 22% owned a gun at the time the survey was completed, and 35% carried a gun at least "now and then."

Similar results have been reported by Callahan and Rivara (1992) for urban high school youths in Seattle. A third of the students surveyed indicated that they had access to handguns (responding that they already owned one or felt they could obtain one "in a few days"). Males and African-Americans reported higher rates of easy access than females or other ethnic groups. More than half the male youths in all social classes have the highest reported easy access to handguns.

Those who perceived access to handguns to be easy were asked how they would go about obtaining one if they felt they needed to. Friends and street sources were the most commonly mentioned potential suppliers; many, of course, already owned one (13%), and more than a few (7%) reported that they would get one at home.

An analysis of inner city high school students by Sheley, McGee, and Wright (1992) suggests that the best predictors of being victimized by gun violence are behavioral, not demographic. High school students who themselves carried guns (either in or out of school), who hung out with other people who carried guns, who used drugs, or who were involved at any level in the drug business were more likely to be victimized by gun violence than other students, net of other factors. These very high-risk health behaviors are now rather commonplace among inner city poor and minority youth.

Risk Behaviors: Alcohol, Tobacco, and Drugs

Abuse of various substances both legal and illegal is an important class of health behaviors about which a great deal has been written. Because the essential facts are well known, our treatment here is perfunctory.

Alcohol

The Homeless. The rate of chronic alcohol abuse among homeless men is reliably estimated to exceed 50% (Wright & Weber, 1987); "in whatever setting homeless adults are studied, alcoholism is the most frequent single disorder diagnosed" (Institute of Medicine, 1988, p. 60), surpassing even chronic mental illness in prevalence. As in the general population, alcohol abuse is correlated with poor health outcomes among the homeless (Wright, Weber, Knight, & Lam, 1987), in that most disorders are more common among the alcohol-abusive homeless than among the nonabusive.

Wright et al. (1993) reported interesting

data on use patterns and histories for a sample of homeless alcoholics in New Orleans. On average the homeless alcoholics in their sample began drinking at age 15, had drunk alcohol to the point of intoxication on 19 of the previous 30 days, and had been doing so more or less continuously for about 15 years. Since the mean age of their sample was 34 years, the implication of this finding is that the average homeless alcoholic has spent virtually his entire adult lifetime drunk on two days out of three.

The Poor.   Alcohol consumption is widespread throughout American society, with approximately three quarters of the population using alcohol at least once in a typical year. The prevalence of alcoholism is unknown (Goodwin, 1992); most alcohol specialists use a "rule of thumb" figure of about 10% of the United States population with a nontrivial drinking problem (Fisk, 1984). It is also unknown whether poor people are more or less likely than the rest of the population to drink or to drink to excess; the literature is simply inconclusive. One review of the epidemiological literature concludes that "the prevalence of drinking problems is greatest among those who are young, male, single, residents of wet regions, urban, less educated, and persons of lower socioeconomic characteristics" (Winick, 1992, p. 25) Another review *in the same volume* (Goodwin, 1992, p. 144) cites evidence (Public Health Reports, 1985) that "heavy drinkers [are] concentrated in the highest income groups and among whites." Goodwin (1992, p. 144) continues, "There is some inconsistency about the social class correlation, since higher rates [of problem drinking] among blue collar workers and urban blacks have been found in other studies."

Tobacco

The health problems associated with cigarette smoking are well known; public concerns over the deleterious health effects of tobacco smoke date back to at least 1604 (Jarvik & Schnei-

der, 1992, p. 337). Cigarettes are the number one preventable cause of premature death in the United States today.

The Homeless.   Precise percentages of the homeless who smoke cigarettes have rarely been published in the literature, but some evidence and the informal sense of most homeless service providers is that smoking is much more common among the homeless than among the general population (Scanlan & Brickner, 1990). In a sample of homeless black men in Miami, 82% were smokers, about 3 times the age-, sex-, and race-adjusted rate (*MMWR*, 1991b). Certainly, smoking-related lung disorders are much more widespread among the homeless than among the domiciled population (Wright & Weber, 1987), reasonably strong evidence in favor of the sense of service providers. To illustrate, in the case of chronic obstructive pulmonary disease, the differential is on the order of 6:1.

The Poor.   Unlike the evidence on alcohol and poverty, the evidence on tobacco and poverty is unambiguous: Poor people smoke more than middle-class or affluent people; moreover, the rate of decline in smoking is slower among disadvantaged groups than among the more advantaged (Jarvik & Schneider, 1992). Estimates in 1991 and 1992 showed that between 31.4% and 38.4% of adults below the poverty line smoke cigarettes, compared to 25% of those at or above the poverty level (*MMWR*, 1994, p. 343). Differences by education are even sharper: Roughly 15% of college graduates but fully a third of high school dropouts smoke. Data from the NHIS for 1990 show equivalent results (National Center for Health Statistics, 1993). The proportion of persons currently smoking in those data varied from 32% among persons with incomes less than $10,000 to 19% of those with incomes of $50,000 or more.

There is a fairly substantial literature on racial differences in smoking behavior, although in the aggregate the differences are not large (e.g., *MMWR*, 1994; National Center for Health Statistics, 1993). There is some evidence, however, that smoking is more widespread among poor, black inner city residents than among the general African-American population (Romano, Bloom, & Syme, 1991), but this seems to be an effect of socioeconomic status, not specifically of race (Manfredi, Lacey, Warnecke, & Buis, 1992).

Drugs

The health effects of substances such as cocaine and heroin are known less certainly than those of alcohol and tobacco, in part because most abusers of these drugs also drink large amounts of alcohol and smoke heavily, making it difficult to separate the effects. Nevertheless, illicit drug use has been linked to a number of physical and psychological dysfunctions.

Probably the most serious health consequences of drug abuse in American society today result less from the direct physiological effects of drugs than from associated patterns of behavior, especially sexual behavior. To illustrate, the classic STDs—gonorrhea, syphilis, and chancroid—have "been increasing at epidemic rates among urban minority populations in the U.S." (Aral & Holmes, 1991, p. 62). What accounts for this epidemic? "Recent studies in urban areas ... have found that transmission of gonorrhea, syphilis, chancroid and HIV infections has been closely associated with the exchange of sex for drugs such as crack. Women, particularly adolescent women, sometimes engage in very large numbers of sexual contacts to support their addiction" (Aral & Holmes, 1991, p. 68). Much of the heterosexual transmission of HIV involves the exchange of sex for drugs or for money to buy drugs; obviously, all of the HIV cases secondary to the use of infected syringes are drug-related.

The Homeless. In numerous studies that were undertaken in the early 1980s—and thus predating the crack cocaine epidemic—between 15% and 30% of the homeless were found to abuse drugs other than alcohol (Shlay & Rossi,

1992). More recent evidence from the mid-1980s onward suggests dramatically higher rates of drug abuse and addiction among the homeless (e.g., Jencks, 1994). Again, Wright et al. (1993) provided interesting details on drug use patterns and histories for a sample of homeless New Orleans substance abusers. On average, program clients started using alcohol and marijuana at about age 15 and first tried hard drugs at about age 21. The average crack user in the data had smoked crack cocaine on 18 of the previous 30 days and had been doing so for about 5 years (i.e., more or less continuously since the first appearance of crack cocaine as a street drug in early 1986 [Akers, 1992, p. 122]).

The Poor. How do patterns of illicit drug use vary by socioeconomic status? In the 1990 National Household Survey of Drug Abuse, annual usage rates of any illicit substance increased from 11% among those with less than a high school education to 14% among high school graduates and to 16% among those with some college, as contrasted with a downturn to 12% among college graduates (National Institute on Drug Abuse, 1991, p. 32). Thus, there is a slight tendency for illicit drug usage to increase with education up through some years of college and then to decline, but differences by education are relatively minor.

Differences in drug use by employment status are rather sharper. Among employed persons in 1990, about 15% reported some use of illicit drugs within the past year; among unemployed persons, the figure was 26%. (Among those not in the labor force, mostly housewives and retired persons, the rate of illicit drug use was only 6%.) The higher rate among the unemployed also held up when looking specifically at marijuana, cocaine, crack, and hallucinogens. Concerning lifetime use patterns, the unemployed show the highest use rates for cocaine, crack, inhalants, hallucinogens, PCP, heroin, stimulants, and tranquilizers; employed persons show the highest use rates for marijuana, sedatives, and alcohol. Although these are the general patterns, none of these drug-specific differences in use rates is especially large.

"Crack cocaine is a major cause of the continuing decline of inner-city communities and is strongly linked to criminal behavior and social turmoil" (McNagny & Parker, 1992, p. 1106). The crack epidemic has also posed a challenge to the health care system. There is evidence that young, urban African-American women are the fastest-growing group of crack users in the United States. Antecedents to crack abuse in this population include alcohol and drug abuse in the families of origin, sexual abuse as children, and early onset of depression and illicit substance use, usually marijuana (Boyd, 1993). As indicated previously, many young crack-addicted inner city women resort to prostitution to support their drug habit; the association between crack use and dramatic increases in the incidence of STDs in this population is incontrovertible (Fullilove, Fullilove, Bowser, & Gross, 1990).

GENDER AND AGE CONSIDERATIONS

Neither the homeless nor the poor are homogeneous social categories, and many of the issues discussed above have differential impacts on various subgroups within these populations, specifically women, children, and the elderly. It is not possible for this chapter to do justice to the full range of relevant subgroups or topics; rather, it briefly notes some of the more common themes that have surfaced in the literature.

Women

That the health professions have not been sufficiently sensitive to women's health issues is now more or less universally accepted. The unique health issues of poor and homeless women are no exception to this pattern.

Women make up an increasingly large share of the homeless population (Burt & Cohen, 1989); likewise, the progressive "feminization of poverty" is a well-described trend (Devine & Wright, 1993). Although all women are at risk for physical

and sexual violence and exploitation, these are exceedingly common elements in the lives of homeless women and are indeed a major precipitating factor for homelessness among women (Hagen, 1987). Wood et al. (1990) compared homeless mothers to poor but housed mothers in Los Angeles and found that homeless mothers more commonly reported spousal abuse (35% versus 16%), child abuse (28% versus 10%), drug use (43% versus 30%), mental health problems (14% versus 6%), and weaker support networks.

The high rate of sexual assault on homeless women and their frequent participation in the sex–drugs commerce also mean that they face elevated risks for STDs and AIDS (Axelson & Dail, 1988). Differences between homeless women and poor women more generally are matters of degree, not of kind.

The increasing numbers of poor and homeless women have led to concerns about their utilization of various preventive health and family planning services. The pregnancy rate among homeless women is known to be high compared to those of other groups of women (Wright & Weber, 1987). Pregnancy risk factors among socioeconomically disadvantaged women include "environmentally induced risk factors such as nutritional inadequacy, excessive stress, life-long medical under-service, inadequate housing and sanitation, and many medical conditions and diseases, both chronic and acute, such as genitourinary tract infections and hypertension" (Geronimus, 1986, p. 1416). Enhanced behavioral risk factors in these populations include elevated rates of alcohol, drug, and tobacco abuse (Bassuk & Weinreb, 1993). The effects of these risk factors on pregnancies among poor and homeless women are evident in the higher proportion of low-birth-weight infants and much higher rates of infant mortality (Combs-Orme et al., 1993). Neglect of routine gynecological and prenatal care is also a common complicating factor. Chavkin et al. (1987) found that 40% of their homeless sample did not receive any prenatal care, compared to 14.5% of public housing residents and 9% of all women in New York during the study period.

Children

There is a very large literature on the physical health status of homeless children, all confirming without exception that "homelessness is not healthy for children and other living things" (Wright 1990, 1991a, b). Several recent studies have compared perceived health status, health-related behaviors, and access to health services among homeless children, poor but domiciled children, and nonpoor children (Miller & Lin, 1988; Wise & Meyers, 1988). The general picture gleaned from these studies is one of lower levels of self-reported health, lower levels of immunization, and fewer checkups coupled with an absence of regular sources of care and insurance coverage.

Miller and Lin (1988) found that parents staying in an emergency shelter were 4 times as likely to report their children to be in "fair" or "poor" health as compared to the general pediatric population in the United States (14% versus 3%) and twice as likely as compared to parents of domiciled children living in poverty (14% versus 6%). Evidence of more serious health problems can also be inferred from the common finding that children in low-income families suffer greater disability, as measured by bed days and higher hospitalization rates, than their higher-income counterparts (Newacheck & Starfield 1988).

Differences in nutrition and preventive health behavior (e.g., immunization patterns) have been found among poor children as compared to the general pediatric population. While there is a need for studies that explicitly document the nutritional intake of poor children, one can infer from the convergence of available evidence that current dietary patterns among poor children are not adequate. Several studies have found a high prevalence of abnormal anthropometry among this group, as well as heightened risk of delayed or stunted growth, iron deficiency, and other health problems (Miller & Lin 1988; Molnar, Rath, & Klein, 1990).

Several studies also highlight a striking difference in immunization patterns among homeless and poor children. Immunization delays ranging from 21% (Miller & Lin, 1988) to 51% (Redlener, 1988) have been found among samples of homeless children. These rates tend to be 3–4 times higher than those reported in samples of poor but domiciled children (Molnar et al., 1990).

Large disparities in access to health care have also been observed. For example, Wise and Meyers (1988) reported that one third of poor children in a national survey conducted in 1986 did not report an ambulatory physician visit in the previous year, a rate 40% higher than that for nonpoor children. They also found that 15% of poor children reported no regular source of care, twice the rate for nonpoor children. While Medicaid has reduced these inequities somewhat, Wise and Meyers (1988, p. 1180) noted that "56% of low-income children in poor or fair health, and 58% of those with chronic activity limitations, lack Medicaid coverage."

The Elderly

Much has been written about the long-term decline in poverty among the elderly, but it is easy to exaggerate the magnitude of this trend (Wright & Devine, 1994). While unmistakable progress has been made, poverty among the elderly has not been eliminated, and among various disadvantaged subgroups, especially women, African-Americans, and the oldest of the old, the rate of poverty among the old continues to exceed that of the general population, frequently by a wide margin.

Recent studies have revealed differences in health status and behaviors between the poor and nonpoor elderly population. Generally speaking, elderly persons in poverty experience both acute and chronic health problems more frequently, experience more limitations in daily activity, and report lower perceived health status than their higher-income counterparts (York, 1992). In terms of health status, 48% of elderly persons in poor families report being in fair or poor health as compared to 22% of the nonpoor elderly (i.e., those with incomes of $20,000 or more) (National Center for Health Statistics, 1990).

In general, health practices of the elderly poor differ from those of the elderly nonpoor (Lubben et al., 1989), almost always in disadvantageous ways. Although little is known about the nutritional needs of the elderly, much of the literature suggests that older poor people are more likely than the nonpoor elderly to consume inadequate diets, placing them at high risk for various nutritional and vitamin deficiency disorders (Brickner, 1985). In at least one study, it was found that "one half of poor elderly persons consume less than two thirds of the recommended daily allowance of vitamin C, calcium, and other nutrients" (York, 1992, p. 89).

Studies of the effects of various health practices among the elderly have produced inconsistent results. For example, Branch and Jette (1984) found no significant relationship between personal health practices and 5-year mortality in a sample of the elderly, whereas Kaplan, Seeman, Cohen, Knudsen and Guralnik (1987) found that being male, smoking, being sedentary, being overweight, and failing to eat breakfast *were* associated with mortality among the elderly, even net of factors such as race and socioeconomic status. Another study of the elderly poor (Lubben et al., 1989) found that smoking, limited social networks, and lack of exercise increased the likelihood of hospitalization. There is also some evidence that older adults with the most serious health problems may become pessimistic about their health, which would obviously limit the effectiveness of health promotion interventions and health-seeking behavior (Ferraro, 1993).

That nearly all poor elderly persons are currently insured through Medicare leads many to underestimate the barriers to medical care that remain for the elderly poor. In 1987, Medicare covered only about one half of medical expenses among noninstitutionalized elderly persons (York, 1992). The elderly nonpoor frequently obtain supplemental coverage to offset costs. Only about 30% of the elderly poor, however, have supplemental coverage.

As of 1990, only about a third of the elderly poor were enrolled in Medicaid (York, 1992, pp. 76–77). Low rates of Medicaid participation seem to result from various factors, including limited program resources, lack of effective outreach, inadequate knowledge among potential recipients, transportation difficulties, and stringent eligibility requirements.

IMPLICATIONS FOR RESEARCH, POLICY, AND PRACTICE

What implications do the findings reviewed in this chapter bear for future research, for health policy, and for the delivery of adequate health care services to poor and homeless people? While health behaviors often have important health consequences, these behaviors are themselves dictated by a range of social, cultural, economic, and political forces that must also be appreciated before one's understanding is complete. In short, understanding the *causes* of various health behaviors is as important as understanding their *effects*. Research on the latter is well developed, but research on the former is not. To the extent that appropriate research exists, it will generally not be found in the medical or public health journals, but in the literature of sociology, criminology, economics, and related cognate disciplines.

It is self evident, for example, that poor and homeless people should "Just Say No" to drugs, alcohol, and tobacco, and there is very little doubt that their health status would improve if they did. The problem with "Just Say No" is not that it is bad advice, but that it ignores the many social and cultural factors that cause people to drink, smoke, or consume drugs in the first place. Too much emphasis on health behaviors and too little on the reasons people behave as they do can divert attention from the real causes of the behaviors of which we rightly disapprove and can all too quickly reframe public issues as private troubles (Hartman, 1989, p. 483). There is a deeply moralistic tone, even a censorious tone, to much of the medical and public health literature on these topics.

Research

Research on the health behavior of the homeless and poor tends to be dominated by small-scale, cross-sectional studies of locally available populations. Thus, external validity or statistical generalizability is routinely problematic. Working mainly with cross-sectional data also means that causal relationships have to be inferred from statistical correlations, always a perilous undertaking. As in practically every other area of social and behavioral research, the need for large-scale studies and longitudinal research is obvious.

Indifference to the need for common definitions across studies is a serious problem. Only rarely is poverty defined in terms congruent with the official federal poverty designation. In many cases, race is used as a proxy for poverty status, a wholly unsatisfactory practice; in other cases, poverty status is inferred from the types of health care institutions from which people receive services (e.g., public health clinics and hospitals). Despite a common misconception, most people seem quite comfortable answering questions about their incomes; likewise, questions about household composition and size are not at all threatening. Thus, income and household composition items should be routinely included in *all* studies of health status and health behaviors, so that persons and households who satisfy the official poverty definition can be isolated in the analysis of the data. A common and agreed-upon definition of homelessness would also be useful in a number of research areas.

There is a related problem of appropriate comparison groups. Often, the homeless are compared to the domiciled poor, and the poor are compared either to some ill-defined "middle class" or to national norms and standards. But homeless, poor, and middle-class people differ in many ways other than income and housing status, and the many ways that they might differ are only rarely held constant in these comparisons. Much of the available research is correlational and bivariate; the need for multivariate analysis of many of the issues discussed here is pressing.

As has been stressed, neither homelessness nor poverty is a monolithic or homogeneous condition; what is true of homeless men is not necessarily true of homeless women, what is true of poor blacks may not be true of poor Hispanics, and so on. Various subgroups *within* the homeless and poverty populations often display markedly different patterns of health behavior, but much of the available research is silent on the question of subgroup differences.

Policy

Many of the behaviors associated with homelessness (and with poverty) are harmful to health. Homeless people often have inadequate personal hygiene, eat insufficient diets, abuse alcohol, engage in unsafe sex, smoke too many cigarettes, and rarely seek health care attention in a timely manner. Given these facts, what is the proper policy response? Should policy attempt to induce behavioral changes among the homeless so as to minimize the health consequences of these unhealthy behaviors? Or should policy seek instead to end homelessness once and for all, so that people are not forced to exist in such degrading, unhealthy conditions? Should the goal be healthy and happy homeless people? Or no homeless people at all?

Although it is frequently convenient to think otherwise, the solution to the health problems of the poor and the homeless is probably not more clinics, better interventions, enhanced access to care, or more functional health behavior. The solution is to reduce and ultimately to eliminate some profound flaws in the human condition. From the viewpoint of national health policy, it is justifiable to look on poverty and homelessness as *remediable* conditions of the environment that place a large and growing portion of the American population at high health risk. Indeed, it is hard to conceive of socially defined "risk factors" that are more consequential for physical well-being.

Unfortunately, there has been no recent progress in eliminating either poverty or homelessness; both the total number of homeless people and the aggregate poverty rate have grown, not declined, in the past decade (Burt, 1992). Among many reasons for the lack of progress are society's ambivalence about the causes of and most appropriate responses to poverty and homelessness, a tendency to stigmatize poor and homeless people as responsible for their own miseries, inappropriate reliance on health and social services to ameliorate poverty and homelessness versus programs to eliminate those conditions and overspecialization, centralization, and bureaucracy within the human services professions themselves. In the words of Halpern (1991, p. 361): "[Social] service reform in the U.S. has been constrained not so much by the lack of good service models and approaches as by a lack of a coherent set of values to guide social problem solving. We still do not know what we want to do about the problems that confront us as a people."

Practice

At the national level, a principal effort to address the health problems of the poor is the Medicaid program and a principal effort to address the health problems of the homeless is the 109-city Health Care for the Homeless clinic system funded under the auspices of the McKinney Act. Since these programs can be considered to represent the "health behaviors" of the entire society towards homeless and impoverished citizens, it is appropriate to conclude this chapter with a brief discussion of them.

Medicaid. There is little doubt that Medicaid has done much to provide health coverage to a large segment of the low-income population, and it is obvious that poor people who received Medicaid benefits have better access and better health outcomes than those who do not. But significant gaps in Medicaid coverage remain. In 1990, there were 25.3 million Medicaid recipients, but 31.5 million persons in poverty, and so about 20% of the poverty population is not covered (Bureau of the Census, 1992). Eligibility re-

quirements vary wildly from state to state; in several states, Medicaid eligibility is tied to AFDC participation.

Fewer and fewer physicians accept Medicaid patients; those who do tend to see only (or mainly) Medicaid patients, creating what are called Medicaid "mills." This practice raises obvious concerns about the quality of care that Medicaid patients receive. Indeed, the patient volume in practices that accept Medicaid patients is 2–3 times the volume in a large mainstream practice (Fossett, Perloff, Peterson, & Kletke, 1990). Also, as more and more of the AIDS burden has been shifted onto Medicaid (Green & Arno, 1990), the system has been further strained.

About 15% of Americans live below the poverty line; nearly a third earn less than $25,000 a year (and are therefore at least near-poor). A reasonably comprehensive health plan for families would cost perhaps $4000–5000 per year. At present, Medicaid (and Medicare) take up a share of the difference between what health insurance costs and what these families can afford to pay, but these systems of public insurance have left tens of millions uncovered. There is no escaping the fact that the provision of health coverage to those now uninsured will require redistribution of income from the top half to the bottom third of the income distribution (Reinhardt, 1994), whether through an expansion of Medicaid coverage or through some other mechanism. Much of the complexity in the recent debate over health reform stemmed ultimately from disingenuousness about this most basic fact.

Health Care for the Homeless. In 1984, recognizing the often unmet health care needs of the homeless population, the Robert Wood Johnson Foundation and the Pew Charitable Trusts announced their National Health Care for the Homeless (HCH) initiative—a 4-year, $25 million demonstration grant program that established Health Care for the Homeless clinics in 19 United States cities. In 1987, motivated by the obvious successes of the Johnson–Pew program, Congress enacted and President Reagan signed the

Stewart B. McKinney Homeless Assistance Act, which extended the HCH clinic system to a total of 109 cities. Literally millions of homeless and near-homeless people have since received care in these clinics.

Funding for the HCH system has been on a year-to-year footing since the system was first established, as though the homeless problem were somehow going to disappear one of these years so that the clinic system would no longer be needed. Every year, there is therefore widespread concern among HCH providers that funding will be sharply curtailed or possibly even eliminated, most of all in an era when deficit reduction is taken as the highest possible political good. So this chapter concludes with the observation that there is more in life worth saving than money. To go forward with the McKinney HCH program and then pull the plug for budgetary reasons would be cruel to homeless people who have come to depend on these clinics for their primary health care. Not incidentally, it would also be incompatible with our national ideals of compassion and social justice.

REFERENCES

Aday, L., Fleming, G. V., & Andersen, R. (1984). *Access to medical care in the U.S.: Who has it, who doesn't?* Chicago: Pluribus Press.

Akers, R. L. (1992). *Drugs, alcohol, and society*. Belmont, CA: Wadsworth.

Altman, D., Bassuk, E. L., Breakey, W. R., Fischer, A. A., Halpern, C. R., Smith, G., Stark, L., Stark, N., Vladeck, B. C., & Wolfe, P. (1989). Health care for the homeless. *Society*, *26*, 4-5.

Annas, G. J. (1986). Your money or your life: "Dumping" uninsured patients from hospital emergency wards. *American Journal of Public Health*, *76*, 74-77.

Aral, S. O., & Holmes, K. K. (1991). Sexually transmitted diseases in the AIDS era. *Scientific American*, *264*, 62-69.

Axelson, L. J., & Dail, P. W. (1988). The changing character of homelessness in the United States. *Family Relations* (October), 463-469.

Bassuk, E. L., & Weinreb, L. (1993). Homeless pregnant women: Two generations at risk. *American Journal of Orthopsychiatry*, *63*, 348-357.

Battle, S. F. (1990). Homeless women and children: The question of poverty. *Child and Youth Services*, *14*, 111-127.

Bowering, J., Clancy, K. L., & Poppendieck, J. (1991). Characteristics of a random sample of emergency food program users in New York. II. Soup kitchens. *American Journal of Public Health*, *81*, 914-917.

Boyd, C. J. (1993). The antecedents of women's crack cocaine abuse: Family substance abuse, sexual abuse, depression and illicit drug use. *Journal of Substance Abuse Treatment*, *10*, 433-438.

Branch, L. G., & Jette, A. M. (1984). Personal health practices and mortality among the elderly. *American Journal of Public Health*, *74*, 1126-1129.

Brickner, P. W. (1985). Health issues in the care of the homeless. In P. W. Brickner, L. K. Scharer, B. Conanan, A. Elvy, & M. Savarese (Eds.), *Health care of homeless people* (pp. 3-18). New York: Springer.

Brickner, P. W., Scharer, L. K., Conanan, B. A., Savarese, M., & Scanlan, B. C. (Eds.) (1990). *Under the safety net: The health and social welfare of the homeless in the United States*. New York: W. W. Norton.

Brown, J. L., & Allen, D. (1988). Hunger in America. *Annual Review of Public Health*, *9*, 503-526.

Browne, A. (1993). Family violence and homelessness: The relevance of trauma histories in the lives of homeless women. *American Journal of Orthopsychiatry*, *63*, 370-384.

Bureau of the Census. (1992). *Statistical abstract of the United States*. Washington, DC: U. S. Government Printing Office.

Burroughs, J., Bouma, P., O'Connor, E., & Smith, D. (1990). Health concerns of homeless women. In P. W. Brickner, L. K. Scharer, B. A. Conanan, M. Savarese, & B. C. Scanlan (Eds.), *Under the safety net: The health and social welfare of the homeless in the United States* (pp. 139-150). New York: W. W. Norton.

Burt, M. R. (1992). *Over the edge: The growth of homelessness in the 1980s*. New York: Sage.

Burt, M. R., & Cohen, B. E. (1989). Differences among homeless single women, women with children, and single men. *Social Problems*, *36*, 508-524.

Callahan, C. M., & Rivara, F. P. (1992). Urban high school youth and handguns: A school-based survey. *Journal of the American Medical Association*, *267*, 3038-3042.

Camasso, M. J., & Camasso, A. E. (1986). Social supports, undesirable life events, and psychological distress in a disadvantaged population. *Social Service Review*, *60*, 378-394.

Chavkin, W., Kristal, A., Seabron, C., & Guigli, P. E. (1987). The reproductive experience of women living in hotels for the homeless in New York City. *New York State Journal of Medicine*, *87*, 10-13.

Cohen, B. E. (1990). Food security and hunger policy for the 1990s. *Nutrition Today* (July-August), 23-27.

Combs-Orme, T., Risley-Curtiss, C., & Taylor, R. (1993). Predicting birth weight: Relative importance of sociodemographic, medical, and prenatal care variables. *Social Service Review*, 67, 617–630.

Conway, G. A., Epstein, M. R., Hayman, C. R., Miller, C. A., Wendell, D. A., Gwinn, M., Karon, J. M., & Petersen, L. R. (1993). Trends in HIV prevalence rates among disadvantaged youth: Survey results from a national job training program, 1988 through 1992. *Journal of the American Medical Association*, 269, 2887–2889.

Devine, J. A., & Wright, J. D. (1993). *The greatest of evils: Urban poverty and the American underclass*. Hawthorne, NY: Aldine de Gruyter.

Egbuonu, L., & Starfield, B. (1982). Child health and social status. *Pediatrics*, 69(5), 550–557.

Elvy, A. (1985). Access to care. In P. W. Brickner, L. K. Scharer, B. Conanan, A. Elvy, & M. Savarese (Eds.). *Health care of homeless people* (pp. 223–231). New York: Springer.

Emmons, L. (1987). Relationship of participation in food assistance programs to the nutritional quality of diets. *American Journal of Public Health*, 77, 856–858.

Federal Task Force on Homelessness and Severe Mental Illness. (1992). *Outcasts on Main Street*. Washington, DC: Interagency Council on the Homeless.

Ferraro, K. F. (1993). Are black older adults health-pessimistic? *Journal of Health and Social Behavior*, 34, 201–214.

Fingerhut, L. A., Ingram, D. D., & Feldman, J. J. (1992a). Firearm and nonfirearm homicide among persons 15 through 19 years of age. *Journal of the American Medical Association*, 267, 3048–3053.

Fisk, N. (1984). Epidemiology of alcohol abuse and alcoholism. *Alcohol Health and Research World*, 9(1), 4–7.

Ford, K., & Norris, A. E. (1993). Knowledge of AIDS transmission, risk behavior, and perceptions of risk among urban, low-income, African-American and Hispanic youth. *American Journal of Preventive Medicine*, 9, 297–306.

Fossett, J. W., Perloff, J. D., Peterson, J. A., & Kletke, P. R. (1990). Medicaid in the inner city: The case of maternity care in Chicago. *Milbank Quarterly*, 68, 111–141.

Franks, P., Clancy, C. M., Gold, M. R., & Nutting, P. A. (1993). Health insurance and subjective health status: Data from the 1987 National Medical Expenditure Survey. *American Journal of Public Health*, 83, 1295–1299.

French, L. (1987). Victimization of the mentally ill: An unintended consequence of deinstitutionalization. *Social Work* (November–December), 502–505.

Fullilove, R. E., Fullilove, M. T., Bowser, B. P., & Gross, S. A. (1990). Risk of sexually transmitted disease among black adolescent crack users in Oakland and San Francisco. *Journal of the American Medical Association*, 263, 851–855.

Furstenburg, F. F., Lincoln, R., & Menken, J. (Eds.). (1981). *Teenage sexuality, pregnancy, and childbearing*. Philadelphia: University of Pennsylvania Press.

Gelberg, L., & Linn, L. S. (1989). Assessing the physical health of homeless adults. *Journal of the American Medical Association*, 262, 1973–1979.

Geronimus, A. T. (1986). The effects of race, residence, and prenatal care on the relationship of maternal age to neonatal mortality. *American Journal of Public Health*, 76, 1416–1421.

Goodwin, D. W. (1992). Alcohol: Clinical aspects. In J. H. Lowinson, P. Ruiz, & R. B. Millman (Eds.), *Substance abuse: A comprehensive textbook* (2nd ed.) (pp. 144–151). Baltimore: Williams & Wilkins.

Gortmaker, S. L. (1981). Medicaid and the health care of children in poverty and near poverty. *Medical Care*, 19(6), 567–582.

Graham, G. C. (1985). Poverty, hunger, malnutrition, prematurity, and infant mortality in the United States. *Pediatrics*, 75(1), 17–125.

Green, J., & Arno, P. S. (1990). The "Medicaidization" of AIDS: Trends in the financing of HIV-related medical care. *Journal of the American Medical Association*, 264, 1261–1266.

Gurin, G., Veroff, J., & Feld, S. (1960). *Americans view their mental health*. New York: Basic Books.

Hadley, J., Steinberg, E. P., & Feder, J. (1991). Comparison of uninsured and privately insured hospital patients: Condition on admission, resource use, and outcome. *Journal of the American Medical Association*, 265, 374–379.

Hagen, J. L. (1987). Gender and homelessness. *Social Work*, 32, 312–316.

Halpern, R. (1991). Supportive services for families in poverty: Dilemmas of reform. *Social Service Review*, 65, 343–364.

Hartman, A. (1989). Homelessness: Public issue and private trouble. *Social Work*, 34, 483–484.

Hilfiker, D. (1989). Are we comfortable with homelessness? *Journal of the American Medical Association*, 262, 1375–1376.

Human Nutrition Information Service. (1982). *Nationwide food consumption survey: Survey of food consumption in low-income households, 1979–1980*. Preliminary Report No. 10 (July). Washington, DC: U.S. Department of Agriculture.

Institute of Medicine. (1988). *Homelessness, health and human needs*. Washington, DC: National Academy Press.

Jarvik, M. E., & Schneider, N. G. (1992). Nicotine. In J. H. Lowinson, P. Ruiz, & R. B. Millman (Eds.), *Substance abuse: A comprehensive textbook* (2nd ed.) (pp. 334–356). Baltimore: Williams & Wilkins.

Jencks, C. (1994). The homeless. *New York Review of Books*, 41, 20–27, 39–46.

Jepson, C., Kessler, L. G., Portnoy, B., & Gibbs, T. (1991). Black–white differences in cancer prevention knowledge and behavior. *American Journal of Public Health*, 81, 501–504.

Joseph, H., & Roman-Nay, H. (1989). The homeless intravenous drug user and the AIDS epidemic. Rockville, MD: National Institute of Drug Abuse.

Kaplan, G. A., Seeman, T. E., Cohen, R. D., Knudsen, L. P., & Guralnik, J. (1987). Mortality among the elderly in the

Alameda County Study: Behavioral and demographic risk factors. *American Journal of Public Health, 77,* 307-312.

Kelly, J. T. (1985). Trauma: With the example of San Francisco's shelter program. In P. W. Brickner, L. K. Scharer, B. Conanan, A. Elvy, & M. Savarese (Eds.), *Health care of homeless people* (pp. 77-91). New York: Springer.

Kerner, J. F., Dusenbury, L., & Mandelblatt, J. S. (1993). Poverty and cultural diversity: Challenges for health promotion among the medically underserved. *Annual Review of Public Health, 14,* 355-377.

Kessler, R., & Neighbors, H. W. (1986). A new perspective on the relationships among race, social class, and psychological distress. *Journal of Health and Social Behavior, 27,* 107-115.

Koop, C. E., & Lundberg, G. D. (1992). Violence in America— A public health emergency: Time to bite the bullet. *Journal of the American Medical Association, 267,* 3075-3076.

Kopanoff, D. E., Snider, D. E., & Johnson, M. (1988). Recurrent tuberculosis: Why do patients develop disease again? A United States Public Health Service Cooperative Survey. *American Journal of Public Health, 78,* 30-33.

Kroll, J., Carey, K., Hagedorn, D., Fire Dog, P., & Benavides, E. (1986). A survey of homeless adults in urban emergency shelters. *Hospital and Community Psychiatry, 37,* 283-286.

La Gory, M., Ritchey, F. J., & Mullis, J. (1990). Depression among the homeless. *Journal of Health and Social Behavior, 31,* 87-101.

Laven, G. T., & Brown, K. C. (1985). Nutritional status of men attending a soup kitchen: A pilot study. *American Journal of Public Health, 75,* 875-878.

Lewis, C. E., Raczynski, J. M., Heath, G. W., Levinson, R., & Cutter, G. R. (1993). Physical activity of public housing residents in Birmingham, Alabama. *American Journal of Public Health, 83,* 1016-1020.

Lubben, J. E., Weiler, P. G., & Chi, I. (1989). Health practices of the elderly poor. *American Journal of Public Health, 79,* 731-734.

Luder, E., Boey, E., Buchalter, B., & Martinez-Weber, C. (1989). Assessment of the nutritional status of urban homeless adults. *Public Health Reports, 104,* 451-457.

Manfredi, C., Lacey, L., Warnecke, R., & Buis, M. (1992). Smoking-related behavior, beliefs, and social environment of young black women in subsidized public housing in Chicago. *American Journal of Public Health, 82,* 267-272.

McArtor, R. E., Iverson, D. C., Benken, D. E., Gilchrist, V. J., Dennis, L. K., & Broome, R. A. (1992). Physician assessment of patient motivation: Influence on disposition for follow-up care. *American Journal of Preventive Medicine, 8,* 147-149.

McBride, K., & Mulcare, R. J. (1985). Peripheral vascular disease in the homeless. In P. W. Brickner, L. K. Scharer, B. Conanan, A. Elvy, & M. Savarese (Eds.), *Health care of homeless people* (pp. 121-129). New York: Springer.

McCord, C., & Freeman, H. P. (1990). Excess mortality in Harlem. *New England Journal of Medicine, 322,* 173-177.

McNagny, S. E., & Parker, R. M. (1992). High prevalence of recent cocaine use and the unreliability of patient self-report in an inner-city walk-in clinic. *Journal of the American Medical Association, 267*(8), 1106-1108.

Meyers, A., Rubin, D., Napoleone, M., & Nichols, K. (1993). Public housing subsidies may improve poor children's nutrition. *American Journal of Public Health, 83,* 115.

Miller, C. A. (1985). Infant mortality in the U.S. *Scientific American, 253*(1), 31-37.

Miller, D., & Lin, E. (1988). Children in sheltered homeless families: Reported health status and use of health services. *Pediatrics, 81*(5), 668-673.

Molnar, J. M., Rath, W. R., & Klein, T. P. (1990). Constantly compromised: The impact of homelessness on children. *Journal of Social Issues, 46,* 109-124.

Monheit, A. C. (1994). Underinsured Americans: A review. *Annual Review of Public Health, 15,* 461-485.

Morbidity and Mortality Weekly Report. (1990). Homicide among young black males, United States, 1978-1987. *Morbidity and Mortality Weekly Report, 39,* 869-873.

Morbidity and Mortality Weekly Report. (1991a). Deaths among homeless persons: San Francisco, 1985-1990. *Morbidity and Mortality Weekly Report, 40,* 877-880.

Morbidity and Mortality Weekly Report. (1991b). Characteristics and risk behaviors of homeless black men seeking services from the Community Homeless Assistance Plan— Dade County, Florida, August 1991. *Morbidity and Mortality Weekly Report, 40,* 865-868.

Morbidity and Mortality Weekly Report. (1993). Prevalence of sedentary lifestyle–behavioral risk factor surveillance system, United States, 1991. *Morbidity and Mortality Weekly Report, 42,* 576-579.

Morbidity and Mortality Weekly Report. (1994). Cigarette smoking among adults: United States, 1992, and changes in the definition of current cigarette smoking. *Morbidity and Mortality Weekly Report, 43,* 342-346.

National Center for Health Statistics. (1985). Health characteristics according to family and personal income. *Vital and Health Statistics, 10*(147).

National Center for Health Statistics. (1990). Americans assess their health: United States, 1987. *Vital and Health Statistics, 10*(174).

National Center for Health Statistics. (1993). *Health, United States, 1992.* Hyattsville, MD: U.S. Public Health Service.

National Center for Health Statistics. (1994). Current estimates from the National Health Interview Survey, 1992. *Vital and Health Statistics, 10*(189).

National Institute on Drug Abuse. (1991). *National household survey on drug abuse: Main findings 1990.* Rockville, MD: National Institute on Drug Abuse.

Navarro, V. (1990). Race or class versus race and class: Mortality differentials in the United States. *Lancet, 336,* 1238-1240.

Newacheck, P. W., & Halfon, N. (1986). Access to ambulatory care services for economically disadvantaged children. *Pediatrics, 78*, 813–819.

Newacheck, P. W., & Starfield, B. (1988). Morbidity and use of ambulatory care services among poor and nonpoor children. *American Journal of Public Health, 78*(8), 927–933.

Novello, A. C., Shosky, J., & Froehlke, R. (1992). A medical response to violence. *Journal of the American Medical Association, 267*, 3007.

Nyamathi, A., Bennett, C., Leake, B., Lewis, C., & Flaskerud, J. (1993). AIDS-related knowledge, perceptions, and behaviors among impoverished minority women. *American Journal of Public Health, 83*, 65–71.

Physician's Task Force on Hunger in America. (1985). *Hunger in America—The growing epidemic*. Middletown, CT: Wesleyan University Press.

Price, J. H., Desmond, S. M., Snyder, F. F., & Kimmel, S. R. (1988). Perceptions of family practice residents regarding health care and poor patients. *Journal of Family Practice, 27*, 615–621.

Public Health Reports. (1985). *Public Health Reports, 101*, 593–598.

Raba, J. M., Joseph, H., Avery, R., Torres, R. A., Kiyasu, S., Prentice, R., Staats, J. A., & Brickner, P. W. (1990). Homelessness and AIDS. In P. W. Brickner, L. K., Scharer, B. A. Conanan, M. Savarese, & B. C. Scanlan (Eds.), *Under the safety net: The health and social welfare of the homeless in the United States* (pp. 215–233). New York: W. W. Norton.

Rask, K. J., Williams, M. V., Parker, R. M., & McNagny, S. E. (1994). Obstacles predicting lack of a regular provider and delays in seeking care for patients at an urban public hospital. *Journal of the American Medical Association, 271*, 1931–1933.

Rauschenbach, B. S., Frongillo, E. A., Thompson, F. E., Andersen, E. J. Y., & Spicer, D. A. (1990). Dependency on soup kitchens in urban areas of New York State. *American Journal of Public Health, 80*, 57–60.

Redlener, I. E. (1988). Caring for homeless children: Special challenges for the pediatrician. *Today's Child, 2* (entire issue).

Reinhardt, U. E. (1994). The Clinton plan: A salute to American pluralism. *Health Affairs, 13*, 161–178.

Reuler, J. B., Bax, M. J., & Sampson, J. H. (1986). Physician house call services for medically needy, inner-city residents. *American Journal of Public Health, 76*, 1131–1134.

Robertson, M. J., & Cousineau, M. R. (1986). Health status and access to health services among the urban homeless. *American Journal of Public Health, 76*, 561–563.

Romano, P. S., Bloom, J., & Syme, S. L. (1991). Smoking, social support, and hassles in an urban African-American community. *American Journal of Public Health, 81*, 1415–1421.

Ropers, R. H., & Boyer, R. (1987). Perceived health status among the new urban homeless. *Social Science and Medicine, 24*, 669–678.

Rosenberg, M. L., O'Carroll, P. W., & Powell, K. E. (1992). Let's be clear: Violence is a public health problem. *Journal of the American Medical Association, 267*, 3071–3072.

Rossi, P. H., Wright, J. D., Fisher, G., & Willis, G. (1987). The urban homeless: Estimating composition and size. *Science, 235*, 1336–1341.

Rotheram-Borus, M. J., & Koopman, C. (1991). Sexual risk behaviors, AIDS knowledge, and beliefs about AIDS among runaways. *American Journal of Public Health, 81*, 208–210.

Rowland, D., & Salganicoff, A. (1994). Commentary: Lessons from Medicaid: Improving access to office-based physician care for the low-income population. *American Journal of Public Health, 84*, 550–552.

Scanlan, B. C., & Brickner, P. W. (1990). Clinical concerns in the care of homeless persons. In P. W. Brickner, L. K. Scharer, B. A. Conanan, M. Savarese, & B. C. Scanlan (Eds.), *Under the safety net: The health and social welfare of the homeless in the United States* (pp. 69–81). New York: W. W. Norton.

Scharer, L. K., Berson, A., & Brickner, P. W. (1990). Lack of housing and its impact on human health: A service perspective. *Bulletin of the New York Academy of Medicine, 66*, 515–525.

Schlosstein, E., St. Clair, P., & Connell, F. (1991). Referral keeping in homeless women. *Journal of Community Health, 16*, 279–285.

Schwarz, D. F., Grisso, J. A., Miles, C. G., Holmes, J. H., Wishner, A. R., & Sutton, R. L. (1994). A longitudinal study of injury morbidity in an African-American population. *Journal of the American Medical Association, 271*, 755–760.

Shah, C. P., Kahan, M., & Krauser, J. (1987). The health of children of low-income families. *Canadian Medical Association Journal, 137*, 485–490.

Shea, S., Misra, D., Ehrlich, M. H., Field, L., & Francis, C. K. (1992). Correlates of nonadherence to hypertension treatment in an inner-city minority population. *American Journal of Public Health, 82*, 1607–1612.

Shekelle, P. G., & Kosecoff, J. (1992). Evaluating the treatment of sexually transmitted diseases at an urban public hospital outpatient clinic. *American Journal of Public Health, 82*, 115–117.

Sheley, J. F., McGee, Z. T., & Wright, J. D. (1992). Gun-related violence in and around inner-city schools. *American Journal of Diseases of Children, 146*, 677–682.

Sheley, J. F., & Wright, J. D. (1993). Gun acquisition and possession is selected juvenile samples. *NIJ Research in Brief* (pp. 1–11). Washington, DC: National Institute of Justice.

Shlay, A., & Rossi, P. (1992). Social science research and contemporary studies of homelessness. *Annual Review of Sociology, 18*, 129–160.

Singer, J. D. (1982). Diet and iron status, a study of relationships, United States. Series 11, Publication No. PHS83-1679.

Washington, DC: National Center for Health Statistics, U.S. Department of Health and Human Services.

Slutkin, G. (1986). Management of tuberculosis in urban homeless indigents. *Public Health Reports, 101*, 481–485.

Stephenson, B. J., Rowe, B. H., Haynes, R. B., Macharia, W. M., & Leon, G. (1993). Is this patient taking the treatment as prescribed? *Journal of the American Medical Association, 269*, 2779–2781.

Stern, R. S., Weissman, J. S., & Epstein, A. M. (1991). The emergency department as a pathway to admission for poor and high-cost patients. *Journal of the American Medical Association, 266*, 2238–2243.

Susser, E. S., Lin, S. P., Conover, S. A., & Struening, E. L. (1991). Childhood antecedents of homelessness in psychiatric patients. *American Journal of Psychiatry, 148*, 1026–1030.

Thompson, F. E., Taren, D. L., Andersen, E., Casella, G., Lambert, J. K. J., Campbell, C. C., Frongillo, E. A., & Spicer, D. (1988). Within month variability in use of soup kitchens in New York State. *American Journal of Public Health, 78*, 1298–1301.

Torres, R. A., Lefkowitz, P., Kales, C., & Brickner, P. W. (1987). Homelessness among hospitalized patients with the acquired immunodeficiency syndrome in New York City. *Journal of the American Medical Association, 258*, 779–780.

Upchurch, D. M., Farmer, M. Y., Glasser, D., & Hook, E. (1987). Contraceptive needs and practices among women attending an inner-city STD clinic. *American Journal of Public Health, 77*, 1427–1430.

Vicic, W. J. (1991). Homelessness. *Bulletin of the New York Academy of Medicine, 67*, 49–54.

Weissman, J. S., & Epstein, A. M. (1993). The insurance gap: Does it make a difference? *Annual Review of Public Health, 14*, 243–270.

Wilton, K. M., & Irvine, J. (1983). Nutritional intakes of socio-culturally mentally retarded children vs. children of low and average socioeconomic status. *American Journal of Mental Deficiency, 88*(1), 79–85.

Winick, C. (1992). Epidemiology of alcohol and drug abuse. In J. H. Lowinson, P. Ruiz, & R. B. Millman (Eds.). *Substance abuse: A comprehensive textbook* (2nd ed.) (pp. 15–29). Baltimore: Williams & Wilkins.

Winick, M. (1985). Nutritional and vitamin deficiency states. In P. W. Brickner, L. K. Scharer, B. Conanan, A. Elvy, & M. Savarese (Eds.), *Health care of homeless people* (pp. 103–108). New York: Springer.

Wise, P. H., & Meyers, A. (1988). Poverty and child health. *Pediatric Clinics of North America, 35*, 1169–1186.

Wood, D. L., Valdez, R. B., Hayashi, T., & Shen, A. (1990). Homeless and housed families in Los Angeles: A study comparing demographic, economic, and family function characteristics. *American Journal of Public Health, 80*, 1049–1052.

Wright, J. D. (1989). *Address unknown: The homeless in contemporary America*. Hawthorne, NY: Aldine de Gruyter.

Wright, J. D. (1990). Poor people, poor health: The health status of the homeless. *Journal of Social Issues, 46*(4), 49–64.

Wright, J. D. (1991a). Children in and of the streets: Health, social policy, and the homeless young. *American Journal of Diseases of Children, 145*(5), 516–519.

Wright, J. D. (1991b). Poverty, homelessness, health, nutrition, and children. In J. Kryder-Coe, L. Salamon, & J. Molnar (Eds.), *Homeless children and youth: A new American dilemma* (p. 71–103). New Brunswick, NJ: Trans-ACTION Books.

Wright, J. D. (1991c). Health and homeless teenager: Evidence from the National Health Care for the Homeless Program. *Journal of Health and Social Policy, 2*(4), 15–35.

Wright, J. D., & Devine, J. A. (1992). Counting the homeless: The Census Bureau's "S-Night" in five U.S. cities. *Evaluation Review, 16*(4), 355–364.

Wright, J. D., & Devine, J. A. (1993). Family backgrounds and the substance-abusive homeless: The New Orleans experience. *Community Psychologist, 26*(2), 35–37.

Wright, J. D., & Devine, J. A. (1994). Poverty among the elderly. *Pride Institute Journal of Long Term Home Health Care, 13*(1), 5–16.

Wright J. D., Devine, J. A., & Joyner, L. M. (1993). *The least of mine: the New Orleans Homeless Substance Abusers Project Final Report*. Washington, DC: National Institute of Alcohol Abuse and Alcoholism.

Wright, J. D., & Weber, E. (1987). *Homelessness and health*. New York: McGraw-Hill.

Wright, J. D., Weber, E., Knight, J. W., & Lam, J. (1987). Ailments and alcohol: Health status among the drinking homeless. *Alcohol Health and Research World, 11*, 22–27.

York, R. L. (1992). Elderly Americans: Health, housing and nutrition gaps between the poor and nonpoor. In: *Old, poor, and forgotten: Elderly Americans living in poverty* (pp. 66–93). U.S. House of Representatives Select Committee on Aging. Washington, DC: U.S. Government Printing Office.

Young, R. F., Waller, J. B., & Kahana, E. (1991). Racial and socioeconomic aspects of myocardial infarction recovery: Studying confounds. *American Journal of Preventive Medicine, 7*, 438–444.

Zee, P., DeLeon, M., Robertson, P., & Chen, C. H. (1985). Nutritional improvement of poor urban preschool children: A 1983–1977 comparison. *Journal of the American Medical Association, 253*(22), 3269–3272.

11

Health Behavior in Persons Living with Chronic Conditions

Eugene B. Gallagher and Terry D. Stratton

OVERVIEW

The historical shift from infectious to chronic disease has tremendous implications for health behavior, attitudes, and expectations concerning health and illness. Exclusive reliance on the prevailing "medical model" of illness, however, tends to perpetuate a health care system that is overly attuned to acute care and intervention, often at the expense of chronic illness and its sufferers. Looking at these inconsistencies, this chapter advances a psychosocial perspective on chronic illness—one that provides a more holistic view of the social processes that take place between the ill person and the illness. Using as examples two modern-day chronic diseases—diabetes and end-stage renal disease—the chapter discusses the potentially diverse behavioral impacts of chronic illness on the illness-bearer within the contexts of the ill person's social networks, the professional medical providers, and society in

Eugene B. Gallagher and Terry D. Stratton • Department of Behavioral Science, University of Kentucky School of Medicine, Lexington, Kentucky 40536-0086.

Handbook of Health Behavior Research III: Demography, Development, and Diversity, edited by David S. Gochman. Plenum Press, New York, 1997.

general. In particular, the chapter advances issues regarding the negotiation of roles and responsibility within the confines of the traditional doctor–patient relationship, as well as those that occur within the broader rubric of social life.

MEDICAL DEMOGRAPHY AND LIFE EXPECTANCY IN THE ERA OF CHRONIC ILLNESS

Life expectancy at birth in the United States was 40 years in 1850, 50 years in 1900, 68 years in 1950, and 75 years in 1989 (Gill, Glazer, & Thernstrom, 1992, p. 22). Even though Americans live longer nowadays than did their forebears, however, they are more likely to suffer and ultimately die from chronic diseases than their forebears were. To illustrate the trend toward chronic disease, consider three major types: heart disease, stroke, and cancer. In 1860, none of these three diseases was among the ten major causes of death, and none accounted for more than 2.0% of total deaths in that year. By 1900, however, heart disease accounted for 8.0% of deaths (fourth leading cause), stroke accounted for 4.2% (seventh leading cause), and cancer accounted for 3.7%

(ninth leading cause). By 1989, the toll of heart disease and cancer had increased to a staggering degree. Heart disease was the leading cause of death, accounting for 34.1% of all deaths, and cancer as the second greatest cause accounted for 23.1% of deaths. Stroke also increased its share to 6.8%, becoming the third greatest cause of death.

The rise of chronic diseases has been accompanied by a decline in infectious diseases. Thus, tuberculosis was the leading cause of death in 1860; in 1900, it was the second leading cause; in 1989, however, it was not even among the first ten causes of death. (The recent resurgence of drug-resistant tuberculosis, while alarming, has not lifted it into the first ten causes.) Similar relative declines can be noted for other infectious diseases: influenza, cholera, diphtheria, diarrhea/enteritis, and scarlet fever (Gill et al., 1992, p. 24). In a different but related reckoning, only 6.0% of all deaths in 1973 were due to the eleven most common infectious diseases: typhoid, influenza, smallpox, scarlet fever, measles, whooping cough, digestive infections, diphtheria, tuberculosis, pneumonia, and poliomyelitis (McKinlay & McKinlay, 1977, p. 414).

This shift from infectious to chronic disease has tremendous implications for public behavior, attitudes, and expectations concerning health and illness.

As noted, the life expectancy at birth was 40 years in 1850. What this simple statement does not say, however, is that various distributions of age-specific mortality can yield the *same* life expectancy. Thus, for the United States in 1850, the 40-year figure did *not* arise because a great many people alive at 35 were dying by age 40 or 45; rather, it arose from the high rates of infant and child mortality. The death of a small number of individuals in infancy or childhood drastically lowers life expectancy for the population as a whole. No doubt parents, doctors, and nurses in that era fought hard to preserve the life of sickly infants, although there was probably also a pervasive fatalism concerning their survival prospects. Many infants succumbed to waterborne disease

vectors, and the proximate cause of death was then commonly listed as "infantile diarrhea."

Many adults also fell prey to epidemics of cholera, typhus, and smallpox during the 19th century. A look at charted death rates in New York City from 1800 to 1910 reveals an irregular pattern clearly differentiating the bad years when outbreaks of disease occurred from the good years when disease was absent (Spiegelman, 1968). People's attitudes toward the prospect of epidemics fluctuated wildly, from active measures to avert danger to passive resignation. There is abundant historical evidence in England of the wiping out of entire villages by waves of the Black Death (bubonic plague) between 1350 and 1450—and of the rapid and permanent abandonment of other villages by people fleeing its rapid advance. Similar behavior occurred in metropolitan areas of the United States. In the main, however, it was not the entire populace of a city that fled in panic in the face of an epidemic (often the mere rumor of an epidemic sufficed), but the upper and middle classes, who had sufficient resources to escape. Thus, those in New York fled to the Catskill Mountains, Philadelphians fled to the Poconos, and the Cincinnati gentry escaped south into Kentucky.

In the past era of infectious disease, morbidity became mortality in mere days or weeks. Survivors, on the other hand, were often not much the worse for having passed through their ordeal; a person could survive influenza or cholera and then, without a lengthy recuperation, be virtually as good as new. Some infectious diseases, however, did leave a residue of disability and disfigurement. Smallpox was dreaded not only for its tormenting rash and fever, but also because it often left its victims with unsightly pockmarks.

Another line of exception occurs in the duration of infectious disease. Not all infections are fast-acting and acute. Leprosy is a well-known example from antiquity of a markedly stigmatized disease for which many victims had to endure social opprobrium and exile to leper colonies for the remainder of a near-normal length of life (Breitha, 1988; Law & Wisniewski, 1988). Syphilis, a major infectious killer in the 19th century, was in fact slow in its progression, often taking decades rather than years to achieve its maximum effect. It was chronic: There was no cure (now it is curable in most patients with antibiotics). In that era, all patients died *with* the disease of syphilis, but not all died *of* the disease. For the latter group—the "lucky" ones who did not suffer such gruesome sequelae as wasting, staggering gait, or paralytic insanity—the infection moved into an indefinitely long plateau of arrest or latency, and another cause of death supervened.

BEHAVIORAL IMPLICATIONS OF CHRONIC ILLNESS

The preceding section set forth the rising impact of chronic disease in society, pointing to the mass fears and panics connected with infectious disease that have become benignly "historical" phenomena, not likely to occur again in modern society. Even the contemporary scourge of AIDS, while widespread and infectious, is a *selective* epidemic; unlike cholera, smallpox, and other historic killers, AIDS does not put at risk everyone who drinks the water or breathes the air or comes near a disease-bearer. Rather, it has specific behavioral routes of etiology, and many segments of the population are at infinitesimal risk. It would be ludicrous, for example, for all the inhabitants of high-incidence geographic areas to flee to "higher ground," in panic akin to that occasioned by cholera, in order to avoid AIDS.

Against this background, the following four features of chronic disease that have important aspects for its treatment and management can be addressed:

1. It is lifelong.
2. It stands in variable but significant relationship to other aspects of the human life span and of individual functioning, such as aging and disability.

3. For its treatment and management, it draws in varying degree upon familial and other lay social networks, as well as professional–medical expertise.
4. Psychological strengths and vulnerabilities of the individual are important, as well as social–situational and social–structural factors that bear upon the individual's ability to cope with the disease.

These features are discussed in the following sections.

Lifelong Duration

Chronic disease is lifelong simply because it is incurable. Semantically, the word *incurable* often has the baleful connotation of "fatal" or "terminal." Literally, however, a person may be incurably deaf, incurably blind, incurably crippled, or incurably afflicted with a superficial but intractable skin infection that will not yield to antibiotic treatment. However unfortunate any of these incurable conditions may be, they lack the finality of being fatal.

Incurability acquires a dark hue—"terminal"– only when the disease or condition portends death within a matter of weeks, months, or perhaps a year or two. Diabetes (which will be discussed at greater length) can truly be said to be a fatal disease. Persons with diabetes have a diminished life expectancy; unless something else supervenes, they can look forward, not pleasantly, to succumbing eventually to one or another of the physiological ravages of the disease, whether renal failure, circulatory impairment, or some other late-stage effect. The key word here, however, is *late-stage*. Since diabetes generally progresses slowly, it is regarded as a chronic disease, not a terminal one.

Cancer as a categorical entity has a predominant meaning not only of incurability but also of a significant probability of death within a matter of months or a few years from the time of diagnosis. Dark stereotypes of cancer are gradually yielding, however, to modulated images of the disease, some of which are more hopeful. With a broader range of early detection and improving treatments, many forms of cancer—leukemias and lymphomas, prostate cancer, breast cancer—are increasingly regarded as chronic diseases with the prospect of extended survival similar to diabetes. Other forms of cancer, e.g., pancreatic and esophageal, are typically so fast-acting (exceptional individual cases of prolonged survival notwithstanding) that they can scarcely be regarded as chronic in most cases.

To sum up, many incurable diseases are chronic rather than terminal. Although many chronic diseases are potentially life-threatening, the feature that distinguishes them from terminal diseases is the degree of predictability of the threat and its remoteness in time (Register, 1987, p. 281). With these distinguishing criteria, it is no surprise that the line between chronic and terminal is rather more a broad zone than a thin line.

The distinction between chronic and terminal is made, it will be recalled, within the more inclusive rubric of lifelong or incurable disease. The psychological tasks and the workings of social support are different for chronic and terminal diseases. The terminally ill person experiences anticipatory grief work over his or her own demise and also, in a more rational, less affective mode, puts his or her affairs in order. Chronic illness, with its implications of "the long haul," calls for a different set of personal and social resources, which will be discussed later.

Life-Span Implications

Although chronic disease stands as a distinct concept and empirical reality, it frequently appears in conjunction with, or as part of, other contingencies of the human organism—arrested or delayed development, handicaps, impairments, and physical limitations. Hovering over these interconnections is the general aging process and the many predictable infirmities that accrue and intensify with the passage of years.

There is broad definitional latitude concerning the delineation of chronic illness as a general category. Hanson (1987, p. 12) defines chronic illness as "any impairment interfering with individual ability to function fully in the environment." Other writers, such as Perdue (Perdue, Mahon, Hawes, & Frik, 1981) and Strauss and Corbin (1988), argue against grouping together chronic conditions and chronic diseases. For them, a critical divide separates *medically pathological* states—i.e., diseases—from *nonpathological but limiting* states, e.g., dwarfism, blindness, quadriplegia arising from accidents, mental retardation, and malnourishment.

These contrasting usages amount to more than a semantic difference. They have far-reaching implications concerning what is to be done by way of therapy, management, and rehabilitation to alleviate the negative states of the organism to which they refer. Broadly speaking, it takes pathology, abnormality, or biological abnormality—in short, disease—to arouse the interest and services of medicine and related paramedical fields; "mere" impairment or limitation of activity does not suffice. Other specialists deal with nonpathological limitations—physical therapists, occupational therapists, rehabilitation counselors, and disability workers. (Sometimes these specialists work on the basis of referrals from physicians, who construct a basis in medical pathology as the ground upon which the referral can be made.)

The provider of services is also in a powerful position to influence, whether wittingly or unwittingly, the self-concept of the recipient—client, patient, customer, claimant, student, trainee, counselee, victim, amputee, service utilizer—as well as the recipient's definition of the objectives to be sought and the work to be carried out. If the deficit state is defined as a chronic disease and treated by a physician, the provider–recipient relationship may well have a different character than if it is defined as a chronic condition and dealt with by a nonmedical specialist.

It should be noted that the term "chronic conditions" in the title of this chapter is intended to be neutral in reference to the foregoing discussion, i.e., devoid of any implication that it refers exclusively to either medical or nonmedical states.

Social Networks and Professional Expertise

Family and extrafamilial social networks and other resources come into play in dealing with chronic conditions: This statement is a virtual corollary of the first proposition, concerning the lifelong, incurable quality of the condition. Only if the patient were confined indefinitely to a hospital or other institutional setting, wholly under professional attendance, could it truly be said that social–familial influence and help were of little importance.

Barring that contingency, families and, usually to a lesser extent, friends of the chronically ill person can help in many ways, some overt and others less so. Food, shelter, and other material needs are obvious outward forms of aid, many of which can also be self-provided. Many adult chronic patients with, for example, manageable diabetes or heart conditions live an independent life, thus engaging in "self-care." If the chronic-illness bearer is not disabled, then that person remains capable of self-care including fully independent, self-sufficient daily life.

The more inward, socioemotional needs of chronic patients may well be greater than those of unafflicted persons, yet they are not easily assessed. Ideally, families can to a large extent meet needs for companionship, expressive outlet, and shared activity; as the carriers of intimate interpersonal memories and traditions, families are uniquely qualified to convey and support the patient's sense of self-continuity and concepts of competence in the face of illness. That said, it must be further said that the family's role in supporting the chronic patient is diffuse and subtle. The family must carefully tread a fine line between two opposing traps: fostering needless dependency in the patient and, in contrast, establishing expectations that are frustratingly difficult or impossible for the patient to meet.

The first trap is well stated by Kleinman (1988), who lays out the notion of "chronicity." For him, chronicity is a socially induced overlay upon the objective limitations that a person's chronic illness imposes (Kleinman, 1988, p. 180):

> Chronicity is not simply a direct result of pathology acting in an isolated person. It is the outcome of lives lived under constraining circumstances with particular relationships to other people. Chronicity is created in part out of negative expectations that come to be shared in face-to-face interactions—expectations that fetter our dreams and sting and choke our sense of self. Patients learn to act as chronic cases; family members and care givers learn to treat patients in keeping with this view.

As a psychiatrist (and anthropologist), Kleinman is attuned to the deep emotional roots of human behavior, yet his view of chronicity rests upon notions of social learning and reinforcement that lie more at the "surface" layer of personality. Family relationships, with their steady daily rhythms, are a prime example of binding expectation systems that can entrap and freeze behavior patterns and self-conceptions.

Another element must be added to Kleinman's picture of chronicity, since other forces are at work besides social reinforcement. Chronicity as an outcome, with both behavioral and intrapsychic aspects, is not simply the patient's yielding to family pressures such as overprotectiveness ("You'll make yourself worse if you try that!") and underexpectation ("In your shape you can't do that, so just forget it!"). Rather, chronicity also feeds and draws upon the patient's dependency needs—the desire to be taken care of, cherished, nurtured, helped—all of which are intensified by the misfortune of illness.

The second, opposite dilemma of overexpectation by the patient is not unknown to behaviorally oriented professionals dealing with chronic illness and disability, but it receives less attention than dependency.

Depending upon the nature and severity of the chronic condition, there are limits to the kinds of physical and social performance that the patient can accomplish. Indeed, many specialized devices and techniques are used to assess physical limits in sensory, motor, and cognitive abilities. In contrast, assessing social potential is more difficult because it depends not only upon the patient's interactive and communicative abilities, but also upon the capacity of participants in a given social environment to accept and respond to the patient.

For many patients, chronic illness interferes with their ability to sustain the poise and project the responsiveness displayed in ordinary social interaction—interactional demands that have been skillfully delineated by Goffman (1963, 1974) in his studies of "presentation of self." Patients may be distracted by interior somatic stimuli or their attention span may be short. They may need to absent themselves in order to monitor their condition or to take medications. Their diet may be restricted. They may require special accommodation for walking, sitting, or eating. Also, being constrained in their own command of social situations, they cannot easily extend themselves to others or take interactional responsibility for sustaining the social performance and "face" of others. Rather, they are on the receiving end of such ministrations.

In his analysis of the development of modern middle-class civilization, Elias (1978) notes that in many aspects of daily life, restraint, moderation, and controlled behavior have replaced earlier modes of greater spontaneity. Natural functions of eating and excretion are today carried out more discreetly than two or three centuries ago. There has been increasing sensitivity to bodily odors, sounds, and displays. "Social demands" are high; chronically ill or impaired persons are likely to lose self-esteem, perhaps already lowered by the awareness of a damaged self, if through overexpectation of family or friends they find themselves in situations that prove frustrating or embarrassing.

Thus, families and caretakers—trying to provide assessment, guidance, and support for chronically ill members—may find themselves challenged to find a tolerable balance between expecting too little and demanding too much.

Psychological Strengths and Vulnerabilities

The patient's psychological strengths and vulnerabilities come into play at virtually every turn in the biological unfolding of chronic illness. Kleinman (1988, p. 8) observes that "the trajectory of chronic illness assimilates to a life course, contributing so intimately to the development of a particular life that illness becomes inseparable from life history." Thus, developmental psychologists who deal with disabled and chronically ill children have noted that the patient, just like a normal child, grows and matures; in other words, chronic illness alters but does not suspend development. Rather, illness and development proceed together, intertwining and affecting each other.

SELF-CARE IN THE HEALTH BEHAVIOR OF THE CHRONIC PATIENT

Professionals, families of patients, and patients themselves substantially agree that self-care—what the patient can do for himself or herself—is a critical element in facing illness and maintaining function and morale.

Among professional care providers, nurses have had perhaps the fullest exposure to the daily stresses and frustrations that patients encounter in chronic illness, including the difficulties of carrying out treatment directives. Being less oriented to the precise pathology of chronic illness than physicians, nurses have also devoted considerable attention and research to the topic of self-care, examining factors that variously facilitate and impede it. In a nursing study of self-care, Connelly (1993, p. 248) makes the following observation: "There is a dearth of empirically based information about the selfcare behaviors of chronically ill adults, with most of the research focused on patient compliance.... By referring only to specific treatment behaviors, compliance neglects the broad range of behaviors essential to promoting and maintaining health." She also notes that many adults have more than one chronic illness, which requires them to consolidate various treatment regimens. She also points out that the clinical status of patients and their general well-being do not correlate strictly with their level of compliance with "doctor's orders." For example, depressive patients may have episodes of instability despite careful adherence to lithium therapy. As will be seen, among diabetic patients, the presence or absence of metabolic control (expressed by the patient's glucose blood level) is not always well-correlated with their dietary adherence.

In search of the other factors that intervene between compliance and the patient's clinical status, investigators of chronic illness have examined a number of variables that describe the patient's emotional state and self-concept, as well as his or her beliefs and knowledge about the illness.

THE HEALTH BEHAVIOR OF "FIGHTING THE ILLNESS"

The issue of "following treatment" is a constant theme in clinical practice and research dealing with chronic illness. If the patient is in a phase of stable equilibrium vis-à-vis the illness, and if treatment requirements are not extensive, then compliance can be placid and unproblematic. During the intermittent exacerbations that occur in many chronic illnesses, however, treatment resources and the patient's adherence to treatment specifics become more critical. During non-critical times, the patient's attitudinal and behavioral stances assume great importance as a kind of reserve to be drawn upon in actual times of crisis. Such stances are important in the variable and often lengthy intervals between crises. These stances include, especially, the qualities of decision, self-commitment, and resolution that come into play in "fighting the illness."

Certain illnesses may lend themselves to the fighting stance more than others. The study by Robinson (1988) of multiple sclerosis patients offers revealing examples of this stance. In this study, one female patient wrote (Robinson, 1988, pp. 55–56):

> I am going to fight you [the disease]; I try to do a little of everything.... I can still drive the car short distances.... I used to love gardening. You should see me [now] balancing my sticks watering the plants, or lying down so I can plant and weed. I can't go on my knees for then I can't get up, but when I lie I can drag myself up. I manage to hang the washing out by holding on to the line.

This posture of gritty defiance can be regarded as a way of negotiating the illness; it is also a form of health behavior in the self-care mode. Accounts of patients who entrench themselves in this mode reveal how they personalize their illness. They view it as an intimate adversary to be tamed and held at bay.

Not all chronic patients put on this particular suit of armor. Certain illnesses seem to invite it more than others—multiple sclerosis, arthritis, Parkinson's disease, amyotrophic lateral sclerosis, and other illnesses that involve motor impairment. The specific locution of "fighting cancer" is employed to describe the attitude of many cancer patients toward their illness. Persons with severe chronic pain also commonly speak of "fighting" it.

This notion of fighting the illness variously means carrying on in daily life with no easy concession to the limitations or discomfort imposed by the illness; engaging in intrapsychic manipulations to distract oneself from awareness of discomfort or constraint; discovering ways to "outwit the enemy" through the material help of mobility aids and sensory devices; adhering rigidly to fixed daily routines; and presenting a deliberately constructed, consistent self-image to others concerning one's pain, impairments, and subjective "battle."

While this stance might not personally suit every patient, it has its own validity for beneficial self-management of the illness. Some experts, however, would question this view, at least when taken to the extreme. Thus, the medical philosopher and essayist Sontag (1989), writing from her own bout with cancer, criticized the military metaphors commonly used to describe cancer. While not contesting the actual behavioral responses of a patient fighting an illness, Sontag sees the warlike imagery conjured up by the "invasiveness" and "colonization" of cancer cells against the body's "defenses" as counterproductive to the curative goal of modern medicine. Such terminology, she observes, has been applied not only to the disease but also to the treatment, e.g., "bombarding" the "infiltration" with toxic rays (radiotherapy) and chemical warfare (chemotherapy) in an effort to "kill" the "invaders." Challenging these verbal images, she argues (Sontag, 1989, p. 183): "We are not being invaded. The body is not a battlefield. The ill are neither unavoidable casualties nor the enemy. We—medicine, society—are not authorized to fight back by any means whatever...."

THE HEALTH BEHAVIOR OF "FOLLOWING THE RULES"

The foregoing health behavior style of fighting the disease centers on behavioral adaptations that attempt to normalize one's accomplishment of ordinary social tasks and role expectations. This form of behavior is not tied to specific routines of treatment (for multiple sclerosis, a case example of which was quoted above, there is no specific treatment); rather, it is tied to the utilization—maximum utilization in the fighting mode, lesser utilization in more passive modes—of one's abilities in the face of illness. Of course, where chronic illness is severe, one's behavioral ability to fight may be drastically curtailed.

The behavior style called "following the rules," in contrast, is focused on the orders, prescriptions, and recommendations propounded by the doctor (or other medical professional), i.e., how the patient deals with and responds to medical directives. Admittedly, the range of ad-

vice and orders that doctors can address to patients is vast; it is concerned variously with diet, medication, exercise, exposure to stress, climatic and environmental elements, sexual behavior, types of work and exertion, and all other aspects of living that can affect somatic health.

Some medical directives are "P.R.N." (Latin *pro re nata*, "as necessary"), or completely at the patient's discretion ("Take one or two of these tablets if you have trouble sleeping"); others are imperative, with the patient's life at stake in the brief span of minutes ("Take two of these whenever you start to feel dizzy; don't wait!") or over a longer time frame ("You must lose fifty pounds in the next nine months to take the strain off your heart!").

In the face of medical advice, patients exhibit a wide range of responses. Though there are many nuances and subtypes, the basic contrast is between two extremes: patients who follow doctors' directives and those who do not. How medically sound the doctors' directives are (for many chronic diseases, medical science does not offer a clear picture of the best management strategies) and how closely the patient adheres to them are important aspects in the life of the chronic illness patient.

The meaning of following the rules as a form of health behavior can be elucidated by looking at two common chronic diseases: diabetes and chronic renal failure (also known as end-stage renal disease [ESRD]).

Diabetes and chronic renal failure have many features in common. They are both incurable and thus chronic. Neither is overtly "behavioral" in the narrow sense of impairing musculoskeletal performance (although both can lead over time to motor function impairment). Both arise as a result of the malfunction of an internal organ. For both, the preferred current treatment is a direct replacement therapy: insulin for the diabetic and hemodialysis or kidney transplantation for the renal patient. In both cases, the replacement therapy establishes a physiological–biochemical equilibrium. It is not, however, a perfect substitute: Over time, the patient is subject to insidious side effects of the treatment. Nevertheless, some ESRD patients have survived with good quality of life for 25 years and more on hemodialysis or transplant, and some diabetic patients have survived longer still.

Behavioral Implications of Diabetes

This discussion deals only with the more severe, insulin-dependent, form of diabetes. "Insulin-dependent" means that the patient cannot manage the disease by behavioral measures alone; the patient is beyond "self-help," no matter how extensive, and external "medicine" is necessary.

The pharmaceutical synthesis of insulin is one of the miracles of modern medicine; before the 1930s, when insulin started to become widely used, all patients whose disease reached the state of insulin dependence died of the disease. Though insulin is a lifesaver, however, the successful management of insulin administration poses a major behavioral challenge that can be understood directly from the nature of the disease.

For brain and muscular activation, the human body requires glucose as carried in the blood circulation. Glucose comes from the digestive metabolism of food. Too much blood glucose (*hyper*glycemia) or too little (*hypo*glycemia) causes dizziness and sensory impairment potentially leading to shock and, at the extreme, death. Insulin is the hormone, secreted in the pancreas, that counteracts excess glucose; glucose deficiency is counteracted by food, especially sweets (which must be avoided except in a glucose-deficiency emergency). Diabetes results when the body's natural capacity to produce insulin is impaired. Glucose levels increase following ingestion of food; lacking self-made insulin, the patient self-injects synthetic insulin, to prevent hyperglycemia. If the patient injects too much insulin, however, then the opposite and more immediately life-threatening state of hypoglycemia ensues. As with many nondiabetics, the diabetic sometimes feels a normal temptation to self-indulge with food—to simply eat too much or to

consume sweets and rich food that raise the glucose level. Too much of the insulin "antidote," however, also leads to trouble.

The task of the patient, then, is to balance insulin administration and food intake in such a way as to keep blood glucose within a safe zone. The diabetic patient is thrust into the position of exercising considerable self-restraint concerning diet; just as difficult as the requisite restraint, however, is the need to continuously monitor one's behavior. A team of social scientists and physicians studying behavioral adaptation to diabetes stated (Peyrot, McMurry, & Hedges, 1987, p. 109) that "... dramatic symptoms occur at both extremes of treatment. This situation is complicated by the fact that a balance between overtreatment and undertreatment requires continual effort and is not necessarily easy to achieve or maintain, even for those who are willing to invest massive effort in doing so."

The long-term danger in diabetes comes from elevated glucose levels, to which clinicians generally ascribe the majority of the complications of diabetes. Avoiding these elevations is therefore the key challenge in diabetes management.

The struggle to maintain glucose control presents other behavioral challenges. One such challenge is the role of the family in helping the patient. The restrictions on the patient's diet have obvious implications for meals and food consumption in the home. Some experts have said that the right diet for a diabetic would be good for anyone; i.e., healthy persons would also benefit by following the patient's diet. That they would does not mean, however, that other family members will be motivated to follow the patient's diet. Clearly, the family food shoppers and preparers have the burden of negotiating the extent to which the patient's regimen will prevail (Kelleher, 1988).

A second important aspect of diabetes is that it is a common disease. Some epidemiologists see it as a "disease of civilization" that is destined to have a gradually increasing incidence in modern society. Despite its severe implications, diabetes is borne successfully by many patients for many years with only moderate inroads into their lives. Usually overshadowed by the medical problems in diabetes management are larger issues concerning quality of life that will become increasingly important in the agenda of social science research on illness.

Behavioral Implications of End-Stage Renal Disease

What are the behavioral implications of ESRD? As with diabetes, the discussion is confined to critical features of treatment, omitting the onset of the disease, behavioral issues in seeking treatment, and the often lengthy trail to definitive diagnosis. More than these other features of the disease, it is treatment that entails a full consideration of "following the rules."

Two radically different treatment modalities exist for ESRD: transplantation and dialysis. Concerning transplantation, the single most important treatment task of the transplant patient is to take the prescribed immunosuppressive (antirejection) medication, such as cyclosporine. All transplant patients must take such medicine throughout their lifetimes (or for the duration of the transplant) to prevent rejection of the acquired kidney. Nephrologists may dream of a single-dose, lifetime-duration immunosuppressive drug, but it has not yet been formulated.

A team of scientists studying renal rehabilitation at Emory University have noted that "cyclosporine's problems are by no means insignificant" (Evans, 1985, p. 81). Cyclosporine and other antirejection drugs have numerous side effects: a moon-faced appearance, enhanced susceptibility to infection, hypertension, and, paradoxically, kidney and liver damage. The patient's physician or treatment coordinator will monitor the side effects and regulate the drug dosage accordingly.

From a behavioral standpoint, it is instructive to compare the self-administration of insulin with that of cyclosporine. Insulin is always taken by injection; cyclosporine is usually taken in tablet form, though injectable forms are available. As

a rule, the diabetic patient is accorded more discretion by the doctor in regard to timing and dosage level than is the transplant patient. Insulin intake is keyed to the steady rhythm of ingestion of food at meals and on other occasions that raises blood glucose level. The patient can self-monitor the need for insulin both by subjective sensation and by blood monitoring. The effects of varying blood glucose levels can be sensed, if only fuzzily, by diabetic patients. The purpose of cyclosporine is to maintain the immune components of blood, especially antibodies, at a sufficiently low level to prevent rejection of the "foreign" kidney by the notably aggressive immune system. Unlike the diabetic patient, the transplant patient cannot subjectively sense this blood-level characteristic. In consequence, the medical requirements for immunosuppressive drugs are more rigid; the patient has less discretion.

Of course, incorrect use of either insulin or immunosuppressive drugs over time works to the medical disadvantage of the diabetic or transplant patient. Further, in a manifestation of the familiar saying that "life is unfair," in both cases patients who "follow the rules" scrupulously may not fare well because of biological processes beyond their control; conversely, resistant or careless patients may escape damage, provided their deviations are not too great.

Similar considerations apply to hemodialysis. Hemodialysis, however, is a more extensive and continuously demanding form of treatment than is transplantation. It takes place via the establishment of an exchange between the patient's blood circulation and a dialyzing machine, whereby the blood is cleansed of metabolic waste products and bodily fluid (mainly water) that, in the normal person, are voided by urination. The patient undergoes dialysis three times weekly for 3–4 hours per session. Although the dialysis process is not painful (except for the needle used initially to draw off and circulate the patient's blood through plastic tubing to the dialyzer), it has uncomfortable periods; e.g., patients often become dizzy due to blood pressure changes as their body fluid is dialyzed off.

Although some patients in the United States carry out home dialysis (with the dialyzer at home and the patient or a family member conducting the treatment), the vast majority of "hemo" patients go to a dialysis center, sit in a chair beside a dialyzer reserved for their treatment session, and turn all treatment responsibility over to professional staff. From a behavioral standpoint, simply by coming to the dialysis center and making themselves available for treatment at the scheduled time, they are following the medical rules laid down for them. Sometimes, however, patients fail to appear on schedule. This missing of an appointment alarms staff on two counts. First, missing a session puts the patient in medical danger. Second, from an administrative standpoint, resources are wasted—professional staff time, supplies, the "empty chair," and infrastructure. Furthermore, the patient cannot simply show up the next day and expect to find an empty dialysis machine waiting.

If the patient's nonappearance is willful and not due to circumstances beyond the patient's control, then it becomes an instance of "health misbehavior"—which is deliberate noncompliance from the standpoint of staff expectations. Such an instance can be viewed in the larger context of health behavior. The following episode occurred at a clinic observed by one of the authors (Gallagher, 1994). It shows that the ramifications of not following the rules can extend well beyond the self-harm that the patient might do.

> Two hemodialysis patients, males ages 25 and 41, were served notice that because of their "uncooperative behavior," Catalpa Clinic would not treat them after a stated date. Each received a registered letter from his own nephrologist to this effect....
>
> What was their uncooperative behavior?
>
> [B]oth patients occasionally missed dialyses without any advance notification to the center and without any explanation when they returned following the missed session. Sometimes each had skipped more than one session and gone elsewhere for an emergency dialysis....
>
> Henry, the 41-year-old patient, had recently reached over from his dialysis chair and switched off an audio-alarm on the dialyzer of the adjacent patient.

The nurses were extremely upset at this. He justified his action by saying that the noise bothered him and that the staff kept letting it ring instead of taking care of it. From his previous training and experience in dialyzing himself at home, he knew—so he claimed—that the staff had set the alarm threshold too low, so that the alarm was giving off many false signals.

The younger patient, George, threatened to sue the clinic for terminating his dialysis.... He also said that he intended to show up for treatment anyway, as if he had not been terminated. This greatly worried the nurse, who regularly came in at 6 A.M. to set up the machines to start dialyzing patients at 7 A.M. She would be there alone and feared that the patient might come in early and aggressively confront her for treatment. The dietician, also female, agreed to go in early with the nurse, for support and protection, on the first day when George would ordinarily appear following the termination. He did not show up. The clinic staff eventually learned that he had gone to the nearby VA dialysis unit for emergency treatment that day and for routine treatment the following week.

The nephrologists assigned the social worker the task of finding another dialysis site for George and Henry following their dismissal. The staff realized that however justified they might feel in terminating the two patients, they could not do so without making alternative arrangements—despite the refusal of both patients to cooperate. (If Catalpa Clinic had been the only dialysis source available, the patients would not have been expelled under any circumstances.)

What other expectations must the dialysis patient meet besides receiving dialysis?

Another important requirement is to observe dietary restrictions on food and fluid intake. It is necessary to monitor fluid intake—for most patients, not more than 1 pint daily—so that the patient does not become "overloaded" between dialyses; if the patient takes in too much fluid, the ensuing dialysis is physiologically difficult, placing strain on the patient's cardiovascular system. Although dialysis can still be carried out, frequent overloading places the patient in long-run medical jeopardy. Like the diabetic patient who engages in dietary overindulgence, the nonobservant dialysis patient risks an acceleration of the degenerative processes that occur cumulatively over months and years of dialysis. Another cautionary note is that approximately 40% of current hemodialysis patients in the United

States are also diabetic; as mentioned, renal failure is a common consequence of diabetes. Diabetic hemodialysis patients are in a position of special jeopardy if they do not follow the rules closely.

CHRONIC ILLNESS: BIOLOGICAL DISEASE AND PSYCHOSOCIAL CONDITION

The foregoing comparison of diabetes and ESRD focused upon these two pathologies in their most sharply etched medical aspect, i.e., as *diseases* that the doctor treats. The comparison revealed some ways in which their behavioral implications were similar and others in which they diverged.

In both cases, the treatment is a replacement therapy, whereby external agents are introduced into the patient's body as a substitute for the patient's own autogenous production, which has been thwarted by a disease process. The notion of a replacement therapy leads directly to another significant behavioral aspect in the treatment of diabetes and renal disease, namely, that the patient must have ongoing, periodic treatment. It is not possible to have a megadose of insulin or a megaintensive dialysis treatment with effects lasting for months or years. Thus, the patient lacks the security of a long-lasting treatment that permits one to put medical care out of mind for an appreciable length of time. Even renal transplantation, which at first blush seems to be the perfect treatment, imposes upon the patient the continuing need for maintenance immunosuppression.

PERSONAL ISSUES

The Patient and the Condition

The foregoing considerations, which focus solely upon the medical aspects of the patient's state, trace out a broad domain of needed medical behavioral research in chronic illness. This domain is mapped by the following questions:

1. What are the objective requirements of treatment for a given chronic illness?
2. To what extent can, or must, patients administer their own treatment? Correlatively, to what extent do professionals perform the treatment? If treatment is performed episodically rather than according to a fixed schedule, who decides when treatment is indicated?
3. What is the behavioral impact of treatment upon the patient's daily life? What restrictions or expectations apply to the patient's behavior in regard to diet, patterns of rest, physical exertion, and social interaction, and to the patient's exposure to environmental stimuli?
4. These questions concern treatment. Many of the same questions apply equally to the disease. Thus, one may ask: What is the behavioral impact of the disease? In chronic disease, treatment is never more than partially successful. Many chronic diseases, such as traumatic spinal cord injury and stroke, have no definitive treatment, although various interventions are possible to assist sensorimotor functions and to improve the patient's quality of life. Questions about the behavioral impact of treatment must therefore always be accompanied by questions about the behavioral impact of the disease itself.

There is a second domain of research endeavor concerning health behavior in chronic illness, an area of study that transcends the purely medical features of the disease and its treatment. This domain regards chronic illness as a *psychosocial condition* that embraces the patient, the illness, the patient's self-concept as modified by both disease and treatment, the patient's ways of coping with the disease and its treatment, and the implications of the illness for the patient's daily life as well as family and social relationships. Taken at its fullest, the psychosocial perspective looks at the patient in totality. It regards the patient not as a pathological organism but as a human being who, although compromised to some extent by a chronic disease, exists, copes, and functions in a full psychosocial space that lies largely outside the concern and cognizance of intervention-minded medical personnel.

The Health Care System

The delineation of a psychosocial perspective in chronic illness both parallels and supports a view of the American health care system that has been expressed in recent years by observers of health care; their view, and criticism, is that the system is too attuned to acute care and intervention, at the expense of chronic illness (Fox, 1993). To be sure, this bias came to prevail for many reasons attributable to the history of biomedical discovery, medical education, and health care financing. Starr (1982), for example, emphasizes the rise of surgery as a mode of intervention in many diseases, leading in turn to the great expansion of hospitals and to a focus upon acute intensive intervention for disease.

Whatever the historical basis for the inability of the modern health care system and health professions to deal holistically with chronic illness, the challenge is to improve the situation—to reverse the bias away from acute care and toward better chronic care. This reversal will require the defining of many new concepts and their introduction into the education of health professionals, together with their application in patient care.

The very notion of health behavior, familiar though it may be to most readers of this *Handbook*, is itself a powerful antidote to the entrenched biomedical paradigm, which sees the patient's disease sheerly at the level of cellular pathology or the dysfunction of particular organs. To study the patient's behavior both as it is affected by and as it responds to disease opens the way for a more systematic, more sustained, and less episodic approach to chronic illness.

The Medical Model

Many of the limitations of the health care system in dealing with chronic illness are captured in criticisms of the so-called "medical model." Important though it may be in targeting specific treatment interventions, the medical model disregards many important parameters of patient behavior and functioning, such as the patient's quality of life (Levine, 1987; Scheuch, 1992/1993; Siegrist & Junge, 1989). Some critics of the medical model employ the term *demedicalization* to denote the process of both recognizing the limitations of an exclusively medical focus and incorporating into treatment the contributions of other professions such as nursing, social work, and rehabilitation (Pope & Tarlov, 1991). Thus, Pope and Tarlov write (pp. 244–245):

> [T]reatment protocols ... would consider not only medical needs but also necessary environmental modifications, the availability of family support, and other nonmedical variables. Thus health care should be viewed as only one component of an array of enabling interventions that have a common aim: whether social, environmental, or medical, the services provided ... should seek to ensure a reasonable quality of life.

THE CHRONIC PATIENT'S TEMPORAL HORIZON AND SELF-CONCEPT

With increasingly precise biochemical assays and imaging "scans" for diagnosis, modern medicine is acquiring the power to assess the staging and progression that characterize many chronic diseases, e.g., cervical and prostate cancer, cystic fibrosis, and chronic renal failure. As suggested, however, medicine has not taken on the task of delineating the psychosocial context of chronic disease. This task has fallen to other health professions and disciplines, such as nursing, social work, and the behavioral sciences dealing with medicine. Some would argue that medicine, through its technological prowess and bureaucratic organizational forms, has "dehumanized" medical care and that it devolves upon other nonmedical professions to humanize medical care (Howard & Strauss, 1975).

Two features of chronic illness that lie in its psychosocial context require review: (1) the time perspective adopted by a patient moving from a pre-illness plane of health into chronic illness and (2) the patient's self-concept as the bearer of chronic illness.

In many chronic illnesses, the definitive diagnosis by a physician comes not with the first appearance of symptoms, but only after a period of weeks or months during which the pattern of the disease crystallizes to a point of diagnostic resolution. That the physician attains cognitive clarity does not necessarily mean, however, that the patient grasps or accepts the reality of the newly diagnosed state and prospects in life. Mental health specialists accustomed to thinking in terms of ego psychology often speak of denial as a typical response to diagnostic bad news. On an overt level, the patient hears the doctor's words and may even express relief that a wrenching uncertainty has now been resolved. On an underlying emotional level, however, the patient also "denies" certain aspects of the diagnosis. Words or actions often reveal that the patient does not comprehend or accept the diagnosis. But the initial reaction is only an early scene in the patient's unfolding temporal horizon. According to Barry (1989, p. 340), the patient gradually learns "to live with the illness and the many changes it is causing and will continue to cause in the lives of all family members." Kubler-Ross's well-known paradigm setting forth the stages by which many dying persons move toward their death—denial, anger, bargaining, depression, and acceptance—has also been adapted, with modification, to chronic illness (Kubler-Ross, 1969).

In the mode of denial, many chronic illness patients start out with a conceptualization of their problem as acute—because their previous illnesses have been of rapid onset, time-limited, and curable. It takes time for the patient's conceptualization, in regard to duration, to shift from acute to chronic (Leventhal & Prohaska, 1986). The patient's self-concept typically undergoes

concomitant shifts. Whether or not there is a feeling of being completely dominated by the illness (a person with mild arthritis, for example, would be unlikely to feel completely dominated even in the face of the gradual realization that it is irreversible), patients feel themselves to be different "selves" or persons, ones who now have an illness that will never go completely away.

Figure 1 is a representation of the illness–self relationship. It presents self and illness as contenders for dominance: To what extent does the illness occupy the psychic space of the self? For the sake of simplicity, this scheme perforce ignores much of the complexity and subtlety in the patient's sense of being ill. Nevertheless, depending upon the nature of the particular illness, its symptomatology, and its tendency toward progression (versus plateau or even regression), Figure 1 offers a graphic means of conceptualizing chronic illness. With it, the patient can be located on the 6-stage continuum.

Stage 1 signifies that the patient (or, more accurately, the prepatient) is healthy, or asymptomatic. Stage 2 signifies the experiencing of symptoms to a minor degree. The transition from the first to the second stage should be regarded as a qualitative shift; i.e., something new has entered the patient's life. Stage 3 signifies an increase in the level of symptoms, indicating a mild to moderate quantitative shift. At stage 4, symptoms are extensive enough to signify a qualitatively different phase, namely, that the patient "has" the disease. The pattern and intensity of symptoms are no longer fragmentary and isolated; instead, they coalesce into the patient's psychic sense, "I have disease X." With a still greater burden of symptoms and concomitant psychic "working through" of their meaning, the patient may arrive at the sense, "I *am* X-ic." At this stage 5, the disease coexists fully with the patient's self; the patient sees no part of the self that is unaffected by disease X. (Another factor that may push the patient into stage 5 is a more extensive treatment or management regimen.) In comparison with stage 5, stage 6 has no greater objective physical magnitudes, such as might appear in

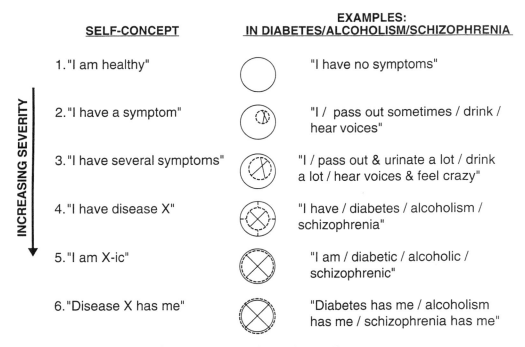

Figure 1. Staging in chronic illness self-concept.

a biochemical assay or CAT-scan; it is included in the schema purely as a hypothetical or asymptotic limit that occurs when, psychically, the patient feels, "X *has* me." It signifies the patient's sense of being dominated by disease X—a state of ultimate victimhood.

The diagram offers a plausible heuristic of a person's possible self-view at different stages or points of being afflicted by a long-term or chronic disease. Although the diagram is laid out in a staged sequence, the patient is not locked into a one-way progression. A patient might move backward, toward lesser severity and a milder self-concept, as well as forward, toward greater severity; some chronic diseases, e.g., lupus erythematosus and multiple sclerosis, are notable for their on-again, off-again quality.

Further, although this schematic "fixes" the balance between self and illness at six different levels, there must be flexibility of interpretation at any level. A greater relative component of illness as reflected in extensiveness of symptoms does not always mean "disease wins/patient loses." Thus a patient with diabetes might put off proper self-care as long as the disease is experienced as a series of discrete, unrelated symptoms (stages 2 and 3); only with the firm cognition "I have diabetes" (stage 4) does the patient, in this example, address energy to the tasks imposed by the illness. In this example, the assertion of the integrated ego of self "over" the disease occurs only when the disease has gained a certain foothold, and not earlier.

GUIDING ISSUES FOR FUTURE EXPLORATION

Most social scientists writing about health behavior have defined it as constituting those activities or regimens that healthy persons perform to maintain their health. They use a complementary term, *illness behavior*, to refer to what "legitimately" ill persons do. This usage suggests, if only implicitly, a sharp dichotomy between health and illness. That dichotomy is—or was—more appropriate to the past era of infectious disease and shorter life expectancy than to the contemporary era of chronic disease, disability, and extended life span. The chronically ill person, though by definition not well or healthy, is neither acutely ill with the promise of recovery ahead nor terminally ill. Chronically ill persons live for decades and engage in many activities, assume many attitudes, and adopt many beliefs that affect their health. Accordingly, this chapter has adopted a broader definitional perspective, acknowledging that it is also possible for already ill persons to engage in health behavior. Diabetic patients, for example, no less than healthy athletes, can carry out actions that affect their health. In fact, some athletes who by any measure are otherwise healthy *are* diabetic. This view is scarcely radical, dissident, or subversive. It is close to, but not identical with, the idea of secondary prevention. Weiss and Lonnquist (1994) write about "health protective behaviors" or primary prevention; they also write about secondary prevention, which includes immunizations to prevent infectious diseases and examinations or screenings for disease, the latter intended to "identify [disease] in a sufficiently early stage so that it is not life-threatening" (Weiss & Lonnquist, 1994, p. 113). Health behavior in chronic illness moves one step further: It occurs past the "early stage" but before a "life-threatening" stage.

As a guide to the study of health behavior in chronic illness, investigators should be urged to adopt a broad stance: Health behavior includes not only overt behavior but also personal beliefs, values, perceptions, and motives as they bear upon health maintenance, health restoration, and illness management.

It is well accepted among epidemiologists, health psychologists, and medical sociologists that industrial societies are moving into an era of chronic disease. A second element of generally accepted knowledge is that the health care sys-

tem took its basic form in an earlier era of infectious disease and shorter life expectancy; only now, however, are the full implications of this second element being recognized. The presuppositions and conceptualizations of the earlier era have powerfully shaped medical care, professional training, popular knowledge about health, and even health care financing in ways that were appropriate for that time, but now must be rethought and expanded.

None of the previous formulations from the infectious disease era can be discarded; smallpox may be gone, but the resurgence of tuberculosis, the proliferation of drug-resistant bacterial strains, and the rise of AIDS tell us that infectious disease is not a thing of the past. The requisite new formulations must be built atop the old, without displacing or burying them.

The general issue posed is how to deal with the foregoing situation—not only in the broadest sense of basic cognitive frames and concepts to reckon with the burden of chronic disease in society, but also, relatedly, how to reframe professional behavior and health manpower organization in a correlative manner.

This general issue can be resolved into four specific, interrelated issues, expressed in the following questions:

1. How can the predominantly intervention-minded, high-action dynamic of medical treatment in the previous era be modified to meet the current needs of the chronic illness patient?
2. Granted that the optimum health behavior of the chronic patient is directed toward maintaining stability and preventing deterioration, what professional roles can best educate and motivate the patient in this direction?
3. What is the optimal balance between medical authority/expertise and nonmedical authority/expertise in dealing with chronic patients?
4. What is the optimal balance between lay authority/expertise (whether that of the

patient or other lay peers) and professional authority/expertise (whether medical or nonmedical)?

The transition from the acute-disease to the chronic-disease era has already begun. Participants in any historical change are never sure what is happening until much later, when confused perception resolves into clearer hindsight. Nevertheless, initiatives for change will in all likelihood approximate the directions traced out in this chapter.

REFERENCES

Barry, D. (1989). *Psychosocial nursing assessment and intervention* (2nd ed.). Philadelphia: J. B. Lippincott.

Breitha, O. R. (1988). *Olivia—My life of exile in Kalaupapa.* Molokai, HI: Pacific Printers.

Connelly, C. E. (1993). An empirical study of a model of self-care in chronic illness. *Clinical Nurse Specialist, 7*(5), 247–253.

Elias, N. (1978). *The civilizing process.* Oxford: Basil Blackwell.

Evans, R. W. (1985). The quality of life of patients with chronic renal disease: Comparison of four treatment modalities, In N. G. Kutner, D. D. Cardenas, & J. D. Bower (Eds.), *Rehabilitation and the chronic renal disease patient.* (pp. 61–83). New York: SP Medical and Scientific Books.

Fox, D. M. (1993). *Power and illness: The failure and future of American health policy.* Berkeley: University of California Press.

Gallagher, E. B. (1994). Quality of life issues and the dialectic of medical progress illustrated by end-stage renal disease patients. In G. Albrecht & R. Fitzpatrick (Eds.), *Advances in medical sociology: Vol. V,* (pp. 67–90). Greenwich, CT: JAI Press.

Gill, R. T., Glazer, N., & Thernstrom, S. A. (1992). *Our changing population.* Englewood Cliffs, NJ: Prentice-Hall.

Goffman, E. (1963). *Stigma: Notes on the management of spoiled identity.* Englewood Cliffs, NJ: Prentice-Hall.

Goffman, E. (1974). *Frame analysis: An essay on the organization of experience.* New York: Harper & Row.

Hanson, S. M. H. (1987). Family nursing and chronic illness. In L. M. Wright & M. Leahey (Eds.), *Families and chronic illness* (pp. 2–32). Springhouse, PA: Springhouse.

Howard, J. & Strauss, A. (Eds.). (1975). *Humanizing health care.* New York: Wiley.

Kelleher, D. (1988). Coming to terms with diabetes: Coping strategies and non-compliance. In R. Anderson & M. Bury (Eds.), *Living with chronic illness: The experience of pa-*

tients and their families, pp. 136–155. London: Unwin Hyman.

Kleinman, A. (1988). *The illness narratives.* New York: Basic Books.

Kubler-Ross, E. 1969. *On death and dying.* New York: Macmillan.

Law, A. V. S., & Wisniewski, A. (1988). *Kalaupapa and the legacy of Father Damien.* Honolulu: Pacific Basin Enterprises.

Leventhal, E. A., & Prohaska, T. R. (1986). Age, symptom interpretation, and health behavior. *Journal of the American Geriatric Society, 34,* 185–191.

Levine, S. (1987). The changing terrains in medical sociology: Emergent concern with quality of life. *Journal of Health and Social Behavior, 28*(4), 1–6.

McKinlay, J. B., & McKinlay, S. M. (1977). The questionable contribution of medical measures to the decline of mortality in the United States in the twentieth century. *Milbank Memorial Fund Quarterly: Health and Society, 55*(3), 405–428.

Perdue, B. J., Mahon, N. E., Hawes, S. L., & Frik, S. M. (1981). *Chronic care nursing.* New York: Springer.

Peyrot, M., McMurry, F., Jr., & Hedges, R. (1987). Living with diabetes: The role of personal and professional knowledge in symptom and regimen management. In J. Roth & P. Conrad (Eds.), *Research in the sociology of health care* (pp. 107–146). Greenwich, CT: JAI Press.

Pope, A. M., & Tarlov, A. R. (Eds.). (1991). *Disability in America—Toward a national agenda for prevention.* Washington, DC: National Academy Press.

Register, C. (1987). *Living with chronic illness: Days of patience and passion.* New York: Free Press.

Robinson, I. (1988). Reconstructing lives: Negotiating the meaning of multiple sclerosis. In R. Anderson & M. Bury (Eds.), *Living with chronic illness: The experience of patients and their families.* (pp. 43–46). London: Unwin Hyman.

Scheuch, E. K. (1992/1993). The puzzle of "quality of life." *Annals of the International Institute of Sociology, 3,* 151–182.

Siegrist, J. & Junge, A. (1989). Conceptual and methodological problems in research on the quality of life in clinical medicine. *Social Science and Medicine, 29*(3), 463–468.

Sontag, S. (1989). *AIDS and its metaphors.* New York: Farrar, Straus and Giroux.

Spiegelman, M. (1968). *Introduction to demography.* Cambridge, MA: Harvard University Press.

Starr, P. E. (1982). *The social transformation of American medicine.* New York: Basic Books.

Strauss, A. L., & Corbin, J. M. (1988). *Shaping a new health care system: The explosion of chronic illness as a catalyst for change.* San Francisco: Jossey-Bass.

Weiss, G. L., & Lonnquist, L. E. (1994). *The sociology of health, healing, and illness.* Englewood Cliffs, NJ: Prentice-Hall.

12

Health Behavior in Persons with Severe Mental Illness

Timothy Hawley

INTRODUCTION

It seems there was a mentally ill man who had a delusion that he was dead. His family, understandably concerned, took him to see a renowned psychiatrist who was known for his ability to treat such problems.

The psychiatrist, after evaluating the man and determining that he did indeed firmly believe he was dead, stood him in front of a full-length mirror. He then instructed him thusly: "I want you to look at yourself in this mirror and repeat 'Dead men don't bleed.'"

So the man stood before the mirror and said over and over and over again, "Dead men don't bleed. Dead men don't bleed. Dead men don't bleed...."

After two hours, the psychiatrist returned and, grabbing the man's hand, stabbed his finger with a needle. Blood spurted from the wound. "Now!" declared the psychiatrist. "What does *that* prove?"

The man looked at his bleeding finger, then replied, with a knowing sidelong glance at the psychiatrist, "Dead men *do* bleed."

People with severe mental illness (SMI)—also referred to as severe and persistent mental illness (SPMI)—represent a very distinct population, albeit one with an extreme degree of heterogeneity. The mental illness of some people with SMI tends to cause their health behaviors to be different from those of people who do not have SMI. The distinctive feature of this population is the epistemological basis upon which their health behaviors are based: What is the basis of their knowledge of, or awareness of, illness? How is this knowledge interpreted? How is the interpretation of this knowledge acted upon?

The introductory humorous example represents some of the features that often characterize people with SMI. The mentally ill man fails to correctly interpret certain aspects of his functioning—he is breathing, for instance, which would normally suggest continuing life—and instead responds to an unknown stimulus or cognition that causes him to develop the belief that he is not alive. When confronted with incontrovertible evidence that he is alive, he simply incorporates this new information into his personal view of the situation. Since he knows he is dead, if he bleeds, then obviously dead men *do* bleed.

Indeed, the body of research on the health behaviors of people with SMI supports the no-

Timothy Hawley • Seven Counties Services, 915 South Third Street, Louisville, Kentucky 40203.

Handbook of Health Behavior Research III: Demography, Development, and Diversity, edited by David S. Gochman. Plenum Press, New York, 1997.

tion that the health behaviors that differentiate this population from others are primarily determined by altered sensations, perceptions, and interpretations of symptoms of physical and mental illness. This body of research has focused on these determinants and their relationship to protective and preventive behaviors, access and utilization of health care, and the development of the sick role.

DEFINITION OF SEVERE MENTAL ILLNESS

It is important at the outset to define the population of people who are considered to have SMI. The *Diagnostic and Statistical Manual of Mental Disorders*, 4th edition (DSM-IV) (American Psychiatric Association, 1994) lists scores of disorders, only a fraction of which would be considered to represent severe mental illnesses. The subset of people with mental disorders who would be considered to have a severe mental illness are usually defined in terms of three criteria, which have been summarized and discussed by Bachrach (1988): diagnosis, duration, and disability.

Diagnosis

People are considered to have a severe mental illness if they have been assigned any diagnosis in the family of schizophrenic disorders, any bipolar disorder, or any other psychotic disorder. People with other diagnoses may be considered to have a severe mental illness if they *also* meet the duration and disability criteria.

Duration

Duration is a broad criterion that quantifies the severity of mental illness on the basis of how long a person has suffered from symptoms, how much treatment—specifically, how much inpatient treatment—the person has received, and how long the symptoms of the disorder are ex-

pected to persist. A person is considered to have SMI by the following criteria: has suffered from the disorder for 2 years, or has been hospitalized for treatment of the disorder more than once in the previous year, or has experienced one psychiatric hospitalization that has lasted for more than 13 days, or the disorder is expected to persist for another 2 years. Obviously, this definition alone would include a large number of people, since people with many different psychiatric disorders would meet one or more of the duration criteria. As Bachrach (1988) explains, however, to be classified as SMI, the disorder must also meet the disability criterion.

Disability

To be considered as having a severe mental illness, a person must have a diagnosis from the *DSM-IV*, must meet the duration criterion, and must also be assessed as being disabled in two or more major life areas. Examples of such areas are employment, self-care, and interpersonal relationships.

Bachrach (1988) goes on to point out that this classification scheme is certainly rife with problems. The definitions for the duration and disability criteria are quite broad, and those people who would not be considered to have SMI on the basis of a diagnosis of a psychotic disorder alone, but who could be included as a result of meeting the duration and disability criteria, are extremely diverse, and certainly unlikely to share etiological factors that might tend to be hypothesized for disorders such as schizophrenia or bipolar illness.

As a result of this diversity, many investigators have focused their studies on diagnostic subcategories that include only those people for whom high agreement would be assumed regarding their being in the category of people with SMI, often limiting participation to people with a diagnosis of schizophrenia or a major affective disorder, such as bipolar illness or major depression.

This chapter focuses on the major areas in which health behaviors of people with SMI have been examined. Studies have assessed the extent to which people with SMI experience physical health problems, their utilization of health care services to treat these problems, and the hypothesized determinants of seeking these services. Some research has focused on protective behaviors among people with SMI and the extent to which they fail to exercise precautions that would protect them from the development of medical problems. A large body of research has focused on the refusal of people with SMI to accept psychiatric treatment and the determinants of this refusal.

INCIDENCE OF PHYSICAL ILLNESS

A number of studies have reported that people with SMI have a high rate of physical health problems, which are often undiagnosed and untreated, leading R. C. Hall, Beresford, Gardner, and Pipkin (1982) to conclude that persons who suffer from SMI are very likely to suffer from physical illness as well. That cause and effect are so inextricably intertwined is one of the enigmas that face researchers trying to evaluate the meaning of some of these findings. Are people with SMI more vulnerable to illness, or to certain types of illness? Harris (1988) reported that there is some evidence to suggest, for instance, that there is an increased risk of breast cancer and cardiovascular disease among people with schizophrenia, and possibly a reduced risk for rheumatoid arthritis and lung cancer—the latter a surprising possibility given the evidence regarding the prevalence of cigarette smoking among people with SMI (e.g., Hughes & Frances, 1995). Or does disruption in perceptual processes tend to prevent people with SMI from seeking medical care, since symptoms may be outside their awareness, thus leading to a higher incidence of more severe illnesses, and illnesses that are found to have been previously untreated?

Regardless of the underlying causes, it is clear that there is overwhelming evidence of high rates of physical illness among people with

SMI and that many illnesses identified during the course of research studies are of a long-standing nature and have failed to be identified for long periods of time. For example, Karasu, Waltzman, Lindemayer, and Buckley (1980) reported that 52% of 200 people with SMI admitted to outpatient mental health treatment were found to have physical illnesses requiring treatment; R. C. Hall, Gardner, Pipkin, LeCann, and Stickney (1981) reported that 80% of their sample of people admitted to a state psychiatric hospital had medical illnesses requiring treatment, of which 46% were unrecognized illnesses that had exacerbated the patients' psychiatric illnesses. Such findings are reflected in the literature over a 50-year period; e.g., from Phillips (1937) to Marticle, Hoffman, Bloom, Faulkner, and Keepers (1987).

Health Care Seeking

The reports of the incidence of medical illnesses would suggest that people with SMI would have a high level of utilization of medical services, with health-care-seeking behavior being abundant and evaluation and identification of illness being commonplace. Such, however, is not the case. As Lally (1989) has pointed out, the process by which people with SMI assume the sick role of "mental patient" involves a near-total "engulfment" of their identify in this role, so that those around them come to perceive them and they come to perceive themselves as being mentally ill first and foremost. There is significant evidence that the illness role of mental patients tends to cause them and the professionals who treat them to focus on their mental illnesses, with an accompanying lack of focus on their physical health care needs.

For example, Freddolino, Moxley, and Fleishman (1988) found, in an interview survey, that nearly three fourths of people with SMI leaving residential treatment settings to return to the community did not express a belief that they would have a need for health care services in the community. Koranyi (1977, 1980) reported that from one third to one half of people with SMI that he studied had physical illnesses that were inadequately diagnosed—and, obviously, inadequately treated—by their referring physicians. These findings were supported by those of other investigators (e.g., Roca, Breakey, & Fischer, 1987).

It could be argued that these findings have much more to do with the fact that the subjects being studied, in addition to having SMI, are typically poor and disenfranchised and are not significantly different from any other impoverished population in terms of health-care seeking. A study of Gelberg and Linn (1988), however, would support a differentiation among people with SMI. In a study of homeless people, these investigators found that homeless people with SMI were significantly less likely to receive needed medical care, even when compared with a control group of similarly disenfranchised individuals, i.e., other homeless people.

Practices of Health Professionals

Much of the problem in identifying and treating physical illnesses among people with SMI lies with the prejudices and practices of the medical profession. Just as people with SMI become "engulfed" in the mental patient sick role, so too are they often perceived within that narrow role by health professionals as well. Professionals often ignore or deemphasize the physical health problems of a patient with SMI because they believe that the patient's mental illness is an overriding concern or that reported physical illness symptoms are either a manifestation of the person's mental illness or an imaginary complaint.

For example, Koranyi (1979) reported a high incidence of failure of physicians to identify physical illnesses in outpatient clinic patients with SMI; psychiatrists were much more likely to fail to diagnose physical illness than were other physicians. Indeed, McIntyre and Romano (1978) reported that only 8% of physicians "frequently" carried out a physical examination of psychiatric patients, even though 94% of their sample of

physicians indicated that they believed such examinations were frequently or sometimes useful. Patterson (1978) reported that *none* of the psychiatrists whom he surveyed routinely performed physical examinations on their patients, and only 16% sought examinations from other physicians.

Thus, the research makes it apparent that despite consistently high reported incidence of physical health problems among people with severe mental illness, there is a very low rate of access to medical treatment, a high rate of undiagnosed and untreated illnesses, and an attitude among health care professionals that tends to support this failure to address psychiatric patients' health care needs.

Pain Insensitivity

One of the determinants of health-care-seeking behavior that has received a significant amount of research attention is pain sensitivity. Dworkin (1994) stated that pain, being a symptom of many illnesses, is an important signal that alerts people to the need to seek health care; an insensitivity to pain can delay recognition of a condition that requires diagnosis and treatment. The literature is replete with reports of diminished pain sensitivity in people with SMI, both with regard to identification of illness or injury and in experimental studies.

Insensitivity to pain was noted in the earliest writings about schizophrenia. Kraepelin (1919, p. 34) indicated that people with schizophrenia are "less sensitive to bodily discomfort." Bleuler (1950) indicated that people with schizophrenia often have analgesia, including both deeper parts of the body and the skin. Marchand (1958, p. 600) stated that "a large proportion of [psychotic] patients offer no complaint when they become physically ill."

A large number of investigators have reported that physical illnesses and injuries in which pain is a cardinal diagnostic indicator do not produce reports of pain at expected rates in people with SMI. The medical conditions include such illnesses as peptic ulcer, fractured femur, and acute appendicitis (Katz, Kluger, Rabinovici, Stein, & Gimmon, 1990; Marchand et al., 1959; West and Hecker, 1952). Similarly, several investigations (Hussar, 1965; Marchand, 1955; Lieberman, 1955) have reported a very low incidence of reports of pain with myocardial infarction among people with SMI.

A number of experimental studies have also been carried out to examine the relative pain insensitivity of people with SMI. These studies have very consistently found significantly decreased sensitivity to a variety of types of induced pain: pinching of the neck (May, 1948), heat applied to the forehead (K. R. L. Hall & Stride, 1954), and electrical shock (Davis, Buchsbaum, & Bunney, 1979).

Bunce, Jones, Badger, and Jones (1982) reported that only 23% of patients sent to an acute medical treatment unit of a psychiatric hospital were capable of adequately communicating the location or intensity of pain associated with medical illness. Somewhat paradoxically, Watson, Chandarana, and Merskey (1981) found that a large number of people with SMI reported complaints of pain that had no determinable physical origin. Thus, while stimuli that should produce pain may not tend to be perceived as being painful by people with SMI, these same people may have a relatively highly likelihood of reporting the experience of pain when the situation would not seem to support the existence of a painful stimulus. It is little wonder, then, that health professionals who treat people with SMI tend to ignore or minimize physical health needs.

RISK BEHAVIOR

Avoidance of risky behaviors is an area that has also been found to be problematic for people with SMI. Persons with SMI engage in risky behaviors such as smoking, use of alcohol and drugs, unprotected sex, and IV needle sharing at high rates.

Smoking

A number of studies have reported that the incidence of cigarette smoking is high among people with SMI. Goff, Henderson, and Amico (1992) reported that 74% of their sample of people with schizophrenia were smokers; Hughes (1993) reported that the incidence of cigarette smoking was reported to vary from 50% to 80% among psychiatric patients, while those with co-occurring alcohol or drug abuse disorders had a rate of smoking of 80–95%, as compared with 28% of the general population. Other investigators have confirmed the unusually high rate of smoking among people with SMI (e.g., Ziedonis, Kosten, Glazer, & Frances, 1994).

It is important to note that factors other than mental illness may contribute to the high incidence of smoking among people with SMI. As Lally (1989) noted, people with SMI are often considered to be disabled and come to depend on public income supports such as Supplemental Security Income and Social Security Disability Income. The typical amount of income from these sources consigns recipients to a decidedly low socioeconomic status. Adler et al. (1994) reported that higher occurrence of smoking is characteristic of people in groups of lower socioeconomic status than in more affluent groups.

Alcohol and Drug Use

Several studies have reported that use of drugs and alcohol occurs at a higher rate in people with SMI. Barry et al. (1995) reported that 41% of 253 subjects with SMI met the criteria in *DSM-IV* (American Psychiatric Association, 1994) for previous or current drug or alcohol disorders. Of this total sample, 35% met the criteria for drug or alcohol disorder during the previous year.

These findings are confirmed by other studies (Barbee, Clark, Crapanzano, Heintz, & Kehoe, 1989; Mueser et al. 1990) that found a high rate of substance abuse among people with SMI. Substance abuse is not only a disorder in and of itself, but also a risk factor for other physical health problems, and the finding that substance abuse is heightened among people with SMI is consistent with findings regarding other health risk behaviors.

HIV and AIDS: Sexual Behavior and Needle Sharing

Perhaps the most clear-cut risk behavior that has emerged in recent years relates to the HIV/AIDS epidemic. This relationship is very clear because transmission of HIV occurs as a result of clearly defined and almost always avoidable behaviors; the extent to which people engage in activities that expose them to risk, or, conversely, take actions to minimize their risk, is a direct reflection of the extent to which they carry out protective and preventive health behaviors.

As might be expected, people with SMI have consistently been found to have a high rate of failure to exercise preventive or protective health behaviors to prevent infection by HIV.

The incidence of HIV infection has been variously reported among groups of people with SMI as being from 4% to nearly 20% (Cournos et al., 1991; Lee, Traven, & Bluestone, 1992; Susser, Valencia, & Conover, 1993). Meyer et al. (1993) reported a lower rate of HIV infection among long-term state hospital patients, who are more closely supervised and have less opportunity to engage in risk behaviors; when new admissions to psychiatric units are studied, the incidence of HIV infection rises dramatically. The highest rate of HIV infection reported (Susser et al., 1993) was among people with SMI who were residing in a New York City men's homeless shelter. In this sample, 19.4% of the subjects were found to be HIV-positive, which may reflect, to some extent, the geographic distribution of the incidence of HIV infection.

A number of investigators have explored specific HIV-related risk behaviors among people with SMI, and their findings are predictably disturbing; as Carmen and Brady (1990, p. 656) point out, "For mentally ill patients, impulsivity

and severe disturbances of self are prominent cofactors in noncompliance with recommendations for risk reduction."

Sacks, Perry, Graver, Shindledecker, and Hall (1990) evaluated people admitted to an acute state psychiatric hospital and found high rates of risky behaviors, such as unprotected anal sex, sharing of needles with other intravenous (IV) drug users, or sex with known HIV carriers. Unfortunately, there was little difference regarding the fear of contracting HIV between those who engaged in risky behaviors and those who did not. All of the subjects studied, regardless of their risk behaviors, reported a low fear of contracting HIV.

Numerous other studies have confirmed the high rate of risk behaviors and the low rate of protective strategies. Kalichman, Kelly, Johnson, and Bulto (1994) reported that nearly one fifth of the people with SMI that they studied reported receiving money or drugs in return for sex. Sacks, Silberstein, Weiler, and Perry (1990) reported that nearly 12% of the subjects they surveyed reported recent heterosexual contact with bisexual individuals, IV drug users, or prostitutes. Cournos et al. (1994) reported that 27% of their subjects with SMI reported multiple sex partners in the previous 6 months, while 12% of those who were sexually active reported having had sex with someone who was HIV-positive or who injected drugs. Kelly et al. (1995) reported that their subjects with SMI used condoms during intercourse less than 25% of the time.

Sacks, Dermatis, Burton, Hull, and Perry (1994) assessed a large number of people with SMI regarding their risk behaviors for HIV. They found that 16% of the 789 subjects surveyed were at high risk for HIV, 35% were at moderate risk, and 49% were at low risk. Of particular interest in this study was the question that was posed to participants regarding the relationship between the acuity of their mental illness and their probable risk behavior. The mentally ill subjects were asked if they were more or less likely to protect themselves from HIV infection during periods of exacerbation of their symptoms of mental illness. About 11% of the subjects reported that they were less likely to protect themselves; they reported that they were less likely to use condoms, more likely to have more sexual partners, and more likely to generally increase their level of sexual activity.

In a related study, Baer, Dwyer, and Lewitter-Koehler (1988) interviewed 90 patients who were being discharged from an inpatient psychiatric unit regarding their knowledge of AIDS. Subjects made about 75% correct responses to the questionnaire, suggesting that knowledge of AIDS and the risk factors for infection was relatively high. As has been reported regarding the attitudes of health care professionals toward people with SMI, however, focus on protective behavior may be lacking in interventions by the mental health care community. Coverdale and Aruffo (1992) surveyed 82 mental health professionals and found that "nearly all" of those surveyed reported that information on AIDS should be provided to people with SMI. They found, however, that only 19% of the patients being served at the community mental health center where the survey was conducted were provided with any information about AIDS. As is so often the case, mental health professionals participate in the mind–body schism and focus almost exclusively on mental health issues, often ignoring important physical health issues.

The preponderance of evidence suggests that people with SMI have a much greater probability of engaging in behaviors that represent high risk for health problems and often fail to take preventive measures to maintain good health.

INSIGHT AND AWARENESS OF ILLNESS

It seems there was a mentally ill man who had a delusion that he was dead ... but he *didn't* believe he was mentally ill.

As mentioned previously, epistemology plays a key role as a determinant of health behaviors of people with SMI. An individual who is unaware of symptomatology is unlikely to engage in health-care-seeking behavior. Protective behavior is likely to be absent if distortions of perception and impairment of judgment prevent an individual from recognizing potential risk. As pointed out in *DSM-IV* (American Psychiatric Association, 1994, p. 275), psychotic disorders involve "gross impairment in reality testing" as well as "delusions ... erroneous beliefs that usually involve a misinterpretation of perceptions or experiences." Psychotic disorders often involve a disorder of "initiation of goal-directed behavior" and "difficulties in performing activities of daily living." Finally, "lack of insight is common."

As noted, research shows that awareness of one of the cardinal physical symptoms that typically alerts people to illness—namely, pain—is often lacking in people with SMI. Lacking, too, is the awareness of those symptoms that would help to identify that a person has a mental illness. This awareness is usually referred to as *insight* and is defined as a psychiatric patient's capacity for understanding his or her problems (Greenfeld, Strauss, Bowers, & Mandelkern, 1989). Much research has been carried out on the phenomenon of insight and its effects on the health behaviors—particularly the health behaviors relating to mental health care—of people with SMI.

In a famous line from the play *Harvey*, Elwood P. Dowd—the apparently hallucinatory and delusional hero—says to a psychiatrist, "Doctor, I wrestled with reality for over forty years, and I am happy to state that I finally won out over it" (Chase, 1944, p. 49). Indeed, mental illness does often seem to "win out" over reality, much to the detriment of the mentally ill patient. Braginsky, Braginsky, and Ring (1969) and Levinson and Gallagher (1964) reported that *most* psychiatric patients they studied in hospitals did not regard themselves as being mentally ill. It would seem that a classic Catch-22 applied to the situation: For a brain to be able to recognize that it is not working properly, it must be working properly. The brains of many people with SMI appear not to function sufficiently well to allow them to recognize their own dysfunction. Amador, Strauss, and Gorman (1991, p. 113) pointed out that "individuals with schizophrenia have been observed to ignore the deficits caused by their illness and the effect their illness has on their lives." Underlying this phenomenon may be what Anscombe (1987) refers to as the *disorder of consciousness*, or an inability to sustain an intentional focus of one's attention. This inability leads to two phenomena that would affect individuals' ability to have insight into their illness: First, stimuli intrude themselves on people with schizophrenia in such a way as to imply greater importance than they warrant, thus tending to create delusions, overshadowing and distorting stimuli that would lead to more accurate self-assessment of internal states.

A number of studies have focused on the role played by insight—or the lack of insight—in accessing or utilizing services. Mulkern and Bradley (1986) surveyed 328 homeless people. They found that while 45% of the people reported having a history of psychiatric hospitalizations, only 24% reported that they perceived themselves as having a need for mental health services, and only 25% actually sought mental health services. Lin, Spiga, and Fortsch (1979) studied 100 people with schizophrenia to determine whether insight related to following prescribed medication treatment regimes. They found that those people who had insight, i.e., those people who expressed a belief that they needed treatment, were more likely to take medications as prescribed. Of those who did not perceive themselves as needing treatment, only 16% (8 of 51 people) adhered to their prescribed medication regimes.

Of course, insight is not a characteristic that remains constant over the course of an individual's life. Insight may be good during periods of stability in an individual's illness, but very poor during periods of exacerbation of the illness. Heinrichs, Cohen, and Carpenter (1985) studied 38 people with SMI to try to determine whether those people who have enough insight to perceive the signs of exacerbation of their illness and an increase in their symptomatology differed

from those who did not have such insight. They found that 63% of their subjects experienced "early insight" that they were experiencing symptoms indicative of the onset of acute symptomatology, while the remaining 37% did not have such insight. Of those who were found to have early insight, only 8% were subsequently hospitalized as a result of their illness; significantly more of those lacking insight—50%—were subsequently hospitalized.

McCandless-Glimcher et al. (1986) interviewed 62 outpatients with schizophrenia regarding their monitoring of their symptoms and the extent to which they associated these symptoms with changes in their illness that required changes in their behavior to manage their illness. A large proportion of the subjects interviewed, 98%, identified symptoms that indicated to them that their illness was getting worse; two thirds of these symptoms were nonpsychotic (e.g., changes in mood, affect, motivation, energy). Further, 82% of those who identified symptoms of worsening of their illness reported that they responded to their perceived change in condition by altering their behavior; they either adjusted their medication, engaged in diversionary activities, attempted to ignore the symptoms (i.e., avoid focusing on them), or sought mental health treatment.

It is generally hypothesized that people who are voluntarily hospitalized for psychiatric care have more insight than are those who must be involuntarily hospitalized, since agreeing to hospital care indicates some recognition that the care is needed. In contrast, involuntary care if it is required is usually necessary only for patients who do not believe that they require hospital care. In a study comparing voluntary with involuntary patients, McEvoy, Applebaum, Geller, and Freter (1989) compared 28 people who were voluntarily admitted to a psychiatric hospital with 24 involuntary patients. They administered an instrument designed to evaluate the level of insight, the Insight and Treatment Attitudes Questionnaire (ITAQ). They found that insight scores for voluntary patients increased significantly from 9.8 at the time of hospital admission to 13.3 at the time of a follow-up evaluation 30 days after hospital discharge; there was no change in insight scores for involuntarily hospitalized patients. Both pre- and posttest ITAQ scores were also significantly higher for voluntary patients than for involuntary patients, reflecting less insight in the latter.

Gove and Fain (1977) reported, however, that of 86 involuntarily committed patients, 75.3% felt that they had been helped by the hospitalization, as compared with 81.4% of those who were hospitalized on a voluntary basis. Thus, while there may be some difference in level of insight between voluntary and involuntary patients, even involuntary patients seem to achieve some level of insight after successful treatment has ameliorated the symptoms of their acute illness.

One of the most problematic iatrogenic disorders in the treatment of SMI is the side effect of tardive dyskinesia (TD) that results from prolonged treatment with certain antipsychotic medications. The most notable symptom of TD is involuntary movements of the facial muscles and extremities. Several studies have focused on the recognition of symptoms of TD among people with SMI. J. M. Smith, Kucharski, Oswald, and Waterman (1979) studied 113 patients with moderate or greater TD. Only 9 subjects (8%) rated their symptoms in such a way as to suggest that they were aware of abnormal movements; of these 9, only 4 expressed distress with the symptoms. Alexopoulos (1979) found that of 19 outpatients showing symptoms of TD, *none* complained about the symptoms to their therapist, and only 8 were aware that they were experiencing symptoms.

Rosen, Mukherjee, Olarte, Varia, and Cardenas (1982) reported that while many patients failed to recognize symptoms of TD, the severity of symptoms increased the probability of recognition. Caracco, Mukherjee, Roth, and Decina (1990) also reported that awareness of psychiatric disorder (i.e., insight) was significantly associated with awareness of involuntary movements. A longer duration of illness was associated with a lack of awareness of symptoms of TD; those who had been ill longer were less likely to be aware of involuntary movements. In this study, awareness of symptoms of TD was not found to be related to severity of symptoms.

As with the findings on studies of physical health behaviors, a primary determinant of failing to seek care seems to be a lack of awareness or knowledge of illness and symptomatology. Just as people with SMI have a deficit in their awareness of the warning signals of pain that would normally cause a person to seek medical attention, they also often fail to have an awareness of the warning signals of a deterioration of their mental illness, which would cause them to seek appropriate care.

ACCEPTANCE VERSUS REFUSAL OF TREATMENT

While seeking treatment for medical illnesses is often impaired among people with SMI as a result of a variety of factors associated with their mental illness, refusal to participate in mental health treatment is itself a common occurrence, and a controversial issue as well. Forced medical treatment is rarely invoked, and the need for medical treatment for people with SMI is often overlooked. Forced mental health treatment is common, however, and the need for mental health treatment for people with SMI is generally apparent. That the need is apparent unfortunately does not always mean that treatment is imposed. As Rose (1988, p. 5), points out, "The unique tragedy of schizophrenia lies in the fact that victims often cannot recognize their illness, refuse treatment, and throw away their lives."

Some people recovering from mental illness have voiced this same sentiment. Bockes (1985, p. 487) wrote, "Unfortunately, the disease affect's one's ability to make the proper decision." Leete (1989, p. 197) described her experience in dealing with mental illness, stating, "Before I came to realize the role medications could play in my illness, I was caught in a vicious circle. When I was off the medication, I couldn't remember how much better I had felt on it, and when I was taking the medication, I felt so good that I was convinced I did not need it."

An ongoing debate has developed as a result of the fundamental dilemma that mentally ill people often recognize after the fact that treatment was necessary. Lucksted and Coursey (1995), for example, found that about half of their subjects felt that the forced treatment they received was in their best interests, and over 90% of the patients supported the use of forced treatment if a person needs help and refuses it. Should they, then, be forced to submit to treatment when they are acutely ill and refuse to participate in treatment? Advocates for the rights of mental patients have argued against forced treatment (Frank, 1986; Rogers & Centifanti, 1988), saying that the right to refuse treatment supersedes society's right to impose treatment, which is based on the belief that the treatment is ultimately in the individual's best interests and on the assumption that the benefit will be recognized as such by the patient when the treatment has had its effect. Faden and Faden (1977) explored the concept of the harm principle to determine whether treatment should be forced. They state that intervention is justified if the "… patient's decision would result in significant harm to other individuals or society." Faden and Faden (1977, p. 135) conclude that "if the patient does not yield to justifiable interventions to change belief, is competent, and the Harm Principle cannot be legitimately invoked, we feel that the physician is obliged to respect the patient's refusal." The determination of competence in this context is based upon making the distinction between a simple delusional belief and complete misunderstanding. If the person has a simple delusional belief, based on information, interpretation, attitude, or other grounds, the person would be considered competent. If the person fails entirely to understand the situation, then the person would be considered incompetent. Obviously, making a distinction between these two circumstances would often require the wisdom of Solomon.

Frequency of Treatment Refusal

Research on cooperation with treatment has focused on several key determinants: the extent to which people with SMI perceive themselves as having symptoms or conditions requiring treatment, the role played by negative side effects of medications, and the types of interventions that have been undertaken to improve cooperation.

Despite reports like that of Kalman (1983), in which people with SMI consistently reported high levels of satisfaction with treatment, other reports reflect a high incidence of refusal of treatment. Such reports have remained consistently high for many years. Atkinson (1971) reported that of 2,529 people discharged from a voluntary psychiatric hospital unit over a 6-year period, 312 (12.3%) were either discharged against medical advice or simply walked away from the hospital.

A number of studies have focused on the extent to which people take the psychiatric medications that are prescribed for the vast majority of people with SMI and the effect that failure to adhere to prescribed medication regimes has on the rate of exacerbation of the illness and the development of acute psychotic symptoms requiring hospitalization. Carpenter, Mulligan, Bader, and Meinzer (1985) compared people with SMI who experienced multiple psychiatric hospitalizations with those who had experienced only one hospitalization. They found that 70% of those with multiple hospital admissions had been noncompliant with their prescribed medications, while significantly fewer, 38%, of those with a single admission had failed to take their medications. Similarly, Green (1988) found that 92% of those with frequent hospitalizations were consistently noncompliant with medications between hospitalizations, while only 36% of those with fewer hospitalizations were noncompliant. Further, Green found that 76% of those with frequent hospitalizations were also noncompliant with other outpatient aftercare plans, failing to follow through with treatment.

In a study of 472 inmates who were committed to a state forensic psychiatric hospital over a

7-year period, L. D. Smith (1989) found that 62% of the inmates had refused medication in prison, leading to their admission to the hospital. This refusal, along with the classic symptoms of psychosis (hallucinations and delusions) and threatened or potential violence toward others, were the three most common reasons cited for hospital admission.

Appelbaum and Gutheil (1980) reported that they found drug refusal among psychiatric hospital inpatients to be "common." In their study of 23 patients who had refused medication during a 3-month period, they concluded that the patients fell into three subgroups. The first subgroup were those referred to as "situational refusers," who occasionally refused their medications for a variety of immediate situational reasons. The second subgroup were those classified as being "stereotypical refusers," who refused medications on the basis of paranoid beliefs relating to the medication, but whose refusal tended to be episodic. The third subgroup were those whom the authors described as being "symptomatic refusers," who simply reported that it was their right to refuse medications and continued their refusal for long periods of time.

Blackwell (1976) reported that nonadherence to treatment is reported in between 25% and 50% of outpatients and in somewhat fewer inpatients. Hogarty, Goldberg, and the Collaborative Study Group (1973) reported that at least 40% of patients stopped taking their prescribed medications within 1 year of hospital discharge. Serban and Thomas (1974) found that 41.9% of a sample of 516 previously hospitalized patients reported that they had not used psychiatric medications between hospitalizations, and 44% did not seek outpatient aftercare. Additionally, 72.3% stated that they believed aftercare would be beneficial, but only 28.3% followed through with any consistency. The authors reported that "... nonuse of prescribed medication appears to be highly related to re-admission, while regular use of medication appears to be highly associated with non-hospitalization ..." (Serban & Thomas, 1974, p. 993).

Clearly, refusal of or failure to participate in and cooperate with treatment is very widespread and results in higher rates of exacerbation of people's illness and resultant rehospitalization.

Perceptions of Symptoms and Conditions

One important determinant of the refusal of people with SMI to participate in prescribed treatment is their perception of their own illness. As noted, many people with SMI have limited insight into their illness and do not recognize that they have a mental illness. This perception often leads to treatment refusal.

Green (1988) found that 44% of those people who were frequently hospitalized for psychiatric care denied their illness; this denial correlated highly with their failure to take medications between hospitalizations and to participate in aftercare services.

Several studies have focused on subgroups within the diverse population of people with SMI to determine whether people with particular patterns of symptomatology vary in their understanding of their illness and their consequent level of refusal. Van Putten, Crumpton, and Yale (1976) compared 29 medication refusers with 30 medication acceptors. They found that while the groups did not differ in the severity of their illness, the medication refusers tended to become grandiose when they were symptomatic, while those who accepted medications tended to become depressed and anxious when symptomatic. Thus, those whose symptoms were more acceptable to themselves were more likely to refuse to accept the medications that removed the symptoms, while those whose symptoms produced more suffering were more likely to accept medications to relieve their distress. Similarly, Wilson and Enoch (1967) reported in their study of 48 people with schizophrenia that those with paranoid delusions tended to reject medications more frequently, possibly because the delusions were of a grandiose nature that was more reinforcing and less noxious than were the symptoms of those without paranoid delusions. Roth, Appelbaum, Sallee, Reynolds, and Huber (1982) and Van Putten (1975) reported similar findings.

Marder et al. (1983) compared 15 voluntary inpatients who refused to consent to medications with 15 who consented. Those who refused received significantly higher scores on the Brief Psychiatric Rating Scale than did those who consented, suggesting that people who refused medications tended to have more severe illness than those who did not. This finding would suggest that people whose illness was more severe had less insight, and consequently less perceived need for medication treatment, a hypothesis that would tend to be confirmed by the fact that the authors found that medication refusers were significantly more likely to believe that they were not ill.

Zito, Routt, Mitchell, and Roerig (1985) examined the diagnoses of people with psychotic disorders who either refused or accepted medication treatment. Of people diagnosed with bipolar illness, 75% refused medications, while only 31% of those diagnosed with schizophrenia refused medications. Of those with a diagnosis of schizoaffective disorder, 62% refused medication. This finding would suggest that those with affective disorders are more likely to refuse medications, which would be consistent with the hypothesis that symptoms that have a less negative impact are less likely to motivate persons to accept treatment to relieve these symptoms.

Side Effects

Another consistent finding relating to treatment refusal is the impact of negative side effects as a determinant. Van Putten (1978) postulated that the development of uncomfortable side effects is a major reason that people stop taking their medications. The side effects of psychiatric medications include tardive dyskinesia, dry mouth, impotence, changes in energy and affect, sedating effects, and depersonalization experiences.

Of course, as Kane (1983, p. 3) points out, "compliance is frequently discussed as an 'all-or-nothing' phenomenon, when in fact it is most often partial. Many patients take less medication than prescribed, take it irregularly, or take excessive amounts at certain times." Van Putten (1974) found that a group of people with schizophrenia took less medication than prescribed over a 2-year period, but did take some medication. He found that the reluctance to take antipsychotic medications was significantly associated with side effects; 89% of those who were "drug-reluctant" had side effects, while only 20% of those who were not drug-reluctant experienced significant side effects.

Cournos, McKinnon, and Adams (1988) reported that 21 patients in a state hospital in New York who refused psychotropic medications were evaluated to determine whether forced medication was justified. In 19 of the 21 cases, negative side effects were cited as being part of the reason for medication refusal; in 11 of these cases, the negative side effects were the sole reason for refusal.

Herz and Melville (1980) and Rodenhauser, Schwenkner, and Khamis (1987) found similar results regarding the role that side effects play in medication refusal, although Rodenhauser et al. (1987) found relatively few medication refusers citing side effects as a major cause of their refusal.

Attitudes toward Treatment

Another determinant of treatment compliance is patients' attitude toward treatment. Shannon (1976) compared 56 voluntary psychiatric inpatients with 44 involuntary patients and found that 50% of the involuntary patients expressed anger about coming to the hospital. The involuntary patients were also more likely to harbor negative expectations of hospital care, expressing beliefs such as that the hospital was a "prison without cells," that it was not the right place for them to be treated, or that they did not require treatment.

Schwartz, Bingiano, and Perez (1988) studied 24 involuntarily medicated patients in a psychiatric hospital. Following forced medication, 17 of the 24 patients expressed the belief that their treatment refusal had been correctly overridden by staff, and they indicated that they would want to be involuntarily medicated should the same circumstances reoccur. Those who continued to disapprove of the involuntary medication were found to be characterized as being highly grandiose, engaging in denial of psychotic proportions, and responding poorly to treatment. Srinivasan, Soundararajan, and Hullan (1980) reported that of 20 patients involuntarily admitted to a psychiatric hospital, 15 subsequently reported that their forced admission was appropriate.

Intervention to Increase Adherence

A number of studies have examined interventions that might improve medication adherence. Seltzer, Roncari, and Garfinkel (1980) studied 67 inpatients at a psychiatric hospital. They divided the subjects into two groups. The experimental group was provided with a series of nine lectures regarding mental illness, including information on medications, symptoms, and other matters. The control group was not provided with this educational series. At 5-month followup after hospital discharge, it was found that 66% of those who had not received the educational series were not taking their medications as prescribed, while only 9% of those in the experimental group were noncompliant. The investigators also found that those people who were living alone were more likely to be noncompliant, although this finding is another one that may confuse cause and effect: Does living alone tend to cause people to be noncompliant, or do noncompliant people tend to end up living alone because they are more likely to be disruptive to others? Seltzer et al. (1980) also found that the subjects in their experimental group were less frightened of side effects and less frightened of becoming

addicted to their medications than were the controls.

Blackwell (1976) reported that adherence to treatment is reduced as treatment regimens become more complex. Brown, Wright, and Christensen (1987) failed to find that a series of educational presentations regarding psychiatric medications and their side effects increased medication compliance in a group of 30 people with severe mental illness, although the study did not use a control group design. They did find, however, that knowledge of medications and side effects was increased by the educational series and that the reporting of side effects was reduced.

Myers and Calvert (1978) studied 66 people with major depression who were receiving outpatient care. They divided the subjects into three groups. Group A were told that they were being given medication to cure depression. Group B were given this same information, but were also given information about side effects. Group C were given the same information as Groups A and B, but were also given written information regarding these topics. The subjects were then evaluated for medication compliance. Group C had 100% compliance, which was significantly greater than that of Group B (68%) or Group A (64%).

Myers and Calvert (1984) studied 120 people with depression, also dividing their subjects into three groups. Group A were given verbal and written information on side effects. Group B were given verbal and written information on the beneficial effects of the medication. Group C were given no information. After 3 weeks, 89.2% of the subjects in Groups A and B were compliant with medication, while compliance in Group C was significantly less at 75%.

Thus, while there is some evidence that certain interventions may produce improvement in treatment compliance, the research has focused only on interventions related to sharing of information, and the results have been relatively modest, though statistically significant.

The Antipsychiatry Movement

Unlike many other special populations, people with SMI have an organized movement that challenges and rejects the health care system that has been developed to serve them. This movement includes primarily people who have SMI themselves, as well as some people in the mental health professional ranks. Most notable among the latter is Thomas Szasz (1974), whose *The Myth of Mental Illness: Foundation of a Theory of Personal Conduct* lashes out at the mental health community and mental health treatment attitudes and beliefs relating to people with SMI. The *Madness Network News*, an antipsychiatry newspaper published in San Francisco, focuses on the mental health profession as a group of oppressors who serve political interests and whose personal motives are often pathologically based on a need for power and control over those with SMI.

While it is tempting for many within the mental health professions to dismiss the antipsychiatry movement as being yet another manifestation of the participants' own mental illness, they are not so easily dismissed. While some of the more virulent rhetoric of the movement attacks all aspects of mental health care, including particularly medication and shock treatment, even the most ardent supporters of the mental health care system must admit that there are many problems inherent in the somatic treatments for mental illness. Furthermore, the argument over forced treatment, which is at the heart of Szasz's writings, has much more to do with the philosophical debate over personal freedom than it does with a challenge to the efficacy of the treatment itself.

The willingness of people with SMI to participate in treatment has a number of clear determinants, among which are insight, negative iatrogenic effects of treatment, and the politics of self-determination and freedom. Regardless of the cause, the preponderance of research evidence supports the fact that failure of people with SMI to fully seek access to and participate in mental health care treatment is a common characteristic of the population.

THE MENTAL PATIENT SICK ROLE

For people with SMI, their identification as "mental patient" often supersedes all other characteristics that they might have, much as is the case with other severely disabled populations. The process by which a person with SMI assumes the role of being a mental patient was characterized by Lally (1989), who described three stages of the process.

In the beginning stage, the individual experiences admission to psychiatric hospitals, which are often accompanied by denial of pathology on the patient's part, a minimizing of symptomatology, and a strong focus on areas of competence. The most commonly reported experience that led mentally ill people to recognize and acknowledge that they were ill was the occurrence of hallucinations at a time when they had enough insight to realize that their experiences were not reflective of actual external stimuli—that they were not actual sensations but were hallucinatory in nature. Rarely did people in the beginning stage of adopting the illness role recognize other symptoms as reflecting pathology. Subsequent and repeated psychiatric hospitalizations, however, tended to contribute to what Lally refers to as the "engulfment" of the people into the mental patient sick role.

The middle stage of the process involves acceptance on the part of the ill individuals that they have psychiatric problems, but some level of unsureness of whether these problems will be permanent or not. Beginning to receive disability benefits from the Social Security Administration—either Supplemental Security Income for people determined to be disabled but with little or no work history or Social Security Disability Income for those with a more significant work history—often leads people to begin to see themselves as being permanently disabled and to further assume, or be engulfed by, the mental patient sick role. Another important event reported by Lally is people's hearing their diagnosis; being labeled with the diagnosis of "schizophrenia" implies permanency, while a more vague label, such as "nerve problems," can be believed to be possibly temporary.

The late stage of the engulfment process is characterized by individuals' coming to view themselves as being mentally ill and the illness becoming the totality of their identity. One important part of this stage is mourning for the lost former identity as a "normal" person.

The adoption of the mental patient sick role is, ironically, an important determinant of the failure of people with SMI to seek out or receive physical health care services. As indicated, people with SMI are often seen by health professionals simply as "mental patients," rather than as people with a heightened set of risk factors for physical illnesses. Since reported symptoms of physical illness often fail to lead to the identification of an illness in a person with SMI, such reports can easily be discounted and ignored. Meanwhile, the symptoms that typically alert the patient and the health professional to an illness are often masked or misinterpreted. Perhaps no special population is as negatively affected by the adoption of the sick role identity as are people with SMI.

RESEARCH METHODOLOGY ISSUES

There are several key issues relating to the methodology of research into health behaviors of people with SMI that create difficulties in interpreting findings and also tend to discourage investigators from carrying out research in the field; the relative dearth of research findings amply testifies to these disincentives.

The first and foremost methodological issue is the question of definition. The population of people with SMI is extremely diverse, including people with a variety of disorders with varying etiological factors related to their illnesses. Studies reported herein have included widely varying subject selection procedures, e.g., studies limiting participation to people with particular diagnoses, studies including all people admitted to an inpatient treatment unit, and studies including all people served in a particular outpatient setting. These subject groups can in no way be considered comparable, and the generalizability of many studies is questionable.

A second methodological issue is the fact that the vast majority of studies have no control groups for comparison purposes. Indeed, the general area of research on the SMI population suffers from the lack of comparison groups and the difficulty of defining and obtaining such groups. Related to these problems is the fact that most of the reports in the literature are not experimental studies at all, but simply postfacto findings, surveys, or what amounts to case reports.

For instance, one might logically conclude from reports of studies on medication noncompliance that the need for hospitalization would be reduced if people with SMI could be convinced to be more compliant with their medication (e.g., Green, 1988; L. D. Smith, 1989). While this may well be the case, an alternative hypothesis might also be considered: People whose illness is more severe, and who might require more frequent hospitalizations, are people who have less insight into their illness and are therefore more likely to be noncompliant with prescribed medications. They might well have a higher need for hospitalization regardless of whether they took their medications or not. Only a study that utilized an experimental design in which patients being discharged from a psychiatric hospital were randomly assigned to a group either receiving psychiatric medications or not receiving such medications could actually clarify this chicken-and-egg conundrum, and such a study would obviously be difficult, if not impossible, to carry out.

Another problem with research on people with SMI is the potential confounding factor of socioeconomic status. Since a very high proportion of people with SMI are also living in poverty, any study of health behaviors must entertain the alternative hypothesis that its findings are simply reflective of the health behaviors of people in lower socioeconomic groups, and not the result of SMI at all. Few studies have adequately addressed this issue.

CONCLUSION

Research on health behavior in people with severe mental illness suggests that this special population has a number of characteristics that make it differ significantly from the general public. People with SMI tend to fail to seek out and utilize health care services, and health professionals tend to ignore the health care needs of the severely mentally ill. People with SMI tend to be impaired in the extent to which they practice protective and preventive behaviors, and they often reject health care and mental health care services that are offered to them.

The determinants of these differentiating behaviors are primarily based on disruptions in sensation, perception, and interpretation of the signs and symptoms of both physical illness and mental illness itself. A common and unifying characteristic of people with SMI is a tendency to be unable to recognize and take appropriate actions relating to illness.

REFERENCES

Adler, N. E., Boyce, T., Chesney, M. A., Cohen, S, Folkman, S., Kahn, R. L., & Syme, S. L. (1994). Socioeconomic status and health: The challenge of the gradient. *American Psychologist, 49,* 15–24.

Alexopoulos, G. S. (1979). Lack of complaints in schizophrenics with tardive dyskinesia. *Journal of Nervous and Mental Disease, 167,* 125–127.

Amador, X. F., Strauss, S. A. Y., & Gorman, J. M. (1991). Awareness of illness in schizophrenia. *Schizophrenia Bulletin, 17,* 113–132.

American Psychiatric Association (1994). *Diagnostic and statistical manual of mental disorders,* (4th ed). Washington: American Psychiatric Association.

Anscombe, R. (1987). The disorder of consciousness in schizophrenia. *Schizophrenia Bulletin, 13,* 241–260.

Appelbaum, P. S., & Gutheil, T. G. (1980). Drug refusal: A study of psychiatric inpatients. *American Journal of Psychiatry, 137,* 340–346.

Atkinson, R. M. (1971). AMA and AWOL discharges: A six-year comparative study. *Hospital and Community Psychiatry, 22,* 293–296.

Bachrach, L. L. (1988). Defining chronic mental illness: A concept paper. *Hospital and Community Psychiatry, 39,* 383–388.

Baer, J. W., Dwyer, P. C., & Lewitter-Koehler, S. (1988). Knowledge about AIDS among psychiatric inpatients. *Hospital and Community Psychiatry, 39,* 986–988.

Barbee, J. G., Clark, P. D., Carpanzano, M. S., Heintz, G. C., & Kehoe, C. E. (1989). Alcohol and substance abuse among schizophrenic patients presenting to an emergency psychiatry service. *Journal of Nervous and Mental Disease, 177,* 400–407.

Barry, K. L., Fleming, M. F., Greenley, J., Widlak, P., Kropp, S., & McKee, D. (1995). Assessment of alcohol and other drug disorders in the seriously mentally ill. *Schizophrenia Bulletin, 21,* 313–321.

Blackwell, B. (1976). Treatment adherence. *British Journal of Psychiatry, 129,* 513–531.

Bleuler, E. (1950). *Dementia praecox, or the group of schizophrenias.* New York: International Universities Press.

Bockes, Z. (1985). First person account: "Freedom" means knowing you have a choice. *Schizophrenia Bulletin, 11,* 487–489.

Braginsky, B. M., Braginsky, D., & Ring, K. (1969). *Methods of madness: The mental hospital as a last resort.* New York: Holt, Rinehart & Winston.

Brown, C. S., Wright, R. G., & Christensen, D. B. (1987). Association between type of medication instruction and patients' knowledge, side effects, and compliance. *Hospital and Community Psychiatry, 38,* 55–60.

Bunce, D. F., Jones, L. R., Badger, L. W., & Jones, S. E. (1982). Medical illness in psychiatric patients: Barriers to diagnosis and treatment. *Southern Medical Journal, 75,* 941–944.

Caracco, G., Muhkerjee, S., Roth, S., & Decina, P. (1990). Subjective awareness of abnormal involuntary movements in chronic schizophrenic patients. *American Journal of Psychiatry, 147,* 295–298.

Carmen, E., & Brady, S. M. (1990). AIDS risk and prevention for the chronic mentally ill. *Hospital and Community Psychiatry, 41,* 652–657.

Carpenter, M. D., Mulligan, J. C., Bader, I.A., & Meinzer, A. E. (1985). Multiple admissions to an urban psychiatric center: A comparative study. *Hospital and Community Psychiatry, 36,* 1305–1308.

Chase, M. (1944). *Harvey: Comedy in three acts..* New York: Dramatists Play Service.

Cournos, F., Empfield, M., Horvath, E., McKinnon, K., Meyer,

I., Schrage, H., Currie C., & Agosin, B. (1991). HIV seroprevalence among patients admitted to two psychiatric hospitals. *American Journal of Psychiatry, 148*, 1225–1230.

Cournos, F., Guido, J. R., Coomaraswamy, M. D., Meyer-Bahlburg, H., Snyden, R., & Horwath, E. (1994). Sexual activity and risk of HIV infection among patients with schizophrenia. *American Journal of Psychiatry, 151*, 228–232.

Cournos, F., McKinnon, K., & Adams, C. (1988). A comparison of clinical and judicial procedures for reviewing requests for involuntary medication in New York. *Hospital and Community Psychiatry, 39*, 851–855.

Coverdale, J. H., & Aruffo, J. F. (1992). AIDS and family planning counseling of psychiatrically ill women in community mental health clinics. *Community Mental Health Journal, 28*, 13–20.

Davis, G. C., Buchsbaum, M. S., & Bunney, W. E. (1979). Analgesia to painful stimuli in affective illness. *American Journal of Psychiatry, 136*, 1148–1151.

Dworkin, R. H. (1994). Pain insensitivity in schizophrenia: A neglected phenomenon and some implications. *Schizophrenia Bulletin, 20*, 235–248.

Faden, R., & Faden, A. (1977). False belief and the refusal of medical treatment. *Journal of Medical Ethics, 3*, 133–136.

Frank, L. R. (1986). The policies and practices of American psychiatry are oppressive. *Hospital and Community Psychiatry, 37*, 497–501.

Freddolino, P. P., Moxley, D. P., & Fleishman, J. A. (1988). Daily living needs at time of discharge: Implications for advocacy. *Psychosocial Rehabilitation Journal, 11*, 32–46.

Gelberg, L., & Linn, L. S. (1988). Social and physical health of homeless adults previously treated for mental health problems. *Hospital and Community Psychiatry, 39*, 510–516.

Goff, D. C., Henderson, D. C., & Amico, B. X. (1992). Cigarette smoking in schizophrenia: Relationship to psychopathology and medication side effects. *American Journal of Psychiatry, 149*, 1189–1194.

Gove, W. R., & Fain, T. (1977). A comparison of voluntary and committed psychiatric patients. *Archives of General Psychiatry, 34*, 669–676.

Green, J. H. (1988). Frequent rehospitalization and noncompliance with treatment. *Hospital and Community Psychiatry, 39*, 963–966.

Greenfield, D., Strauss, J. S., Bowers, M. B., & Mandelkern, M. (1989). Insight and interpretation of illness in recovery from psychosis. *Schizophrenia Bulletin, 15*, 245–252.

Hall, K. R. L., & Stride, E. (1954). The varying response to pain in psychiatric disorders: A study in abnormal psychology. *British Journal of Medical Psychology, 27*, 48–60.

Hall, R. C., Beresford, T. P., Gardner, E. R., & Popkin, M. K. (1982). The medical care of psychiatric patients. *Hospital and Community Psychiatry, 33*, 25–34.

Hall, R. C., Gardner, E. P., Popkin, M. D., LeCann, A. F., &

Stickney, R. N. (1981). Unrecognized physical illness prompting psychiatric admission: A prospective study. *American Journal of Psychiatry, 138*, 629–635.

Harris, A. E. (1988). Physical disease and schizophrenia. *Schizophrenia Bulletin, 14*, 87–96.

Heinrichs, D. W., Cohen, B. P., & Carpenter, W. T. (1985). Early insight and the management of schizophrenia decompensation. *Journal of Nervous and Mental Disease, 173*, 133–138.

Herz, M. I., & Melville, C. (1980). Relapse in schizophrenia. *American Journal of Psychiatry, 137*, 801–805.

Hogarty, G. E., Goldberg, S. C., and the Collaborative Study Group. (1973). Drug and sociotherapy in the aftercare of schizophrenic patients. *Archives of General Psychiatry, 28*, 54–63.

Hughes, J. R. (1993). Possible effects of smoke-free inpatient units on psychiatric diagnosis and treatment. *Journal of Clinical Psychiatry, 54*, 109–114.

Hughes, J. R., & Frances, R. J. (1995). How to help psychiatric patients stop smoking. *Psychiatric Services, 46*, 435–436.

Hussar, A. E. (1965). Coronary heart disease in chronic schizophrenic patients: A clinicopathologic study. *Circulation, 31*, 919–929.

Kalichman, S. C., Kelly, J. A., Johnson, J. R., & Bulto, M. (1994). Factors associated with risk for HIV infection among chronic mentally ill adults. *American Journal of Psychiatry, 151*, 221–227.

Kalman, T. P. (1983). An overview of patient satisfaction with psychiatric treatment. *Hospital and Community Psychiatry, 34*, 48–53.

Kane, J. M. (1983). Problems of compliance in the outpatient treatment of schizophrenia. *Journal of Clinical Psychiatry, 44*, 3–6.

Karasu, T. B., Waltzman, S. W., Lindenmayer, J., & Buckley, P. J. (1980). The medical care of patients with psychiatric illness. *Hospital and Community Psychiatry, 31*, 463–472.

Katz, E., Kluger, Y., Rabiniovici, R., Stein, D., & Gimmon, Z. (1990). Acute surgical abdominal disease in chronic schizophrenic patients: A unique clinical problem. *Israel Journal of Medical Sciences, 26*, 275–277.

Kelly, J. A., Murphy, D. A., Sikkema, K. J., Somlai, A. M., Mulry, G. W., Fernandez, I., Miller, J. G., & Stevenson, L. Y. (1995). Predictors of high and low levels of HIV risk behavior among adults with chronic mental illness. *Psychiatric Services, 46*, 813–818.

Koranyi, E. K. (1977). Fatalities in 1070 psychiatric outpatients: Preventive features. *Archives of General Psychiatry, 34*, 1137–1142.

Koranyi, E. K. (1979). Morbidity and rates of undiagnosed physical illnesses in a psychiatric clinic. *Archives of General Psychiatry, 36*, 414–419.

Koranyi, E. K. (1980). Somatic illness in psychiatric patients. *Psychosomatics, 21*, 887–891.

Kraepelin, E. (1919). *Dementia praecox and paraphrenia*. Edinburgh, Scotland: E. & S. Livingstone.

Lally, S. J. (1989). "Does being in here mean there is something wrong with me?" *Schizophrenia Bulletin, 15*, 253–265.

Lee, H., Travin, W., & Blustone, H. (1992). HIV-1 in inpatients. *Hospital and Community Psychiatry, 43*, 181–182.

Leete, E. (1989). How I perceive and manage my illness. *Schizophrenia Bulletin, 15*, 197–200.

Levinson, D. J., & Gallagher, E. B. (1964). *Patienthood in the mental hospital.* Boston: Houghton-Mifflin.

Lieberman, A. L. (1955). Painless myocardial infarction in psychotic patients. *Geriatrics, 10*, 579–580.

Lin, I. F., Spiga, R., & Fortsch, W. (1979). Insight and adherence to medication in chronic schizophrenia. *Journal of Clinical Psychiatry, 40*, 430–432.

Lucksted, A., & Coursey, R. D. (1995). Consumer perceptions of pressure and force in psychiatric treatments. *Psychiatric Services, 46*, 146–152.

Marchand, W. E. (1955). Occurrence of painless myocardial infarction in psychotic patients. *New England Journal of Medicine, 253*, 51–55.

Marchand, W. E. (1958). The practice of medicine in a neuropsychiatric hospital. *Archives of Neurology and Psychiatry, 80*, 599–611.

Marchand, W. E., Sarota, B., Marble, H. C., Leary, T. M., Burbank, C. B., & Bellinger, M. J. (1959). Occurrence of painless acute surgical disorders in psychotic patients. *New England Journal of Medicine, 260*, 580–585.

Marder, S. R., Mebane, A., Chien, C., Winslade, W. J., Swann, E., & Van Putten, T. (1983). A comparison of patients who refuse and consent to neuroleptic treatment. *American Journal of Psychiatry, 140*, 470–472.

Maricle, R. A., Hoffman, W. F., Bloom, J. D., Faulkner, L. R., & Keepers, G. A. (1987). The prevalence and significance of medical illness among chronically mentally ill outpatients. *Community Mental Health Journal, 23*, 81–90.

May, P. R. A. (1948). Pupillary abnormalities in schizophrenia and during muscular effort. *Journal of Mental Science, 94*, 89–98.

McCandless-Glimcher, L., McKnight, S., Hamera, E., Smith, B. L., Petersen, K., & Plumlee, A.A. (1986). Use of symptoms by schizophrenics to monitor and regulate their illness. *Hospital and Community Psychiatry, 37*, 929–933.

McEvoy, J. P., Appelbaum, P. S., Geller, J. L., & Freter, S. (1989). Why must some schizophrenic patients be involuntarily committed? The role of insight. *Comprehensive Psychiatry, 30*, 13–17.

McIntyre, J. S., & Romano, J. (1978). Is there a stethoscope in the house (and is it used)? *Archives of General Psychiatry, 34*, 1147–1151.

Meyer, I., McKinnon, K., Cournos, F., Empfield, M., Bavli, S., Engel, D., & Weinstock, A. (1993). HIV seroprevalence among long-stay patients in a state psychiatric hospital. *Hospital and Community Psychiatry, 44*, 282–284.

Mueser, K. T., Yarnold, P. R., Levinson, D. R., Singh, H., Bellack, A. S., Kee, K., Morrison, R. L., & Yadalam, K. G. (1990). Prevalence of substance abuse in schizophrenia: Demographic and clinical correlates. *Schizophrenia Bulletin, 16*, 31–56.

Mulkern, V., & Bradley, V. J. (1986). Service utilization and service preference of homeless persons. *Psychosocial Rehabilitation Journal, 10*, 23–29.

Myers, E. D., & Calvert, E. J. (1978). Knowledge of side effects and perseverence with medication. *British Journal of Psychiatry, 132*, 526–527.

Myers, E. D., & Calvert, E. J. (1984). Information, compliance and side effects: A study of patients on antidepressant medication. *British Journal of Clinical Pharmacology, 17*, 21–25.

Patterson, C. W. (1978). Psychiatrists and physical examinations: A survey. *Amerian Journal of Psychiatry, 135*, 967–968.

Phillips, R. J. (1937). Physical disorder in 164 consecutive admissions to a mental hospital. *British Medical Journal, 1937(2)* 363–366.

Roca, R. P., Breakey, W. R., & Fischer, P. J. (1987). Medical care of chronic psychiatric outpatients. *Hospital and Community Psychiatry, 38*, 741–745.

Rodenhauser, P., Schwenkner, C. E., & Khamis, H. J. (1987). Factors related to drug treatment refusal in a forensic hospital. *Hospital and Community Psychiatry, 38*, 631–637.

Rogers, J. A., & Centifanti, J. (1988). Madness, myths and reality: Response to Roberta Rose. *Schizophrenia Bulletin, 14*, 7–15.

Rose, R. (1988). Schizophrenia, civil liberties, and the law. *Schizophrenia Bulletin, 14*, 1–16.

Rosen, A. M., Mukherjee, S., Olarte, S., Varia, V., & Cardenas, C. (1982). Perception of tardive dyskinesia in out-patients receiving maintenance neuroleptics. *American Journal of Psychiatry, 139*, 372–373.

Roth, L. H., Appelbaum, P. S., Sallee, R., Reynolds, C. F., & Huber, G. (1982). The dilemma of denial in the assessment of competency to refuse treatment. *American Journal of Psychiatry, 139*, 910–913.

Sacks, M., Dermatis, H., Burton, W., Hull, J., & Perry, S. (1994). Acute psychiatric illness: Effects on HIV-risk behavior. *Psychosocial Rehabilitation Journal, 17*, 5–18.

Sacks, M. H., Perry S., Graver, R., Shindledecker, R., & Hall, S. (1990). Self-reported HIV-related risk behaviors in acute psychiatric inpatients: A pilot study. *Hospital and Community Psychiatry, 41*, 1253–1255.

Sacks, M. H., Silberstein, C., Weiler, P., & Perry, S. (1990). HIV-related risk factors in acute psychiatric inpatients. *Hospital and Community Psychiatry, 41*, 449–451.

Schwartz, H. I., Bingiano, W., & Perez, C. B. (1988). Autonomy and the right to refuse treatment: Patients' attitudes after involuntary medication. *Hospital and Community Psychiatry, 39*, 1049–1054.

Seltzer, A., Roncari, I., & Garfinkel, P. (1980). Effect of patient education on medication compliance. *Canadian Journal of Psychiatry, 25*, 638–645.

Serban, G., & Thomas, A. (1974). Attitudes and behaviors of

acute and chronic schizophrenic patients regarding ambulatory treatment. *American Journal of Psychiatry, 131,* 991–995.

Shannon, P. J. (1976). Coercion and compulsory hospitalization: Some patients' attitudes. *Medical Journal of Australia, 2,* 798–800.

Smith, J. M., Kucharski, L. T., Oswald, W. T., & Waterman, L. J. (1979). A systematic investigation of tardive dyskinesia in inpatients. *American Journal of Psychiatry, 136,* 918–922.

Smith, L. D. (1989). Medication refusal and the rehospitalized mentally ill inmate. *Hospital and Community Psychiatry, 40,* 491–496.

Srinivasan, D. P., Soundararajan, P. C., & Hullin, R. P. (1980). Attitudes of patients and relatives to compulsory admission. *British Journal of Psychiatry, 136,* 200–201.

Susser, E., Valencia, E., & Conover, S. (1993). Prevalence of HIV infection among psychiatric patients in a New York City men's shelter. *American Journal of Public Health, 83,* 568–570.

Szasz, T. (1974). *The myth of mental illness: Foundation of a theory of personal conduct.* New York: Harper & Row.

Van Putten, T. (1974). Why do schizophrenic patients refuse to take their drugs? *Archives of General Psychiatry, 31,* 67–72.

Van Putten, T. (1975). Why do patients with manic–depressive illness stop their lithium? *Comprehensive Psychiatry, 16,* 179–183.

Van Putten, T. (1978). Drug refusal in schizophrenia: Causes and prescribing hints. *Hospital and Community Psychiatry, 29,* 110–112.

Van Putten, T., Crumpton, E., & Yale, C. (1976). Drug refusal in schizophrenia and the wish to be crazy. *Archives of General Psychiatry, 33,* 1443–1446.

Watson, G. D., Chandarana, P. D., & Merskey, H. (1981). Relationships between pain and schizophrenia. *British Journal of Psychiatry, 138,* 33–36.

West, B. M., & Hecker, A. O. (1952). Peptic ulcer: Incidence and diagnosis in psychotic patients. *American Journal of Psychiatry, 109,* 35–37.

Wilson, J. D., & Enoch, M. D. (1967). Estimation of drug rejection by schizophrenic in-patients, with analysis of clinical factors. *British Journal of Psychiatry, 113,* 209–211.

Ziedonis, D. M., Kosten, T. R., Glazer, W. M., & Frances, R. J. (1994). Nicotine dependence and schizophrenia. *Hospital and Community Psychiatry, 45,* 204–206.

Zito, J. N., Routt, W. W., Mitchell, J. E., & Roerig, J. L. (1985). Clinical characteristics of hospitalized psychotic patients who refuse antipsychotic drug therapy. *American Journal of Psychiatry, 142,* 822–826.

13

Health Behavior of Caregivers

Lore K. Wright

INTRODUCTION

Approximately 8 million adult Americans provide personal care to an older, ill family member or close friend (Harper, 1991). These adults are known as "informal caregivers," and many studies have documented that caregiving responsibilities put them at risk for emotional and physical health problems (Schulz, Visintainer, & Williamson, 1990; Wright, Clipp, & George, 1993).

Health behaviors of informal caregivers, however, are far less well documented than their risks for health problems. In this chapter, available evidence of health-promoting and health risk-taking behaviors by caregivers is documented and barriers to engaging in health behaviors are explored. Special attention is given to the impact of cultural factors on health behaviors of minority caregivers. Throughout the chapter, researchers' and clinicians' lack of attention to health behaviors is pointed out, and the need for a paradigm shift is argued.

THE NATURE OF CAREGIVING

Caregiving often begins with providing limited assistance to an elder person to meet basic needs for transportation, shopping, hygiene, dressing, and nourishment. The need for assistance tends to escalate, however, until caregivers assume total responsibility for an impaired spouse, parent, or other relative. Responsibilities include bathing, feeding, toileting, and day and night supervision of activities to assure the elder's safety. These responsibilities become especially great when elders with memory impairment display agitated behaviors and aimless and restless wandering or when they have cognitive deficits that prevent them from managing their own affairs, or when both circumstances arise. Often, caregivers also assume financial and legal responsibilities for the impaired elder.

Caregiving, in summary, is time-consuming, labor-intensive, and stressful (Wright et al., 1993). Caregiving responsibilities can extend over many years, and it is precisely because caregivers are faced with never-ending demands that their own health and health-seeking behavior are threatened. C. H. Connell and Schulenberg (1990) found in analyzing spouse caregivers' health diaries and simultaneous recordings of caregiving responsibilities that spouse caregivers neglected their own self-care needs whenever the demands

Lore K. Wright • Department of Mental Health/Psychiatric Nursing, School of Nursing, Medical College of Georgia, Augusta, Georgia 30912-4220.

Handbook of Health Behavior Research III: Demography, Development, and Diversity, edited by David S. Gochman. Plenum Press, New York, 1997.

of caregiving increased. The same pattern held for adult children as caregivers. They deprived themselves of "needed medical care and rest periods because of their responsibilities to the parent" (Archbold, 1980, p. 83).

It is therefore surprising that very few studies provide detailed information about health behaviors of informal caregivers. In contrast, there are extensive data on caregivers' health status.

A NATIONAL PROFILE OF CAREGIVERS

Demographic Characteristics

Who are the informal caregivers, and what can be inferred from their demographic characteristics? The data clearly show that they are a population at risk for health problems.

While the average age of caregivers is 57 years, 25% are between 65 and 74 years old, and at least 10% are over the age of 75 (Stone, Cafferata, & Sangle, 1987). Of these older caregivers, approximately 80% are spouses, and wives are 2–3 times more likely to be caregivers than husbands (Stommel, Given, & Given, 1990; Stone et al., 1987). Approximately one third of older spouse caregivers report their incomes as poor or near-poor. Many have their own increasing health problems, yet most provide care to the ill spouse every day of the week.

An important characteristic to keep in mind is that 72% of all caregivers are women, of whom 23% are wives, 29% adult daughters, and 20% other females. By contrast, only 28% of all caregivers are men, of whom 13% are husbands, 8% sons, and 7% other males (Stone et al., 1987). Based on the 1982 National Long-Term Care Survey and Informal Caregivers Survey, 44% of caregiving daughters and 55% of caregiving sons are in the labor force (Stone et al., 1987). Some community surveys report higher employment rates for adult children as caregivers: 88% of sons and 62% of daughters are working (Horowitz, 1985), although women are much less likely than men to hold full-time jobs (Boaz & Muller, 1992).

A survey of major corporations highlights the issue of female caregivers in the labor force: While 1 in 4 employees reported having caregiving responsibilities for an elderly parent, 75% of these employees were women (Dussell & Roman, 1989). Among these women, 40% simultaneously cared for an elder person and raised their own children. Their caregiving "career" spanned many years: an average of 17 years caring for their children and 18 years caring for an elderly parent. One would anticipate these women to have different health needs and different patterns of health behaviors than older spouses in the caregiver role (Dussell & Roman, 1989; Suitor & Pillemer, 1990). Brody (1981) has called caregiving daughters and daughters-in-law "women in the middle" whose lives are characterized by role overload. The lives of caregiving spouses, on the other hand, are more intensely focused on one person: the ill spouse. The close bond between husband and wife and the caregiver's own failing health with increasing age add to the strain (Cantor, 1983).

Health Status

Numerous studies have documented that the stress or "burden" associated with caregiving has negative emotional and physical health consequences for caregivers (for comprehensive reviews on this subject, see Baumgarten, 1989; Schulz et al., 1990; Wright et al., 1993). Caregiving undoubtedly differs depending on the elder's type and severity of illness. Yet in most studies, type of illness, level of impairment, and length of illness correlate not at all or only weakly with caregivers' ill health (Deimling, Bass, Towsend, & Noelker, 1989; Holbrook, 1982; Pruchno, Kleban, Michaels, & Dempsey, 1990; Silliman, Fletcher, Earp, & Wagner, 1986; Snyder & Keefe, 1985; Stetz, 1987; Stommel et al., 1990). The exception is poorer *physical* health in caregivers of aphasic (left hemisphere stroke) persons and those with cancer (Artes & Hoops, 1976; Clipp & George, 1993).

Type of kin relationship does show differences, to some extent, in caregivers' health status. Based on standardized measures of *depression*, caregiver wives have the highest level of depression, followed by daughters, then other female caregivers, then sons, and then husband caregivers (Gallagher, Rose, Rivera, Lovett, & Koin, 1989). The pattern of poorer emotional health in women than in men holds among caregivers of cognitively and physically impaired, stroke, heart disease, and cancer patients (Biegel, Sales, & Schulz, 1991; Gallagher et al., 1989; Schulz, Tompkins, & Rau, 1988; Tennstedt, Cafferata, & Sullivan, 1992; Young & Kahana, 1989).

Rates of depression in caregivers range from 28% to 55%, while comparable rates for the general population are 14–16% (Blazer & Williams, 1980; Miller, 1987; Stommel et al., 1990; Tennstedt & McKinlay, 1989). Depression in caregivers may have been overestimated, however, since many suffer from transient dysphoric moods but do not show extreme depression scores that would indicate severe depression (Brody, Dempsey, & Pruchno, 1990; C. M. Connell, 1994; Kiecolt-Glaser, Dyer, & Shuttleworth, 1988; Neundorfer, 1991; Pruchno et al., 1990). Sample bias may also contribute to the reported high rates of depression, since many researchers recruit subjects from support groups or evaluation clinics. For example, Gallagher et al. (1989) showed that 68% of caregivers who volunteered to participate in "Coping with Caregiving" classes had depressive symptomatology, yet only 36% of caregivers who did not seek professional help could be classified as such.

Findings regarding *physical health* show similar trends: Spouses, compared to others in the caregiver role, have poorer health, and many attribute physical decline to caregiving responsibilities (Cantor, 1983; Deimling et al., 1989; George & Gwyther, 1986; Pruchno & Potashnik, 1989; Stommel et al., 1990; Stone et al., 1987; Tennstedt & McKinlay, 1989). Differences between spouses and caregiving daughters, however, are often small and not statistically significant (Deimling et al., 1989).

There is conflicting evidence regarding the physical health of husband versus wife caregivers; some data suggest that females are more negatively affected by caregiving (Fitting, Rabins, Lucas, & Eastham, 1986; Miller, 1987; Miller, McFall, & Montgomery, 1991; Pruchno & Potashnik, 1989), while others document greater negative health impact for male spouses (Eagles, Beattie, Blackwood, Restall, & Ashcroft, 1987; Moritz, Kasl, & Berkman, 1989; Moritz, Kasl, & Ostfeld, 1992).

Regardless of whether the focus is emotional or physical health, the caregivers' income is an important consideration. High income and other financial resources can promote health-seeking behavior, while low income and poor resources create barriers. Indeed, several studies showed that lower income and financial concerns other long periods of caregiving contribute to emotional illness (Clipp & George, 1990a; Moritz et al., 1989; Schulz et al., 1988; Tennstedt et al., 1991), while high income and education seem to lower the risk of depression in caregivers (Gallagher-Thompson, Walsh, Lovett, & Koin, 1991; Walsh, Yoash-Gantz, Rinki, Koin, & Gallagher-Thompson, 1991).

For physical health, the data are less clear. High income is associated with better health in some studies (Gallagher-Thompson et al., 1991; Walsh et al., 1991), but other studies show that even caregivers with incomes above that of community controls report poor health (Kiecolt-Glaser et al., 1987). Yet another study reports that not income but high out-of-pocket expenses for caregiving are associated with poor health (Stommel et al., 1990).

Undoubtedly, caregivers are a population at risk. But to what extent do they engage in health behaviors?

HEALTH BEHAVIOR OF CAREGIVERS

Definition and Measures of Health Behaviors

Following the definition that guides this *Handbook*, the term *health behavior* refers to personal attributes, overt behavior patterns, actions, and habits "that relate to health maintenance, to health restoration, and to health improvement" (Gochman, 1983, p. 3). Very few caregiver studies use this conceptualization, and pertinent questions regarding health behaviors are not included in the National Informal Caregivers Survey.

The limited data available on this subject have to be extracted from studies that focused on caregiver stress and illness and the mediating variables of coping and social support. A notable exception is the work by C. M. Connell (1994), who questioned caregivers about changes in health behavior in the time since they assumed care for a cognitively impaired spouse. Connell's study, which includes data on nutritious meals, exercise, smoking, and alcohol intake, will be discussed in more detail later.

The most frequently cited indicators of health behavior in the caregiving literature are number of doctor visits in the past year, number of days sick in bed at home or in the hospital, the use of psychotropic medications, and coping and stress reduction activities. Interestingly, however, researchers rarely refer to these indicators as behaviors aimed at maintaining, restoring, or improving health (a notable exception being, again, the work of Connell [1994]). In the majority of caregiver studies, behaviors are conceptualized as stress responses to the caregiving situation, and whether the caregivers' actions were intended to restore or improve health is not addressed.

For example, in the study of Gallagher et al. (1989) mentioned earlier, a large percentage of depressed caregivers volunteered to participate in "Coping with Caregiving" classes. While caregivers did not seek treatment for depression, they nevertheless engaged in health-seeking behavior: They recognized the need to learn effective coping strategies. In caregiving research, however, this motivation becomes an issue of "sample bias" and is not conceptualized as health-seeking behavior.

The example points to another important issue: Caregivers themselves define their actions mostly in relation to the elders' illness and the demands caregiving makes on their time and energy. Many caregivers (76%) worry about their own health, but engaging in health behavior tends not to be the focus of their thinking and coping strategies (Barusch, 1988). It is possible, however, that this situation will change as caregiving research moves from predominantly descriptive studies to testing the efficacy of intervention programs.

Evidence of Health Behaviors

Use of Formal Health Services.   Given the large percentage of older caregivers and the high rate of depressive symptoms and physical health problems among caregivers, one would expect a high degree of health behavior such as spending more days in bed to get some rest and frequent utilization of formal health care services. In the general population, older persons and those with more physical health problems see physicians significantly more often than those who are younger and healthier (Mutran & Ferraro, 1988). Depressed persons have more frequent doctor visits than those who are physically ill (Katon, 1985). Epidemiological surveys also show that persons with depressive symptoms seek physician services at higher rates than those with a formal diagnosis of clinical depression. The services sought by people with depressive symptoms include emergency department use, medical counseling for emotional problems, requests for sleeping pills or psychotropic medications, and treatment for suicide attempts (Johnson, Weissman, & Klerman, 1992).

Caregivers, however, do not follow this pattern. Instead, caregivers report fewer days in the hospital, fewer days sick in bed at home, and physician visits less frequent or about as frequent as age-matched community controls (Pruchno & Potashnik, 1989). Specifically, caregiver spouses, daughters, and other family members report an average of 2 physician visits per year, while comparable community groups report 3–5 yearly visits (George & Gwyther, 1986). Even when the data are broken down for specific age groups of 45–64, 65–74, and 75 years and older, spouse caregivers in each group visit the physician less frequently than age-matched groups in the general population (Pruchno & Potashnik, 1989).

In two studies, a control group design was used instead of comparing findings to national or community norms. The researchers found that spouses and other family caregivers reported more frequent doctor visits than controls obtained through local senior citizen centers, other groups, and newspaper advertisements. Controls were matched with the caregivers on demographic variables such as age, gender, race, education, and marital status (Haley, Levine, Brown, Berry, & Hughes, 1987; Kiecolt-Glaser, Dura, Speicher, Trask, & Glaser, 1991). When the caregiver doctor visits in these two studies were compared to other community norms, however, the caregivers' mean number of physician visits in 1 year was again lower (Haley, Levine, Brown, Berry, & Hughes, 1987; Kiecolt-Glaser et al., 1991).

The data support the finding of C. H. Connell and Schulenberg (1990) that caregivers neglect their own health. It appears that they seek health care for themselves only when they think it is absolutely necessary.

Use of Medications. While caregivers report fewer physician office visits, 30% use psychotropic medications, a significantly higher rate than the 20% found in comparable community controls (Brocklehurst, Morris, Andrews, Richards, & Laycock, 1981; Clipp & George, 1990; George & Gwyther, 1996). In a group of highly educated, high-income caregivers, however, psychotropic drug use was only 8% (Gallagher-Thompson et al., 1991; Walsh et al., 1991).

Looking at types of psychotropic drugs, caregivers use predominantly antianxiety agents (19%) and sedatives/hypnotics (18%) and relatively few antidepressants (4%). These percentages include only prescription drugs; over-the-counter medications were excluded from the analysis (Clipp & George, 1990a).

In addition to psychotropic medications, between 20% and 34% of caregivers use alcohol as a way to cope with stress, although only 4% of caregivers report increasing their alcohol consumption since assuming the caregiving role (C. M. Connell, 1994; George, 1991).

The high rate of prescription psychotropic medications and the use of alcohol as a way of coping suggests simultaneous health-seeking and health risk-taking behavior. A puzzling observation, however, is the caregivers' low rate of physician office visits together with high use of medications. Perhaps caregivers request a prescription for themselves at the same time they bring their impaired elder to the physician's office; yet when researchers ask health questions, caregivers may not count that particular visit as pertaining to themselves (Wright et al., 1993).

As Clipp and George (1990a) have commented, there is no empirical knowledge of the process by which decisions to prescribe psychotropic medications are made. Studies investigating the caregiver–patient–professional relationship tend to focus on communication patterns and power/authority issues between the impaired elder, the caregiver, and the physician (Hasselkus, 1988, 1992; Haug, 1994). While some caregivers voice their own health needs when questioned, concerns about their health needs and behaviors are rarely initiated by clinic personnel (Hasselkus, 1992).

Over the past decade, there has been a steady increase in the number of professional articles and television documentaries on family caregiving. In 1993, the Council on Scientific Affairs (1993) of the American Medical Association made an explicit recommendation to physicians to enter into a "partnership" with caregivers of their patients and to attend to the needs of caregivers. Thus, many primary physicians are cognizant of caregiver stress. This awareness may explain the higher rate of antianxiety agents and hypnotics and lower rate of antidepressants. Stress and sleep disturbances are expected, while other depressive symptomatology may or may not be assessed during office visits intended for the impaired elder (Wright et al., 1993).

Nutrition, Exercise, and Smoking. C. M. Connell's (1994) study is enlightening, since it details specific health behaviors of caregivers. Her data on nutrition, exercise, and smoking show that approximately half of all caregivers did not change their health-seeking or risk-taking behaviors (range for no change in behaviors: 43–58%). After assuming caregiving responsibilities, however, 39% ate less nutritiously, 32% decreased their exercise routines, and 43% increased the amount they smoked. By contrast, only 7% reported eating more nutritiously, 10% increased their exercise, and 14% decreased the amount they smoked.

Objectively, the data show that health risk-taking behaviors outweigh health-seeking behaviors in response to caregiving. Yet for caregivers, even health risk-taking behaviors seem to represent attempts at reducing stress: Caregivers frequently report that they find "comfort in food" and that smoking reduces tension or anxiety (C. M. Connell, 1994). Interestingly, however, Moritz et al. (1992) found that neither smoking nor drinking nor the use of psychotropic medications among caregivers was related to an ill spouse's severity of cognitive impairment. Moritz and colleagues did not question whether these behaviors had changed in response to caregiving demands.

Coping Strategies. Caregivers' most frequently reported coping strategies are problem solving, help seeking, and trying to change the situation (Barusch, 1988; Quayhagen & Quayhagen, 1988). These strategies again reflect the caregivers' primary focus: the impaired elder. Nevertheless, the strategies can be interpreted as health behaviors, since problem-solving coping and a perceived sense of mastery decrease the likelihood of emotional and physical ill health (Folkman & Lazarus, 1980; Pruchno & Resch, 1989; Quayhagen & Quayhagen, 1988), while the use of emotion-focused coping is more often related to depression in caregivers (Cohen & Eisdorfer, 1988; Haley, Levine, Brown, & Bartolucci,

1987; Neundorfer, 1991; Pagel, Becker, & Coppel, 1985; Pruchno & Resch, 1989).

Some change in coping behaviors over time have also been observed. During the early phases of a spouse's illness, wife caregivers are more emotionally involved than husband caregivers. As the illness progresses, wife caregivers adopt problem-solving coping strategies similar to those used by husband caregivers (Miller, 1987; Zarit, Todd, & Zarit, 1986).

Another frequently used coping strategy among caregivers is information seeking: They read anything they can find and watch all TV programs that provide them with knowledge about their impaired elders' condition and problems (Wright, 1993a). As these information sources increasingly stress the importance of the caregivers' own health and suggest strategies to maintain, restore, or improve health, there is hope that these suggestions will motivate caregivers to increase their health behaviors. C. M. Connell (1994, pp. 33–34) observed that some caregivers do indeed perceive maintaining their health as both "an investment in personal well-being and the ability to provide full-time care at home for as long as possible." C. M. Connell (1994) suggests that this view could serve as a powerful incentive for other caregivers to engage in health-promoting behaviors and decrease risk behaviors.

Barriers to Health Behaviors

The reasons for caregivers' low rate of health behaviors are most likely to be found in role overload and, possibly, some denial that they are at risk. Spouse caregivers and adult children voice similar ethical obligations to provide care (Miller, 1989; Pratt, Schmall, & Wright, 1987), but adult children, most of whom are daughters, experience far greater conflict with other obligations. This conflict in turn may prevent them from engaging in health behaviors.

In spouse caregivers, altruism and feelings of reciprocity as expressed in such statements as "He is more important than I" or "She would do the same for me if I were sick" are sometimes encountered (Pratt et al., 1987; Wright, 1993a). Extreme altruism may take the form of passive suicidal behaviors, as can be exemplified by two clinical cases: One wife caregiver refused cancer treatment because she did not want to deplete the couple's financial resources; she explained that the money would be needed for her cognitively impaired husband's long-term care. Another wife caregiver deliberately neglected her diabetic condition. Her reasoning was that her life insurance would pay for her memory-impaired husband's long-term care.

In these cases, barriers to health behavior were created by our present health care system. As yet, neither Medicare nor private health insurance covers the type of care the majority of these elders need. Families bear most of the costs (ADRDA, 1993). Medicaid will pay for long-term care, but only after couples have depleted their own resources (Wright, 1993a).

SOCIAL SUPPORT AND HEALTH BEHAVIOR

Caregivers seldom function in social isolation. Even though one person is the primary caregiver who assumes most of the caregiving responsibilities, other individuals and social agencies provide assistance to a greater or lesser extent. Help from family members, friends, and neighbors is generally referred to as "informal social support," while help from agencies (e.g., respite services, day care, home health) is referred to as "formal social support."

Informal and formal social support are important considerations in this context. They not only reduce demands on the caregivers' time and energy, but also make it logistically possible for caregivers to engage in health-promoting or -restoring behaviors. Social support research provides for now the best longitudinal perspective on caregivers' health behaviors, covering time periods from primary caregiving responsibilities

at home, to becoming a former or secondary caregiver following the elder's nursing home placement, and, finally, to bereavement.

Support-Mobilizing Behavior of Caregivers

Especially relevant to this discussion is the "support-mobilizing" hypothesis found in caregiver research. It is thought that stressful life situations encountered by caregivers will motivate them to elicit support (Bass, Tausig, & Noelker, 1988/1989). For the purpose of this discussion, therefore, eliciting support is conceptualized as a form of health behavior.

But evidence for the support-mobilizing hypothesis is not strong. Overall, older caregivers have fewer contacts with family members and friends than do age-matched community controls, and caregivers whose demented elders are at home have less social support than those whose elders are in nursing homes (George & Gwyther, 1986; Wright, 1993a).

Certainly, structural barriers such as the size of the caregivers' social network and the driving distance between the caregivers' and other relatives' homes need to be considered. Eliciting social support also depends, however, on certain caregiver characteristics (Robinson, 1988, 1990). Those with high self-esteem and good social skills have adequate social support, which in turn seems to lower stress; the opposite pattern was found in caregivers with poor self-esteem and poor social skills (Robinson, 1988, 1990). Good social skills may be particularly important for eliciting informal social support.

Friends, Neighbors, and Family Members. How caregivers communicate their needs to friends or neighbors and other family members can either elicit the desired help or create barriers. For example, in the early phases of dementia, it is quite common for the primary caregiver to cover up the elder's memory problems and hide the existence of something wrong—perhaps out of a sense of shame or because close family members do not know how to tell others (Wright, 1993a). Sooner or later, however, friends and neighbors will notice that "something is wrong." Not telling others creates barriers to social support. Friends and neighbors do not know how to act, what to say, or how to be supportive, and so they keep their distance.

Open, assertive communication, on the other hand, will elicit the needed support. Examples are friends running requested errands for the caregiver or neighbors being alert to the possibility that a memory-impaired elder may wander off (Robinson, 1988).

Assertive communication is also necessary in interactions between family members. A caregiver spouse may sigh and say to a grown daughter who comes to visit, "You have no idea what it's like to stay with your dad 36 hours a day." Certainly, the caregiver is trying to communicate her distress, but only implies that she needs help. To the daughter, the mother's words communicate an accusation: She does not really understand her mother's difficulties. Consequently, the mother's words arouse feelings of helplessness in the daughter (Robinson, 1988; Wright, 1993a).

In contrast, a direct request such as "Can you stay with your dad on Saturday from 4 'til 7 P.M. while I ...?" will elicit the kind of help the caregiver wants. The daughter can provide the requested support herself or make other arrangements (Wright, 1993a).

Given these dynamics when eliciting support, it is perhaps not surprising that *perceived* adequacy and *perceived* quality of support have been shown to be more important to caregivers than quantity of social support (Clipp & George, 1990b; Haley, Levine, Brown, & Bartolucci, 1987; Robinson, 1989). High quantity, i.e., high levels of support, can actually be detrimental to caregivers of functionally impaired elders (Bass, Tausig, & Noelker, 1988/1989). A likely explanation for this observation is that caregivers find it difficult to coordinate different types of help or services; each is likely to have a different time schedule and even a different approach to caregiving.

But smaller helping networks are more manageable and are less likely to experience interpersonal conflicts (Bass et al., 1988/1989).

Support Groups. Many caregivers attend support groups offered through local Alzheimer's Disease and Related Disorders Associations or other community groups. At these meetings, specific information about the elder's illness is provided, difficult and frustrating caregiving experiences are shared, and tips on handling stressful situations are exchanged. In addition, caregiver support groups provide companionship with other adults and a sense of being understood. Thus, attending such support groups could be viewed as health seeking behavior, as attempts to reduce stress and increase coping skills.

Caregivers indicate that they like the groups, but there is little empirical evidence that support groups and other psychosocial interventions actually reduce stress, depression, or increase morale (Knight, Lutzy, & Macofsky-Urban, 1993; Toseland & Rossiter, 1989). In fact, Winogrond, Fisk, Kirsling, and Keyes (1987) found that caregivers repeatedly resisted efforts by group leaders to include psychotherapy in support group discussions. Attempts to examine the meaning of behaviors, to "induce insight and self-awareness were thoroughly rebuffed" (Winogrond et al., 1987, p. 388). This result again points to the observation that caregivers do not see themselves as "patients." By keeping the focus on the impaired elder, they can suppress their own feelings.

Formal Social Services Support. Home health, respite, and day care are the most common types of formal social support. Home health and respite care are provided in the caregivers' home; the impaired elder receives physical care or supervision or both. Day care is provided in the community; the elder participates in structured group activities offered daily or several times a week. Transportation to and from day care may be either the caregiver's responsibility or part of the program offering.

Formal social support frees caregiver time

that could be used to engage in health behaviors. Using such services when caregiver responsibilities escalate would make sense. The data, however, do not provide consistent evidence for this assumption. Rather, those who have been caregivers the longest are least likely to use social services (Snyder & Keefe, 1985). Furthermore, the elders' severity of cognitive impairment, length of illness, and the caregivers' emotional state do not influence the amount of social support received by caregivers, which led Clipp and George (1990b) to conclude that need does not necessarily mobilize support. Poor physical health in caregivers and higher levels of physical impairment in elders have been shown, however, to *predict* increased use of formal social support services (Noelker & Bass, 1989). Again, it seems that caregivers engage in health-promoting behavior only when absolutely necessary, although financial barriers such as inadequate resources to purchase formal support are also contributing factors.

Nursing Home Placement. The most intense and comprehensive formal social support occurs when the impaired elder is placed in a nursing home. Nursing homes provide care 24 hours a day, 7 days a week. The primary caregiver now becomes a former or "secondary" caregiver, freed of 24-hour responsibilities for the elder. But to what extent does this gain in time translate into health behavior?

The number of physician visits does indeed increase after the primary caregiver role is relinquished, but so does the use of psychotropic medications (Colerick & George, 1986; Wright, 1994a). Interactions between caregivers and physicians change once impaired elders are no longer part of the office visits; caregivers can finally focus on their own health needs. But it is also important to recognize that in many cases, the elder's nursing home placement was precipitated by the caregiver's declining health. Thus, more frequent visits to a physician may be a necessity at this time as caregivers seek to restore their health.

Only limited data are available on other health behaviors by caregivers following an elder's institutionalization. Moss, Lawton, Kleban, and Duhamel (1993) studied time use by caregivers before and after nursing home placement. Their data give some indications of increased health-maintaining and health-promoting behaviors following the elder's institutionalization. The average time gained per day by caregivers was 1 hour and 47 minutes (Moss et al., 1993). Some of the specific gains were increased interactions among family members of the same household, a net gain of 26 minutes per day. Caregivers also gained 23 minutes per day for recreational activities and, in general, spent more time away from home (Moss et al., 1993). The researchers concluded that, overall, there was a gain in "quality time" for the former caregivers. The preponderant percentages of time, however, continued to be used in much the same way as before nursing home placement.

King, Collins, Given, and Vredevoogd (1991) took a slightly different approach and questioned whether the negative impact on the caregivers' schedule had been reduced following an impaired elder's nursing home placement. Impact on schedule included curtailment of leisure activities and elimination of visits with friends. King et al. (1991) provided information on spouses, adult child, and other former primary caregivers. Institutionalization of the elder resulted in less negative impact on daily schedules for all caregivers, but this decrease was less for spouses than for the other caregiver groups; spouses still had a significantly higher negative impact on their schedules than daughters and other caregivers (King et al., 1991).

The conclusion to be drawn from these observations is that very few spouse caregivers are able to redefine their role following a mate's nursing home placement (Ade-Ridder & Kaplan, 1993). Spouses' self-perception continues to be that of a wife or husband; they visit the nursing home almost daily (King et al., 1991), and their perception of the ill spouse as a unique person increases following nursing home placement (Wright, 1993b).

Perhaps it is not surprising, therefore, that spouse caregivers' emotional and physical health continues to decline after nursing home placement, while the health of others stabilizes (King et al., 1991; Wright, 1994a). It seems that the close bond between a husband and wife and the commitment undertaken "for better or for worse" become barriers to health behavior for these caregivers.

Bereavement.   Final relief from caregiving responsibilities occurs with the impaired elder's death. George and Gwyther (1984) found that compared to predeath scores, bereaved family members as a group showed increased participation in voluntary organizations, increased satisfaction with social and recreational activities, decreased stress, and decreased use of psychotropic drugs. Thus, despite reports of grief and mourning, there was improvement in the caregivers' quality of life and health-promoting behavior.

Others have argued that following lengthy and stressful periods of caregiving, family members (i.e., daughters and spouses) have limited reserves left to deal with bereavement; hence, they will experience heightened bereavement. Indeed, Bass and Bowman (1990) found that family members who experienced caregiving as highly stressful assessed bereavement as difficult and reported high postdeath strain for the family.

Assistance with adjustment to bereavement is seldom offered by community agencies, since they tend to view cases as closed with the death of the elder (Bass & Bowman, 1990). Nevertheless, bereaved caregivers seem to be able to elicit adequate family support, and the majority adjust to a spouse's or parent's death without serious consequences (Bass, Bowman, & Noelker, 1991). Jones and Martinson (1992, p. 173) reported that 77% of caregivers stated that the death of the elder was a relief, and 31% were "ready to get on with life."

Another important finding is that surviving caregivers' perceptions of the elder's care prior to death are more important to their adjustment than support given to them during bereavement (Bass et al., 1991). This finding would again suggest the importance of caregivers' ability to elicit quality social support during the time of primary caregiving responsibilities.

Caregivers' health status and health-seeking behavior during the bereavement phase is not solely a consequence of past responsibilities, but is closely linked to prior health status and health behavior. Wright (1994b) followed a group of caregiver spouses for 2 years. At baseline, all impaired spouses were in the early to middle phases of Alzheimer's disease, and all were cared for at home by their spouses (Wright, 1991). At follow-up, those caregivers whose spouses had died reported significantly poorer emotional and physical health and more frequent visits to a physician's office than nonbereaved caregivers. When comparing baseline assessments of all three groups (widowed, nursing home placement, ill spouse still at home), however, the subsequently widowed spouses' health had been poorer and doctor visits had been higher even at the beginning of the study. The impaired spouses' illness characteristics and demographic factors could not explain these differences.

These findings suggest that caregivers in poor health do not have sufficient energy to interact effectively with a memory-impaired spouse (Wright, 1994b). The importance of interactions has been previously observed with other highly dependent, vulnerable individuals. Spitz (1945) and Spitz and Wolf (1946) documented that infants who lacked nurturing touch and interactions with the environment died for no apparent physical reason. This now classic work on maternal–child deprivation may have some parallels to Alzheimer's disease caregiving: Afflicted spouses who lack interactions with a "nurturing" caregiver may sense abandonment and withdraw; subsequently, such spouses may die just like the infants in Spitz's studies (Wright, 1994b).

The findings also suggest, however, that there is a subgroup of caregivers with initial poor health and high rates of use of formal health services; their poor health can influence reported averages (means) in research reports. It could be that other caregivers' health is less negatively affected than currently ascertained, but this would make their rates of health-seeking behavior even lower.

CULTURAL FACTORS AND HEALTH BEHAVIORS OF CAREGIVERS

Culture and ethnicity are known to influence health behaviors (Yee & Weaver, 1994). People's beliefs, attitudes, and values influence not only their perceptions of what is normal and what is sickness, but also how often they will engage in self-care versus seeking formal health services, how many medications they take, how often they rest and exercise, and what type of foods they consume (Wykle & Haug, 1993). Patterns of health behavior among African-American, Hispanic, and Asian caregivers could thus be substantially different. Unfortunately, caregiver research is based predominantly on white subjects, and ethnic differences are rarely analyzed. Further, very few studies focus specifically on minority caregivers.

Demographic Differences

Among minority caregivers, kin relationship to the impaired elder shows a different pattern compared to whites: Minority caregivers are less likely to be spouses; more often, they are adult children and grandchildren, siblings, cousins, and nonrelatives (or "fictive kin") (Haley et al., 1995; Stone et al., 1987; Taylor & Chatters, 1986; Wykle & Segall, 1991). Just as among whites, however, these caregivers are predominantly women. They care for more impaired elders, and mean income levels tend to be substantially lower than those of white caregivers (Haley et al., 1995; Wykle & Segall, 1991; Wood & Parham, 1990).

Health Status Differences

Caregivers from different ethnic backgrounds show different patterns of health. For example,

despite caring for elders with higher levels of impairment, minority caregivers have reported lower levels of stress than whites (Haley et al., 1995; Mintzer & Macera, 1992; Wood & Parham, 1990). The data, however, are not consistent. Wykle and Segall (1991) found very similar patterns of stress among African-American and white caregivers, and Valle (1994) found higher stress among Hispanic than among white caregivers.

Lawton, Rajagopal, Brody, and Kleban (1992) identified a crossover effect with socioeconomic status (SES) in that stress (burden) was greater among higher-income than among lower-income African-American caregivers, while the opposite pattern was observed for white caregivers. This intriguing finding has spurred a number of interpretations such as the role of religiosity, respect for elders, disappointed aspirations due to financial impact of caregiving, or other cultural moderating factors (Hartung, 1993; Lawton et al., 1992; Wright & Mintzer, 1993).

Data on caregiver depression, the other important health status variable, show that African-Americans are less depressed than whites (Haley et al., 1995; Mintzer & Macera, 1992); African-Americans are also less depressed than Hispanic caregivers (Cox & Monk, 1990).

Data on physical health status of minority caregivers are inconsistent. Some studies show no racial differences in self-reported physical health (Lawton et al., 1992; Wykle & Segall, 1991); others report that black caregivers have poorer health (Haley et al., 1995; Mui, 1992), and that Hispanic caregivers' health is most negatively affected by caregiving (Cox & Monk, 1990; Valle, 1994).

Culture-Fair Assessments

Given such differences and inconsistent findings in reported stress, depression, and physical health, one needs to question whether assessment tools are culturally sensitive or "culture-fair" (Valle, 1994). Hernandez (1991) has argued that stress or burden scales have especially questionable content validity for minority populations. For example, behaviors associated with dementia are interpreted differently by various cultures, and hence caregiver reactions would be different.

During clinical evaluations, African-American spouse caregivers have been observed to be reluctant to admit just how stressful the impaired spouse's behaviors are. Caregivers often qualify their answers with "but I love her/him." Similarly, Hispanic caregivers try to keep others from knowing how bad the caregiving situation really is (Valle, 1994). Denial of problems may also influence these caregivers' self-assessed moods and physical health.

Evidence of Health Behaviors in Minority Caregivers

Formal Services. Minority caregivers report fewer physician visits, less use of prescription medications, and less use of psychotropic drugs than whites (Cox & Monk, 1990; Haley et al., 1995). Lower use of formal services may be a cultural phenomenon, or it may result from barriers such as language, income, and local availability of services. A recent study by Haley et al. (1995) sheds some light on this issue. Haley and associates simultaneously evaluated groups of black and white caregivers and black and white *non*caregivers matched on socioeconomic variables. While ethnic differences observed in other studies remained (i.e., less use of health services by black caregivers), black *non*caregivers reported more physician visits, fewer prescription medications, and less use of psychotropic medications than black caregivers. It appears that the lower rate of physician visits yet higher use of medications by African-American caregivers (when compared to African-American controls) is similar to the pattern observed among white caregivers (when compared to white controls). Within the same culture, overwhelming caregiver responsibilities rather than economic and other social factors may be the underlying cause for using fewer formal health services.

Exercise and Nutrition. Only limited information about health-promoting behaviors such as exercise and nutrition is available. Hispanic caregivers exercise or engage in sports significantly less often than whites; Hispanics also eat significantly less nutritious meals (Valle, 1994).

Since Hispanic caregivers in Valle's study were lower in income, age, and education than white caregivers, these potential confounds were analyzed; statistically, they did not change the findings. Valle (1994) concluded that the observed differences do not appear to be based on social status differences but on different ethnocultural values and perceptions. Exercise and nutritious meals, as defined by the majority culture, are not valued health behaviors among Hispanics.

Coping Strategies. Interesting patterns of coping were observed by Valle (1994) when comparing Hispanic and white caregivers. Hispanics were consistently less likely to seek assistance from others (including talking to someone about the situation or getting professional help); however, they were significantly more likely than white caregivers to rely on prayer and faith. Similarly, Wykle and Segall (1991) found that black caregivers' predominant coping strategies were prayer, faith, and religion, while white caregivers were more likely to seek help from professionals. These differences seem to be culturally determined. But regardless of type of coping strategy used, the caregivers' aim was to decrease stress. Hence, all coping strategies can be viewed as health-promoting or health-restoring behavior.

Social Support for Minority Caregivers

Informal Social Support. Compared to whites, minority caregivers tend to maintain larger caregiver households, use greater numbers and a wider range of informal social supports, and especially rely on volunteers from their local churches (Advisory Panel, 1993; Wood and Parham, 1990).

While Bass et al. (1988/1989) reported that larger helping networks can lead to interpersonal stress, perhaps the culturally determined larger caregiver households and networks help to decrease stress among minority caregivers. Whatever the case, it does not appear that the wider availability of help leads to increased health behaviors; even leisure activities do not increase for black caregivers with the presence of more caregivers (White-Means & Thornton, 1990; Wykle & Segall, 1991).

Another important finding is that informal support declined significantly over a period of 6 months for African-American and Hispanic caregivers (Cox & Monk, 1990). Despite initially larger helping networks, minority caregivers may find it difficult to keep others engaged in providing informal support over longer periods of time.

Formal Social Support.   Given the decline in informal support over time, it does make some sense that more African-American than white caregivers voiced a need for respite services (Wykle & Segall, 1991). Indeed, use of formal social support has been shown to increase significantly for African-American and Hispanic caregivers over a period of 6 months (Cox & Monk, 1990). But a relationship between use of respite care and increased health behavior among minority caregivers can only be inferred. Availability of "substitute" caregivers increased leisure time for African-American caregivers (White-Means & Thornton, 1990); the term "substitute" is ambiguous, however, since it included formal and informal helpers. The most comprehensive form of social support, nursing home placement, is used far less often by minority caregivers than by whites (McFall & Miller, 1992; Morycz, Malloy, Bozich, & Martz, 1987; Advisory Panel on Alzheimer's Disease, 1993). Cultural factors such as respect for elders and greater tolerance of disoriented and dependent behaviors may be contributing factors. Socioeconomic and systemic factors (poverty, absence of insurance, maldistribution of services), however, also play a role. It is not known whether nursing home placement,

when it does occur, increases health behavior in minority caregivers.

SUMMARY AND DIRECTIONS FOR RESEARCH

Despite two decades of caregiving research, little is known about health behaviors of informal caregivers to impaired elders. Bits of information from over a hundred sources were pieced together to paint this beginning profile. There is no doubt that caregivers experience high stress and are a population at risk for emotional and physical health problems; few caregivers, however, engage in health-maintaining, -restoring, or -promoting behaviors, while health risk-taking behaviors such as alcohol consumption, smoking, and denial of problems are fairly common. Caregivers attend to their own health needs only when absolutely necessary. Their time, energy, and thinking are predominantly focused on the ill elder.

The most common indicator of health behavior reported in the literature is use of formal health services. Caregivers see physicians less frequently than community controls, but somehow they are able to gain access to more psychotropic medications. This beginning profile is based on studies using a high percentage of white subjects. Even less information is available on health behaviors of minority caregivers. They use formal health care services less often than whites, and compared to ethnically matched controls, they show the same pattern of fewer doctor visits but higher use of medications. Many minority caregivers seek to reduce stress through prayer.

Confirming the accuracy of these profiles requires further research. A major reason for the current lack of knowledge is researchers' and clinicians' inattention to health behaviors. Simply put, researchers have not asked the right questions. With the notable exception of C. M. Connell's (1994) work, almost all caregiver research uses a stress–illness paradigm; health-maintaining, -restoring, and -promoting or risk-taking behaviors, if questioned at all, are part of general health–illness scales or assessments. Researchers need a paradigm shift, Kuhn (1970) would once again have stated. Yes, caregivers are under tremendous stress, but researchers have failed to focus on what caregivers can do or are doing to maintain, restore, or promote health. Even one simple question (which incidentally is part of every clinical nursing assessment) can provide a wealth of information: "What do *you* do to make it better?"

Currently, health behavior questions are not part of the National Informal Caregiver Survey; only one survey item alludes to this issue: "Taking care of … limits my social life or free time": True or False? Again, the conceptualization is negative impact rather than questioning whether caregivers actively engage in health behaviors. It is hoped that future national surveys will include succinct questions about health behaviors.

Lack of knowledge about caregiver health behavior creates opportunities for research and clinical interventions. As this review has documented, most caregivers focus their thinking and energy on the ill person and neglect their own health. It is also well documented that health varies according to age, closeness of the relationship, financial resources, and cultural background. But little is known about actual health-seeking or health-risk-taking practices among caregivers. Thus, researchers could build on existing knowledge but make a paradigm shift and narrow their focus to health behaviors.

Following are examples of questions that need answers:

1. Is there consensus on what constitutes health behaviors among caregivers?
   a. How do caregivers define health behaviors?
   b. Does health behavior vary by age, kinship, SES, and cultural background?
   c. Are caregivers' definitions of health behavior similar to or different from those used by researchers and clinicians?
2. What motivates caregivers to engage in

health behaviors, and does motivation vary across subgroups of caregivers?
3. What are barriers to health behaviors for caregivers, and do barriers vary across subgroups or caregivers?
4. Are currently used standardized scales "culture-fair"; i.e., are they valid and reliable when used with minority caregivers?
5. Does cultural competence of a researcher/interviewer significantly affect the caregivers' answers?

Seeking answers to these questions is not simply academic. How researchers conceptualize the world determines what they find and influences the design of intervention programs. Robinson (1988, 1990) used social skills training to help caregivers mobilize social support. Adequate social support in turn allows caregivers to engage in health behaviors.

Another important issue, however, is the readiness of health professionals to encourage health behaviors of caregivers, even though the identified patient may be the ill elder. Addressing the caregiver's stress and role overload may be just as important as providing medical care to the elder. Professionals in office or clinic settings could play a powerful role in promoting health behaviors of caregivers.

Interventions therefore need to be guided by the following question: What can be done to increase health behaviors among caregivers? Following are examples of suggested intervention programs, programs that could at the same time be designed as efficacy or effectiveness studies:

1. Educating caregivers about the benefits of maintaining their own health together with teaching specific health-promoting strategies.
2. Providing incentives/rewards (perhaps even cash payments) to caregivers for engaging in health behaviors.
3. Providing unsolicited physician support/health restoration to caregivers during office visits at which the identified patient is the impaired elder (Haug, 1994).

4. Conducting health assessments in the caregiver's home followed by recommendation and facilitation of specific health-promoting behaviors.
5. Making respite available specifically for health-maintaining activities.

A paradigm shift from stress response to health behavior will empower caregivers. But are researchers and clinicians ready to embrace the zeitgeist of active participation and self-determination when the focus is caregiver health?

REFERENCES

Ade-Ridder, L., & Kaplan, L. (1993). Marriage, spousal caregiving, and a husband's move to a nursing home. *Journal of Gerontological Nursing, 19*(10), 13–23.

ADRDA (Alzheimer's Disease and Related Disorders Association, Inc.). (1993). *Alzheimer's disease: Statistics*. Chicago: ADRDA.

Advisory Panel on Alzheimer's Disease. (1993). *Fourth report of the Advisory Panel on Alzheimer's Disease, 1992*. NIH Publication No. 93-3520. Washington, DC: Superintendent of Documents, U.S. Government Printing Office.

Archbold, P. G. (1980). Impact of parent caring on middle-aged offspring. *Journal of Gerontological Nursing, 6*(2), 78–85.

Artes, R., & Hoops, R. (1976). Problems of aphasic and non-aphasic stroke patients as identified and evaluated by patients' wives. In Y. Lebrun & R. Hoops (Ed.), *Recovery in aphasics* (pp. 31–45), Amsterdam: Swets & Zeitlinger.

Barusch, A. S. (1988). Problems and coping strategies of elderly spouse caregivers. *Gerontologist, 28*, 677–685.

Bass, D. M., & Bowman, K. (1990). The transition from caregiving to bereavement: The relationship of care-related strain and adjustment to death. *Gerontologist, 30*, 35–42.

Bass, D. M., Bowman, K., & Noekler, L. S. (1991). The influence of caregiving and bereavement support on adjusting to an older relative's death. *Gerontologist, 21*, 32–42.

Bass, D. M., Tausig, M. G., & Noelker, I. S. (1988/1989). Elder impairment, social support and caregiver strain: A framework for understanding support's effects. *Journal of Applied Social Science, 13*, 80–115.

Baumgarten, M. (1989). The health of persons giving care to the demented elderly: A critical review of the literature. *Journal of Clinical Epidemiology, 42*, 1137–1148.

Biegel, D. E., Sales, E., & Schulz, R. (1991). *Family caregiving in chronic illness* (pp. 62–163). Newbury Park, CA: Sage.

Blazer, D., & Williams, C. D. (1980). Epidemiology of dysphoria and depression in an elderly population. *American Journal of Psychiatry, 137*, 439–444.

Boaz, R. F., & Muller, C. F. (1992). Paid work and unpaid help by caregivers of the disabled and frail elders. *Medical Care, 30*(2), 149–158.

Brocklehurst, J. C., Morris, P., Andrews, K., Richards, B., & Laycock, P. (1981). Social effects of stroke. *Social Science and Medicine, 15A*, 35–39.

Brody, E. M. (1981). "Women in the middle" and family help to older people. *Gerontologist, 21*, 471–480.

Brody, E. M., Dempsey, N. P., & Pruchno, R. A. (1990). Mental health of sons and daughters of the institutionalized aged. *Gerontologist, 30*, 212–219.

Cantor, M. H. (1983). Strain among caregivers: A study of experience in the United States. *Gerontologist, 23*, 597–604.

Clipp, E. C., & George, L. K. (1990a). Psychotropic drug use among caregivers of patients with dementia. *Journal of the American Geriatrics Society, 38*, 227–235.

Clipp, E. C., & George, L. K. (1990b). Caregiver needs and patterns of social support. *Journal of Gerontology, 45*, S102–S111.

Clipp, E. C., & George, L. K. (1993). Dementia and cancer: A comparison of spousal caregivers. *Gerontologist, 33*(4), 534–541.

Cohen, D., & Eisdorfer, C. (1988). Depression in family members caring for a relative with Alzheimer's disease. *Journal of the American Geriatrics Society, 36*, 885–889.

Colerick (Clipp), E. J., & George, L. K. (1986). Predictors of institutionalization among caregivers of patients with Alzheimer's disease. *Journal of the American Geriatrics Society, 34*, 493–498.

Connell, C. M., & Schulenberg, J. (1990). *Daily variation in the physical and mental health impact of caregiving*. Paper presented at the Gerontological Society of America, Boston, November.

Connell, C. M (1994). Impact of spouse caregiving on health behaviors and physical and mental health status. *American Journal of Alzheimer's Care and Related Disorders and Research* (January/February), 26–36.

Council on Scientific Affairs, American Medical Association. (1993). Physicians and family caregivers: A model for partnership. *Journal of the American Medical Association, 269*(10), 1282–1284.

Cox, C., & Monk, A. (1990). Minority caregivers of dementia victims: A comparison of black and hispanic families. *Journal of Applied Gerontology, 9*(3), 340–354.

Deimling, G. T., Bass, D. M., Towsend, A. L., & Noelker, L. S. (1989). Care-related stress: A comparison of spouse and adult-child caregivers in shared and separate households. *Journal of Aging and Health, 1*, 67–82.

Dussell, C., & Roman, M. (1989). The elder care dilemma. *Generations, 13*(3), 30–32.

Eagles, J. M., Beattie, J. A. G., Blackwood, G. W., Restall, D. B., & Ashcroft, G. W. (1987). The mental health of elderly couples. I. The effects of a cognitively impaired spouse. *British Journal of Psychiatry, 150*, 299–303.

Folkman, S., & Lazarus, R. S. (1980). An analysis of coping in a middle aged community sample. *Journal of Health and Social Behavior, 21,* 219-239.

Fitting, M., Rabins, P., Lucas, M. J., & Eastham, J. (1986). Caregivers for dementia patients: A comparison of husbands and wives. *Gerontologist, 26,* 248-252.

Gallagher, D., Rose, J., Rivera, P., Lovett, S., & Thompson, L. W. (1989). Prevalence of depression in family caregivers. *Gerontologist, 29,* 449-456.

Gallagher-Thompson, D., Walsh, W., Lovett, S., & Koin, D. (1991). The relationship among indices of physical and psychological distress in family caregivers. Paper presented at the Gerontological Society of America, 44th Annual Scientific Meeting, San Francisco, November. *Gerontologist, 31* (Special Issue II), 90.

George, L. K. (1991). *Social support and caregiving roles of aging women: Health implications.* Paper presented at the National Institutes of Health Seminar Series on Women's Health and Behavior on the theme of Women's Quality of Life: The Cost Benefits of Living Longer. Bethesda, MD, April 3.

George, L. K., & Gwyther, L. P. (1984). The dynamics of caregiving burden: Changes in caregiver well-being over time [Special Issue]. *Gerontologist, 24,* 249.

George, L. K., & Gwyther, L. P. (1986). Caregiver well-being: A multidimensional examination of family caregivers of demented adults. *Gerontologist, 26,* 253-259.

Gochman, D. S. (1988). Health behavior: Plural perspectives. In D. S. Gochman (Ed.), *Health Behavior: Emerging research perspectives* (pp. 3-17). New York: Plenum Press.

Haley, W. E., Levine, E. G., Brown, S. L., & Bartolucci, A. A. (1987). Stress, appraisal, coping and social support as predictors of adaptational outcome among dementia caregivers. *Psychology and Aging, 2,* 323-330.

Haley, W. E., Levine, E. G., Brown, S. L., Berry, J. W., & Hughes, G. H. (1987). Psychological, social, and health consequences of caring for a relative with senile dementia. *Journal of the American Geriatrics Society, 5,* 405-411.

Haley, W. E., West, C. A. C., Wadley, V. G., Ford, G. R., White, F. A., Barrett, J. J., Harrell, L. E., & Roth, D. L. (1995). Psychological, social, and health impact of caregiving: A comparison of black and white dementia family caregivers and noncaregivers. *Psychology and Aging, 10,* 540-552.

Harper, M. S. (1991). An overview: mental disorders of the elderly. In M. S. Harper (Ed.), *Management and care of the elderly)* (pp. 3-23). Newbury Park, CA: Sage.

Hartung, R. (1993). On black burden and becoming nouveau poor. *Journal of Gerontology and Social Science, 48*(1), S34.

Hasselkus, B. R. (1988). Meaning in family caregiving: Perspectives on caregiver/professional relationships. *Gerontologist, 28,* 686-691.

Hasselkus, B. R. (1992). Physician and family caregiver in the medical setting: Negotiation of care? *Journal of Aging Studies, 6,* 67-80.

Haug, M. R. (1994). Elderly patients, caregivers, and physicians: Theory and research on health care triads. *Journal of Health and Social Behavior, 35,* 1-12.

Hernandez, G. G. (1991). Not so benign neglect: Researchers ignore ethnicity in defining family caregiver burden and recommending services. *Gerontologist, 31,* 271-272.

Holbrook, S. E. (1982). Stroke: Social and emotional outcomes. *Journal of the Royal College of Physicians of London, 16,* 100-104.

Horowitz, A. (1985). Sons and daughters as caregivers to older parents: Differences in role performance and consequences. *Gerontologist, 25*(6), 612-617.

Johnson, J., Weissman, M. M., & Klerman, G. L. (1992). Service utilization and social morbidity associated with depressive symptoms in the community. *Journal of the American Medical Association, 267*(11), 1478-1483.

Jones, P. S., & Martinson, I. M. (1992). The experience of bereavement in caregivers of family members with Alzheimer's disease. *Image: Journal of Nursing Scholarship, 24,* 172-176.

Katon, W. (1985). Somatization in primary care. *Journal of Family Practice, 21,* 257-258.

Kiecolt-Glaser, J. K., Dura, J. R., Speicher, C. E., Trask, J., & Glaser, R. (1991). Spousal caregivers of dementia victims: Longitudinal changes in immunity and health. *Psychosomatic Medicine, 53,* 345-362.

Kiecolt-Glaser, J. K., Dyer, C. S., & Shuttleworth, E. C. (1988). Upsetting social interactions and distress among Alzheimer's disease family care-givers: A replication and extension. *American Journal of Community Psychology, 16,* 825-837.

Kiecolt-Glaser, J. K., Glaser, R., Shuttleworth, E. F., Dyer, C. S., Ogrocki, P., & Speicher, C. E. (1987). Chronic stress and immunity in family caregivers of Alzheimer's disease patients. *Psychosomatic Medicine, 49,* 523-535.

King, S., Collins, C., Given, B., & Vredevoogd, J. (1991). Institutionalization of an elderly family member: Reactions of spouse and nonspouse caregivers. *Archives of Psychiatric Nursing, 5*(6), 323-330.

Knight, B. G., Lutzky, S. M., & Macofsky-Urban, F. (1993). A meta-analytic review of interventions for caregiver distress: Recommendations for future research. *Journal of Gerontology, 33*(2), 240-248.

Kuhn, T. S. (1970). *The structure of scientific revolutions* (2nd ed.) Chicago: University of Chicago Press.

Lawton, M. P., Rajagopal, D., Brody, E., & Kleban, M. H. (1992). The dynamics of caregiving for a demented elder among black and white families. *Journal of Gerontology, 47*(4), S156-S164.

McFall, S., & Miller, B. H. (1992). Caregiver burden and nursing home admission of frail elderly people. *Journal of Gerontology, 47*(2), S73-S79.

Miller, B. (1987). Gender and control among spouses of the cognitively impaired: A research note. *Gerontologist, 27,* 447-453.

Miller, B. (1989). Adult children's perceptions of caregiver stress and satisfaction. *Journal of Applied Gerontology, 8*, 275–293.

Miller, B., McFall, S., & Montgomery, A. (1991). The impact of elder health, caregiver involvement, and global stress and satisfaction. *Journal of Gerontology, 46*, S9–19.

Mintzer, J. E., & Macera, C. A. (1992). Prevalence of depressive symptoms among white and African-American caregivers of demented patients. *American Journal of Psychiatry, 149*(4), 575–576.

Moritz, D. J., Kasl, S. V., & Berkman, L. F. (1989). The health impact of living with a cognitively impaired elderly spouse: Depressive symptoms and social functioning. *Journal of Gerontology, 44*, S17–S27.

Moritz, D. J., Kasl, S.V., & Ostfeld, A. M. (1992). The health impact of living with a cognitively impaired elderly spouse: Blood pressure, self-rated health, and health behaviors. *Journal of Aging and Health, 4*, 244–267.

Morycz, R. K., Malloy, J., Bozich, M., & Martz, P. (1987). Racial differences in family burden: Clinical implications for social work. *Gerontological Social Work, 10*, 133–154.

Moss, M. S., Lawton, M. P., Kleban, M. H., & Duhamel, L. (1993). Time use of caregivers of impaired elders before and after institutionalization. *Journal of Gerontology, 48*(3), S102–S111.

Mui, A.C. (1992). Caregiver strain among black and white daughter caregivers: A role theory perspective. *Gerontologist, 32*(2), 203–212.

Mutran, E., & Ferraro, K. F. (1988). Medical need and use of services among older and men and women. *Journal of Gerontology, 43*, S162–S171.

Neundorfer, M. M. (1991). Coping and health outcomes in spouse caregivers of persons with dementia. *Nursing Research, 40*, 60–265.

Noelker, L. S., & Bass, D. M. (1989). Home care for elderly persons: Linkages between formal and informal caregivers. *Journal of Gerontology, 44*, S63–S70.

Pagel, M. D., Becker, J., & Coppel, D.B. (1985). Loss of control, self-blame, and depression: An investigation of spouse caregivers of Alzheimer's disease patients. *Journal of Abnormal Psychology, 94*, 169–182.

Pratt, C., Schmall, V., & Wright, S. (1987). Ethical concerns of family caregivers to dementia patients. *Gerontologist, 27*, 632–638.

Pruchno, R. A., Kleban, M. H., Michaels, J. E., & Dempsey, N. P. (1990). Mental and physical health of caregiving spouses: Development of a causal model. *Journal of Gerontology, 45*, 192–199.

Pruchno, R. A., & Potashnik, S. L. (1989). Caregiving spouses: Physical and mental health in perspective. *Journal of the American Geriatrics Society, 37*, 697–705.

Pruchno, R. A., & Resch, N. L. (1989). Mental health of caregiving spouses: Coping as mediator, moderator, or main effect? *Psychology and Aging, 4*, 454–463.

Quayhagen, M. P., & Quayhagen, M. (1988). Alzheimer's stress: Coping with the caregiving role. *Gerontologist, 28*, 391–396.

Robinson, K. M. (1988). A social skills training program for adult caregivers. *Advances in Nursing Science, 10*(2), 59–72.

Robinson, K. M. (1989). Predictors of depression among wife caregivers. *Nursing Research, 38*, 359–363.

Robinson, K. (1990). The relationships between social skills, social support, self-esteem and burden in adult caregivers. *Journal of Advanced Nursing, 15*, 788–795.

Schulz, R., Tompkins, C. A., & Rau, M. T. (1988). A longitudinal study of the psychosocial impact of stroke on primary support persons. *Psychology of Aging, 3*, 131–141.

Schulz, R., Visintainer, P., & Williamson, G. M. (1990). Psychiatric and physical morbidity effects of caregiving. *Journal of Gerontology, 45*, 181–191.

Silliman, R. A., Fletcher, R. H., Earp, J. L., & Wagner, E. H. (1986). Families of elderly stroke patients: Effects of home care. *Journal of the American Gerontological Society, 34*, 643–648.

Snyder, B., & Keefe, K. (1985). The unmet needs of family caregivers for frail and disabled adults. *Social Work in Health Care, 10*, 1–14.

Spitz, R. (1945). Hospitalism: An enquiry into the genesis of psychiatric conditions in early childhood. *Psychoanalytic Study of the Child, 1*, 53–174.

Spitz, R., & Wolf, K. M. (1946). Anaclitic depression. *Psychoanalytic Study of the Child, 2*, 313–342.

Stetz, K. M. (1987). Caregiving demands during advanced cancer. *Cancer Nursing, 10*, 260–268.

Stommel, M., Given, C. W., & Given, B. (1990). Depression as an overriding variable explaining caregiver burden. *Journal of Aging and Health, 2*, 81–102.

Stone, R., Cafferata, G. L., & Sangle, J. (1987). Caregivers of frail elderly: A national profile. *Gerontologist, 27*, 616–626.

Suitor, J. J., & Pillemer, K. (1990). Transition to the status of family caregiver: A new framework for studying social support and well being. In S. Stahl (Ed.), *The legacy of longevity: Health, illness and long-term care in later life* (pp. 310–320). Newbury Park, CA: Sage.

Taylor, R. J., & Chatters, L. M. (1986). Patterns of informal support to elderly black adults: Family, friends, and church members. *Social Work* (November-December), 432–438.

Tennstedt, S., Cafferata, G. L., & Sullivan, L. (1992). Depression among caregivers of impaired elders. *Journal of Aging and Health, 4*, 58–76.

Tennstedt, S. L., & McKinlay, J. B. (1989). Informal care for frail older persons. In M. G. Ory & K. Bond (Eds.), *Aging and health care* (pp. 145–166). New York: Routledge.

Toseland, R. W., & Rossiter, C. M. (1989). Group interventions to support family caregivers: A review and analysis. *Journal of Gerontology, 29*, 438–448.

Valle, R. (1994). Culture-fair behavioral symptom differential assessment and intervention in dementing illness. *Alzheimer Diseases and Associated Disorders, 8*(3), 21–45.

Walsh, W. A., Yoash-Gantz, R., Rinki, M., Koin, D., & Gallagher-Thompson, D. (1991). The use of alcohol, exercise, smoking and psychotropic drugs among female caregivers. Paper presented at the Gerontological Society of America, 44th Annual Scientific Meeting, San Francisco, CA, November. *Gerontologist, 31* (Special Issue II), 90.

White-Means, S. I., & Thornton, M. C. (1990). Ethnic differences in the production of informal home health care. *Gerontologist, 30*(6), 758–768.

Winogrond, I. R., Fisk, A. A., Kirsling, M. S., & Keyes, B. (1987). The relationship of caregiver burden and morale to Alzheimer's disease patient function in a therapeutic setting. *Gerontologist, 27,* 336–339.

Wood, J. B., & Parham, I. A. (1990). Coping with perceived burden: Ethnic and cultural issues in Alzheimer's family caregiving. *Journal of Applied Gerontology, 9*(3), 325–339.

Wright, L. K. (1991). The impact of Alzheimer's disease on the mental relationship. *Gerontologist, 31,* 224–237.

Wright, L. K. (1993a). *Alzheimer's disease and marriage.* Newbury Park, CA: Sage.

Wright, L. K. (1993b). *Commitment to an Alzheimer's disease afflicted spouse: A longitudinal perspective.* Paper presented at the Southern Nursing Research Society, Birmingham, AL, February 1991.

Wright, L. K. (1994a). AD spousal caregivers: Longitudinal changes in health, depression, and coping. *Journal of Gerontological Nursing, October,* 33–48.

Wright, L. K. (1994b). Alzheimer's disease afflicted spouses who remain at home: Can human dialects explain the findings? *Social Science Medicine, 38*(8), 1037–1046.

Wright, L. K., Clipp, E. C., & George, L. K. (1993). Health consequences of caregiver stress. *Medicine, Exercise, Nutrition, and Health, 2,* 181–195.

Wright, L. K., & Mintzer, J. E. (1993). Ethnicity, culture and mental health in the elderly. *Association for Geriatric Psychiatry Newsletter* (May/June/July/August), 14–15.

Wykle, M., & Haug, M. R. (1993). Multicultural and social-class aspects of self-care. *Generations* (Fall), 25–28.

Wykle, M., & Segall, M. (1991). A comparison of black and white family caregivers experience with dementia. *Journal of the Black Nurses' Association, 5,* 29–41.

Yee, B. W. K., & Weaver, G. D. (1994). Ethnic minorities and health promotion: Developing a "culturally competent" agenda. *Generations, 18*(1), 39–44.

Young, R. F., & Kahana, E. (1989). Specifying caregiver outcomes: Gender and relationship aspects of caregiving strain. *Gerontologist, 29,* 660–666.

Zarit, S. H., Todd, P., & Zarit, J. M. (1986). Subjective burden of husbands and wives as caregivers: A longitudinal study. *Gerontologist, 26,* 260–261.

IV

HEALTH BEHAVIOR IN STRUCTURED COMMUNITIES

Some populations live in "structured communities"—communities that are relatively closed and separated from the larger society by well-marked physical and social boundaries and that define or influence the lives of their members through a sharing of housing, household and occupational tasks, and explicit behavioral norms. Extreme examples of such communities include cloistered monasteries and convents in which entrance and egress are carefully guarded and in which membership is usually voluntary. Other extreme examples where entrance and egress are also carefully guarded are correctional facilities in which membership is involuntary and mental hospitals where membership typically—but not always—is involuntary. Structured communities also include collectives such as communes and Kibbutzes, the military, and residential schools, all of which are less rigidly bounded than cloistered communities but in which the totality of life is lived for defined periods and in which freedom of movement and behavior is often far more limited than in the larger society.

Other structured communities would include populations working in offshore oil rigs, and those sequestered in biospheres and spacecraft. Very little research has been done on the health behaviors of persons living in such communities, particularly in relation to their perceptions of symptoms and use of services.

The military, correctional facilities, and religious orders are three major types of structured communities for which some health behavior data exist.

MILITARY COMMUNITIES

Data from a naval sample suggest that age, rank, marital status, perceived health status, and whether one is shore-based were related to a higher level of health-promoting behaviors (Simmons, 1993). These behaviors included self-actualization, health responsibility, interpersonal support, exercise, nutrition, and stress management, but not disease-reducing behaviors such as smoking cessation or weight reduction. Simmons suggests that health promotion strategies be based on appropriate knowledge and "targeted both to individual behavioral changes and to supportive social policies that provide the context for health attitudes and behaviors" (p. 597).

The rise of HIV infection, coupled with the risk of pregnancy, has focused attention on contraceptive and other risk-reducing behaviors in female military personnel. Data from a study of female marines suggest that they underestimate their vulnerability to these health risks—that they suffer an illusion of "unique vulnerability" arising from their selective focusing on their own

285

risk-reducing behaviors to the exclusion of others' risk-reducing behaviors and of their own risk-increasing behaviors (Gerrard, Gibbons, & Warner, 1991). Although respondents generally underestimated their risks for HIV infection and pregnancy, their perceptions of vulnerability were found to be mediated by perceived efficacy and the undesirability of the negative outcome.

The population living in military communities includes not only service personnel but also their families. Military families in the United States and elsewhere, as in Israel (e.g., Anson, Rosenzweig, & Shwarzmann, 1993), often are subject to residential changes over which they have no control and that impede their maintaining social networks, developing spousal careers, and other presumably health-enhancing activities. Data from an Israeli sample showed that despite these negative factors, the wives of Israeli career soldiers did not perceive their health status any differently than a comparable control group, nor did they consume more medications (Anson et al., 1993).

Utilization patterns of prenatal and child health services are of considerable interest to the military, since they are presumed to be related to the morale of personnel. In a study of child health knowledge of mothers using military well baby clinics, 86% of the mothers reported use of professional sources of information beyond that provided at the clinics and 55% reported use of nonprofessional sources such as family or neighbors (Ellwood & Rack, 1982). The data also revealed that a large proportion of the mothers had inappropriate expectations about infant behavior, feeding, socialization, and immunization.

In other military populations, negative relationships were observed between optimal use of prenatal services and levels of family dysfunction. Kugler, Yeash, and Rumbaugh (1993) observed that families with lower levels of cohesion and of overall family functioning were less likely to use prenatal care. In addition, wives whose husbands had lower ranks, and who themselves had less education, were less fully employed, and had difficulties with transportation, were more likely to enroll in the prenatal services provided at an obstetrical clinic than to get their care within a family practice clinic. Transportation and child care problems, income, and educational level were all observed to be risk factors in obtaining adequate prenatal care.

CORRECTIONAL COMMUNITIES

Health issues in correctional communities often involve questions of volunteerism and choice. In a study of male prison inmates in Wisconsin, Hoxie et al. (1990) noted no differences in levels of volunteering for HIV screening between those who admitted to being intravenous drug users and thus presumed to be at higher risk for HIV infection and inmates who did not admit to such use.

Mental health and criminal justice issues are sometimes interwoven in correctional communities. Data indicate that in comparison with males, female residents of correctional communities were disproportionately diagnosed with mental illnesses if their behavior appeared to be inappropriate for their gender role (Baskin, Sommers, Tessler, & Steadman, 1989). In such instances, the encounter between the patient and health professionals reflects the way in which diagnosis and sick role are used as means of social control through psychiatrization. At the same time, the rights of prisoners to refuse mental health treatment are considered to be identical to those of persons in mental hospitals, especially when the treatment is actually a punishment, e.g., certain forms of aversive therapy (Alexander, 1988). In Chapter 14, Anno discusses a broad range of health behaviors in correctional facilities, focusing on risk and nutritional behaviors and on the use of sick call.

RELIGIOUS COMMUNITIES

In considering religious communities, it is difficult to find literature that addresses closed communities alone and that deals with health behavior rather than with illness or treatment. Much of the health-related literature is based on clergy—priests, rabbis, ministers—as an occupational category rather than as a community, and deals with issues of their health status and medical needs. Literature reviews show a large number of studies on the stresses inherent in the clerical role, on the use of alcohol and drugs by clergy, and on programs to deal with these problems. In Chapter 15, Duckro, Magaletta and Wolf discuss health behavior in several religious communities, including nuns, as well as among the clergy as an occupational group.

REFERENCES

Alexander, R., Jr. (1988). Mental health treatment refusal in correctional institutions: A sociological and legal analysis. *Journal of Sociology & Social Welfare, 15*(3), 83-99.

Anson, O., Rosenzweig, A., & Shwarzmann, P. (1993). The health of women married to men in regular army service: Women who cannot afford to be ill. *Women and Health, 20*(1), 33-45.

Baskin, D. R., Sommers, I., Tessler, R., & Steadman, H. J. (1989). Role incongruence and gender variation in the provision of prison mental health services. *Journal of Health and Social Behavior, 30*, 305-314.

Ellwood, L. C., & Rack, R. V. (1982). The influence of military well baby clinics on maternal knowledge and health care practices. *Military Medicine, 147*, 485-488.

Gerrard, M., Gibbons, F. X., & Warner, T. D. (1991). Effects of reviewing risk-relevant behavior on perceived vulnerability among women marines. *Health Psychology, 10*, 173-179.

Hoxie, N. J., Vergeront, J. M., Frisby, H. R., Pfister, J. R., Golubjatnikov, R., & Davis, J. P. (1990). HIV seroprevalence and the acceptance of voluntary HIV testing among newly incarcerated male prison inmates in Wisconsin. *American Journal of Public Health, 80*, 1129-1131.

Kugler, J. P., Yeash, J., & Rumbaugh, P. C. (1993). The impact of sociodemographic, health care system, and family function variables on prenatal care utilization in a military setting. *Journal of Family Practice, 37*, 143-147.

Simmons, S. J. (1993). Explaining health-promoting lifestyles of Navy personnel. *Military Medicine, 158*, 594-598.

14

Health Behavior in Prisons and Correctional Facilities

B. Jaye Anno

INTRODUCTION AND BACKGROUND

The Correctional Environment

Incarceration for wrongdoers began in America in the 1820s. The penitentiary was conceived as a means of reforming criminals and was considered by its founders to be less harsh and more humane than traditional corporal punishments such as the stocks, whipping, or the gallows. The intent was to rehabilitate offenders by removing them from all sources of corruption, providing them with a well-disciplined routine, and isolating them from one another so they could become penitent (hence the name) for their misdeeds (Rothman, 1971).

At the end of the 20th century, while most correctional officials have abandoned any notion of rehabilitating offenders, incarceration remains the most popular punishment for those accused and convicted of serious crimes. Most cities and

counties in the United States have a jail for pretrial detention of those accused of felonies (i.e., serious crimes such as murder, arson, robbery, rape, or grand theft) who cannot make, or are denied, bail. These same local facilities often serve as places of confinement for individuals convicted of misdemeanors and usually sentenced to a year or less. Those convicted of felonies generally serve their time in state or federal prisons, of which there are an estimated 1500 at present. While felons often are sentenced to lengthy prison terms, the average time served is only about 2 years.

For lawbreakers who are considered juveniles (under age 18 in most jurisdictions), larger cities have separate youth detention centers that serve the same purpose as adult jails, namely, to hold the youth until a court hearing or some other disposition of the case has been made. Youngsters who are adjudicated delinquent may be placed in a juvenile confinement center, which is usually operated by the state.

While detention and correctional facilities for juveniles and adults may differ in architecture, size, stated purpose, and other characteristics, they all share a similar function—to remove individuals from the community and hold them for

B. Jaye Anno • Consultants in Correctional Care, 54 Balsa Road, Santa Fe, New Mexico 87505.

Handbook of Health Behavior Research III: Demography, Development, and Diversity, edited by David S. Gochman. Plenum Press, New York, 1997.

specified periods of time. In doing so, federal, state, and local governments assume responsibility for meeting inmates' basic needs. They must provide housing, clothes, food, safety, and health care.

In a 1976 case, *Estelle v. Gamble*, the United States Supreme Court ruled that correctional facilities were responsible for meeting inmates' serious medical needs. The Court reasoned that because the kept are not free to seek care on their own, the responsibility must lie with the keepers. With this decision, inmates became the only group of Americans who have a constitutional right to health care. It was several more years, though, before most prisons and jails had an adequate delivery system in place to meet their inmates' serious health needs (see Anno, 1991).

At the end of the 20th century, the typical correctional health delivery system provides basic ambulatory care on site and makes arrangements with community providers for secondary and tertiary care. Most facilities use a reactive sick call model (patterned after the military) to provide services, rather than a proactive preventive care model. Generally, inmates who have a health complaint sign up for sick call, their requests are reviewed and triaged by a health professional, and they are then called in to be seen by the appropriate health provider (e.g., nurse, physician, dentist, mental health worker, optometrist).

In some ways, the process is similar to making an appointment with a health provider in the community, but there are some important differences. For one thing, inmates have no choice of health providers; they must see whoever is employed by the facility or no one. Inmates also have no say regarding the appointment time or how long they must wait to be seen. In the community, of course, patients and providers work out appointment times together, and a patient who feels that 2 days or 2 weeks or 2 months is too long to wait is free to seek out another caregiver.

While inmate patients generally retain the right to refuse care, they have no right to determine the scope of services that may be offered. In the community, persons are entitled to health care if they can get to it and pay for it. In confinement, inmates generally can get to health services, but have to take what is offered or do without.

The Population Defined

The United States incarcerates more people per capita than any other country in the world (Mauer, 1991). In 1992, the United States incarceration rate for adults in jails and prisons reached 684 per 100,000 adults (Snell, 1995). For juveniles, the rate was 221 per 100,000 juveniles in 1991 (Maguire & Pastore, 1994, p. 583). On any given day, there are over a million and a half people behind bars, including approximately 1,013,000 in state and federal prisons (Beck & Bonczar, 1994), an estimated 442,000 in local jails (Snell, 1995, p. iii), and another 58,000 or so in public juvenile facilities (Maguire & Pastore, 1994, p. 584). During the course of a year, there are over 22 million admissions and discharges to and from United States correctional facilities, of which an estimated 1.36 million are juveniles (Maguire & Pastore, 1994, p.582), about 1 million are state and federal prisoners (pp. 604–605), and 20.3 million are from local jails (Snell, 1993, p. 9).

Most of those incarcerated are young. Over half of the federal prisoners (Maguire & Pastore, 1994, p. 628) and more than three fourths of the state prisoners (p. 624) and jail inmates (p. 592) are between the ages of 18 and 35. Most are male. Females represent less than 10% of admissions to any type of correctional facility (Snell, 1992; Snell & Morton, 1994). Inmates also are disproportionately minorities. Blacks constitute a third of all federal prisoners (Maguire & Pastore, 1994, p. 628), more than half of all state prisoners (p. 624), and almost half of all jail inmates (p. 592).

The individuals incarcerated in United States jails, prisons, and juvenile facilities are overwhelmingly poor. Fewer than half of the adults have finished even high school (Maguire & Pastore, 1994, pp. 592 and 624). Their socioeconomic status and their lifestyle choices (e.g., tobacco use, drug and alcohol abuse, multiple sexual partners) make them among the least likely to have had access to preventive care or regular health services and among the most susceptible to serious illness, violence, and debilitating conditions (Anno, 1993).

When it comes to health care, the inmates in United States prisons, jails, and juvenile facilities are very much a forgotten population. They are seldom mentioned in discussions of the uninsured or underinsured, and they are ignored or excluded from debates on health care reform. They are, after all, politically powerless. They cannot vote, and they have no national organization to lobby for them, yet those behind bars are a substantial number of Americans and are among the nation's neediest in terms of health care resources, owing, in part, to their health behaviors.

HEALTH BEHAVIORS OF INMATES BEFORE AND DURING CONFINEMENT

In terms of understanding the population it deals with, correctional medicine is significantly behind other health care fields. Data regarding the health status and health behaviors of inmates are very hard to obtain. Occasionally, a study is published that presents data on a specific disease, condition, or behavior in a particular jail, prison, or juvenile facility at a given time. Few correctional systems, however, routinely collect morbidity and mortality data; if they do, they do not publish them in a readily accessible format. There is no national agency or organization that serves as a repository for correctional health information.

As a result, what is known often is based on individual studies in particular locales that may or may not be generalizable to the entire population of inmates. Consequently, the information presented in this chapter regarding inmates' health behaviors should be viewed with this caveat in mind.

Tobacco Use

The vast majority of inmates in all types of correctional facilities smoke. Studies conducted over the past 20 years consistently show that incarcerated individuals smoke at rates 2–3 times those of people in the "free world." For example, a 1974 study of 413 males and 45 females residing in seven prisons in Michigan found that 82% of the males and 90% of the females were cigarette smokers (Office of Health and Medical Affairs, 1975). A study of 987 men admitted to the Cook County Jail in Chicago during a 10-day period in December 1980 found that over 84% were tobacco users (Raba & Obis, 1983). Similar results were obtained in a cohort of 366 male inmates at the Middlesex County House of Correction in Massachusetts, 86% of whom indicated that they were current cigarette smokers (Fitzgerald, D'Atri, Kasl, & Ostfeld, 1984). Another study of female inmates in Michigan revealed that over 70% smoked (Gold, 1984), and one conducted in a women's prison in Illinois in 1990 found that 81% smoked cigarettes, of whom 73% smoked at least a pack per day (Coe, Kwasnik, & Shansky, 1991).

Available evidence indicates that inmates' smoking behavior starts at an early age. The National Commission on Correctional Health Care (NCCHC) undertook a survey in 1991 to determine health risk behaviors of delinquent adolescents (Morris, Harrison, Marquis, & Watts, 1995). Ultimately, 1801 adolescents (12.2% of whom were female) responded from 39 juvenile facilities in five states. More than a fourth of these individuals reported that they had started smoking by the age of 9 or 10. By the time they were 13 or 14, over two thirds smoked. Only 19.2% of the respondents denied smoking at the time of the survey. In contrast, a national survey of about 18,000 high school students conducted by the Centers for Disease Control and Prevention (CDC) that same year revealed that only 12.7% identified themselves as frequent cigarette users (defined as smoking cigarettes on 20 or more of the 30 days preceding the survey), ranging from 8.4% of those in grade 9 to 15.6% of those in grades 11 and 12 (Kann et al., 1993).

Most inmates continue to use tobacco while incarcerated. A telephone survey of 18 state prison systems as well as the federal prison system in 1986 revealed that 10 of them still provided tobacco free to at least some of their residents (Romero & Connell, 1988). At that time, none of the state systems had nonsmoking areas in any of the inmate living units and only three systems offered smoking cessation programs.

More recently, some institutions have banned tobacco on the premises for both residents and staff. Juvenile facilities are the most likely not to allow smoking, since it is illegal in most states for people under the age of 18 to purchase tobacco. Among adult institutions, there is a growing trend for jails to become smoke-free (e.g., see Mendelson, 1991; Talkington, 1992), although the majority of jails in this country still permit smoking by both inmates and staff in at least some designated areas. Long-term adult facilities have been the slowest to develop nonsmoking policies (see Skolnick, 1990). In the mid-1990s, only a handful of prisons are smoke-free.

There appear to be at least two reasons that correctional administrators may be reluctant to ban smoking in their facilities. One is their fear that if cigarettes were contraband, some visitors or even correctional staff would begin smuggling them in to give or sell to inmates. A black market would thus be created on the inside for a substance that adults can purchase legally on the outside. Another is that cigarettes in prison can be used by the administration to control inmate behavior. Smoking is a privilege that can be withdrawn for disciplinary reasons. With so many inmates addicted to tobacco, the threat of loss of smoking privileges can be a compelling reason to follow institutional rules.

Alcohol and Drug Use

All studies, regardless of setting, consistently show that inmates are heavy users of alcohol and illicit drugs. For example, in two studies of 30 jails in six states conducted a year apart in the 1970s, it was found that 50% of 641 inmates (Anno, 1997) and 44% of 548 inmates (Anno, 1978) were *daily* users of alcohol on the outside. Over two thirds of the individuals in both studies reported daily use of alcohol or illicit drugs or both prior to their incarceration. It should be noted that marijuana use was excluded from these percentage calculations, since its use was almost universal with these samples.

The drug use forecasting reports of the National Institute of Justice (NIJ) for 1993 showed that from 18% to 54% (median: 33%) of juvenile male arrestees/detainees in 12 selected sites tested positive for at least one drug (NIJ, 1994b), as did 54–81% (median: 63%) of adult male arrestees in 23 sites and 42–83% (median: 67.5%) of female arrestees in 20 sites (NIJ, 1994a). A summary report of the Bureau of Justice Statistics (1994) surveys revealed that about four fifths of the inmates in jails, state prisons, and public juvenile facilities had used drugs at some point in their lives, with two fifths of the juveniles, a quarter of the jail inmates, and a third of the state prisoners admitting that they were under the influence of an illegal drug at the time of their offense.

As with tobacco use, there is some evidence that alcohol use starts at a very early age with correctional populations. The NCCHC study (Morris et al., 1995) revealed that 20% percent of the juveniles in confinement reported starting drinking before age 9, 57% were drinking by age 12, and by age 15, alcohol use was almost universal. About a third of these youths reported more than 100 days of drinking in their short lifetimes. Unfortunately, comparable data are not available for nonincarcerated adolescents. While about 51% of the high school students in the CDC study said that they had had at least one drink in the past 30 days (ranging from 41% of the 9th graders to 60% of the seniors), lifetime alcohol use was not calculated (Kann et al., 1993).

Illicit drug use starts early as well among correctional populations. In fact, in the NCCHC survey, marijuana use paralleled tobacco use; two thirds of the incarcerated adolescent respondents had used marijuana by the age of 13 or 14, and only a fifth denied having used marijuana by the time of the survey. Results regarding other illicit drug use also were discouraging; 11% of girls and 6.6% of boys in this study said they had used cocaine by age 12. In all, 42% of the girls and 30% of the boys had used cocaine, and 20% of the girls and 10% of the boys had used intravenous drugs (Morris et al., 1995). An earlier, smaller study of juveniles in a detention center had similar findings of both early onset and extensive use of alcohol and illicit drugs by this population (Dembo, Dertke, Schmeidler, & Washburn, 1986–1987).

Such extensive drug and alcohol use and abuse contribute to inmates' incidence of HIV seropositivity/AIDS, tuberculosis, sexually transmitted diseases (STDs), and other illnesses at rates much higher than comparable populations in the community (Anno, 1991; Glaser & Greifinger, 1993; Hammett & Harrold, 1994; Hammett, Harrold, Gross, & Epstein, 1994; Weiner & Anno, 1992). The good news, though, is that unlike the case of tobacco, no correctional facility permits consumption of alcohol even though it is a legal substance. As well, of course, all illicit drugs are prohibited in all types of detention and correctional institutions. While illegal drugs or alcohol may occasionally be smuggled into a correctional facility, or inmates may try to make some "home brew," for the most part those incarcerated are drug- and alcohol-free during their confinement. In this sense, many of them are healthier when inside than when outside.

Unfortunately, however, inmates' healthier lifestyles may be short-lived, since most are drug- and alcohol-free because of institutional rules rather than personal choice. The absence of sufficient alcohol and drug treatment programs for inmates (e.g., see Chaiken, 1989; Wellisch, Prendergast, & Anglin, 1994) means that many of them will return to a life of substance abuse when they are released to the community.

Exercise and Nutrition

Very little is known about offenders' exercise and nutrition choices while in the community. Given that most inmates live in poverty and most are heavy users of tobacco, alcohol, and illicit drugs on the outside, it can be inferred that they have poor nutrition and exercise only on a limited basis. Again, their lifestyles often are healthier once confined, since virtually all detention and correctional facilities offer a nutritionally adequate basic diet as well as therapeutic medical diets as needed, and most inmates have the opportunity to exercise at least a few times a week. Standards set by national professional organizations (e.g., see American Correctional Association, 1990; NCCHC, 1992a–c) as well as inmate litigation have put an end to "bread and water" diets and 24-hour per day cell time.

Not all inmates take advantage of the good nutrition and exercise opportunities available to them, though. Pop, chips, candy bars, and other fats and sweets are available for purchase at commissaries in most institutions, even for those on special diets such as diabetics. Legally, institutions cannot force inmates to choose only nutritionally balanced diets any more than they can force them to exercise. Unfortunately, there are no studies that define the nutrition and exercise choices of those behind bars.

Sexual Activity

Most of what is known regarding offenders' sexual activity on the outside is inferred from their lower socioeconomic status, their criminal histories of sex offenses including prostitution, their heavy substance abuse, and their medical conditions. In addition to HIV/AIDS noted previously, studies show that inmates have higher rates of other STDs than the community at large. Of 987 male jail inmates in Chicago, 1.2% said they had a history of syphilis and 15.4% reported having had gonorrhea. On examination, 5.15% of these males had positive cultures for gonorrhea (at that time 11.2 times the United States rate), and 3% were found to have syphilis of undetermined stage (Raba & Obis, 1983). This later figure is consistent with that reported for a sample of New York City male prisoners (Novick, Della Penna, Schwartz, Remmlinger, & Lowenstein, 1977). Raba and Obis (1983) also found that 8.3% of this group had genital abnormalities, mirroring the findings of two earlier examinations of male jail inmates, which identified genital abnormalities in 8.9% (Anno, 1977) and 8.2% (Anno, 1978).

Rates of STDs and abnormalities of the reproductive organs are even higher among female offenders. Resnik and Shaw (1980) reported that 10% of the incoming women at Rikers Island Correctional Facility in New York City had untreated syphilis and 8% had untreated gonorrhea. In her studies of jail inmates over a 2-year period, Anno (1977, 1978) found that between a fifth and a third of the females examined had abnormalities of the cervix or uterus. Ingram-Fogel (1991) stated that in the studies she reviewed, the reported incidence of STDs for female offenders ranged from 10% to 50%. A quarter of the women prisoners in her study reported a history of STDs, and more than 40% had abnormal pelvic findings upon intake examination.

Four more studies contribute to an understanding of inmates' sexual activity in the community. In their study of arrestees at the Lake County Jail in Indiana, Minshall, Dickinson, and Fleissner (1993) found that 2.5% had serological evidence of syphilis, which was significantly associated with the female gender (rate: 13.6% versus 0.73% for males) and with a reported history of prostitution.

In their study of HIV seroprevalence among male New York State prison inmates, Lachance-McCullough, Tesoriero, Sorin, and Lee (1993) reported an overall rate of 7.5% for their sample of 4151 inmates. As part of their study, Lachance-McCullough and colleagues looked at risk behaviors of this population. Of the total sample, 45% reported having had an STD, 20.5% said they were intravenous (IV) drug users, 15.5% said they

had a sex partner who was either an IV drug user or HIV-positive, 3.1% said they were homosexual or bisexual, 4.7% reported being prostitutes, and 15.2% said they had sought the services of a prostitute. For those who were HIV-positive, the rates of risk behaviors were higher for all categories except having had a history of STDs and having sought the services of a prostitute.

Some members of this same group of researchers looked at HIV seroprevalence among a sample of 219 female New York State prison inmates and found an overall rate of 13.4% (Lachance-McCullough, Tesoriero, Sorin, & Stern, 1994). In their review of risk behaviors of this female sample, 31% admitted to IV drug use, 40.7% had had sex with an IV drug user or someone known to be HIV-positive, 36.1% said they had engaged in homosexual or bisexual activity, 20.8% admitted to prostitution, and 58.8% said they had a history of STDs. Interestingly, the reported risk behavior rates of the HIV-positive women were lower than those of the HIV-negative women for all categories except IV drug use.

Finally, Inciardi, Lockwood, Martin, Pottieger, and Scarpitti (1994) looked at HIV infection among 679 prison releasees in Delaware. They found an overall seropositivity rate of 10.2% (9% for males and 16% for females). A little over half of the sample admitted to using injectable drugs, and the vast majority reported having had multiple sex partners over a period of 10–13 years: 9.2% said they had had over 100 sex partners; 53.3%, 11–100 sex partners; 27%, 4–10; and only 10.5% reported 0–3 sex partners.

As with other risk behaviors, there is some evidence to indicate that prisoners begin sexual activity at earlier ages than most people. Over a third of the juvenile delinquents in the NCCHC study (Morris et al., 1995) said that they had had their first sexual intercourse by age 9 or 10. By the age of 13 or 14, over three fourths of these juveniles had had sexual intercourse, and by age 15 or 16, sexual intercourse was reported by almost everyone. What is more, at least two thirds of the incarcerated youths in all ethnic groups had had 4 or more sexual partners, and from 15% (whites) to 45% (blacks) of each ethnic group said they had had 20 or more sexual partners. In contrast, in the CDC study, a little more than half of the high school students said they had ever had sexual intercourse (ranging from 39% of the 9th graders to 67% of the seniors), and only about 19% of all high school students said they had had 4 or more partners (Kann et al., 1993).

Unfortunately, almost nothing is known about the sexual activity of prisoners while they are incarcerated. One can infer that they are considerably less sexually active while behind bars, since they live in a controlled environment and virtually all sexual activity is prohibited. Available sex partners usually are inmates of the same gender, since the overwhelming majority of state correctional institutions are sex-segregated, and even in coed facilities like most jails, males and females are held in separate areas and are not allowed to interact. Occasionally, one hears of a staff member such as a female nurse becoming involved with a male inmate or of male correctional officers having sex with female prisoners. Such occurrences are the exception, though, since staff members who engage in sex with inmates do so at the risk of losing their jobs and would not be hired by another correctional facility.

Methodological Issues. It seems unlikely that the extent of sexual activity of inmates while they are incarcerated will ever be known. While those who work in corrections are aware that consensual situational homosexuality is not uncommon (particularly in long-term institutions), and that coerced sexual activity occurs in all types of correctional settings, it would be methodologically difficult to gather accurate information about such occurrences. Assuming one could obtain permission from correctional administrators to conduct such a study, there are only two sources of data: official incident reports kept by the administration (which would reflect sexual behavior only when inmates were caught) and the inmates themselves, who may be reluctant to

report any sexual activity both because they do not want to be labeled homosexual and because they fear disciplinary action should their behavior become known to the facility administration.

Self-Mutilation and Suicide Behavior

Individuals who are incarcerated commit suicide at rates much higher than for the population at large. This is true in all types of correctional settings, including juvenile institutions (Brown, 1993), jails (Danto, 1973; Hayes & Kajdan, 1981; Hayes & Rowan, 1988; King & Whitman, 1981; Steadman, McCarty, & Morrissey, 1989), and state prisons (Anno, 1985; Danto, 1973; Jones, 1976; Salive, Smith, & Brewer, 1989).

There is also evidence that those incarcerated attempt suicide at greater rates than those in the community (Peters, Kearns, Murrin, & Dolente, 1992; Steadman et al., 1989). This is true even for juveniles. The NCCHC study found that more than a fifth of the youths reported suicidal ideation, while 15.5% (13% of the male and 35% of the female adolescents) said they had made one or more suicide attempts (Morris et al., 1995).

Less is known about inmates' self-mutilating behavior, particularly the frequency with which it occurs. While little has been written on this topic, there is a sense that it is not uncommon. Inmates' self-mutilating behavior can run the gamut from the relatively benign, such as crude, self-inflicted tattoos, usually denoting gang membership, to the extremely serious. Thorburn (1984) identified 14 different categories of prisoners' self-injury methods, including swallowing foreign objects such as razor blades, ingesting toxic substances, puncturing skin or body parts, and cutting wrists, necks, and tendons.

The etiology of intentional self-injurious behavior in prison is not well understood. Part of the difficulty is in trying to sort out whether such behavior is attributable to an underlying psychiatric illness, represents a genuine suicide attempt, is a self-reinforcing behavior, or is a manipulative gesture for safety reasons or convenience (Quijano, 1991). E. H. Johnson (1973) suggests that self-mutilation is a correlate of stress in prison. Regardless of what triggers such self-injurious behavior, it is clearly necessary to learn more about it.

Violence Behavior

It is only since the early 1990s that violence has been identified as a public health problem and even more recently that correctional health professionals have begun to study violence behavior among their patients. As a group, inmates are among those at highest risk of participating in (and being victimized by) violence behavior. In the NCCHC survey, Morris et al. (1995) stated that just under half of the juvenile delinquents (girls as well as boys) reported being members of a gang. Over two thirds of these respondents said they had been in one or more fights during the past year, and a third said they had been in four or more fights during that time,with about a fifth reporting fight-related injuries. Fewer than a fourth of these youths had *never* used a weapon during a fight.

Bell and Jenkins (1995) reported that juveniles between the ages of 12 and 15 have the highest simple assault rate and those between 16 and 19 years old have the highest assault with weapon rate of any age groups. Black youths are the most likely to die from violence as a result of arguments with family, friends, and strangers, whereas Hispanic youths are at the greatest risk of gang-related killings. May, Ferguson, Ferguson, and Cronin (1995) note that in large urban areas, a third to almost a half of homicide victims have prior criminal records. In May and colleagues' study of 582 detainees at the Cook County (Chicago) jail, over half of the respondents stated that they had sought treatment at a hospital for injuries sustained as a result of a fight, stabbing, or gunshot.

Violence behavior does not stop once individuals are incarcerated. Bell and Jenkins (1995) reported that in 1991, per 100 juveniles in custody, there were 3.1 incidents of juvenile-on-juvenile injuries in a 30-day period, and 1.7

juvenile-on-staff injuries. A survey of adult state and federal prisons revealed that during 1993, 42 jurisdictions reported a total of 47 inmates killed by other inmates. The same survey found that in that year, there also were 4829 assaults on staff by inmates resulting in injury (38 jurisdictions reporting), and 8295 inmate-on-inmate assaults resulting in injury (37 jurisdictions reporting) (Maguire & Pastore, 1994, p. 665).

HEALTH CARE
UTILIZATION PATTERNS

Comparison of Correctional versus Community Utilization

Virtually all correctional institutions record the number of sick call visits by inmates per month. By all accounts, inmates use ambulatory health services at rates far exceeding those of comparable populations in the community, particularly in long-term institutions (Anno, 1991; Fitzgerald et al., 1984; Fitzgerald, D'Atri, Kasl, & Ostfeld, 1985; L. J. Johnson, 1989; Reed, 1981; Sheps, Schechter, & Prefontaine, 1987). It is not at all unusual for 5–10% of the inmate population to turn out for sick call every day. Since sick call usually is available 5 days per week in all but the smallest or least progressive facilities, the number of times inmates seek care on an annual basis can be quite astonishing.

Paris (1994) reported an average of 21.6 nursing sick call visits per year per inmate for the Florida Department of Corrections in 1992. This totals 1.7 million contacts annually for a population of about 48,000 prisoners. Similar results have been found in previous studies. Fitzgerald et al. (1984) reported an average of 19.5 outpatient visits per year among a cohort of male jail inmates (18.5 if dental reasons were excluded). Twaddle (1976) noted an average of 17.8 visits annually among residents of a Midwestern prison, and Ingram-Fogel (1991) found an average of 12.5 sick call visits over a 6-month period in her study of a women's prison.

Factors That Affect Utilization

The extensive utilization of ambulatory health services by inmates is affected by a number of factors unique to the correctional setting as well as by those common to all individuals seeking care. The extent of inmates' health needs, the correctional environment, institutional rules, system-mandated visits, inefficiencies in the health delivery system, unrestricted access to care, manipulation for secondary gains, and psychological factors all play a part in increasing inmates' utilization of health services.

Extent of Need. It is clear that inmates, despite their relatively young age, have substantial health needs and manifest a number of risky health behaviors. Contributing to their greater need of health services are the higher rates of HIV/AIDS, STDs, tuberculosis, and other infectious diseases among prisoners as well as their lifestyle choices (e.g., tobacco use, drug and alcohol abuse, sexual activity) discussed earlier.

Inmates also are subject to a number of acute and chronic diseases and conditions that require ongoing medical services (see Anno, 1991). Raba and Obis (1983) noted that over 17% of jail inmates at intake were on medications for chronic conditions, and these individuals would average four visits per year apiece just for follow-up care of their existing chronic problems. In his study using health hazard appraisals to compare prison and community populations, Smith (1982) found that inmates' appraised age (i.e., their projected age based on risk factors such as gender, ethnicity, heredity, and lifestyle) averaged 11.5 years more than their chronological age.

The Correctional Environment. Living in a jail or prison can be hazardous to your health. The overcrowding found in many institutions contributes to the spread of infectious diseases such as tuberculosis as well as less serious conditions such as the common cold or flu. Faulty ventilation systems, lack of temperature control, and unsanitary conditions also can lead to increased morbidity in correctional populations (Anno, 1991).

Further, correctional management practices can increase inmates' utilization of health services. Failure to provide a safe environment can lead to increased injuries from fights with or without weapons. Nathan (1985) notes that institutions that do not provide inmates with adequate nutrition, or sufficient work or recreation, or whose policies are too restrictive, can anticipate greater demands on their health services.

Institutional Rules. In many correctional systems, inmates are required to go on sick call to obtain certain products and services that are only marginally medically related. They must make at least one sick call visit to obtain permission not to shave, or to obtain an extra mattress or blanket, or to receive a different type of shoe than the regular prison-issued one. Similarly, inmates in many areas must go on sick call to obtain special products such as dandruff shampoo, lotion soaps, and other toiletries that are not provided without a determination that they are "medically necessary." Periodic revisits are then required to replenish these products or to continue permission to deviate from institutional rules such as the requirement to remain clean-shaven (Anno, 1991).

System-Mandated Visits. There also are a number of visits to the health unit required by the institution's policies rather than initiated by the patients themselves. Examples include intake examinations, periodic reexaminations, annual tuberculosis screening, HIV testing, chronic disease clinic visits, obtaining vital signs or lab samples periodically for persons on certain medications, medical clearance for certain jobs in the institution, and medical review prior to transfer, discipline, or discharge of the inmate.

Inefficiencies in the Health Delivery System. In many institutions, all medications, including over-the-counter (OTC) preparations, must be distributed by health staff. Additionally, inmates are not allowed to keep any drugs (even

OTCs) on their person or in their housing units. Thus, an individual who has a cold, the flu, a headache, menstrual cramps, indigestion, or constipation must come to the health unit to receive an individual dose of an OTC.

Further, few facilities have established any means of communication between patients and health care providers other than through a sick call visit. For security reasons, inmates are not told the dates of their appointments with community providers, but even the schedule for diagnostic or follow-up care within the institution may not be communicated to the patient. Thus, individuals who saw a nurse at sick call with a dental complaint, or requested to see a mental health provider or to have their eyes checked, or who were told they would be put on the list to see the physician or a specialist or to have lab work done, may never be informed when (or whether) their appointments are scheduled. These individuals must then put in another sick call request to obtain information about follow-up care.

Owing to scheduling difficulties, an inmate may have to make several trips to the health unit to resolve a particular problem. Usually, on the first visit, the inmate sees a nurse. If the nurse cannot resolve the problem, the patient is scheduled for another visit to see the physician. If the physician orders lab work or X rays or a specialty consultation, each would require a separate visit to the health unit. Rarely can an inmate get everything done on the same day.

Access to Care.   At the end of the 20th century, in most institutions, inmates have almost unlimited access to care. National standards require that inmates' health requests be picked up and triaged 7 days a week and that sick call be offered in accordance with the size of the population. In juvenile facilities with more than 100 residents, jails with more than 200 inmates, and all prisons, sick call must be available at least 5 days per week (NCCHC, 1992a–c). Litigation, or the fear of litigation, associated with restricting access to care (see Boney, Dubler, & Rold, 1991) has resulted in these liberal sick call policies.

In the modern correctional environment, there usually are few disincentives to seeking care. The care generally is free, the health professionals are nice, and an inmate cannot be punished for going. The wait to see a health professional may be long and boring, but it may be preferable to the usual daily prison routine. Besides, there are a number of secondary gains to be made by putting in a sick call request.

Manipulation for Secondary Gains.   Inmates have few "perks" in prison, so little things can mean a lot. As an example, they are not entitled to a certain number of "sick days" like many workers in the community. If they want a day off from work, they must go to the health unit and obtain a "lay-in" from the physician. Paris (1994) notes a number of other perks that inmates may be seeking when they exhibit illness behavior, including different diets, job changes, restricted duty, or special products as already discussed.

Goldsmith (1975) describes other secondary gains that can accrue to inmates by adopting the sick role. For one thing, the medical unit contains medications, syringes, and other items that can be used to get high or to sell to other inmates for goods or services. For another, inmates may attain increased status by reason of their ability to "con" health professionals into giving them what they want.

The health unit also provides an opportunity for inmates in different parts of a facility to meet and talk with one another. In fact, in facilities in which inmate movement is restricted, the health unit may be the only place where individuals in different housing units are mixed. Further, if an inmate can convince a physician that a condition requires additional medical workup not available within the facility, a trip to a community provider may be ordered. This may be simply diversion for the inmate or an attempt to enhance the opportunity for escape from the institution.

Psychological Factors. Finally, psychological factors may underlie inmates' requests for sick call. Megargee and Carbonell (1991, p. 21) stated that "somatic responses to stress and individual differences in a person's willingness to adopt the 'sick role' " are two of the psychological elements that influence sick call utilization. Zamble and Porporino (1988) found that 30% of the sick call visits initiated by inmates were stress-related complaints. Fitzgerald et al. (1985) noted that younger inmates and those in the system for shorter periods of time were the most likely to exhibit illness behavior as a coping mechanism. In their study, Suls, Gaes, and Philo (1991) found that negative life events influenced inmates' physical symptomatology and thus increased their utilization of the health clinic.

The study by Megargee and Carbonell (1991) supports the notion that increased health care utilization is associated with psychological factors for some individuals. These workers divided inmates into Nonusers, Occasional Users, and Frequent Users of sick call and administered a number of psychological tests. Frequent Users scored significantly higher on stress, anxiety, and depression scales; were significantly more likely to express their emotions somatically; and reported significantly more nurturing relationships with parents and others than Occasional Users or Nonusers.

PATIENT COMPLIANCE AND SATISFACTION

Almost nothing is known about patient compliance with medical orders or patient satisfaction with health services received in correctional facilities. No published studies dealing with either of these topics showed up in literature searches. Measures of patient compliance would be readily available in many facilities, since "no shows" for clinic appointments are tracked and refusals of care are documented. In addition, the controlled environment in which inmates live makes it easier to determine patient compliance with medication and treatment regimens and the extent to which they have altered their behavior on medical advice (e.g., stopped smoking).

Until recently, the concept of determining patient satisfaction with the health care received in a correctional facility would have been laughable. Inmates are notorious complainers and very litigious. In her survey of grievances in state prisons, Manny (1995) found that health-related grievances ranged from 5% to 50% of all of the grievances filed within the 26 state prison systems responding. The mean number of health-related grievances filed during 1993 was 2375 per state system.

That same year, over 35,000 petitions were filed in federal courts by state and federal prisoners (Maguire & Pastore, 1994, pp. 550–551). This figure does not include the thousands of cases filed in state courts by state prisoners or jail inmates or on behalf of juvenile offenders. While there is no breakdown to indicate how many of these cases might be health-related, suits alleging inadequate health care are common (Anno, 1991).

The filing of a health-related grievance or lawsuit may be a measure of the patient's lack of satisfaction with the care received, but of course it does not mean that the inmate's complaint is valid. Most grievances and lawsuits are resolved in favor of the institution. Inmates often want treatment, services, and medications that the facility is not obligated to provide. Thus, the concept of "patient satisfaction" is somewhat different in corrections than in the community. On the outside, unhappy clients take their business elsewhere. On the inside, they file grievances and lawsuits.

Still, some correctional health administrators have begun to apply concepts borrowed from the continuous quality improvement movement. They have found that administering patient satisfaction questionnaires to inmates can serve as a gross measure of the adequacy of the health delivery system and can help identify areas in which the efficiency or effectiveness of health services can be improved. It would be interesting to track whether early identification of problems through regular patient satisfaction surveys has any impact on reducing the number of health-related grievances and lawsuits filed by inmates.

CONCLUSIONS

Available evidence suggests that inmates' health behaviors in the community contribute to their substantial need for health resources while confined. Drug and alcohol abuse, tobacco use, multiple sex partners, risky sexual practices, violence behavior, and intentional self-injurious behavior put this population at high risk for a host of debilitating diseases and conditions.

There also is evidence that inmates utilize health services at much higher rates than their counterparts in the free world. At present, however, such comparisons are not useful, since much of inmates' utilization of health care is driven by factors unique to the correctional environment. Institutional rules, health care policies, and inefficiencies in the health delivery system inflate utilization patterns for correctional patients.

True comparisons of health care utilization between correctional and community populations should focus only on those factors common to both groups in seeking care, namely, extent of need, illness behavior as a coping mechanism, and manipulation for secondary gains. In all likelihood, though, such studies still would show higher inmate utilization of health care, owing to inmates' risky health behaviors, the stressful environment in which they live, and their greater motivation to manipulate the system.

Some facilities have had success in reducing inmate utilization of sick call by eliminating some of their institutional requirements prohibiting self-care and rescinding policies requiring medical permission to obtain special products and services. Making OTCs readily available and allowing inmates to purchase soaps, shampoos, lotions, and other hygiene products through the commissary are steps that have helped to reduce sick call visits. A number of correctional administrators also have begun to realize that it does not make sense to use expensive health resources to make decisions such as who gets an extra mattress or blanket or a different pair of shoes.

Staff at other facilities are experimenting with therapeutic measures to reduce stress, such as relaxation training (Lutz, 1990) or aerobic exercise (Genovese, Libbus, & Poole, 1995), in the hope of decreasing illness behavior among inmates. Still others are trying to reduce sick call lines by instituting an inmate copayment for medical services. The constitutionality of this latter practice, however, has not been decided (see Lopez & Chayriques, 1994). It is likely that if copayments are determined to limit inmates' access to care for serious medical needs, the courts will not allow their continued imposition.

In many respects, inmates may be better off healthwise while incarcerated, since they have an opportunity to eat good food, exercise, and avoid alcohol and illicit drugs. They also have access to health care on a regular basis. It may be, though, that inmates change only those health behaviors that are prohibited behind bars and continue to engage in other behaviors (such as smoking and eating fats and sweets) that are not prohibited. Further, there is no assurance that inmates will not resume their unhealthy lifestyles when they return to the community.

Too little is known about prisoners' health behaviors while they are confined. Even less is known about why they take the health risks that they do. It should not be assumed that they always do so out of ignorance. Most correctional facilities provide some health education, especially on high-profile diseases like HIV/AIDS (Hammett et al., 1994), and inmates may know as much as people in the community about such diseases (Celentano, Brewer, Sonnega, & Vlahov, 1990; Setzer et al., 1991). They have a number of other health education needs, however, such as smoking cessation programs and self-care for chronic conditions, that go unmet (Coe et al., 1991; Kruzich, Levy, Ellis, & Olson, 1984), and treatment programs for substance abuse as well as wellness programs often are lacking.

Perhaps inmates feel that they have little control over their own health (Zehner Moore, McDermott, & Cox, 1988) or their health behaviors (Voermans & Keller, 1995). Perhaps family and environmental factors have a negative influence on inmates' health risk taking (Dembo et al., 1990; Stevens et al., 1995). Perhaps it is their low self-esteem that contributes to their self-destructiveness, or perhaps they feel that they will not live to a ripe old age anyway, given the dangerous environments in which they reside, both on the inside and in the community.

Clearly, there is a need to learn more about inmates' health behaviors and their reasons for taking the health risks that they do. Only then will we be able to establish effective education and treatment programs to assist them to alter such practices on a permanent basis. It is to society's benefit to do so, since the health costs of imprisonment are great, and behaviors left unchecked on the inside are a threat to the public when inmates are released. Given a captive audience in a controlled environment, what better time is there to try to develop healthier lifestyles in a high-risk population?

REFERENCES

American Correctional Association. (1990). *Standards for adult correctional institutions*. Laurel, MD: American Correctional Association.

Anno, B. J. (1977). *Analysis of inmate/patient profile data*. Chicago: American Medical Association.

Anno, B. J. (1978). *Analysis of inmate/patient profile data—Year two*. Chicago: American Medical Association.

Anno, B. J. (1985). Patterns of suicide in the Texas Department of Corrections 1980–1985. *Journal of Prison and Jail Health*, 5(2), 82–93.

Anno, B. J. (1991). *Prison health care: Guidelines for the management of an adequate delivery system*. Chicago: National Commission on Correctional Health Care.

Anno, B. J. (1993). Health care for prisoners: How soon is soon enough? *Journal of the American Medical Association*, 269(5), 633–634.

Beck, A. J., & Bonczar, T. P. (1994). State and federal prison populations tops one million [press release]. Washington, DC: Bureau of Justice Statistics, U.S. Department of Justice.

Bell, C. C., & Jenkins, E. J. (1995). Violence prevention and intervention in juvenile detention and correctional facilities. *Journal of Correctional Health Care*, 2(1), 17–38.

Boney, J. M., Dubler, N. N., & Rold, W. J. (1991). The legal right to health care in correctional institutions. In B. J. Anno (Ed.), *Prison health care: Guidelines for the management of an adequate delivery system* (pp. 33–52). Chicago: National Commission on Correctional Health Care.

Brown, R. T. (1993). Health needs of incarcerated youth. *Bulletin of the New York Academy of Medicine*, 70(3), 208–218.

Bureau of Justice Statistics. (1994). *Drugs and crime facts, 1993* (NCJ-146246). Washington, DC: U.S. Department of Justice.

Celentano, D. D., Brewer, T. F., Sonnega, J., & Vlahov, D. (1990). Maryland inmates' knowledge of HIV-1 transmission and prevention: A comparison with the U.S. general population. *Journal of Prison and Jail Health*, 9(1), 45–54.

Chaiken, M. R. (1989). *In-prison programs for drug-involved offenders*. Washington, DC: National Institute of Justice.

Coe, J., Kwasnick, P., & Shansky, R. M. (1991). Health promotion and disease prevention. In B. Jaye Anno (Ed.), *Prison health care: Guidelines for the management of an adequate delivery system* (pp. 165–184). Chicago: National Commission on Correctional Health Care.

Danto, B. L. (1973). *Jail house blues: Studies of suicidal behavior in jail and prison*. Orchard Lake, MI: Epic Publications.

Dembo, R., Dertke, M., Schmeidler, J., & Washburn, M. (1986–1987). Prevalence, correlates and consequences of alcohol and other drug use among youths in a juvenile detention center. *Journal of Prison and Jail Health*, 6(2), 97–127.

Dembo, R., Williams, L., LaVoie, L., Berry, E., Getreu, A., Kern, J., Genung, L., Schmeidler, J., Wish, E. D., & Mayo, J. (1990). Physical abuse, sexual victimization, and marijuana, hashish and cocaine use over time: A structural analysis among a cohort of high risk youths. *Journal of Prison and Jail Health*, 9(1), 13–43.

Fitzgerald, E. F., D'Atri, D. A., Kasl, S. V., & Ostfeld, A. M. (1984). Health problems in a cohort of male prisoners at intake and during incarceration. *Journal of Prison and Jail Health*, 4(2), 61–76.

Fitzgerald, E. F., D'Atri, D. A., Kasl, S. V., & Ostfeld, A. M. (1985). Predicting ambulatory medical care utilization in prison. *Journal of Prison and Jail Health*, 5(2), 70–81.

Genovese, J. A., Libbus, M. K., & Poole, M. J. (1995). Organized aerobic exercise and depression in male county jail inmates. *Journal of Correctional Health Care*, 2(1), 5–16.

Glaser, J. B., & Greinfinger, R. B. (1993). Correctional health care: A public health opportunity. *Annals of Internal Medicine*, 118(2), 139–145.

Gold, E. B. (1984). *The changing risk of disease in women: An epidemiologic approach.* Lexington, MA: Collamore Press.

Goldsmith, S. B. (1975). *Prison health.* New York: Prodist.

Hammett, T. M., & Harrold, L. (1994). *Tuberculosis in correctional facilities.* Washington, DC: National Institute of Justice.

Hammett, T. M., Harrold, L., Gross, M., & Epstein, J. (1994). *1992 Update: HIV/AIDS in correctional facilities.* Washington, DC: National Institute of Justice.

Hayes, L. M., & Kajdan, B. (1981). *And darkness closes in ...: National study of jail suicides.* Alexandria, VA: National Center on Institutions and Alternatives.

Hayes, L. M., & Rowan, J. R. (1988). *National study of jail suicides: Seven years later.* Alexandria, VA: National Center on Institutions and Alternatives.

Inciardi, J. A., Lockwood, D., Martin, S. S., Pottieger, A. E., & Scarpitti, F. R. (1994). HIV infection among Delaware prison releasees. *Prison Journal, 74*(3), 364–370.

Ingram-Fogel, C. (1991). Health problems and needs of incarcerated women. *Journal of Prison and Jail Health, 10*(91), 43–57.

Johnson, E. H. (1973). Felon self-mutilation: Correlate of stress in prison. In B. L. Danto (Ed.), *Jail house blues: Studies of suicidal behavior in jail and prison* (pp. 237–272). Orchard Lake, MI: Epic Publications.

Johnson, L. J. (1989). Health status of juvenile delinquents: A review of literature. *Journal of Prison and Jail Health, 8*(1), 41–61.

Jones, D. A. (1976). *The health risks of imprisonment.* Lexington, MA: D. C. Heath.

Kann, L., Warren, W., Collins, J., Ross, J., Collins, B., & Kolbe, L. J. (1993). Results from the national school-based 1991 youth risk behavior survey and progress toward achieving related health objectives for the nation. *Public Health Reports, 108*(1), 47–55.

King, L., & Whitman, S. (1981). Morbidity and mortality among prisoners: An epidemiologic review. *Journal of Prison Health, 1*(1), 7–29.

Kruzich, J. M., Levy, R. L., Ellis, J., & Olson, D. G. (1984). Assessing health education needs in a prison setting. *Journal of Prison and Jail Health, 4*(2) 107–116.

Lachance-McCullough, M. L., Tesoriero, J. M., Sorin, M. D., & Lee, C. (1993). Correlates of HIV seroprevalence among male New York State prison inmates: Results from the New York State AIDS Institute Criminal Justice Initiative. *Journal of Prison and Jail Health, 12*(2), 103–134.

Lachane-McCullough, M. L., Tesoriero, J. M., Sorin, M. D., & Stern, A. (1994). HIV infection among New York State female inmates: Preliminary results of a voluntary counseling and testing program. *Prison Journal, 74*(2), 198–219.

Lopez, M., & Chayriques, K. (1994). Billing prisoners for medical care blocks access. *National Prison Project Journal, 9*(2), 1, 2, 17.

Lutz, S. J. (1990). The effect of relaxation training on sleep, state anxiety, and sick call in a jail population. *Journal of Prison and Jail Health, 9*(1), 55–71.

Maguire, K., & Pastore, A. L. (Eds.). (1994). *Sourcebook of criminal justice statistics—1993.* Washington, DC: Bureau of Justice Statistics, U.S. Department of Justice.

Manny, B. (1995). *Comparative study of grievance processes in prison systems.* Unpublished master's thesis. Finch University of Health Sciences, Chicago.

Mauer, M. (1991). *A comparison of international rates of incarceration.* Washington, DC: Sentencing Project.

May, J. P., Ferguson, M. G. Ferguson, R., & Cronin, K. (1995). Prior nonfatal firearm injuries in detainees of a large urban jail. *Journal of Health Care for the Poor and Underserved, 6*(2), 162–175.

Megargee, E. I., & Carbonell, J. L. (1991). Personality factors associated with frequent sick call utilization in a federal correctional institution. *Journal of Prison and Jail Health, 10*(1), 19–42.

Mendelson, D. (1991, April). Another jail goes smoke free. *CorrectCare, 5*(2), 4.

Minshall, M. E. Dickinson, D. J., & Fleissner, M. L. (1993). Prevalence of syphilis, hepatitis B virus (HBV), and human immunodeficiency virus (HIV) infection in new arrestees at the Lake County Jail, Crown Point, Indiana. *Journal of Prison and Jail Health, 12*(2), 135–155.

Morris, R. E., Harrison, E. A., Marquis, D. K., & Watts, L. L. (1995). Health risk behavior of delinquent adolescents. *Journal of Adolescent Health, 17*, 330–344.

Nathan, V. M. (1985). Guest editorial. *Journal of Prison and Jail Health, 5*(1), 3–12.

National Commission on Correctional Health Care. (1992a). *Standards for health services in jails.* Chicago: National Commission on Correctional Health Care.

National Commission on Correctional Health Care. (1992b). *Standards for health services in juvenile detention and confinement facilities.* Chicago: National Commission on Correctional Health Care.

National Commission on Correctional Health Care. (1992c). *Standards for health services in prisons.* Chicago: National Commission on Correctional Health Care.

National Institute of Justice. (1994a). *Drug use forecasting 1993 annual report on adult arrestees* (NCJ 147411). Washington, DC: National Institute of Justice.

National Institute of Justice (1994b). *Drug use forecasting 1993 annual report on juvenile arrestees/detainees* (NCJ 150709). Washington, DC: National Institute of Justice.

Novick, L. F., Della Penna, R., Schwartz, E. S., Remmlinger, E. E., & Lowenstein, B. (1977). Health status of New York City prison population. *Medical Care, 11*, 205–216.

Office of Health and Medical Affairs. (1975). *Key to health for a padlocked society.* Lansing: Michigan Department of Corrections.

Paris, J. E. (1994). Inmate over-utilization of health care—Is there a way out? *Journal of Correctional Health Care, 1*(1), 73–90.

Peters, R. H., Kearns, W. D., Murrin, M. R., & Dolente, A. S. (1992). Psychopathology and mental health needs among drug-involved inmates. *Journal of Prison and Jail Health*, *11*(1), 3–25.

Quijano, W. Y. (1991). Special populations: Self-mutilation and explosive disorders. In B. J. Anno (Ed.), *Prison health care: Guidelines for the management of an adequate delivery system* (pp. 148–150). Chicago: National Commission on Correctional Health Care.

Raba, J. M., & Obis, C. B. (1983). The health status of incarcerated urban males: Results of admission screening. *Journal of Prison and Jail Health*, *3*(1), 6–24.

Reed, W. (1981). The prison milieu and health problems. *Journal of Prison Health*, *1*(2), 144–153.

Resnick, J., & Shaw, N. (1980). Prisoners of their sex: Health problems of incarcerated women. In I. Robbins (Ed.), *Prisoners' rights sourcebook: Theory, litigation, and practice: Volume II*. New York: Clark Boardman.

Romero, C. A., & Connell, F. A. (1988). A survey of policies regarding smoking and tobacco. *Journal of Prison and Jail Health*, *7*(1), 27–36.

Rothman, D. J. (1971). *The discovery of the asylum*. Boston: Little, Brown.

Salive, M. E., Smith, G. S., & Brewer, T. F. (1989). Suicide mortality in the Maryland state prison system, 1979 through 1987. *Journal of the American Medical Association*, *262*(3), 365–369.

Setzer, J. R., Scott, A. A., Balli, J., Rodriguez-Aragon, G., Mangos, J. A., Flynn, C., Castillo, J. E., & Sherman, J. O. (1991). An integrated model for medical care, substance abuse treatment and AIDS prevention services to minority youth in a short-term detention facility. *Journal of Prison and Jail Health*, *10*(2), 91–115.

Sheps, S., Schechter, M., & Prefontaine, R. (1987). Prison health services: A utilization study. *Journal of Community Health*, *12*(1), 23–30.

Skolnick, A. (1990). While some correctional facilities go smoke-free, others appear to help inmates light up. *Journal of the American Medical Association*, *264*(12), 1509, 1513,

Smith, B. C. (1982). The use of health hazard appraisal in a prison population. *Journal of Prison and Jail Health*, *2*(1), 58–66.

Snell, T. L. (1992). *Women in jail 1989* (NCJ-134732). Washington, DC: Bureau of Justice Statistics, U.S. Department of Justice.

Snell, T. L. (1993). *Correctional populations in the United States, 1991* (NCJ-142729). Washington, DC: Bureau of Justice Statistics, U.S. Department of Justice.

Snell, T. L. (1995). *Correctional populations in the United States, 1992* (NCJ-146413). Washington, DC: Bureau of Justice Statistics, U.S. Department of Justice.

Snell, T. L., & Morton, D. C. (1994). *Women in prison* (NCJ-145321). Washington, DC: Bureau of Justice Statistics, U.S. Department of Justice.

Steadman, H. J., McCarty, D. W., & Morrissey, J. P. (1989). *The mentally ill in jail*. New York: Guilford Press.

Stevens, J., Zierler, S., Dean, D., Goodman, A., Chalfen, B., & De Groot, A. S. (1995). Prevalence of prior sexual abuse and HIV risk-taking behaviors in incarcerated women in Massachusetts. *Journal of Correctional Health Care*, *2*(2), 137–149.

Suls, J., Gaes, G., & Philo, V. (1991). Stress and illness behavior in prison: Effects of life events, self-care attitudes, and race. *Journal of Prison and Jail Health*, *10*(2), 117–132.

Talkington, M. V. (1992, November/December). Smoke-free county jails in Illinois. *American Jails*, 27.

Thorburn, K. M. (1984). Self-mutilation and self-induced illness in prison. *Journal of Prison and Jail Health*, *4*(1), 40–51.

Twaddle, A. C. (1976). Utilization of medical services by a captive population: An analysis of sick call in a state prison. *Journal of Health and Social Behavior*, *17*, 236–248.

Voermans, P., & Keller, M. L. (1995). Incarcerated adolescents' ideas about the reasons for risky and non-risky sexual behavior. *Journal of Correctional Health Care*, *2*(2), 113–135.

Weiner, J., & Anno, B. J. (1992). The crisis in correctional health care: The impact of the national drug control strategy on correctional health services. *Annals of Internal Medicine*, *117*(1), 71–77.

Wellisch, J., Prendergast, M. L., & Anglin, M. D. (1994). *Drug-abusing women offenders: Results of a national survey* (NCJ-149261). Washington, DC: National Institute of Justice.

Zamble, E., & Porporino, F. (1988). *Coping behavior and adaptation in prison inmates*. New York: Springer-Verlag.

Zehner Moore, J. E., McDermott, D., & Cox, J. (1988). Health locus of control of female inmates from the Virginia Correctional Center for Women (VCCW) measured by the Multidimensional Health Locus of Control (MHLC) scale. *Journal of Prison and Jail Health*, *7*(2), 98–108.

15

Health Behavior in Religious Communities

Paul N. Duckro, Philip Magaletta, and Ann Wolf

INTRODUCTION

The focus of this chapter is health behavior, as defined for this *Handbook*, among members of religious communities. Relevant literature was culled from the domain of empirical psychology and medicine and from the discursive writings of theologians and leaders of religious communities. Topics include both ideal and actual practice of health behavior, as well as the effects of such behaviors on health status.

A chapter on health behavior in religious communities is subject to certain unavoidable limitations. First, there is little research available (cf. Shelton, 1992). Although there have been many articles on the importance of physical health and care of the body from religious perspectives, there are relatively few empirical studies of health behavior *per se* among members of religious communities. Many of the existing studies focus on mortality rates and the epidemiology of particular disease states among members of religious communities, but do not measure directly the health behaviors of these groups.

Second, although religious communities may be found in many religious traditions, they are most clearly represented and systematically organized in the Roman Catholic Christian tradition. Perhaps for that reason, the bulk of the theoretical and empirical articles published deal with Roman Catholic religious communities. This chapter will reflect that emphasis, adding references to other communities when available. Religious communities discussed are to be assumed to be Roman Catholic unless specifically stated to be otherwise. Theological underpinnings will largely reflect those of the Judaic and Judeo-Christian tradition.

Third, many of the male religious communities are clerical. When studies are done on priests, they typically include both diocesan priests (i.e., priests serving a diocese) and religious priests (i.e., priests who are members of religious communities). The chapter, therefore, includes studies of priests that evaluated both diocesan and religious priests.

Finally, religious congregations do not con-

Paul N. Duckro, Philip Magaletta, and Ann Wolf • Department of Community and Family Medicine, School of Medicine, St. Louis University Health Sciences Center, St. Louis, Missouri 63104.

Handbook of Health Behavior Research III: Demography, Development, and Diversity, edited by David S. Gochman. Plenum Press, New York, 1997.

stitute a monolithic entity. Individual congregations are actually quite variable in culture, lifestyle, and religious practice (Rooney, 1991). Individual members of "local communities" of any given congregation vary within the common culture of the broader congregation (Shelton, 1992). Generalization of findings from any particular study or essay must be considered as very tentative. Nevertheless, this chapter does contribute an otherwise unavailable compilation of relevant research on health behaviors of religious communities as a source for researchers, clinicians, and leaders of religious communities.

FOUNDATIONS FOR HEALTH BEHAVIORS

Health is not an unfamiliar subject in the teachings that underlie the faith traditions of religious communities. Many faith traditions view the body as a gift from God that is to be cared for with all the reverence due the Giver (Grundfast, 1988). Dualism, with its suspicion toward the body, was certainly widespread in late antiquity; early Christianity was certainly affected by this philosophy (Bokenkotter, 1990). Nevertheless, the Judeo-Christian ethic, reflected in the varied writings of the Bible, also embodies many teachings that encourage the promotion of health and wellness (Grundfast, 1988). There is a particular emphasis on the relationship of physical health and mental or spiritual well-being. Health in the Biblical sense implies wholeness: "not only physical, but spiritual and psychological; not only individual, but also social and institutional wholeness" (National Conference of Catholic Bishops, 1981). In Judaism, fasting and abstinence are designed to call attention to the holy, rejecting any idea that pain itself effects holiness or atonement (Dorff, 1988). Jews are asked to maintain health to allow accomplishment of their individual purposes in life and to live a life of holiness.

The idea that physical and mental health is a necessary prerequisite to fulfilling apostolic ministry of any type is also found in the teachings of

many founders of religious communities (Shelton, 1992). In the several major traditions that form the basis of the large majority of Roman Catholic religious communities, one finds many references to the importance of health behaviors. Ignatius of Loyola, founder of the Jesuits, noted that ascetics who neglected the body "ran the risk of ruining the only vehicle for work that the soul has" (Lockington, 1913). He saw ill health as an opportunity to grow spiritually, but neglect of the body as a willful disregard of the instrument that God provides for the soul to render active service to others. Francis of Assisi, founder of the Franciscan communities, punished his body severely in the early part of his life, but is said after experiencing the stigmata to have asked his body's "forgiveness for punishing it instead of embracing it" (Bodo, 1984). Francis held the opinion that it was sinful to deprive the body of needed nourishment. Augustine is also said to have intended interior and sensory mortification, eschewing heavy physical penances (Zumkeller, 1986).

Horden (1985) notes that even early Byzantine monks were not as a group ascetic to the extreme. Their use of secular medicine was seen as compatible with their monastic life. He suggests that those who practiced the most rigorous asceticism were singled out by hagiographers, thus creating an illusory image of the "horrifyingly inventive" ascetic. Although corporal discipline remained a part of the religious life, Western monasticism turned clearly from the extreme forms of asceticism with the Rule of Benedict (McManners, 1992). Chittister (1990) states that Benedictine spirituality calls for "harmony, awareness and balance" rather than deprivation.

While vocation is recognized as broader than any one issue, most communities today recognize the importance of selecting candidates who are psychologically and physically healthy (Shelton, 1992). Physical health is a prerequisite for entry into candidacy for priesthood and religious life in the Roman Catholic Code of Canon Law (Canon Law Society Trust, 1983).

As a whole, then, the teachings of the major

religious traditions can be used profitably to confirm and encourage the importance of personal health (cf. National Conference of Catholic Bishops, 1981). On the other hand, it must be acknowledged that some religious communities have not maintained a culture in which individual health care is valued. For example, Ryan (1992) recently reflected, on the basis of her clinical experience, that many women religious, from years of dedication to serving others and the commitment to simplicity in life style, have avoided caring for themselves preventively.

ATTITUDES TOWARD SICKNESS

Attitudes toward illness would also seem to play an important role in health behaviors. In principle, it would seem that a person in religious life would be predisposed to understand illness holistically. In fact, the traditions that underlie most religious communities do offer their members great support in understanding illness in terms of the spiritual, social, and psychological factors that affect it and result from it.

Early ascetic monks understood illness as having the utmost spiritual significance (Horden, 1985). Although illness might be understood as the result of sin or possession, it was the individual's response to illness that was the important spiritual act. Of course, the language used by the ascetics seems foreign, but their ideas are not incompatible with 20th-century thought regarding individual responsibility for prevention and treatment of disease. Many of the great monks taught that prayer and secular medicine were entirely compatible in healing, consistent with their view that disease was not exclusively a spiritual event, especially in its treatment (Horden, 1985).

The Talmud forbade a Jew to live in a town in which there was no physician (Dorff, 1988). Physicians were seen as God's partners in healing. Again, illness was not seen as an unqualified evil; in some ways, illness could be seen as a teacher or even as a gift (Lockington, 1913). In such cases, it

was to be borne with patience so that its lessons could be absorbed.

Many founders and other leaders of religious have recognized the effect of adverse health behaviors on the body. A dominant theme bearing on prevention of illness is balance. For example, overindulgence or overexertion is as great a problem as excessive abstinence or inactivity in the Benedictine Rule (Chittister, 1990). Ignatius understood the importance of prevention in avoiding illness. Noting that many men were dying shortly after entry into the community, he accepted the advice of physicians who urged a more balanced lifestyle, including adequate sleep, recreation, and exercise (Ganss, 1970). In most cases, it was understood that the responsibility lay with the individual member to decide, with sufficient reflection, what constituted appropriate self-care (O'Malley, 1993).

In most traditions, there is also a strong reverence for healing and care of the sick. Visiting the sick is "one of the ten ethical duties rehearsed in the daily morning liturgy" in Judaism. Three times daily, the Jewish liturgy includes a communal prayer for the sick (Dorff, 1988). Religious communities founded on Christian principles have carried out this reverence in many forms, including healing ministries. One of the most visible actualizations of this impetus has been the founding of hospitals, most often by women religious (J. P. Dolan, 1992).

Care of their own sick has also been a priority in religious communities. The *Jesuit Constitutions* encourage the assignment of one member to oversee the preservation and restoration of health (Ganss, 1970). In the major communal traditions, those who are ill are excused from duties that might prevent or slow their recovery, and members who are well are enjoined to care for ill members as they would wish to be treated in similar circumstances (Bonaventure, 1922; Kestens, 1962; Zumkeller, 1986).

Persons with long-standing or terminal illness are not to be resented, nor is their care to be slighted. Francis enjoined other members of the community not to form a judgment regarding the seriousness of such illnesses. Bonaventure (1922) encouraged the community's superior to be generous even if it was thought that an individual might be exaggerating a disability.

SEEKING HEALTH CARE

Selection of care providers is not a casual matter for anyone and is no more so for members of religious communities. It is an important health behavior in its own right, with implications for availability and quality of health care. In addition to questions of the provider's competence and manner, members of religious communities may also be concerned about, and want to know, the provider's spirituality and religious commitment, especially when the health matter involves psychological or sexual issues. Discussing the reasons that women religious have not sought out regular physical examinations, Ryan (1992) included reticence to discuss "sensitive health concerns" with male physicians. She noted that many are not comfortable in discussing such issues in any type of mixed-gender group. Women religious share the desire of women in general to be treated with sensitivity by those physicians who examine and treat their reproductive organs.

Many religious are concerned about, and want to identify, providers who are comfortable with the choice of religious life in general and with the choice of celibacy in particular. Uneasiness with celibacy or condescension regarding religious life is quickly evident in the casual aspects of the medical examination. Discomfort with spirituality as an aspect of the person being treated is perhaps even more prevalent among providers than discomfort with psychological factors. In most patient care interactions, spirituality simply is not addressed. The absence of discussion of spirituality or issues related to community life may be more often tolerated in the evaluation and treatment of physical disease, although decision making regarding prolongation of life in the face of serious disease is only one example of the many instances in which spiritual beliefs significantly affect medical care.

On the other hand, the absence of attention to spirituality or religious community is often painfully evident in psychological and psychiatric treatment. It might be suggested that insensitivity to the client's spirituality in mental health care is as serious a breach of practice standards as is insensitivity to the client's ethnicity or culture. It is likely to be particularly so in dealing with persons who have committed themselves to a religious vocation (e.g., Duckro, Busch, McLaughlin, & Schroeder, 1992). A clinical vignette illustrates the point: A priest was reviewing his previous participation in a program to reduce overeating and overweight. He described the process of treatment, which was very comprehensive in its coverage of psychological, social, and physiological elements. It was temporarily effective, but he recalled wondering at the time whether his destructive pattern of eating did not also have implications for his spiritual beliefs. He noted that there was no opportunity to introduce his spirituality or to consider the meaning of his overeating in the context of the values central to his profession and his life. For example, what did it mean to him to overeat in light of his commitment to a simple way of life? What "hunger" was driving his addictive pattern of eating? How could he use his practice of regular prayer to bolster the effects of psychological treatment? If, in fact, attention to spiritual dimensions of religiously committed patients leads to enhanced compliance and outcomes (Martin & Carlson, 1988), ignoring this material in treatment of members of religious communities is even more unfortunate.

Individuality is a highly prized aspect of adulthood in Western culture. It is reflected in common attitudes regarding selection of health care providers and choices regarding health behaviors. Even in this culture, however, there is an ongoing national debate concerning the balance of individual rights and the common good of the community. Consider, for example, the issues surrounding cigarette smoking and use of seat belts.

Even more than in Western society as a whole, the conflict between individual rights and community needs becomes a "turning point" in religious life, with the potential to generate creative resolutions or bitter resentment. In the selection of health care providers (largely in the area of mental health) and the maintenance of health, there is an ongoing effort to balance involvement of concerned leadership (representing the common purpose) with confidentiality or privacy for the individual. The tensions are witnessed in members of the community and treatment teams alike.

RESPONSE TO TREATMENT

For some subgroups in religious communities that did not allow secular medicine to play any role in treating disease, illness was to serve as an aid to salvation through self-discipline (Horden, 1985). To treat disease medically was seen by such monks as spiritually damaging. This attitude was not dominant, however, even among ascetic monks. It is certainly not the prevalent attitude among members of religious communities today. Then and now, the ideal was and is the combination of doing what can be done medically while enduring, and even growing as a result of what cannot be avoided. Giving oneself over, whether to a medical regimen or to God's work in healing, may be associated with improved response to treatment (Martin & Carlson, 1988).

Attitudes toward psychological care are not always as positive. In part, this difference can be attributed to cultural influences, reflecting divergent attitudes toward physical and "mental" illness. The former has been seen more often as out of the individual's control. On the positive side, this perception has led to little shame being associated with most physical diseases, an attitude that has not always been true among persons of religious faith. On the negative side, it has contributed to a reduced sense of individual responsibility for prevention, identification, and treat-

ment. Nevertheless, there have been many advances toward bringing personal and social responsibility as well as impersonal factors into an integrated disease model (Rosenstock, 1990).

In contrast, early conceptualizations of psychological distress and psychiatric illness were overweighted in the direction of individual responsibility. Consequently, shame regarding "mental" illness was quite prevalent (Pincus, Lyons, & Larson, 1991). This was no less true among members of religious communities. Mental health treatment very often was not undertaken unless symptoms were very severe or embarrassed the community. Even then, treatment might be arranged under conditions of great secrecy, unintentionally compounding the shame. The stigma was enduring. There is little anonymity in religious community, and the "community memory" perdures, whether or not the memory is balanced, just, or kind. Reputations, in turn, affect assignments and autonomy. McAllister and Vander Veldt (1961, 1965) found that clergy and religious often felt forced to accept psychological care, seeing it almost as a punishment. This being the case, it is not surprising that they also more often sought symptomatic relief than lasting resolution of their problems.

Since the early 1960s, attitudes toward psychological care have changed remarkably and for the better. There has been a great outpouring of writing from theologians and other spiritual teachers attempting to integrate their faith with psychological science. Great attention has been given to those schools of psychology that are most interested in a broad and deep understanding of human experience. Relatively less attention has been given to more molecular approaches, such as cognitive–behavioral therapy. More recently, there has been attention within the psychological community to the importance of sensitivity to the religious beliefs of clients and to the role of spirituality in human development.

In many ways, religious commitment can itself be considered a positive health behavior. Over the last decade, reviews of empirical research have found a surprisingly robust relationship between various measures of religiosity and health (D. G. King, 1990; Levin & Shiller, 1987). These effects may be mediated by many aspects of religious faith and practice, including diet, presence of hope, and social support (Jarvis & Northocott, 1987). For example, McIntosh and Shifflett (1984) found among elderly religious a weak but statistically significant association of religious commitment with healthy dietary behaviors. One may assume that religious practice and commitment in members of religious communities, considered as a group, will be equal to or greater than in persons in general.

Physical cure is not the only positive contribution of religious commitment. Just as the ancient ascetics taught, founders of religious communities and other religious teachers also affirmed that illness may be transformed and transforming when experienced in the context of one's spiritual beliefs (Etter, 1891; Ganss, 1991; Kestens, 1962). In this context, accommodation to illness comprises a discipline in which all things are turned to good. It may coexist with, but does not require, full trust that all is "God's will"; certainly, however, it does not inevitably lead to passivity or "quietism." On the contrary, a spiritually rooted accommodation to illness can and often does encourage creative productivity over discouragement and is likely to interact positively with medical efforts to heal disease (e.g., Martin & Carlson, 1988).

Articles from the Protestant and Jewish faith communities suggest that this approach to illness continues in religious life. Spaeth (1978) described the results of interviews she conducted with clergy from a variety of Christian denominations who had been ill. Amid the brokenness and loss that she found, there was also a creative energy for life that emerged from the coping, leading to new directions in ministry and spiritual growth. Cutter (1991) wrote of his experience as a rabbi dealing with heart disease. He found greater appetite for living and compassion toward others in the experience. Vanderwell (1986) found that questions regarding his capacity for pastoral leadership after he fell ill with

cancer were more from himself than from his congregation. In the process, he found new courage in his willingness to struggle with trust and hope as he battled his illness. In these ways, persons in religious communities are also likely to find their religious commitment to be a resource when dealing with illness and discomforting medical treatment.

HEALTH AND PERCEIVED HEALTH IN RELIGIOUS COMMUNITIES

Madigan (1958), reviewing the history of thinking about health in religious communities, conjectured that prior to 1900, most persons would have said that the health of Catholic clergy and religious was poorer than that of the population at large. Even educated persons proposed that their presumed state of health was due to their "peculiar" way of living and particularly to their commitment to celibacy (Fecher, 1970).

Later research indicated that the higher death rate was due to more concrete causes and associated with an identifiable set of illnesses. In particular, many religious worked in hospitals; consequently, their exposure to communicable disease was much greater. In addition, diseases such as tuberculosis were easily passed from one member to another in the closeness of community life. As these causes were identified and remedied, quality and length of life became comparable to or greater than those of relevant comparison groups. For example, Fecher (1970) reported on studies of that era indicating that nuns had lower mortality rates than other American women. Madigan (1962) found that mortality rates of priests from some religious orders compared favorably to those of men in general, despite what were perceived to be the greater stresses to which this group was exposed. He suggested that the high role satisfaction reported by these religious may have had a protective effect. By way of comparison, H. King and Locke (1980) found low overall mortality rate in relation to men in general for "white Protestant clergy" in the 1950s; they suggested that the difference might be a reflection of higher social class and its attendant health-related benefits. In another form of religious community, life expectancy of members of Israeli kibbutzim was found to be greater than that of the overall Jewish population of Israel (Leviatan, Cohen, & Jaffe-Katz, 1986). The authors attributed this difference to enhanced social support and medical care common to kibbutzim.

Perceived Health Status. Although mortality may be reduced in religious communities that encourage members to live prudently, Mackenbach, Kunst, de Vrij, and van Meel (1993) made clear the difference between mortality and morbidity, particularly in relation to perceived health status. In their comparison of self-reported morbidity rates between a sample of monks and the general population of males, perceived morbidity for chronic conditions and perceived general health were found to be similar. Disability for activities of daily living, however, was also much higher among the monks, in consequence of the likelihood that as mortality is reduced, disability associated with age may increase. Unfortunately, their sample of monks combined two groups (Benedictines and Trappists) that other studies found to have significant differences in health habits and cardiovascular mortality, limiting the interpretation of their findings.

Nevertheless, in an extensive survey conducted by Fichter (1985a, 1987), the majority of Catholic priests reported their health to be excellent or good. Their perception seemed to be confirmed by more objective data, including days of illness. Overall, the results suggested that clergy have "lower rates of morbidity, both generally and specifically." Primary causes of death were cardiovascular disease and cancer. Catholic sisters also rated themselves as healthy in a study reported by Meurer, McDermott, and Malloy (1990).

Assessment of mental health produced less optimistic data. A substantial proportion of the priests studied by Fichter (nearly 40%) reported

"severe personal, behavior, or mental problems" in the year prior to the survey. The greatest strain was noted among younger clergy, in the first 25 years of ministry. The most common causes appeared to be both psychological and spiritual in nature: overextension, questions of meaning in their work, inadequate personal and organizational resources, groping for relevant religious faith, and a sense of lack of accomplishment. A high proportion of Catholic sisters also reported high perceived stress in every day life, in contrast to their self-reported good physical health (Meurer et al., 1990).

PREVENTIVE BEHAVIORS

Foundations

As in the United States generally, more attention is being given to the role of the individual members of religious communities in maintaining their own health. It is recommended that priests hold themselves individually accountable for their personal health (Fichter, 1985a, 1987). Proper care of the body is evident, however, in the long and varied traditions of religious communities. As a corrective to their culture, early Christians may have stressed more the avoidance of the cult of the body, but there was a corresponding emphasis on maintaining good health, using both spiritual and physical methods. Lockington (1913) observed that although biographers may choose to emphasize the deprivations endured by the saints, they certainly must have had very well trained and healthy bodies to endure such penances without contracting mortal illness. It is written in the *Constitutions of the Society of Jesus* that "just as an excessive preoccupation over the needs of the body is blameworthy, so too a proper concern about the preservation of one's health and bodily strength for the divine service is praiseworthy ..." (Ganss, 1970), p. 167). Although the body was understood by Augustine to be a "lesser good" than the soul, nevertheless it was good, and he enjoined his followers not to mistreat it (Zumkeller, 1986). Franciscan spirituality also places love of the body equal to love of the spirit in the desire to be a complete human being (Bodo, 1984). In the end, most of the great souls behind the development of religious communities agreed that if the body were ruined, no other good work could be done.

Judaism also incorporates clear admonitions to maintain the health of the body (Dorff, 1988). It is a religious duty to care for the body as God's creation, on loan, as it were, until the time of death. Dorff shares a story of Hillel in which he ended a lesson saying he must now perform a religious duty. When questioned as to which religious duty he was going to perform, he answered, "To bathe in the bath-house." His comment clearly indicates the importance that he attributed to care of the body.

The most common admonition in the rules of religious communities is keep to simplicity and moderation in all things. Many specific prescriptions for health behaviors, however, may be found in their rules. It is sometimes forgotten, in this age of science, that many things regarding health promotion were known already to our predecessors, perhaps not with the same precision regarding mechanisms, but with attention to the whole person and with the desired effect of promoting health. Nevertheless, Ryan (1992) found that among religious women, those in communities not associated with a health care apostolate or mission were not well aware of preventive health care.

Among the specific areas addressed are proscriptions against the overuse of alcohol, tobacco, and drugs. The major concern of many writers in the past was drunkenness and associated sinful behavior. There is again, however, the concept that the use of substances that harm the body by causing disease constitutes a sin against the gift of God (Bodo, 1984; Dorff, 1988; National Conference of Catholic Bishops, 1981). Bodo (1984) draws from Franciscan spirituality an invitation to relaxation and a slower pace of life as a way of charity toward the self. The Priests' Senate

of the Diocese of Charlotte, North Carolina (1983), stated that regular time off to cultivate social support systems and recreational opportunities resulted in a better pastor. The welfare of the priest and the vitality of the parish were seen as inseparable. Other areas addressed in rules of religious communities include overeating, food selection, living quarters, clothing, personal hygiene, and exercise (Gill, 1980; Jackson, 1981; Lockington, 1913; National Conference of Catholic Bishops, 1981; O'Malley, 1993). Maimonides published a code of laws with an entire section on health behaviors; he wrote that even sleep, to prevent illness, was in the service of God (Dorff, 1988).

Community Policies and Norms

Given the strong mandate for health promotion in the religious tradition underlying religious communities, an informal survey to compare actual practices to the ideal was conducted for this chapter (and not published elsewhere). Leaders responsible for coordinating the health care plans for 15 of the largest religious communities in the St. Louis area were contacted for telephone interviews. They were questioned regarding their policies on physical examinations, selection of providers, insurance coverage, and preventive education. In this survey, 10 of the 15 leaders reported policies that encouraged or required physical examinations for their active members. One group, a nursing order, had a very specific schedule of suggested examinations for their women, e.g., breast examination and Pap smear. Almost all the communities were self-insured, using government- and employer-provided insurance plans when available to the individual member. (In 1984, Neal [1984] reported that more than 90% of sisters surveyed were participating in the Medicare system). Some communities had established larger risk pools by combining resources with other communities. Costs incurred beyond the limits of the plan or with outside providers were covered by the communities. None indicated that needed care could not be provided. Note, however, that Ryan (1992) found that costs have affected the willingness of some religions to seek preventive care.

Educational programs can play a large role in promoting preventive health behaviors, early identification of disease, and collaboration in treatment. The survey indicated that educational programs were scheduled regularly by 6 of the 15 communities; the rest had no regular plan. Many recognized the need to establish a more concrete plan of illness prevention. Much more attention was given to elderly or retired members than to active members in terms of prevention. Regular examinations were more commonly prescribed. Health education programs were more often carried out on a regular, even monthly, basis.

Prevalence and Effects

The large-scale survey by Fichter (1985a, 1987) of religious and diocesan Roman Catholic priests is a major source of health behavior data. His findings—based, like so many others, on self-reports—are a major framework for this section and are interwoven with the findings of others.

Lifestyle. More than three fourths of the 4660 respondents in Fichter's study reported that they did not smoke cigarettes; almost half of the senior priests reported that they had used tobacco regularly earlier in their lives. Stellman, Boffetta, and Garfinkel (1988) also found that male and female clergy had a low rate of tobacco smoking. Almost none of the women in the Meurer et al. (1990) study were smokers. Consistent with these reports, lung cancer or emphysema or both have been found to be relatively infrequent among priests and religious (Kaplan, 1988; Kinlen, 1982; Nix, 1957; Taylor, Carroll, & Lloyd, 1959). Nix (1957) noted, however, that the close living arrangements of those in communities made transmission of contagious diseases, including respiratory diseases, particularly likely. (The problems with tuberculosis earlier in this century have already been noted.)

Although nearly 40% of the respondents to Fichter's study said they did not drink alcoholic beverages, almost 20% used alcohol daily. Other studies suggest that if alcohol overuse is not a problem for the majority of priests and religious, when it occurs it has serious consequences. McAllister and Vander Veldt (1961, 1965) found that alcoholism was the most common reason for psychiatric admission in their sample of clergy. In addition, a cohort of diocesan priests were found to have a higher prevalence of mortality from cirrhosis of the liver (Kaplan, 1988). On the other hand, Nix (1957), in a review of medical records in his own practice, found cirrhosis of the liver to be uncommon among religious women of the time, most of whom used alcohol very sparingly, if at all. Meurer et al. (1990) also found that few women in their sample used alcohol frequently. Nix found the risks for overuse of alcohol and its consequences to be much greater among male religious and clergy.

Of Fichter's sample, about 40% reported themselves to be overweight, and approximately one third neglected regular exercise. These figures are similar to those generated in an earlier report by Madigan (1962), who found that most of the priests in the religious community he studied gave up regular exercise shortly after ordination. In that study, about one third were overweight by at least 10%. Meurer et al. (1990) also reported that regular exercise was taken by fewer than 60% of the sisters studied; 69% identified themselves as overweight.

Diet may also play a role in excessive body weight and associated disorders. Nix (1957) suggested that diet was responsible for a higher prevalence of gastrointestinal disorders among women religious. He was concerned with the types of food that were typically eaten, including high fat intake. At that time, he believed that many women religious essentially ate a diet typical of low-income families, with the same adverse health consequences. He also commented on the lack of special diets for particular needs, lack of knowledge of dietetics, and poor habits of food preparation. In many communities, there has been tremendous progress in diet over the last three decades. Small local communities allow for individualized food preparation. In a more recent study of two religious communities that eat little or no red meat, however, Kinlen (1982) found no benefit of this dietary restriction in terms of cancer mortality, including colorectal or breast cancer. On the other hand, endometrial cancer was more common. Kinlen noted that the sisters ate a high-carbohydrate diet and that obesity was common. In a study of diocesan priests, Kaplan (1988) found a higher rate of mortality from diabetes. Nevertheless, it is important to recall how much variation there is from community to community and from person to person within a community. Harland and Peterson (1978) studied the nutritional status of a group of Trappist monks who followed a lacto-ovo vegetarian diet. They found that body weights and heights were normal and that planned menus provided sufficient nutrients. Some monks, however, because of their food choices, had low intake of some nutrients. Harland and Peterson recommended careful education for communities that adhere to severe dietary restrictions.

Madigan (1962) found that nearly 30% of a religious community of men reported less than 7 hours of sleep most nights. Meurer et al. (1990) found that more than 80% of their sample of women felt that they got adequate sleep. Hoch et al. (1987) pointed out that mild sleep deprivation is not an unmitigated evil. Comparing the sleep architecture of ten elderly Catholic sisters to that of a control group, the former fell asleep more quickly, wakened less during the early morning, and enjoyed greater REM sleep time. The authors suggested that the improved sleep reflected the effects of attention to sleep hygiene over time, including careful entrainment of sleep schedule and modest habitual sleep restriction. Incidentally, the authors noted that the sisters had "exceptional health habits," with no tobacco use, minimal alcohol intake, balanced diet, and preventive health care.

Preventive Medical Care. Physical examinations are recommended every 1 or 2 years in the policies of many religious communities. More than half of the priests responding to Fichter's survey, however, had not had a physical examination in the last year. The rates of those not obtaining various preventive physical examinations were similar to those for men in general. Those reporting better health were less likely to have had a physical examination in the last year, suggesting that physical examinations are used more often to respond to symptoms than to prevent illness. Nix (1957) found that only a minority of communities, as a type of spiritual discipline, ignored early signs of illness.

More recently, Ryan (1992) and Meurer et al. (1990) reported a "precarious" lack of preventive/screening physical examinations among women religious. Of a group participating in a health forum, up to 20% had not sought a physical examination over the previous 4 or more years. Similar statistics were presented for breast and pelvic examinations. Fewer than half performed regular self-examination of their breasts. There were many reasons offered, including lack of knowledge, reticence to speak with male physicians, reluctance to spend community funds, and a sense of their not being worth the expense unless truly ill. Nursing staff indicated that routine mammography was not recommended for sisters under their care because of perceived cost. In response, a consortium of women's religious communities began a series of annual health forums that have served a large number of women religious. The focus has been on increased awareness of health care options, including self-care and screening. Follow-up surveys indicated positive changes in health habits and increased sense of personal responsibility for health (Meurer et al., 1990; Ryan, 1992).

Sexual Behavior. A unique aspect of the lifestyle of Roman Catholic religious communities is the commitment to celibacy. There have been many studies of the relationship of this behavioral commitment to prevalence of reproductive organ disease. Nix (1957), Taylor et al. (1959), Fecher (1961), and Fraumeni, Lloyd, Smith, and Wagoner (1969) reported that women religious had frequent cancer of the breast in later years (with one report also finding higher incidence of ovarian, uterine, and large intestine cancer), but less frequent cancer of the cervix. Other studies since that time continued to suggest that celibate religious women are protected against cervical cancer (Levin & Schiller, 1987), with cancer rates consistent with those of unmarried women. However, Skrabanek (1988) and Griffiths (1991) argued against accepting the latter conclusion, suggesting that the data were based on weak studies that were at best inconclusive. The most reliable finding is the higher incidence of breast cancer, the risk factor presumed to be not having either delivered or nursed children. Despite this finding, Ryan (1992) and Meurer et al. (1990) found disturbingly low rates of breast-screening examinations among women in religious communities. Snowden, Gonzalez, O'Leary, and Ostwald (1989) reported an even lower rate of screening for breast cancer in their study of a group of elderly sisters.

Among male clergy and religious, rates for prostate cancer have been found to be equivalent to or somewhat lower than those for men in general (Kaplan, 1988; Michalek, Mettlin, & Priore, 1981; Ross, Deapen, Casagrande, Paganini-Hill, & Henderson, 1981). Celibacy appears to be at worst a neutral factor with regard to prostate cancer and at best to provide a slightly protective effect.

Psychological Factors. Psychological health is more problematic among religious than physical health. In Fichter's survey, about 40% reported "severe personal, emotional, behavioral, or mental problems" in the last 12 months. In fact, about 6% of priests exhibited a variety of characteristics that were judged to be risk factors for a "nervous breakdown." Those who experienced frequent depressed mood or reported high levels of emotional stress also reported higher rates of various physical ailments. These characteristics were most evident in the younger priests, especially in the first 25 years of service.

Only about 20% sought professional help despite their perception of these problems as severe; the rest "managed" the problem themselves. This finding echoes earlier observations that psychiatric care is often delayed or avoided because of cost, time, and embarrassment (cf. Nix, 1957).

McAllister and Vander Veldt (1965) presented data suggesting that clergy and religious presenting for hospitalization were admitted more frequently than lay groups for problems involving alcohol, drugs, sexual behavior, obsessive-compulsive disorders, and personality disorders. The data did not imply that such problems were more prevalent among religious and clergy, but pointed to those problems most likely to lead to hospitalization among clergy and religious at that time. They may reflect both the particular standards held for them by their leadership and unique representations of psychosocial problems within that group.

The report of the Priests' Senate of the Diocese of Charlotte, North Carolina (1983), associated much of the risk for psychological distress among clergy with the lack of boundaries between work and home. The difficulty with boundaries between home and work is likely to be true of nonclergy in religious communities and for clergy of other denominations and faith traditions. In the Fichter study, however, only about 20% of the priests felt overburdened by their work. About 60% reported taking one day off per week. More than three fourths took their annual vacation, typically 3 weeks or more. On the other hand, younger priests, among whom was found the greater psychological distress, reported working more hours than their seniors. Many of the priests reported being "on duty" more than 60 hours per week. Poor health was associated with taking less time off. Among women religious, Meurer et al. (1990) found that perceived daily stress was high. This stress was not entirely associated with time demands, but there was an inverse relationship between time to relax and perceived stress.

Bangs (1986), among many others, has written about the many potential sources of psychosocial stress in religious life in addition to the work role. There were suggestions outside Fichter's formal database that many of the stressors affecting the respondents might be associated with the religious organizations themselves, rather than with the duties of ministry.

Community Practices. There have been many effects of the renewal initiated in religious life beginning with the 1960s. McCann (1977–1978) noted that women religious (and men as well) have been asked to relate interpersonally more intensely, without many of the formal common activities that previously provided structure to daily interactions. The increased social ambiguity and attendant emotions that this practice introduced into religious life cannot be overemphasized. Aggressive anger has become more prominent as an acknowledged feature of women religious (Dolan, Meier, & Dill, 1993). Frustration with church organizations and colleagues is less masked (Kenel, 1988).

Ostini (1990) suggests that another effect of these changes has been the emphasis on ministry rather than on community. Many religious now have primary identification with their job rather than with their community. In some cases, the religious may have found the worst of both worlds. In addition to the erosion of comfort in the home community, there are all the tensions of daily work. Without the obligations of families, religious are seen and see themselves as having more time to devote to their apostolates, as being persons who can work long hours and many years. Many elderly religious think of themselves as persons who never retire. As the number of elderly disabled has increased, those who can work feel even more pressure. The work becomes not only an apostolate, but also a means of financially supporting strapped communities. Ostini worries that members of religious communities are now commonly overworking, citing this a risk factor for disease and psychological distress.

On the other hand, Rayburn, Richmond, and Rogers (1986) reported that in a sample of men and women religious, seminarians, and clergy (including a sample of Protestant ministers),

those in religious life exhibited lower overall occupational stress and personal strain than a control group (not otherwise described). The Protestant ministers were noted to experience the highest occupational stress of the religious sample subgroups.

Behavioral factors are related to disease in a number of studies. Building on previous studies, Caffrey (1969) compared several subgroups of monks. One subgroup, with the highest rate of myocardial infarction, could be differentiated from the other groups on the presence of Type A behavior and "role conflict" in their lives, beyond what could have been predicted from dietary factors and serum cholesterol alone. In a specific assessment of 644 monks, Caffrey (1970) reported that a set of six factors (derived from an initial pool of 57 variables), including a "Type A" factor, could discriminate monks who had suffered myocardial infarction. The association of Type A behavior pattern with heart disease has been the subject of many studies in the general population, with conflicting results.

Caffrey's results may be further considered in the light of a study in which the blood pressures of Italian sisters of a "secluded monastic order" were compared to those of a group of lay women living in communities surrounding the monastery (Timio et al., 1988). Despite similar increases over 20 years in body weight, body mass, serum cholesterol, and triglycerides, blood pressures increased only in the lay group. Urinary sodium excretion was similar in the two groups, and neither used tobacco or oral contraceptives. The authors noted that the lifestyle of the sisters was characterized by silence, meditation, and prayer. In Fichter's survey as well, there were significant relationships among positive health habits, physical well-being, and psychological well-being. Positive health habits included abstinence from tobacco, adequate hours of sleep, regular exercise, normal body weight, and minimal or no alcohol use.

The obstacles to discussing the psychological health of communities include an unwillingness to disclose "family secrets" (Shelton, 1992). Another obstacle is shame, in that communities hold high ideals that are difficult to meet. Still another obstacle is limited skill at resolving conflict, so that healthy anger cannot be entertained. This limitation results in the suppression of anger or the development of unhealthy hostility, often tied to illness or greater disability (Duckro, Chibnall, & Tomazic, 1995; Tschannen, Duckro, Margolis, & Tomazic, 1992; Williams & Williams, 1994). Isolation, another obstacle, results in loneliness and depression, which in turn lead to other health risks and increased risk of acting in ways unacceptable or hurtful to the community. Shelton encouraged more preventive behaviors to enhance the quality of community life, including mechanisms to enhance communication, sense of shared spiritual commitment, and psychological intervention without stigma. Sperry (1991) also suggested that although the emphasis in many reports is on the priest as individual, greater emphasis is due the "structure or culture" of individual communities or dioceses.

Of historical interest, Fecher (1961) suggested that the choice of "headgear ... and other full-flowing garments" worn by women religious could not be discounted as an influence in the rate of accidents in the home and on the highway. Nix (1957) also singled out religious garb as a risk factor for some types of diseases, injuries, and postural anomalies. In most communities, religious garb now so closely approximates conservative lay garb in style that it is not likely to be a problem. Nix also found that prepatellar bursitis (housemaid's knee) was common among young women religious, particularly novices; he seldom encountered it among priests.

Other Religious Communities. Among the few studies considering non-Catholic religious communities, Ogata, Ikeda, and Kuratsune (1984) studied Zen priests. They noted that although not all monks now live celibate lives or eliminate all tobacco, alcohol, or animal foods, they continue as a group to honor the traditional precepts. The monks live during at least several months of their training in an atmosphere of strict discipline in a monastery and afterward continue to try to live a simple life with time for meditation. Particular health behaviors typically include a high proportion of vegetables in the diet, minimal tobacco use, and moderation in all activities. The authors found that Zen priests had lower mortality rates in general and for a variety of specific diseases as well. Jarvis and Northcott (1987) cited two studies of Hutterites, a group that lives communally and conservatively. Hutterites are physically active, abstinent from tobacco, and make full use of health care facilities. Female members of this religious community had lower mortality from cancer. Men had lower rates of lung cancer, consistent with the prohibition of smoking, but higher rates of stomach cancer.

In considering these studies, one must bear in mind that religious communities vary widely with respect to their health habits, with predictable variations in health status. It is very difficult to generalize any particular finding to religious communities as a whole. In addition, members within each group vary in their behaviors. Fonnebo (1985) found that male members of the Seventh-Day Adventist church considered to be actively following the prescriptions of their church had more favorable total cholesterol and systolic blood pressure than those who were not. Enstrom (1978) reported analogous data in studying active Mormon males (High Priests and Seventies [elders ordained for missionary work under the 12 Mormon Apostles]), compared with men in general and Mormons as a whole. The active Mormons had greater life expectancy, and reduced mortality from cancer, especially at smoking-related sites. The differences were attributed to adherence to prohibition of the use of alcohol, tobacco, and caffeine. Gardner and Lyons (1982) reported similar findings with regard to rates of several types of cancer among Mormon priests who were most adherent to the practices of their faith.

FUTURE DIRECTIONS

Research

Many implications arise from consideration of the data on health behaviors among religious communities. Clearly, further research could be profitably conducted in this area. In many communities, there are coherent databases regarding disease and community lifestyle that lend themselves to retrospective study of the relationship of health behaviors and disease. In most cases, the resulting findings would have implications for persons not living in religious communities. Fecher (1961) provided an example of such research by way of the discovery that the high mortality rate among women religious was due in part to the prevalence of tuberculosis, which spread quickly in their close living situations. This finding was important not only to changing the practices of religious communities, but also to the understanding of preventive health behaviors in the larger population.

In addition, there may be much to be learned with regard to maintaining quality of life among the elderly in religious communities. Perhaps because of the overall positive health behaviors found in religious communities, there are many "superannuated" members whose past and present health behaviors and needs might contribute significantly to the betterment of the elderly in general.

It might be instructive to compare communities that differ with regard to common practice of given health behaviors to determine the effect on physical and psychological health. Within a given community, systematic study of the changes in such variables before and after the radical changes of the 1960s may be possible. Religious communities are obvious sites for study of the relationship of religious commitment and health.

Religious communities are also ideal settings in which to study the efficacy of educational efforts to change health attitudes and practices and the effects of such changes. Dietary and exercise practices may be a needed focus, and preventive care among active adults is inconsistent. Such studies might be of mutual benefit, in that communities would also receive free care associated with the studies in a time of limited financial resources.

The declining numbers living in religious communities should not discourage further study of these groups for their own sake. The current declines do not indicate that religious communities are inevitably doomed. From the long-range perspective, the current reductions in size may be part of a larger cyclic movement, returning to the smaller numbers that were common prior to the middle of this century.

Finally, there are lacunae in the research literature. Nix (1957) postulated that "an entire thesis" could be written on the subject of neglect of "colored" religious by Catholic medical facilities and practitioners of this time. The need remains. There are few or no data on ethnic minorities in religious communities. In addition, more research is needed on the nature of religious communities of other denominations and faith traditions and on their health behaviors. Overall, there are far more data on disease states than on health behaviors; this imbalance must be corrected in the interest of disease prevention and health promotion.

Clinical Care

Clinically, two areas stand out. First, Fecher's (1961) three-way model and Nix's (1960) community physician model continue to be debated in their modern forms, particularly with regard to mental health care (e.g., Duckro et al., 1992; Harris, 1992; Moore, 1990; Tortorici, Grame, & Coyne, 1993). Recognizing the quasi-familial nature of religious communities, Fecher (1961) tried to formalize a "three-way" model of health maintenance, including the physician, community superior, and individual member. Nix (1960), reporting the work of a committee studying health care of religious, suggested use of a "community physician" who was aware of the particular community's culture and trusted by the community's superior.

In practice, there are many difficulties in carrying out such a plan. Members of religious communities may resist being attended by a health care provider who works collaboratively with leadership. Although the ideal of religious community is relationship and trust, members in some communities fear the kind of "paper trail" that can be established when medical records or summaries are shared with leadership. Particularly in mental health or psychosomatic medicine, there is the often realistic fear of being "labeled" (e.g., Greer, 1994). In addition, leadership itself changes regularly. Community leaders are commonly admonished to treat their members well because one of them may well be their superior in the next term. These changes contribute to renewal of community life, but they also result in an inherent instability. Leaders usually have been actively involved in their congregations; they bring a history of friendship or animosity with many other individual members, with whom they now may be asked to share, as leader, in some of the most personal aspects of the individual members' lives.

Nevertheless, the collaborative model still seems to be most compatible with the actual and ideal structure of religious life. It has the potential to contribute fruitfully to planful and effective preventive health care. Given the inherent tensions, effective mechanisms for conflict resolution must be part of the plan. Resolution must be carried out in the context of shared respect for the motives if not the behaviors of fellow members, and especially leaders of the community.

Further professional consideration of these collaborative models would be fruitful. They are quite different from the models of treatment on which current professional ethics codes are based. Professionals working with religious communities find themselves having to make many judgment calls. From the other side of the issue, some members of religious communities find the collaborative model of care to be intrusive. While some of these reactions may in fact reflect prior problems in relationship to authority or issues that gave rise to personal shame or resentment, there is also much to be learned from these reactions. The primary question is whether it is possible to implement such a collaborative model, seemingly so well suited to the unique nature of religious community, without sacrificing due privacy and autonomy of the individual. Ground rules for informed consent, preservation of confidentiality, and avoidance of "secrets" may be critical aspects of successful implementation.

The overall "social health" of the community being served may be an important issue. The psychological health of religious communities is an area ripe for study and clinical work. Stress is reported by men and women religious alike, and there seems to be more common difficulty in this area than in the maintenance of physical health.

When the problem for which the member is referred involves distress to the community as well as or instead of to the individual member, the issues are more complex. In some cases, it may be that psychological intervention is not appropriate or possible and that the community must decide the issue according to its own procedures and policies. In such cases, the best psychological consultation may be to community leadership, to assist in applying consequences naturally, dispassionately, clearly, and consistently. Overall, encouragement of community cultures in which individual and group needs are balanced, and in which conflicts are resolved openly, will be essential underpinnings for any collaborative model.

The second salient area in clinical care is the aging of members, which is an important clinical and social issue for religious communities as well as a potential area of study. Religious communities must provide for the health of their members, which requires personal, physical, and financial resources for their care. Of necessity, provision of care will require innovative approaches to preventive health care, encouragement of self-care to the extent possible, and development of a positive social environment.

There seems to be a solid base on which to build programs for the elderly religious, despite the daunting numerical projections. Fichter (1985b) found that among religious and diocesan priests who had reached the age of retirement, about two thirds claimed excellent or good health. Those who had retired more often reported only fair or poor health, although about two thirds of both groups reported no sick days in the last year. Fichter concluded that many priests retire because of age rather than illness. On psychological factors, retirees reported much less emotional tension and worry.

Duckro, Hay, and Smith (in press) reviewed many ways in which religious communities are trying to increase the quality of life for senior members. Among these means were programs designed to help the elders continue to feel part of the community. For persons who have given themselves to community life, this feeling is a critical aspect of quality of life. The different types of reminiscence therapies were discussed in detail as a method benefiting not only the elderly, but also the younger members who conducted them.

Manasse (1994) described programs offered by two Sisters of Mercy. Sister Marie Shefckik teaches senior members an ancient Chinese system of exercise and meditation, t'ai chi, as a way of reducing stress and enhancing health and subjective well-being. She teaches a modified form of the discipline, with simpler movements that can be done even sitting down. Sister Mary Chistelle Macaluso promotes the health-giving effects of laughter. This idea, popularized by Norman Cousins (1979) in the story of his own healing, is perhaps one of the most pleasing and painless methods of preventive health care.

The attention to elders is entirely consistent with the beliefs of many religious communities, even though the actualization of these beliefs may be strained on difficult days. Chit (1989) noted that the Buddha also taught high respect for the seniors in his Order of Monks. Describing Buddhist communities in Burma, he noted that living in Buddhist monasteries can be a source of emotional and physical support to those elderly who have prepared themselves by regular retreats and religious studies over the years of their active life. Maintaining specific homes for the elderly is another way the Buddhist community cares for medical and psychosocial needs, growing from the desire to give. Chit (1989, p. 58)

recalled these words from the discourses of the Buddha: "He who wishes to serve and attend on the Buddha, such a one should serve and attend on the sick and the aged."

REFERENCES

Bangs, A. J. (1986). The application of the cognitive therapy model to the treatment of burnout among members of active religious communities. *Journal of Pastoral Counseling*, *21*, 9–21.

Bodo, M. (1984). *The way of St. Francis*. Garden City, NY: Doubleday.

Bokenkotter, T. (1990). *A concise history of the Catholic church*. New York: Image Books (Doubleday).

Bonaventure. (1922). *A Franciscan view of the spiritual and religious life* [translated by D. Devas]. London: Thomas Baker.

Caffrey, B. (1969). Behavior patterns and personality characteristics related to prevalence rates of coronary heart disease in American monks. *Journal of Chronic Diseases*, *22*, 93–103.

Caffrey, B. (1970). A multivariate analysis of sociopsychological factors in monks with myocardial infarctions. *American Journal of Public Health*, *60*, 452–458.

Canon Law Society Trust. (1983). *Code of canon law* [in English translation]. Grand Rapids, MI: Eerdmans Publishing.

Chit, D. K. M. (1989). Add life to years the Buddhist way. In W. M. Clements (Ed.), *Religion, aging, and health: A global perspective* (pp. 39–67). New York: Haworth Press.

Chittister, J. (1990). *Wisdom distilled from the Daily: Living the Rule of St. Benedict today*. New York: HarperCollins.

Cousins, N. (1979). *Anatomy of an illness*. New York: W. W. Norton.

Cutter, W. (1991). Growing sick: Thoughts on months as a heart patient, years as a rabbi. In L. Meier (Ed.), *Jewish values in health and medicine* (pp. 29–40). New York: University Press of America.

Dolan, J. P. (1992). *The American Catholic experience: A history from Colonial times to the present*. South Bend, IN: University of Notre Dame Press.

Dolan, S. A., Meier, M. M., & Dill, C. A. (1993). The changing image of Catholic women. *Journal of Religion and Health*, *32*, 91–106.

Dorff, E. (1988). Judaism and health. *Health Values*, *12*, 32–36.

Duckro, P. N., Busch, C., McLaughlin, L., & Schroeder, J. (1992). Psychotherapy with religious professionals: An aspect of the interface of psychology and religion. *Psychological Reports*, *70*, 304–306.

Duckro, P. N., Chibnall, J. T., & Tomazic, T. J. (1995). Anger, depression, and disability: A path analysis of relationships in a sample of chronic post-traumatic headache patients. *Headache, 35,* 7-9.

Duckro, P. N., Hay, L., & Smith, D. (in press). Caring for elderly clergy and religious. In P. Szwabo, K. Solomon, & G. Grossberg (Eds.), *Psychosocial needs of special populations of elderly.* New York: Springer.

Enstrom, J. E. (1978). Cancer and total mortality among active Mormons. *Cancer, 42,* 1943-1951.

Etter, J. W. (1891). Editorial: Sickness better than health. *United Brethren Review, 2,* 260-268.

Fecher, C. J. (1961). Health and longevity of today's sisters. *Social Compass, 8,* 347-354.

Fecher, C. J. (1970). History of health studies. In J. T. Nix & C. J. Fecher (Eds.), *Stamina for the apostolate* (pp. 3-14). Washington, DC: Center for Applied Research in the Apostolate.

Fichter, J. H. (1985a). *A study of the health of American Catholic priests.* Washington, DC: United States Catholic Conference.

Fichter, J. H. (1985b). The dilemma of priest retirement. *Journal for the Scientific Study of Religion, 24,* 101-104.

Fichter, J. H. (1987). Life-style and health status of American Catholic priests. *Social Compass, 34,* 539-548.

Fonnebo, V. (1985). The Tromso heart study: Coronary risk factors in Seventh-Day Adventists. *American Journal of Epidemiology, 122,* 789-793.

Fraumeni, J. F., Lloyd, J. W., Smith, E. M., & Wagoner, J. K. (1969). Cancer mortality among nuns: Role of marital status in etiology of neoplastic disease in women. *Journal of the National Cancer Institute, 42,* 455-468.

Ganss, G. E. (Ed.) (1970). *Saint Ignatius of Loyola: The Constitutions of the Society of Jesus.* St. Louis: Institute of Jesuit Sources.

Ganss, G. E. (Ed.) (1991). *Ignatius of Loyola: The spiritual exercises and selected works.* New York: Paulist Press.

Gardner, J. W., & Lyons, J. L. (1982). Cancer in Utah Mormon men by law priesthood level. *American Journal of Epidemiology, 116,* 243-257.

Gill, J. (1980). Apostolic health. *Human Development, 1,* 38-47.

Greer, J. M. (1994). Needed: An ethic of memories. *Review for Religious, 53,* 200-206.

Griffiths, M. (1991). "Nuns, virgins, and spinsters": Rigoni-Stern and cervical cancer revisited. *British Journal of Obstetrics and Gynaecology, 98,* 797-802.

Grundfast, S. H. (1988). Editorial: To life. *Health Values, 12,* 27.

Harland, B. F., & Peterson, M. (1978). Nutritional status of lacto-ovo vegetarian Trappist monks. *Journal of the American Dietetic Association, 72,* 259-264.

Harris, J. (1992). Therapy for religious: The troublesome triangle. *Review for Religious, 51,* 282-288.

Hoch, C. C., Reynolds, C. F., III, Kupfer, D. J., Houck, P. R., Berman, S. R., & Stack, J. A. (1987). The superior sleep of healthy elderly nuns. *International Journal of Aging and Human Development, 25,* 1-9.

Horden, P. (1985). Monks, hermits and the ascetic tradition. *Studies in Church History, 22,* 41-52.

Jackson, E. (1981). *The role of faith in the process of healing.* Minneapolis, MN: Winston Press.

Jarvis, G. K., & Northcott, H. C. (1987). Religion and differences in morbidity and mortality. *Social Science and Medicine, 25,* 813-824.

Kaplan, S. (1988). Retrospective cohort mortality study of Roman Catholic priests. *Preventive Medicine, 17,* 335-343.

Kenel, M. E. (1988). Religious women and the problem of anger. *Journal of Religion and Health, 27,* 236-244.

Kestens, A. (1962). *Spiritual guidance: Fundamentals of ascetical theology based on the Franciscan ideal.* Paterson, NJ: St. Anthony Guild.

King, D. G. (1990). Religion and health relationships: A review. *Journal of Religion and Health, 29,* 101-112.

King, H., & Locke, F. B. (1980). American white Protestant clergy as a low-risk population for mortality research. *Journal of the National Cancer Institute, 65,* 1115-1124.

Kinlen, L. J. (1982). Meat and fat consumption and cancer mortality: A study of strict religious orders in Britain. *Lancet, 1*(April 24), 946-949.

Leviatan, U., Cohen, J., & Jaffe-Katz, A. (1986). Life expectancy of kibbutz members. *International Journal of Aging and Human Development, 23,* 195-205.

Levin, J. S., & Schiller, P. L. (1987). Is there a religious factor in health? *Journal of Religion and Health, 26,* 9-36.

Lockington, W. J. (1913). *Bodily health and spiritual vigor.* New York: Longmans, Green.

Mackenbach, J. P., Kunst, A. E., de Vrij, J.H., & van Meel, D. (1993). Self-reported morbidity and disability among Trappist and Benedictine monks. *American Journal of Epidemiology, 138,* 569-573.

Madigan, F. C. (1958). Do religious die younger? *America, 98,* 562-564.

Madigan, F. C. (1962). Role satisfactions and length of life in a closed population. *American Journal of Sociology, 67,* 640-649.

Manasse, D. (1994). Positive outlooks to maintaining health. *VITA* (newsletter), January, 8.

Martin, J. E., & Carlson, C. R. (1988). Spiritual dimensions of health psychology. In W. R. Miller & J. E. Martin (Eds.), *Behavior therapy and religion* (pp. 57-110). Beverly Hills, CA: Sage.

McAllister, R., & Vander Veldt, A. J. (1961). Factors in mental illness among hospitalized clergy. *Journal of Nervous and Mental Disease, 132,* 80-88.

McAllister, R., & Vander Veldt, A. J. (1965). Psychiatric illness in hospitalized Catholic religious. *American Journal of Psychiatry, 121,* 881-884.

McCann, M. (1977-1978). The best—worst of times: A reflection on stress as it affects religious women. *Journal of Pastoral Counseling, 12,* 61-64.

McIntosh, W. M., & Shifflett, P. A. (1984). Dietary behavior, dietary adequacy, and religious social support: An exploratory study. *Review of Religious Research, 26*, 158–175.

McManners, J. (Ed.). (1992). *The Oxford illustrated history of Christianity*. New York: Oxford University Press.

Meurer, J., McDermott, R. J., & Malloy, M. J. (1990). An exploratory study of health practices of American Catholic nuns. *Health Values, 14*, 9–17.

Michalek, A. M., Mettlin, C., & Priore, R. L. (1981). Prostate cancer mortality among Catholic priests. *Journal of Surgical Oncology, 17*, 129–133.

Moore, M. E. (1990). Therapist, client, and superior. *Review for Religious, 49*, 539–544.

National Conference of Catholic Bishops. (1981). U.S. bishops' pastoral letter on health and health care. *Origins, 11*, 396–401.

Neal, M. A. (1984). *Catholic Sisters in transition*. Wilmington, DE: Michael Glazier.

Nix, J. T. (1957). Introduction to study of occupational diseases of religious. *Linacre Quarterly, 24*, 115–121.

Nix, J. T. (1960). Health care of clergy and religious. *Linacre Quarterly, 27*, 90–97.

Ogata, M., Ikeda, M., & Kuratsune, M. (1984). Mortality among Japanese Zen priests. *Journal of Epidemiology and Community Health, 38*, 161–166.

O'Malley, J. W. (1993). *The first Jesuits*. Cambridge: Harvard University Press.

Ostini, A. H. (1990). Are religious working themselves to death? *Review for Religious, 49*, 714–718.

Pincus, H. A., Lyons, J. S., & Larson, D. B. (1991). The benefits of consultation–liaison psychiatry. In F. K. Judd & G. D. Burrows (Eds.), *Handbook of studies in general hospital psychiatry* (pp. 43–52). New York: Elsevier.

Priests' Senate, Diocese of Charlotte, North Carolina. (1983). Tensions over a priest's time off. *Origins, 12*, 505–509.

Rayburn, C. A., Richmond, L. J., & Rogers, L. (1986). Men, women, and religion: Stress within leadership roles. *Journal of Clinical Psychology, 42*, 540–546.

Rooney, J. J. (1991). Psychological studies of nuns. *Research in the Social Scientific Study of Religion, 3*, 115–134.

Rosenstock, I. M. (1990). Personal responsibility and public policy in health promotion. In S. Schumaker, E. Schron, & J. Ockene (Eds.), *The handbook of health behavior* (pp. 424–445). New York: Springer.

Ross, R. K., Deapen, D. M., Casagrande, J. T., Paganini-Hill, A., & Henderson, B. E. (1981). A cohort study of mortality from cancer of the prostate in Catholic priests. *British Journal of Cancer, 43*, 233–235.

Ryan, M. J. (1992). Health forum for women religious. *Human Development, 13*, 5–8.

Shelton, C. M. (1992). Toward healthy Jesuit community living. *Studies in the Spirituality of Jesuits, 24*(4) (entire issue).

Skrabanek, P. (1988). Cervical cancer in nuns and prostitutes: A plea for scientific continence. *Journal of Clinical Epidemiology, 41*, 577–582.

Snowden, D. A., Gonzalez, N., O'Leary, B. M., & Ostwald, S.K. (1989). Making mammography a habit [letter]. *Journal of the American Medical Association, 262*, 207.

Spaeth, M. (1978). Personal illness: A creative force in pastoral care. *Bulletin of the American Protestant Hospital Association, 43*, 40–43.

Sperry, L. (1991). Determinants of a minister's well-being. *Human Development, 12*, 21–26.

Stellman, S. D., Boffetta, P., & Garfinkel, L. (1988). Smoking habits of 800,000 American men and women in relation to their occupations. *American Journal of Industrial Medicine, 13*, 43–58.

Taylor, R. S., Carroll, B. E., & Lloyd, J. W. (1959). Mortality among women in 3 Catholic religious orders with special reference to cancer. *Cancer, 12*, 1207–1223.

Timio, M., Verdecchia, P., Venanzi, S., Gentilli, S., Ronconi, M., Francucci, B., Montanari, M., & Bichisao, E. (1988). Age and blood pressure changes: A 20-year follow-up study in nuns in a secluded order. *Hypertension, 12*, 457–461.

Tortorici, J. S., Grame, C. J., & Coyne, L. (1993). Psychiatric treatment of Roman Catholic religious patients: A pilot follow-up study. *Bulletin of the Menninger Clinic, 57*, 517–522.

Tschannen, T., Duckro, P., Margolis, R., & Tomazic, T. (1992). The relationship of anger, depression, and perceived disability among headache patients. *Headache, 32*, 501–503.

Vanderwell, H. D. (1986). Turning weakness into strength. *Leadership, 7*, 122–127.

Williams, R., & Williams, V. (1994). *Anger kills*. New York: HarperCollins.

Zumkeller, A. (1986). *Augustine's ideal of the religious life*. New York: Fordham University Press.

V
INTEGRATION

16

Demography, Development, and Diversity of Health Behavior

An Integration

David S. Gochman

This chapter provides an integration of major points and findings presented in Volume III. Although its contents primarily reflect the contributions to this volume, rather than the larger body of scholarship about how health behaviors are distributed across and within populations, they are consistent with such knowledge. The section on future directions is the major exception to this statement concerning content, including as it does some additional perspectives. The chapter's organizing framework is a "work in progress" and is intended to become the foundation for a future synthesis and integration of this larger body of knowledge.

Unlike Volumes I and II, in which authors wrote primarily on specific levels of personal, social, or health care systems as determinants, contributors to Volume III focused on selected populations. Yet, in a fashion similar to that of the integrating chapters in Volumes I and II, a major part of this chapter is organized around categories of health behaviors, presenting them with some modest reframing and in a different order to reflect the major thrusts of the volume: risk behaviors; responses to illness, including sick role and adherence; care seeking; lifestyle; preventive, protective, and safety behaviors; and health-related cognitions, such as definitions of health and illness.

Each of these categories of health behavior is then considered in terms of the relevant personal (including developmental), family, social, institutional, organizational, and community determinants used in Volume I, plus the health provider determinants identified in Volume II. The chapter continues with an analysis of some common themes and concludes with some directions for future research.

David S. Gochman • Kent School of Social Work, University of Louisville, Louisville, Kentucky 40292.

Handbook of Health Behavior Research III: Demography, Development, and Diversity, edited by David S. Gochman. Plenum Press, New York, 1997.

SELECTED HEALTH BEHAVIORS

Risk Behaviors

Personal Determinants

Not surprisingly, risk behaviors increase during the life-span transitions in childhood and adolescence. Use of tobacco and alcohol and other drugs and sexual activities are initiated and often maintained as the young person grows older and deals with the transitions into puberty (Prohaska & Clark, Chapter 2; Cowell & Marks, Chapter 4). Prohaska and Clark note that non-school-attenders are more likely to smoke and use alcohol and to carry weapons than school attenders, and early maturers—both male and female—are more likely to use substances (alcohol, marijuana, cigarettes) within a year of puberty than are late maturers. Furthermore, they report that smoking may also be linked to levels of testosterone in interaction with the smoking status of the same-sex parent. Sexual risk taking is only weakly related to the transition to puberty. Hormonal levels are not by themselves good predictors of sexual activity in adolescents. Moreover, there may be only a low level of stability for risk behaviors over the years from childhood through adolescence and into the early adult years.

While women reduce their alcohol intake and smoking during pregnancy, due to a fear of adverse pregnancy outcomes, many of them relapse within the immediate postpartum period. Little is known about how the transition to parenthood affects risk behaviors in the father. Some evidence indicates that alcohol use increases after the child is born and that problem drinkers are less comfortable sharing feelings about parenthood (Prohaska & Clark).

In children, peer pressure and fears of being teased may be related to failure to use helmets, and increasing developmental autonomy seems to be related to the assumption by young persons of greater responsibility for use of abusable substances (O'Brien & Bush, Chapter 3). A sense of

invincibility may exist in children and adolescents in relation to injuries and risks. Children aren't able to anticipate the future consequences of their actions; their awareness of other persons' accidents seems to have no impact on their own risk behaviors (O'Brien & Bush).

In adolescents, increased cognitive awareness of reproduction and contraception is related to increased contraceptive use, yet adolescents have limited knowledge of services available (Cowell & Marks). Behavioral intentions seem to be good predictors of having intercourse, or an abortion, and of smoking marijuana, having multiple sex partners, and using condoms. For adolescent males, skills in talking to partners about condoms predicted condom usage. For both adolescent males and females, past use and ability to enjoy sex with condoms also predicted condom usage. While contraceptive self-efficacy beliefs were the most important determinant of condom use in college-age students, no clear-cut conclusions concerning self-efficacy beliefs and risk-reduction behaviors can be drawn (Cowell & Marks).

Young persons who are academically successful and have high educational and life goals are less likely to engage in intercourse and are more likely to use contraception (Cowell & Marks). Older adolescents, moreover, are more likely to use more effective methods of contraception than younger ones. Earlier initiation of sexual behaviors seems to be related to engaging in other adult risk behaviors, such as smoking and drinking, and in drug use. The predictive value of self-efficacy, however, is unclear in relation to risk reduction in adolescents; some data suggest that high levels of self-efficacy are related to higher levels of sexually transmitted diseases and, by inference, to unprotected or risky sexual behaviors.

School transitions are linked to self-concept and drug use (Cowell & Marks). Drug use in adolescents seems to be related to job instability, cigarette smoking in males and marijuana use in females being related to higher rates of unemployment. Alcohol use in adolescents is also related to poor social skills and to positive expectancies about the effects of its use. Substance abuse in adolescents appears to be related to low cognitive competence and to a history of academic difficulties.

Rakowski (Chapter 5) notes that older persons are less likely to smoke or drink than younger ones, raising questions about whether those who do not engage in risk behaviors have increased survival rates. Moreover, in older populations, each risk behavior appears to have its own set of correlates, although there is some clustering of smoking and drinking behaviors.

Gay men may become sexually active at earlier ages and may engage in sexual risk behaviors more frequently than other population groups (Kauth & Prejean, Chapter 6). Moreover, among gay men, condom use may lapse after a while. Further, while it is often assumed that substance abuse increases the likelihood of unsafe sex practices, Kauth and Prejean raise questions about the strength of this linkage. Gay men struggling with identity issues are more likely to experience substance abuse, eating disorders, and risky sexual activities than gay men not dealing with these issues. Some personal factors such as coming out early or low self-concepts may also increase depression and suicidal behavior.

Merely being gay may also elicit violent behavior from others and lead to a sense of victimization. Overall, Kauth and Prejean note that being gay puts people's safety at risk. Drinking behavior and use of illicit substances are assumed to be 2–3 times more prevalent in gay men than in the general population and are viewed as providing relief from loneliness and the stress and anxiety of being gay. Kauth and Prejean note that these findings, along with most others in this population group, can be readily critiqued on methodological grounds. Thomason and Campos (Chapter 8) note that psychosocial factors such as alcohol and drug use, negative emotional states, dysfunctional beliefs, and the denial of seropositive status in persons with HIV infection also appear to be linked to continuation of risk behaviors such as needle sharing and unsafe sex,

as are personal perceptions of risk, beliefs about self-efficacy, and coercion resistance.

High rates of sexual risk behavior are also noted in the homeless and poor (J. D. Wright & Joyner, Chapter 10). Poor persons may be less likely than the nonpoor to use contraception. Women are becoming an increasingly larger percentage of the homeless, leading to the "feminization of poverty." Pregnancy rates may be higher among the homeless and the poor, with additional pregnancy risk factors such as nutritional inadequacy, less medical care, and infections.

Homeless and poor people are also at greater risk for violence. Violence often shows up in the life stories of the homeless, and inner city youth have high rates of carrying guns, which itself increases their risks for violence. Homeless persons have higher rates of alcohol use, but there is no conclusive evidence on alcohol use rates among the poor. It is possible that there is less alcohol abuse among the poor than among the rich.

Persons who are homeless and in poverty are also more likely to smoke than the general population, and the rate of smoking decline is lower among the poor (J. D. Wright & Joyner). The homeless are more likely to use and abuse drugs than the general population, but drug use may increase slightly with increased socioeconomic status and education. Employed persons, however, are less likely to use drugs than the unemployed. Among those not in the labor force (women working at home, retired persons), drug usage was lower than among the employed or the unemployed.

Persons with severe mental illness are more likely than the general population to engage in risk behaviors such as smoking, use of alcohol and drugs, unprotected sex, and needle sharing in IV drug use (Hawley, Chapter 12). Caregivers are more likely than the general population to use psychotropic medications and to increase their smoking after assuming caregiving responsibilities (L. K. Wright, Chapter 13).

Anno (Chapter 14) reports that prisoners have higher rates of smoking, use of alcohol and drugs, and (inferred) higher rates of unsafe sexual activities than the general population and that they begin smoking and drinking at earlier ages. They also have higher rates of mutilative and suicidal behavior and are at risk for violence.

Family Determinants

Parental smoking may be related to initiation of smoking behavior at the transition to puberty (Prohaska & Clark, Chapter 2). Although the family is a major source of information about AIDS (O'Brien & Bush, Chapter 3), findings attempting to link the concept of family aggregation to smoking are inconclusive. Parents appear to be less active than is appropriate in injury prevention and safety instruction behaviors. Family use of alcohol and abusable substances is apparently related to a child's use of—and intentions to use—these substances (O'Brien & Bush). Kauth and Prejean (Chapter 6) note that disclosure of being gay to families may have put some gay men at risk for violence.

Cowell and Marks (Chapter 4) note that the adolescent female's decision to initiate sexual activity is linked to her mother's sexual and fertility experience; the earlier the mother engaged in sex or gave birth, the earlier the daughter initiated the activities. Parental substance abuse is linked to the adolescent's substance abuse and use of psychoactive drugs. Parents who use drugs may possibly lack parenting skills and family management skills. These parental deficiencies also may encourage use of psychoactive substances.

Some types of family structures may protect families' adolescent children against drug use (Cowell & Marks). Authoritative families and families with confident structures and some nontraditional beliefs fostered high levels of competence in their adolescent children and low levels of drug usage; "democratic" families, however, fostered high levels of competence but heavy levels of marijuana use. Family who provided directive environments and higher control had children who avoided drug use but were less competent. In addition, parental and sibling

smoking was associated with adolescent smoking behavior.

Social Determinants

Peer Influence. O'Brien and Bush (Chapter 3) note the consistent impact of peer pressure on substance abuse and risk and safety behaviors and on the increasing rates of smoking among young girls. They also note the inverse relationship between peer pressure to abuse and the social acceptability of the substance; the less acceptable the substance was, the higher was the pressure to use it. The overall impact of peer pressure declined, however, as children moved through higher grades.

Perception of peer sexual activity is related to sexual activity in adolescents, but the impact of these perceptions is mediated by age and gender. Younger white adolescent females appear to be more susceptible to peer pressure than other groups. Peer smoking and use of psychoactive drugs were consistent predictors of these behaviors in adolescents. Strong peer affiliation also seems to be related to higher levels of sexually transmitted diseases and, by inference, to unprotected or risky sexual behaviors (Cowell & Marks, Chapter 4).

In gay men, social support and social integration may reduce the risk of suicidal behavior (Kauth & Prejean, Chapter 6). On the other hand, disclosure of victimization to other persons may lead others to view the gay man as deserving of the violence.

Social Roles. Pol and Thomas (Chapter 1) note social determinants of risk behaviors in terms of gender role effects. For example, there are pervasive gender differences in smoking behavior; although the gap is narrowing, males consistently smoke at higher rates than females at all ages. Gender role influences are also noted in the differential relationships between peer smoking and an individual's initiation of smoking during the puberty transition (Prohaska & Clark, Chapter 2). During pregnancy, the transition to the role of mother, women reduce their smoking and alcohol consumption (Prohaska & Clark). In developing countries, women's role behaviors place them at greater risk than men for AIDS, as well as for some waterborne diseases (Coreil, Chapter 9).

Gender role influences were also observed in eating behavior in adolescents; young women were more at risk for engaging in dangerous weight control behaviors, young men at greater risk for eating foods high in fat content. The older an adolescent woman is at the time of her first sexual activity, the higher the likelihood of her using contraception, but this linkage is not observed among young men (Cowell & Marks, Chapter 4).

Institutional and Community Determinants

Community antigay sentiments or norms may lead young gay men to run away from their hometowns, thus increasing their risks for substance abuse, prostitution — with its risks for unsafe or risky sex behavior — and suicidal behavior (Kauth & Prejean, Chapter 6). Rural communities are more likely to stigmatize gay men and thus make it difficult for them to find social support. If runaways do not find social support within one or two weeks, they are at increased risk for substance abuse and unsafe sex practices. The availability and accessibility of gay bars in a community provides elements of social support; at the same time, the major role of these bars as meeting places in the social life of the gay community may be a factor in the higher rates of use of alcohol among gay men.

On a more optimistic note, the use of key community members as targets of preventive efforts has led to positive community-wide changes in levels of sexual risk behaviors in the gay community (Thomason & Campos, Chapter 8).

O'Brien and Bush (Chapter 3) note that the media have been the major source of children's information on AIDS. However, the messages children receive about drug abuse from the me-

dia, their families, and the wider community are mixed. The availability of "user-friendly" on-site clinics in schools is seen as an effective way of reducing alcohol consumption, smoking, sexual activity, and pregnancy.

Institutional factors such as the availability of free tobacco to inmates in certain states naturally increases or maintains the level of smoking behavior (Anno, Chapter 14). Moreover, few prisons offer smoking cessation programs, and few if any have a no-smoking section. At the mid-1990s, there are some attempts to initiate bans on tobacco use and to increase smoke-free areas. In other structured communities, there is evidence of decreased rates of smoking among priests; there is virtually no smoking among female clergy. Priests, however, have higher levels of problems with alcohol use than the general population (Duckro, Magaletta, & Wolf, Chapter 15).

Cultural Determinants

There is some evidence that ethnicity or race may have an impact on risk behaviors. Black adolescent females become sexually active earlier than whites; whites smoke more than blacks and Hispanics (Cowell & Marks, Chapter 4). Moreover, Coreil (Chapter 9) notes that cultural stigmatization of AIDS is a barrier to reducing risk behaviors in developing countries.

Health Provider Determinants

As Thomason and Campos (Chapter 8) affirm, many health education and health promotion risk-reduction efforts are based primarily on increasing knowledge and are thus overly simplistic. Health education must be viewed as only a first stage in AIDS prevention. Interventions directed at reducing sexually risky behaviors must include efforts at changing specific risk behaviors (e.g., Thomason & Campos). Risk prevention is increased when explicit messages, clear in relation to sexual and IV drug use behavior, are incorporated into the intervention, and when vague and often misunderstood terms such as "engaging in intercourse" are avoided and replaced by culturally appropriate and lay language (Thomason & Campos).

An important communication role for health professionals emerges from O'Brien and Bush's observations (Chapter 3). Children perceive health professionals as preferable to families and the media as sources of information about AIDS.

Responses to Illness, Adherence

Personal Determinants

Sex and marital status are related to keeping appointments with health professionals (Pol & Thomas, Chapter 1). The development of personal autonomy in children is linked to adherence, although personality variables as such are not (O'Brien & Bush, Chapter 3). Perceived benefits of use of a medicine are related to the frequency of its use by children (O'Brien & Bush). Fear is a primary factor in acceptance of, and of returning for results in, HIV screening; both those who returned for results and those who do not had fears, but those who returned believed knowledge would empower them to deal with their fears, while those who did not return feared they wouldn't be able to deal with seropositivity (Thomason & Campos, Chapter 8).While denial is the most immediate reaction to a diagnosis of HIV infection, such denial can be an adaptive defense. A person's repertoire of coping skills may be critical to participation in the screening process. Fears associated with HIV and HIV screening include anticipation of worsening health, discrimination, and loss of resources. Among persons with positive HIV status, improving and protecting health were, by contrast, critical reasons for being tested. Younger persons and African-Americans were less likely to return for testing results than other older and white persons; homosexuals were more likely to return than others. Among IV drug users, those with longer histories of sobriety and those who sought methadone treatment were more likely to return for results.

Moreover, having faith in Eurocentric, scientific biomedicine and in standard prescribed treatment increases adherence to drug regimens for persons with HIV (Thomason & Campos). Beliefs that *Pneumocystis carinii* pneumonia (PCP) prophylaxis and antiviral medications delayed the onset of illness and increased longevity were associated with increased adherence to HIV regimens. On the other hand, having little faith in Eurocentric biomedicine and being acceptant of alternative therapies were related to decreased adherence to prophylactic treatments. Younger, less educated, and *healthier* persons were less likely to adhere. Data on adherence in African-Americans are inconclusive. A history of IV drug use is associated with poor adherence; those in recovery, however, show adherence levels similar to those with no history of substance abuse. Being homeless may complicate adherence (Thomason & Compos). Relapse into risky behaviors may reflect emotional or affective status, either positive or negative.

Homeless persons are less likely to accept dietary regimens and often have no refrigeration to keep insulin supplies, making it difficult for them to manage diabetic regimens (J. D. Wright & Joyner, Chapter 10). Homeless persons, almost by definition, also lack a "routine" to serve as a frame of reference for adherence to medical regimens.

As J. D. Wright and Joyner observe, homeless persons with mental illness and substance abuse problems also often have severe memory problems that impede adherence to a regimen. Problems in adhering to hypertension medications among the poor are often also linked to increased use of emergency rooms. Poverty is also a barrier to adherence to regimens for tuberculosis and AIDS.

Among persons living with chronic illness, issues of adherence are related to personal skills and self-care ability, particularly skills in self-restraint and self-monitoring, and to a behavioral style of following the rules (Gallagher & Stratton, Chapter 11). Among persons living with severe mental illness (SMI), the illness itself serves as a barrier to adherence; it affects the persons' perceptions that they are ill as well as the memory necessary to adhere (Hawley, Chapter 12). Persons with SMI also have a high incidence of refusing treatment, often based on their refusal to accept that they are in fact ill and in need of treatment. Their responses to illness reflect altered sensations, perceptions, interpretations of physical and mental signs, analgesia, and diminished pain sensitivity. Both clinical and experimental evidence indicates that conditions and injuries that produce pain in others do not generate reports of pain in persons with SMI. Conversely, persons with SMI may perceive pain where there are no determinable physical origins. Patients fail to recognize the dramatic symptoms of tardive dyskinesia and have problems in perceptions of illness and in recognizing their own symptoms as indicative of mental illness.

Hawley further observes that persons who become *grandiose* with severe mental illness are more likely to refuse treatment than those who become *depressed* when symptomatic. Grandiosity is presumed to be more acceptable or comfortable for the patient than depression. Persons with a paranoid component are more likely to refuse treatment than those without paranoia; persons with more severe conditions are more likely to refuse than those with less severe conditions, possibly reflecting their decreased insight about their condition. Persons with bipolar conditions are more likely to refuse than those with schizoaffective disorders. The experience of side effects also affects refusal. Patients who believe that their treatment is inappropriate, or that they were wrongly hospitalized, are more likely to refuse treatment.

Family Determinants

Parental medicine use influences a child's medicine use during illness; moreover, adherence behavior for chronic conditions in children improves with support from families (O'Brien & Bush, Chapter 3). Support from family and significant others also increases adherence behavior for HIV treatment (Thomason & Campos, Chapter 8). In chronic illness, the family plays a more diffuse and subtle role; it must avoid traps of fostering needless dependence and of establishing nonrealistic expectations (Gallagher & Stratton, Chapter 11). The family's ability to adapt to the patient's dietary needs is also a factor in adherence, as is its role in food preparation. Having to engage in a caregiving role within a family increases the likelihood of using psychotropic, antianxiety, and sedative medications, but not antidepressants (L. K. Wright, Chapter 13).

Social Determinants

Race and social class are related to appointment breaking (Pol & Thomas, Chapter 1). Within the context of the relatively high overall rates of adherence in the HIV community (80–90%), Thomason and Campos (Chapter 8) note that the impact of social norms is reflected in the greater rates with which homosexuals return for HIV testing results and treatment; norms within the homosexual community presumably support and encourage such behavior. Intervention programs that increase social support lead to increased adherence to treatment (Thomason & Campos).

People with severe mental illness living alone are more likely to be noncompliant than those not socially isolated (Hawley, Chapter 12). There is virtually no information concerning compliance or satisfaction with care in prison populations (Anno, Chapter 14).

Institutional and Community Determinants

The lives of domiciled persons, i.e., persons with adequate housing in the community, are far more tightly determined by routines of family and work than are the lives of the homeless. Without these routines, the lives of homeless people are too chaotic for adherence in terms of keeping appointments or taking medication. Nor do the homeless have places in which to store medications safely, with the result that they are often stolen.

Nuns, despite being very adequately housed, have inappropriately low rates of acceptance of breast screenings (Duckro et al., Chapter 15).

Presumably, the norms of their communities about bodily privacy and sexuality inhibit their participation.

The prevalence and strength of antipsychiatry movements in communities, together with increased questioning of the legitimacy of many mental illness diagnoses, are all barriers to acceptance of medication for severe mental illness (Hawley, Chapter 12). On the other hand, the availability of disability benefits serves to legitimate the condition and may increase adherence.

Cultural Determinants

The cultural constructions of disease, including lay beliefs about etiology, may be factors in acceptance of treatment for certain conditions, such as diarrhea (Coreil, Chapter 9). Yet acceptance of treatment or prevention does not depend on the existence of complete congruence between lay beliefs and scientific beliefs.

Health Provider Determinants

Interactional Determinants. Support from health professionals, particularly from primary care nurses, increases adherence to medical treatment for HIV (Thomason & Campos, Chapter 8). On the other hand, providers fail to give standard levels of care to the poor, often stereotyping them as more likely to miss appointments without calling. This neglect in turn increases the likelihood that the poor will not adhere (J. D. Wright & Joyner, Chapter 10). Moreover, providers may influence the self-concept of the chronically ill patient in a way that has implications for adherence (Gallagher & Stratton, Chapter 11). Providers' acceptance of their patients' spirituality and the spiritual dimensions of illness is a factor in acceptance of treatment and continuing in care in religious communities (Duckro et al., Chapter 15).

Structural Determinants. Policies and guidelines relating to anonymity and confidentiality have eliminated many barriers to HIV testing, but fears about institutional violations of anonymity and confidentiality remain strong and serve as deterrents to being tested (Thomason & Campos, Chapter 8).

Uneven promotion of HIV testing in communities, particularly among ethnic and minority communities, is a barrier to community-wide participation in screening (Thomason & Campos). The provision of pre- and posttest counseling in a supportive environment by qualified professionals can enhance patients' ability to cope with the stress of testing and the emotional outcomes of the HIV diagnosis. This counseling maximizes returning for test results and initiates the process of health maintenance and improvement. Lack of institutional patient education programs increases nonadherence in persons with severe mental illness, as does the complexity of the medical regimen (Hawley, Chapter 12).

Thomason and Campos further observe that proximity and familiarity with testing sites were important determinants of returning for test results by IV drug users. Providing comprehensive medical care in a centralized, accessible site reduces adherence problems with HIV regimens in IV drug users. Respect and sensitivity by medical staffs also increase rates of participation in clinical trials. Moreover, the availability of social service support increases adherence to HIV treatment.

Care Seeking

Personal Determinants

With increasing age, adults are more likely to obtain more general medical examinations, while younger adults are more likely to have had a specific screening such as a Pap smear or mammogram (Pol & Thomas, Chapter 1). In rural communities, the likelihood of using a local rather than a regional hospital increases with age and decreases with income (Pol & Thomas). In children, allowing for autonomy and participation seems to be a factor in appropriate seeking of care from school health personnel (O'Brien & Bush, Chapter 3). For adolescents, financial and insurance factors can deter care-seeking behavior (Cowell & Marks, Chapter 4). Moreover, as Cowell and Marks note, adolescent perceptions of health and medical needs are different from those of physicians, which may make the care-seeking process frustrating. Illicit drug use in adolescents may also be a determinant of care seeking for mental health issues.

The elderly appear to be less likely to make dental visits than other groups in the adult population (Rakowski, Chapter 5). The stress of "coming out" may be a determinant of care-seeking behavior in gay men (Kauth & Prejean, Chapter 6). VanScoy (Chapter 7) notes that lesbians do not experience any particular health issues around their identity, but underlying their care-seeking behaviors is a wish to be viewed "holistically," to be given correct information about prevention, diagnosis, and treatment for legitimate health concerns, and to receive respectful and sensitive service from providers.

Denial of HIV status may result in the refusal of seropositive persons to take appropriate care-seeking steps. Fears may impede care seeking in the same way that they impede HIV screening (Thomason & Campos, Chapter 8). Concern for the health status of one's sexual partner is a factor in seeking testing. Moreover, an appreciable percentage of persons with HIV use at least one form of alternative therapy. Money is often a factor underlying seeking of alternative treatments. While there are no consistent data on who among those with seropositivity seek alternative therapies, having lived longer with the condition seems to be related to seeking alternative care, the more so among gay men than among other HIV groups. Thomason and Campos point out that there is a high use of alternative therapies by persons with HIV, indicating that 31–60% seek out at least one of the more than 100 types of alternative therapies available.

The homeless and the poor are less likely to have regular sources of care, and most have no medical insurance (J. D. Wright & Joyner, Chapter 10). Their basic survival needs distract the homeless from health concerns. Furthermore, delay in care seeking usually means that care is more likely to be sought in emergency rooms.

Children of the homeless and those living in poverty have fewer checkups in the absence of insurance and regular sources of care. Problems in adhering to hypertension medications among the poor are often also linked to increase use of emergency rooms.

Total "engulfment" by severe mental illness (SMI) interferes with care seeking for medical illnesses (Hawley, Chapter 12). Persons with SMI often do not perceive their somatic symptoms in terms of physical illness, but relate them instead to their identities as mental patients (Hawley). While the most commonly reported symptom leading to care seeking was experiencing a hallucination at a time when the person had enough insight to realize it was not attributable to physical stimuli, other somatic symptoms are not appropriate recognized and processed. This failure is further abetted by "lack of insight" and poor reality checking. Moreover, Hawley notes, the homeless with SMI are less likely to seek care than the homeless without mental illness.

Among caregivers, extreme altruism is a barrier to care seeking (L. K. Wright, Chapter 13). In addition, an analog—or alternative form—of care-seeking behavior is support-seeking behavior, and "support mobilization" is an important concept in caregiver research (L. K. Wright). No evidence exists showing that caregivers engage in appropriate levels of support mobilization on their own behalf. However, high levels of personal and social skills and high self-esteem are linked to having high levels of social support. Caregivers also tend to deny the degree of illness in the patient for whom they are caring, which is a barrier to mobilizing social support; they also tend to overestimate the level of social support they receive. Moreover, the longer a person serves as a caregiver, the less likely that person is to use social support.

Prison inmates use ambulatory health care services at rates far exceeding comparable groups in the general population (Anno, Chapter 14). Although much of this use is dictated by their substantial medical needs, a considerable part of their use of "sick call" may reflect ways of stress management and negative life events. Frequent users of prison health services have higher levels of stress, anxiety, and depression than occasional users or nonusers and are more likely to express emotions somatically and to report more nurturing parents.

Family Determinants

Unmarried persons and members of nontraditional households are less efficient users of health services and often have less ability to pay (Pol & Thomas, Chapter 1). Cowell and Marks (Chapter 4) observe that mothers and adult children share a common factor in care seeking, suggesting some common understandings of illness.

Within the family, caregivers often define health needs largely in terms of an identified patient's illness and demands; depressed caregivers thus seek help in *coping* with the identified patient's needs rather than help for their own depression (L. K. Wright, Chapter 13). Moreover, caregiving reduces the time available to deal with their own health (Prohaska & Clark, Chapter 2), days spent in hospitals, sick days in bed at home, and physician visits (L. K. Wright). Becoming a secondary caregiver after the identified patient has been placed in a nursing home leads to an increase in the number of physician visits and an increase in the use of psychotropic medications, even though the nursing home placement had little impact on changing the caregiver's roles or other behaviors.

Social Determinants

The impact of gender role on care seeking can be seen early in life: Girls use the school nurse more than boys (O'Brien & Bush, Chapter 3). On the other hand, women in religious communities are often reluctant to seek care from male physicians (Duckro, Chapter 15).

The awareness of social support through counseling may improve the likelihood of following up after notification of seropositivity (Thomason & Campos, Chapter 8). Peers and HIV literature inform persons about the availabil-

ity of alternative therapies. Extensive and sophisticated social networks have evolved to meet the unaddressed needs of the HIV/AIDS community. There are no consistent gender effects in use of alternative care. One study showed that none of the female HIV respondents reported use of alternative therapies; another study showed that use of alternative treatments was popular among women, a finding consistent with VanScoy's (Chapter 7) observations.

The absence of supportive social networks is a barrier to care seeking among the poor (J. D. Wright & Joyner, Chapter 10). Finally, among gay men, relationship issues often underlie care seeking for psychotherapy (Kauth & Prejean, Chapter 6).

Institutional and Community Determinants

Demographic changes resulting in an increasingly elderly population, and variation in fertility leading to an increase in births after the year 2000, will change the mix of health service needs in communities in the first part of the 21st century (Pol & Thomas, Chapter 1). Older persons will have increased needs for specialized services such as cardiology, oncology, and rheumatology; baby-boomers will need more "adult" services, such as urology, gynecology, and chronic disease management.

Older, pre-World War II generations, according to Pol and Thomas, had different views, emphasizing security, authority, and the sanctity of society's health care institutions. They bought indemnity insurance, didn't question their physicians, complied with medical regimens, and believed that the route to health lay essentially through the formal health care system. The post-World War II cohort is different. They believed that they had more control over their destinies and sought participation in the health care process. They moved from indemnity insurance to enrollment in HMOs, took an active role in health care, questioned their physicians, and sought innovation in the health care system.

In adolescents, access to care may be affected by insurance barriers, lack of acceptable providers, laws requiring parental consent, and lack of information about appropriate services. Even where finances are not an issue, laws about confidentiality and anonymity may deter adolescents from seeking sex-related and emotion-related services (Cowell & Marks, Chapter 4).

Lack of a community transportation system is a critical barrier to care seeking for those living in poverty. Lack of community resources such as respite services and day care also impedes care seeking for caregivers (L. K. Wright, Chapter 13). The media in a community also play a role in informing persons about alternative therapies for HIV/AIDS (Thomason & Campos, Chapter 8).

The correctional community environment is hazardous to health. It fails to provide safety to prisoners, and it increases injuries to them (Anno, Chapter 14). Policies require that prisoners use sick call to obtain products and services that are only marginally medically related, such as permission not to shave, extra blankets or mattresses, a different type of shoe, dandruff shampoo, and lotion soaps. Subsequent sick call visits are required to replenish supplies of products or to continue permissions. In addition, sick call visits are mandated by the intake, discharge, and transfer processes, and by periodic screenings for tuberculosis, HIV, and chronic disease monitoring, as well as for clearance to work at certain institutional jobs. Because inmates are prohibited from keeping over-the-counter medications in their cells, they must continue to go on sick call for additional dosages of nonprescription medications for colds, headaches, menstrual cramps, and the like. Due to institutional security policies, inmates must also make sick call visits merely to obtain information about future appointments with health professionals. Sick call also provides some secondary gains for inmates, such as time off from required work details or chances to socialize with other inmates.

Many religious communities, even ascetic ones, support health behaviors (Duckro et al., Chapter 15). The Talmud, for example, forbids living in a town that has no physician. Care of the sick is often recognized as a community priority, and Judaism mandates, as an ethical imperative, caregiving activities such as visiting the sick. Few ascetic communities adhere to extreme denial of somatic issues, but some communities avoid caring for themselves preventively.

Religious communities want caregivers to be comfortable with religious lifestyles. According to Duckro et al., some religious communities see the medical treatment of disease as spiritually damaging and avoid secular medicine in favor of self-discipline, but for most communities, the ideal is a combination of both spiritual and medical care seeking. Some religious communities, however, are not as positive toward psychological therapy as they are toward somatic care; the shame and stigma attached to symptoms of mental illness are barriers to care seeking, as is an unwillingness to "share family secrets." Priests tend not to seek sufficient help for psychological symptoms.

Cultural Determinants

Pol and Thomas (Chapter 1) note cultural influences in data showing that immigrant groups are likely to be apprehensive about formal health care or about related social institutions such as day care. Coreil (Chapter 9) observes that cultural constructions of diseases, e.g., of diarrhea, have an impact on care seeking. In addition, in many developing countries, cultural beliefs consider birth to be a natural event, best managed at home with the care of loved ones and a midwife and avoiding care seeking in hospitals.

Minority caregivers report fewer physician visits than white caregivers and show less use of prescription medications and psychotropic drugs (L. K. Wright, Chapter 13). Blacks and whites appear similar in caregiver/noncaregiver differences in care-seeking behavior. Among caregivers, however, whites are more likely to seek care from other persons, particularly from professionals, while Hispanics and blacks are more likely to rely on religion, faith, and prayer. Finally, the less positive attitudes toward psychological care among religious communities (Duckro et al., Chapter 15) should be viewed as reflections of larger cultural attitudes that differentiate physical and mental illness.

Health Provider Determinants

Interactional Determinants. Provider statements to parents are likely to be actively listened to and accurately recalled by children, who are very interested in information about their health. But children's developmental stages may not permit appropriate processing of such information (O'Brien & Bush, Chapter 3). Ironically, pediatricians spend very little time on providing guidance and are unwilling to treat adolescents' health problems, are often unable to do so, and tend to focus more on narrow biomedical definitions of problems than on what young persons perceive their problems to be (Cowell & Marks, Chapter 4). The refusal of some providers to see Medicaid patients limits care seeking for a number of young persons.

Other provider obstacles to care seeking can be observed in the homophobia of some physicians, which shows up in their refusal to treat gay men (Kauth & Prejean, Chapter 6). Such homophobia can make gay men fear the humiliation of having their gay identities recognized and thereby impede careseeking from traditional mental health sources. It also can lead to some gay men experiencing a lack of support when they do disclose their identities and to their being encouraged to change their identities.

Many health providers also assume that all of their patients are heterosexual and may not even ask about sexual orientation (Kauth & Prejean, Chapter 6; VanScoy, Chapter 7), which impedes the flow of appropriate information even when care is sought. Moreover, negative attitudes may be conveyed even unintentionally. Providers' degree of comfort with spirituality has an affect on care-seeking behavior of members of religious communities (Duckro, Chapter 15).

Health professionals frequently define the homeless and indigent as unworthy or as undesirable clients (J. D. Wright & Joyner, Chapter 10), which serves as a barrier to successful care seeking. Health professionals can also become so "engulfed" by severe mental illness, seeing it as an overarching concern, that they view their treatment role in a very narrow way and pay little or no attention to somatic symptoms (Hawley, Chapter 12). Thus, physical illnesses in persons with severe mental illness are likely to be undiagnosed and untreated. A similar narrowness in focusing is found in providers so exclusively concerned with the identified patient that they rarely take initiatives in relation to the health of the caregiver (L. K. Wright, Chapter 13).

Structural Determinants. Even adolescents with insurance coverage face barriers to access to care in the form of limitations on many of the services of greatest use to them: care for mental health, substance abuse, abortion, and preventive screenings (Cowell & Marks). Moreover, private insurance coverage often excludes care by nonphysicians such as social workers and psychologists, who are often the most appropriate professionals to provide these needed services. There is still often a long wait for treatment, even where such limitations do not exist in institutional policies. While Medicaid reduces some barriers, the degree of such reduction varies from state to state.

System barriers also impede care seeking for lesbians and gay men (VanScoy; Kauth & Prejean). The health care system is patriarchal, dominated by men, and often oppressive of women, both ignoring and inappropriately medicalizing women's health concerns (VanScoy). As VanScoy notes, virtually no time is allocated to issues of homosexuality in medical school training, and lesbian encounters with the health care system reflect this situation. This lack has a significant impact on lesbian care-seeking behavior, since lesbians see the system as doubly devaluing them because they are not potential partners for men and because they do not follow the traditional rules for women. The documented homophobia of the system is especially apparent in mental health, substance abuse, sex education and therapy, gynecological and obstetrical care, and adolescent and geriatric health. For lesbians, this attitude often results in either negative experiences or anticipated negative experiences based on what others report, and thus, in turn, in disproportionate avoidance of the traditional care system, reliance on alternative providers, delay in care seeking, nondisclosure of lesbianism, choice of lesbian or other female providers, and increased use of mental health and substance abuse services, programs, and groups.

Thomason and Campos (Chapter 8) also convey the continuance of rejecting, hostile health care environments for persons living with HIV infections. The potential for rejection by dental professionals is a barrier to the seeking of dental care; disclosure of HIV status led to denial of care for an appreciable number of persons.

Thomason and Campos further report the importance of the counseling process for maximizing the process of health maintenance among persons living with HIV. Alternative practitioners are apparently more likely to encourage persons with HIV to be proactive in their treatment regimens and to elevate their patients' sense of empowerment and self-control.

The unfriendliness of health care environments is also noted in developing countries, where hospitals are often stark, with dirty wards and beds, and the technologically invasive procedures of modern obstetrical care become a barrier to using hospitals for childbirth (Coreil, Chapter 9). In the United States, a developed country, inadequacies in the health care environment include the lack of public health facilities, lack of sufficient providers for Medicaid patients, distance and other geographic and locational issues, and "the forbidding and often unfriendly institutional settings in which care is typically delivered" (J. D. Wright & Joyner). These barriers impede care seeking in the homeless. Moreover, the uninsured poor receive worse care than the nonpoor when they do seek treatment. Even with insurance, the elderly poor face barriers in

terms of limited resources available, stringent eligibility requirements, and lack of effective institutional outreach.

Lifestyle

Personal Determinants

Developmental changes can be observed in the decrease in exercise behaviors in adolescents, and in the increase in adults of certain appropriate behaviors such as limiting alcohol intake and eating breakfast regularly (Prohaska & Clark, Chapter 2). Younger adults are more likely to participate in vigorous physical activity than are other groups; nearly half of older adults have no leisure time activities, although about one third engage in moderate physical activities and 10% in vigorous physical activities. Elderly persons are more likely to avoid salt, have regular sleep patterns, and a balanced diet, and are less likely to exercise (Prohaska & Clark; Rakowski, Chapter 5). While only a low level of consistency is found across lifestyle behaviors in childhood or in the early years of adolescence, increased consistency is observed in adults.

O'Brien and Bush (Chapter 3) note the development and socialization of lifestyle behaviors in relation to dental and sleep and exercise behaviors, and the developmental increases in autonomy for hygiene behaviors and food decisions. Increased autonomy, however, was related to increased fat and sodium consumption. Cowell and Marks (Chapter 4) note that adolescents develop to a point where health and illness can be perceived as existing together, which allows young persons to adopt a healthy lifestyle despite having acute or chronic health conditions. Moreover, children's nutritional behavior seems to predict adolescents' nutritional behavior. In adolescents, perceived benefits coupled with perceived competence are linked to levels of physical activity.

Among elderly persons, internal locus of control may possibly be linked to better health-promoting behaviors (Rakowski). An "information-seeking" cluster of items was found to be related to levels of physical activity, having emergency numbers handy, regular seat belt use, asking to sit in a nonsmoking section, and breast self-examination. Rakowski suggests that such information seeking is a generic process that underlies behavior change.

Among gay men, involvement in "fitness" is seen as a sign of health and strength; it also counters a sense of vulnerability to HIV infection and at the same time reclaims the "myth" of masculinity (Kauth & Prejean, Chapter 6). Knowledge of HIV status, either positive or negative, may lead to an increase in healthy lifestyle behavior (Thomason & Campos, Chapter 8). Decreased use of substances, dietary change, rest and exercise, and stress management are some of the basic tactics used by gay men to cope with HIV (Thomason & Campos).

There are no data on dietary adequacy among those homeless who do not use shelters or soup kitchens, nor are there data on physical activity among the homeless. Diets of food stamp recipients were more adequate than those of persons who were eligible for stamps but who were nonrecipients. Participation in emergency food assistance programs did not improve nutritional status. Iron deficiency is inferred to be more likely in poor children than in nonpoor children, but is not measured directly through assessments of diet. The elderly poor are less likely to have an adequate diet than other elderly.

Little is also known about the lifestyle choices of prison inmates when they lived in the community. Poor nutrition and exercise can be inferred, but has not been measured directly (Anno, Chapter 14).

Family Determinants

Loss of a spouse may be related to changes in nutritional intake and grief to adverse eating behavior (Prohaska & Clark, Chapter 2). Many elderly who live alone lack the ability to prepare food. O'Brien and Bush (Chapter 3) report no linkages between parental physical activity or fitness levels and those of their children, and they note inconsistent findings about family aggregation and eating and exercise behavior. Nutritious food must be available in the home, however, if it is to be consumed. Moreover, mothers make fewer statements to children about exercise and fitness than about food and hygiene. To the degree that a child has responsibilities for food purchase or preparation, the child's diet will be higher in sodium and fat.

Cowell and Marks (Chapter 4) suggest the importance of role modeling in the acquisition of lifestlye behaviors in adolescents. Moreover, father's education, mother's age, and the child's own motivation were significant predictors of nutritional behavior. Older mothers were more likely than younger ones to provide balanced meals and to make appropriate use of the food pyramid. Where families showed greater concern for dietary intake, children were given more choice in food decisions. Parental activity levels and involvement also were determinants of adolescent's physical activity.

In developing countries, the role of the mother in premature introduction of supplementary foods and liquids was associated with suboptimal nutrition and exposure to infection. The mother's decision to introduce supplementary food is related to her beliefs about the adequacy of her milk supply (Coreil, Chapter 9).

While about half of caregivers do not change their lifestyle behaviors, many reported that they ate less nutritiously, decreased their exercise routines, and increased their smoking contingent upon undertaking the caregiver's role (L. K. Wright, Chapter 13). Caregivers report less time available for exercise and rest (Prohaska & Clark).

Social Determinants

Better lifestyle health practices are linked to socioeconomic resources and to social support (Rakowski, Chapter 5). Among caregivers, even large social support networks, however, fail to lead to increased leisure activities for blacks (L. K. Wright, Chapter 13). Social determinants in the form of gender role effects are seen in the disproportionately higher rates of women who try to lose weight compared with men (Pol & Thomas, Chapter 1). Women are also less likely to exercise or play sports or to drive under the influence of alcohol (Pol & Thomas). In childhood, girls report more positive health behaviors than boys, such as eating more healthful foods; they also exercise less and are more concerned about weight (O'Brien & Bush, Chapter 3). Among adolescents, males are more likely to exercise than females (Cowell & Marks, Chapter 4), and peer activity level influences adolescents' physical activity. Among the elderly, women continue to report more health-promoting behaviors than men and men report more vigorous activity (Rakowski).

Institutional and Community Determinants

The availability of transportation and facilities may be more relevant than parental activity level to children's exercise behaviors (O'Brien & Bush, Chapter 3). Media attention to low-nutrient foods increases children's recall, purchase, and consumption of these foods. Coreil (Chapter 9) notes that in developing countries, bottle feeding was linked to urban residence and exposure to the media.

Poverty and homelessness have appreciable impact on all aspects of lifestyle. There is evidence that homeless persons have nutritional deficits; they generally do not eat three meals a day, and their diets deviate from nutritional recommendations (J. D. Wright & Joyner, Chapter 10). Some evidence exists that increased income level improves dietary intake and that housing subsidies improve diet. In addition, relatively high levels of sedentary behavior are observed among low-income, low-educational-level groups (J. D. Wright & Joyner). The availability of formal services does not appear to be linked to greater leisure time for black caregivers, but this is more an inference than a finding (L. K. Wright, Chapter 13).

Many religious communities emphasize a "balance" between overexertion and inactivity and between overindulgence and abstinence. Religious commitments themselves are somewhat linked to healthy diet behaviors (Duckro et al (Chapter 15). Zen Buddhist monks eat a high proportion of vegetables, use alcohol and tobacco minimally, and show moderation in all their activities. Hutterite religious communities place a high premium on physical activity, abstain from tobacco, and make full use of health care facilities.

There is an emergence in religious communities of concern for relaxation and cultivating group support, linking the welfare of the clergy with the welfare of the congregation, and policies that encourage rather than discourage a healthy lifestyle (Duckro et al.). Evidence remains of lack of exercise and dietary problems, however, particularly among women religious who eat a poverty-level diet. In contrast, incarceration improves nutritional and exercise behavior for prison inmates (Anno, Chapter 14).

Cultural Determinants

Race and ethnicity were found to be linked to exercise behavior, with less such behavior occurring in Hispanic and Asian children (O'Brien & Bush, Chapter 3). White adolescents were less likely to be enrolled in physical education than blacks (Cowell & Marks, Chapter 4). Hispanic caregivers exercise and engage in sports less than non-Hispanic whites and eat less nutritious meals (L. K. Wright, Chapter 13). Socioeconomic status was not a contributing factor in this, but ethnocultural values and perceptions were. Rakowski (Chapter 5) observes that some ethnic profiles show better lifestyle behaviors than white non-Hispanics.

Health-Related Cognitions

Personal Determinants

O'Brien and Bush (Chapter 3) show how children's conceptions of health and illness can be understood with a Piagetian framework of developmental stages, progressing with increased grasp of time and space through understanding the consequences of actions and increasing ability to consider unobservables, e.g., germs. Cowell and Marks (Chapter 4) also show how the meaning of health changes developmentally in adolescents. Although much of this research has focused on cognitive development as such, more recent findings deal with the meaning of health in positive terms: health being able to do what you want to do. When adolescents present to physicians, they focus on physical illness. Adolescents are able to grasp that health and illness can exist simultaneously.

When gay men's experiences with violence leads to "profound life disruption" and posttraumatic stress, these have an impact on a range of health-related cognitions. Such experiences interfere with the gay man's basic assumptions about safety and security, about people being trustworthy and the world being an orderly and meaningful place (Kauth & Prejean, Chapter 6).

Perceived health status among the homeless, measured through self-reports, is poorer than among comparable domiciled low-income groups, and especially lower for those homeless with chronic conditions, those who had recently seen a physician, and those with chronic depression (J. D. Wright & Joyner, Chapter 10). Parents reported lower levels of health among homeless children than were reported in the general pediatric population and in domiciled children living in poverty. Increased income is related to improved perceptions of health status. At the other end of the developmental cycle, elderly living in poverty were also more likely than the nonpoor elderly to report poorer health status.

The existence of chronic illness, with its lifelong but not necessarily life-threatening aspects, presents difficulties in personal definitions of health and illness (Gallagher & Stratton, Chapter 11); the stages of the illness have an impact on how it is defined. The personalization of illness may sometimes be reflected in attitudes such as "I'm going to fight you" (Gallagher & Stratton).

Similarly, Hawley (Chapter 12) notes that persons living with severe mental illness base their definitions of health and illness on altered or distorted sensations, perceptions, and interpretations of physical and mental symptoms. As a result of their conditions, they experience grossly impaired reality testing, delusions, and perceptions, coupled with lack of insight. The mental illness consistently wins over reality. Many such persons do not define themselves as ill; the brain does not recognize its own dysfunctioning. Those with more severe illness had less insight and were more likely to believe they weren't ill.

Family Determinants

Parents living in homeless shelters were more likely to report their children to be in fair or poor health than parents in the general population and domiciled parents living in poverty (J. D. Wright & Joyner, Chapter 10).

Social Determinants

Health cognitions are also affected by components of the social role/sick role of being a mental patient. Hawley (Chapter 12) notes that during the early stages of the mental patient role, when hallucinations bring people into hospital settings, patients are inclined to deny that they have a mental illness. Eventually, as a result of some period of treatment, of receiving disability payments, and of social labeling, they enter the middle stage of the role, where they are more likely to define themselves as being sick. In the late stage, they become totally engulfed by their condition and their identity as a mental patient. At this point, their identity transcends all other aspects of their experience and leads to their defining themselves as the illness. Adherence to regimens is, in turn, affected by these health cognitions.

Institutional and Community Determinants

Kauth and Prejean (Chapter 6) note that community antigay harassment, which links being gay with being assaulted, may lead to a heightened sense of vulnerability and at the same time reinforce negative beliefs about homosexuality. Repeating material already mentioned in another context, the community's ability to provide home and shelter is linked to perceived health status; persons with homes perceive themselves to be in better health than the homeless (J. D. Wright & Joyner, Chapter 10).

In most religious communities, illness is defined in terms of spiritual, social, and psychological functioning. Ascetics might see illness as a result of sin or possession, but also recognize individual responsibilities for treatment and prevention (Duckro, Chapter 15). Illness can also be perceived as a teacher or a gift or as a transforming event. While religious communities are likely to perceive physical illness as being less of a personal responsibility, or even beyond it, they are likely to perceive psychological illness as related to personal responsibility, often with concomitant shame and stigma. Although clergy seem to have positive perceptions of their own physical health status, many priests report depression.

Cultural Determinants

The stigmatizing effects of cultural determinants of definitions of illness are clearest in the chapters dealing with gay men and lesbians. Kauth and Prejean (Chapter 6) discuss the issue of cultural definitions of homosexuality as a disease or a crime, with attendant stigma. VanScoy (Chapter 7) elaborates on how such cultural ideologies are reflected in medical constructions of illnesses.

Coreil (Chapter 9) discusses how culturally constructed theories of sickness in developing countries are reflected in personal perceptions of their etiologies and these, in turn, determine care-seeking behavior and choices of treatment. Although early studies dichotomized conceptions of illness into biomedical and supernatural, among many cultures conceptions of disease reflect both of these perspectives. Finally, white persons perceive themselves to have better health status than African-Americans (J. D. Wright & Joyner, Chapter 10).

Health Provider Determinants

Gallagher and Stratton (Chapter 11) show the impact of health care providers on the construction of perceptions of chronic conditions. If the provider defines the condition as a disease and then treats it medically, the implications for the individual's self-concept are different than if the provider defines the condition as chronic, but not as a disease.

Definitions of health or illness may also be changed or deconstructed by vote within certain health institutions themselves. In 1973, the American Psychiatric Association, acted to remove homosexuality as a disorder after it had voted it to be such in 1942 (Kauth & Prejean, Chapter 6; VanScoy, Chapter 7). Medical construction has also led to the medicalization of lesbian identities, with a considerable amount of research by allopathic physicians, and psychiatrists in particular, devoted to establishing lesbianism as a medical disorder, and medical theories pathologizing lesbians as a group. Similar institutional construction can be observed in the evolution of *DSM* diagnoses, which are used as the basis for classifying persons as severely mentally ill or not (Hawley, Chapter 12).

Preventive, Protective, and Safety Behaviors

Personal Determinants

Prohaska and Clark (Chapter 2) report that younger adults are more likely to have had a preventive screening than older adults. Cowell and Marks (Chapter 4) note that behavioral intentions predict use of condoms and that adolescents who are academically successful are more likely than others to use contraceptives consistently. Older adolescents, moreover, are more likely to use more effective methods of contraception than younger ones. The older an adolescent female is at her first sexual interaction, the more likely she is to use contraception. Females with clear academic aspirations and good school performance are more likely to use contraception. Rakowski (Chapter 5) notes that older women are less likely than younger women to have clinical breast examinations, Pap testing, flu shots, and mammography screening.

In developing countries, maternal age, number of children, and education are positively related to contraceptive use. In countries where the fertility transition is well advanced, however, education has much less of an impact (Coreil, Chapter 9).

Poor and homeless children have lower levels of immunization than nonpoor and domiciled children (J. D. Wright & Joyner, Chapter 10). Furthermore, immunization delay was greater for homeless than for domiciled poor children. Finally, among gay men, being less open was related to greater fear of harassment in college students; concealing gay identity thus becomes a protective behavior (Kauth & Prejean, Chapter 6).

Family Determinants

Coreil (Chapter 9) notes that competing time demands on mothers in developing countries were linked to their failure to have their child immunized. The mother's age and number of children in the family were inversely related to her use of antenatal care and other types of preventive care.

Social Determinants

Cowell and Marks (Chapter 4) note the impact of social determinants on preventive behaviors in observations that adolescents in steady relationships are more likely to use contraception than those not in steady relationships.

Institutional and Community Determinants

O'Brien and Bush (Chapter 3) note that Head Start Programs provided material about prevention in preschool classrooms. Presumably this material had positive impacts on preventive behaviors. Duckro (Chapter 15) note that some religious communities are so committed to car-

ing for others that they avoid preventive actions on their own behalf. Religious commitment itself is sometimes viewed by these communities as a positive health behavior. Christianity and Judaism both support preventive behaviors, but some women in religious orders are not aware of prevention and do not make appropriate use of preventive services. Although policies are emerging in some religious communities that emphasize the need for prevention, there is still insufficient use of preventive physical examinations, as well as low rates of screening for breast cancer among nuns, who are at high risk (Duckro et al.).

Cultural Determinants

Black adolescent females were less likely to use contraception than whites, except for those whose parents had high educational levels. Blacks were more likely than poor whites to use a prescription form, such as a diaphragm or pill (Cowell & Marks, Chapter 4). Questions arise about whether this finding reflects some "learned helplessness" among the poor whites or whether "internal motivation" on the part of poorer whites may initiate over-the-counter sales. Possibly black females have higher access to formal family planning services.

Health Provider Determinants

Accessibility, availability, acceptability, and affordability of services and the educational communication of service providers are highly linked to immunization levels in developing countries (Coreil, Chapter 9). This situation is very similar to system factors that serve as barriers to care in other countries.

COMMON THEMES

Conceptual Issues

Conceptual issues that emerge from the chapters in Volume III include transition concepts, the role of theory, and stigma.

Transition Concepts

Transition concepts dominate a number of chapters in this volume. Transitions in the characteristics of the population, such as changes in fertility levels and mortality rates, have important implications for health behavior. Pol and Thomas (Chapter 1) observe a transition in the differences between the pre–World War II and post–World War II generations' attitudes toward insurance, as well as in levels of consumerism and use of services. These demographic transitions are not yet clearly understood. Coreil (Chapter 9) notes how demographic, epidemiological, and health status transitions affect health behaviors in developing countries and observes the impact of education on the transition to an expanded world view that makes persons more receptive to new ideas and ways of responding to life situations. The impact of education on women's transitions to more empowered status is particularly relevant.

Transitions in individual personal and social growth and development are used or implied throughout this volume. For example, the role transitions of the life cycle, especially those of puberty, parenthood, caregiving, and loss of a spouse, are linked to the potential for risk behavior, as is the concept of whether the transition occurs at the normative time or whether its occurrence deviates from the norm (Prohaska & Clark, Chapter 2). Models of gradual developmental transitions attempt to relate the transitions to changes in children's health cognitions and risk behaviors (O'Brien & Bush, Chapter 3). The biological, cognitive, emotional, and social transitions that underlie puberty in adolescence, including school transitions and peer group transitions, can be seen as related to risk behaviors and care seeking (Cowell & Marks, Chapter 4).

The transition toward greater autonomy is also discussed in relation to selected health behaviors in children and adolescents (O'Brien & Bush; Cowell & Marks). Kauth and Prejean (Chapter 6) raise questions about how the transitions involved in aging affect the health behaviors of gay men. Moreover, the value or importance of the same health behavior may vary as transitions are made throughout the life cycle, and the same behavior may be determined by different factors as these transitions are made (Prohaska & Clark). Questions also arise of whether changes in health behavior are attributable to some intervention or to the transition itself, and little is known about how some of these transitions, particularly moving into parenthood, caregiving, and experiencing the death of a spouse, affect health behavior (e.g., Prohaska & Clark; L. K. Wright, Chapter 13).

Role of Theory

Virtually all of the theoretical models covered in Volume I are employed to some degree in this volume in examining health behaviors in diverse populations. The health belief model, social learning theory, social cognitive theory, behavioral intention theory (theory of planned behavior/theory of reasoned action), transtheoretical/stages of change models, and locus of control frameworks are shown to have differential value in understanding health behaviors at different ages and in different populations. Questions arise, for example, about whether the predictive value of different components of the health belief model varies with development (O'Brien & Bush, Chapter 3) or whether it has overall predictive value throughout the life cycle (Prohaska & Clark, Chapter 2). The transtheoretical model is thought to be more congruent with transition concepts (Prohaska & Clark). The children's health belief model and children's locus of control for health model are attempts to reformulate the health belief and locus of control models for younger populations (O'Brien & Bush).

While no single variable in any of these theoretical formulations is assumed to be important for all persons, at least one psychosocial variable would be expected to be important for most persons (Rakowski, Chapter 5). Rakowski proposes a model for predicting health behavior in older persons that combines behavioral epidemiology and psychosocial epidemiology and thus integrates a number of the "psychosocial" variables with physiological status, laboratory measures, and external variables such as demographic factors, health status, income, and residential isolation. In addition, information seeking is proposed as a critical variable in understanding health behavior (Rakowski; L. K. Wright, Chapter 13). Rakowski argues that information seeking as a generic process may transcend factors that underlie diverse health behaviors, and thus may be a common foundation underlying a large number of behaviors that, on the surface, do not show any commonality. L. K. Wright urges that information seeking be viewed as a critical strategy underlying the health behavior of caregivers.

Coreil (Chapter 9) observes, however, that while health behavior research in the United States draws heavily on conceptual frameworks, much of the work on health behavior in developing countries is not conceptually driven. Coreil discusses health communication models that deal with the impact of communications on acculturation and behavior change, and ecological models that examine health behaviors as adaptive responses to physical, biological, and sociocultural environments.

Stigma

Several of the populations discussed in this volume have been devalued or stigmatized by either their culture, their communities, or their families, or by all of these. Unhappily, such devaluation also occurs at the hands of health professionals and health institutions. The negative implications of such stigma on care seeking and on interactions with health professionals are readily seen in gay men (Kauth & Prejean, Chapter 6), lesbians (VanScoy, Chapter 7), persons living with HIV/AIDS (Thomason & Campos, Chapter 8), the poor and the homeless (J. D. Wright & Joyner, Chapter 10), and persons with severe mental illness (Hawley, Chapter 12). Health behavior research shows that the stigma of these conditions impedes initiation of appropriate care seeking and adherence to regimens. Furthermore, the stigma increases the likelihood of per-

sons engaging in risk behaviors such as alcohol consumption, smoking, or inappropriate eating. To the degree that health institutions and professionals exacerbate or reinforce community and cultural biases, they are counterproductive to the achievement of their missions and in violation of professional oaths and commitments.

Methodological Issues

The methodological issues presented in this volume can be dealt with using the same broad categories used in the integrating chapters for Volume I and II: measurement, sampling, and procedure. Again, in many instances, these are "boilerplate" concerns—criticisms that can be made of nearly any corpus of research.

Measurement

As was observed in Volumes I and II, there is great lack of clarity and consistency in definitions and measures of health behaviors in diverse populations, as well as within single population groups (e.g., Prohaska & Clark, Chapter 2; Cowell & Marks, Chapter 4; Rakowski, Chapter 5; VanScoy, Chapter 7; Hawley, Chapter 12), and great concern about the psychometric properties, i.e., validity and reliability of a number of measures (e.g., O'Brien & Bush, Chapter 3). These shortcomings impede generalizations about health behavior in diverse populations as well as comparisons of the effectiveness of interventions designed to change behaviors. One telling example is the use of the phrase "usual care," which appears in some research. It is very difficult to determine what, if anything, this phrase means either in its own right or in relation to some control or comparison (Rakowski).

Particular problems exist in obtaining information from and about young populations. Caregiver reports of children's health behaviors may be influenced unduly by their concerns about appearing to be responsible in their roles and having necessary caregiving or parenting skills (O'Brien & Bush). In addition, parents and caregivers are often less informed about children's behavior than they assume, and children may be better informants about their own actions (O'Brien & Bush).

Self-report can be a problem in relation to assessing risk and sexual behaviors, and behavioral change (Cowell & Marks; Thomason & Campos, Chapter 8). Persons who have attempted to change a behavior, for example, but who had a hard time adopting it, may report that they do not engage in it (Rakowski).

Sampling

Most life-cycle or developmental data come from samples that are disproportionately white, motivated, and middle class (Prohaska & Clark, Chapter 2). Studies of the elderly also have disproportionately fewer persons with less than a high school education, which is also related to the paucity of persons of color (Rakowski, Chapter 5). Moreover, there are virtually no data on Catholic clergy of "color" (Duckro, Chapter 15). Men are also undersampled in studies of the elderly (Rakowski). Much research is based on nonprobability, convenience samples (e.g., Cowell & Marks, Chapter 4). Some national cross-sectional surveys are based on probability sampling, but these surveys deal largely with demographic variables and rarely, if ever, with psychological or social ones (e.g., Rakowski).

Most studies of health behavior are household-based and thus tend to exclude the homeless; additionally, data from special studies conducted at shelters, soup kitchens, or special clinics for the homeless present problems in external validity and cannot be used to generalize to the entire homeless population (J. D. Wright & Joyner, Chapter 10). It is also difficult to generalize about health behavior from data based on caregivers participating in support groups, since these groups may disproportionately include persons seeking support for depression and related problems (L. K. Wright, Chapter 13).

Other sampling issues involve the representation of stigmatized groups and raise questions about many existing databases. In some instances, e.g., lesbians, the population is not readily defined by external sources (VanScoy, Chapter 7). Among gay men (Kauth & Prejean, Chapter 6), the data reflect their connectedness to the gay community and their openness about being gay; convenience sampling overrepresents patrons of bars, members of gay community centers or organizations, participants in support groups, and recipients of formal services. Among lesbians (VanScoy), data additionally reflect "snowball" and convenience sampling. Attempts to increase the diversity of such samples—through use of newspaper ads, for example—prevents limiting responses exclusively to gays or lesbians or both (Kauth & Prejean). Often, studies confound gay men and male bisexuals. In addition, gay men themselves may be more open to reporting drug and alcohol use than the general population, which may make these behaviors appear disproportionately prevalent among gay men. Neither the community of gay men nor the lesbian community is homogeneous, and the diversity within each group needs to be included in sampling. Similar diversity exists in the HIV/AIDS community.

Procedure

Most health behavior research on populations or subpopulations is cross-sectional rather than longitudinal, providing data about prevalence of a behavior but limiting conclusions about behavioral change. Some regional surveys (e.g., Alameda County, Framingham) are longitudinal, as is at least one national survey (National Survey of Personal Health Practices), but these are the exceptions rather than the rule. Longitudinal studies in elderly persons themselves offer problems in external validity, since they disproportionately reflect the selective survival of those with presumably better health practices (Prohaska & Clark, Chapter 2). The absence of longitudinal research to separate age, transitions, the effects of interventions, and other correlates of health behavior is especially noted in children

(O'Brien & Bush, Chapter 3), in the elderly (Rakowski, Chapter 5), and in gay men (Kauth & Prejean, Chapter 6). Without longitudinal study, it is impossible to interpret some of the observed linkages between social support, health problems, and health behaviors; health problems could themselves lead to increased social support and family contact (Rakowski).

The absence of comparison or controls is pervasive in research on diverse populations. This lack is made especially clear by Rakowski's observation that there appear to be no standard lists of covariates to be controlled in studies of the elderly and by Hawley's (Chapter 12) similar observation about research on persons with severe mental illness. Moreover, there are few if any controlled multicultural studies of responses to the same condition in different developing countries (Coreil, Chapter 9).

VanScoy (Chapter 7) observes that many reports on lesbian health-related behaviors are not scientifically based and are nonstatistical; she further observes that much of the research is nonconnected, i.e., studies don't link to one another. VanScoy also points out that rigorous qualitative research can be a source of strength in the literature on lesbian health behavior. Similarly, following Coreil's observations that much of the work done in developing countries is qualitative and not conceptually driven, use of ethnographic methods can be critical sources of insights into the family and community contexts of health behavior in such countries.

Professional versus Phenomenological Perspectives

The increased use of psychosocial epidemiology in conjunction with classic epidemiology and behavioral epidemiology (e.g., Rakowski, Chapter 5) can be viewed as a way of integrating the phenomenological with the professional. Psychosocial epidemiology recognizes the importance of subjective perspectives in understanding health behavior, i.e., of discovering the reasons for engaging in health-related actions.

The distinction between professional and phenomenological perspectives is given a different twist in Pol and Thomas's (Chapter 1) observations of the demographic correlates of formal and informal care. Formal care involves externally identified and legitimated services and professionals such as hospital admissions, emergency room use, and visits to physicians; informal care involves actions that do not involve the formal system, such as self-care, the purchase and use of over-the-counter drugs and home diagnostic kits, self-prescribed physical therapy, diets, exercise programs, and so forth.

On the other hand, the dominance of the professional perspective is seen in providers whose views on health and illness are often at variance with those of laypersons. VanScoy (Chapter 7) discusses the attempts of providers to over-medicalize many issues of concern to lesbians, and L. K. Wright (Chapter 13) discusses providers whose views of health behavior, especially care-seeking behavior, are at variance with those of caregivers, and who overlook the caregiver's health issues by focusing solely on the health and medical needs of the identified patient.

Role of Affect

Although cognitive models have dominated the field of health behavior research, questions arise about their validity across the life span (Prohaska & Clark, Chapter 2). The concept of transition may imply a period of strong emotional arousal during which cognitions may have little predictive value. Persons going through puberty may be so strongly influenced by hormonal changes and powerful feelings that their beliefs and rationality are overcome (Prohaska & Clark).

Fear rather than rationality may play a critical role in the health behavior of persons with HIV/AIDS. Fears of being diagnosed as seropositive may impede a person from participating in screening, as well as from returning to discover the results (Thomason & Campos, Chapter 8). Similarly, fear of being victimized may be a barrier to care-seeking behavior in gay men and lesbians (Kauth & Prejean, Chapter 6; VanScoy, Chapter 7).

Range of Focus

In a number of areas, health behavior researchers are encouraged to enlarge their focus. For example, research on children's health behavior needs to recognize that children often participate actively in their own care and that their health and health behaviors are not solely the responsibilities of parents and caregivers (O'Brien & Bush, Chapter 3).

There is also a need to broaden the range of behaviors studied. Rakowski (Chapter 5) suggests that suicide be included in a list of risk behaviors. Cowell and Marks (Chapter 4) indicate the need to study a wide range of risk behaviors in adolescents rather than simply one or two. The importance of studying the *antecedents* of sexual risk behaviors, the cues that drive the risk behaviors, is emphasized by Thomason and Campos (Chapter 8).

At the same time, Cowell and Marks note that it is important to move beyond risk behaviors, particularly in adolescence, to the study of issues related to access, and to examine more positive health behaviors rather than focus almost solely on negative ones. A similar theme is voiced by Kauth and Prejean (Chapter 6), who suggest that research on health behavior in gay men should move beyond a narrow range of questions about risk behaviors, increasingly asked in relation to AIDS, toward examining behaviors that foster positive gay identities. These behaviors might include health-promoting behaviors as well as the coping skills necessary to deal with the stress of living in a heterosexist society. Adding coping skills to the range of health behaviors studied by health behavior researchers is also endorsed by L. K. Wright (Chapter 13), who views such skills as encompassing problem solving, help seeking, and trying to change the situation. L.K. Wright suggests that the seeking of social support identified as a health behavior, despite the observation that caregivers seldom seek it. The issues of caregiving also relate to the role of mothering. Coreil (Chapter 9) suggests that maternal time constraints need to be recognized and included in studied of the determinants of health-related behaviors both on the mother's own behalf and on behalf of her children.

FUTURE RESEARCH DIRECTIONS

Future directions for research on the demography, development, and diversity of health behavior include those relating to methodology, conceptual models, the search for meaning, the origins and development of health beliefs and actions, provider behaviors, and a framework for organizing knowledge.

Methodological Directions: The "Boilerplate"

A discussion of future directions for health behavior research would be remiss if it did not include a restatement of "boilerplate" themes, although many of these themes are the mirror images of the earlier discussion of methodological issues. Future research on diverse populations (as in any of the dimensions of social/behavioral science) must be increasingly longitudinal to disentangle age, time period, and cohort effects on behavioral change and to determine developmental life-cycle changes (Prohaska & Clark, Chapter 2), despite some of the issues of selective survival. Future research must:

1. Embrace more diverse samples, including greater probability sampling of young persons and adolescents (Cowell & Marks, Chapter 4) and persons of color (e.g., Rakowski, Chapter 5; Duckro et al., Chapter 15), as well as creative methodology (Kauth & Prejean, Chapter 6) to include hard-to-reach populations such as gays and lesbians who are not "out" (Kauth & Prejean; VanScoy, Chapter 7), persons with HIV/AIDS

(Thomason & Campos, Chapter 8), and homeless persons who do not use shelters (J. D. Wright & Joyner, Chapter 10).

2. Use more appropriate, valid, and reliable measures, and multiple methods of studying a behavior (O'Brien & Bush, Chapter 3); employ consensually identical or comparable measures across diverse studies and samples; and eliminate errors of subject recall.

3. Incorporate developmentally sensitive (Cowell & Marks) and prospective designs (Thomason & Campos).

4. Encourage a combination of idiographic and nomothetic approaches to see which specific psychosocial variables operate for a particular person (Rakowski).

Some of these future studies might then shed light on whether there are common factors associated with transitions (Prohaska & Clark) or whether there are patterns of change in some of the variables that seem to be antecedents of behavioral or outcome changes (Rakowski). As Pol and Thomas (Chapter 1) note, demographic transitions indicate that in the future more patients will be women; that numbers of dental visits have already increased, and then decreased, and are likely to increase again. These transitional changes raise important research questions about what communities and their institutions, especially health institutions, will look like in the 21st century and how they will affect care-seeking behavior.

Future culturally sensitive research could reveal the degree to which the cultural competence of the researcher affects responses, especially in caregivers (L.K. Wright, Chapter 13). Appropriately conducted cross-cultural studies of persons with same-sex attractions could reveal the degree to which culture affects the health behaviors of gay men and lesbians (Kauth & Prejean).

A Common Frame of Reference   Crosscutting these proposals, and most critically needed for the future, is increased awareness of and agreement about some common frame of reference. The cluster of questions raised in Part I provide the beginning of such a framework:

1. How are health behaviors (or a particular type of health behavior) and their determinants and correlates distributed within a population?

2. What accounts for changes in health behaviors within a population?

3. What accounts for demographic differences within a population?

4. How are health behaviors and their determinants and correlates distributed across different populations (or population subgroups)?

5. What accounts for differences in health behaviors between populations (and population subgroups)?

Addressing these questions, however, require consensus—or at least greater uniformity and standardization—about the behaviors and their correlates to be studied and the ways they will be measured. Use of such a framework would increase the comparability of findings and add to knowledge about genuine similarities and differences between populations.

Conceptual Models

Future research should explore the relevance of the health belief and other conceptual models to understanding the development of health behaviors in young populations (O'Brien & Bush, Chapter 3). It should examine the relationship between the transtheoretical model, transitions, and the life cycle; the linkages of concepts such as self-efficacy and social learning to health behaviors throughout the life span; and the differential predictive value of the several available conceptual models across the life span (Prohaska & Clark, Chapter 2). In addition, future research should focus on how maturation variables operate in conjunction with these conceptual predictors (Cowell & Marks, Chapter 4).

The Search for Meaning

The issue of the meaning of health and its relation to beliefs and actions continues to arise whether health behavior research findings are examined in terms of different levels of determinants or in terms of diverse populations. For example, in relation to the elderly, Rakowski (Chapter 5) stresses the importance of understanding a person's "reasons to get out of bed in the morning"—a person's reasons for being actively involved in life—as important internal motivations for engaging in health behaviors. Meanings need to be sought in relation to perceived control and social linkages. Rakowski raises the incisive question of what meaning, if any, is attached to perceived control over health or having social support; whether it is tenable to assume that these are *subjectively* meaningful; and whether and how these personal, phenomenological experiences are related to health behaviors and to positive views of health status.

Within the context of transitions, future research should also determine the meanings that life-span transitions have for individuals and how such meanings are related to health behavior. Movement into parenthood and losing a spouse (e.g., Prohaska & Clark, Chapter 2) are each experienced individually, and each has differential meaning. What impacts do the meanings of such transitions have for changed likelihoods of risk or health-promoting behavior?

Traumatic events convey meanings of a different nature. Future health behavior research should also explore the meanings attached to being victimized as a member of a stigmatized group and the implications of these meanings for risk behaviors as well as for health-protective behaviors (Kauth & Prejean, Chapter 6).

Finally, the subjective meanings of caregiving should be explored in order to understand the linkages between caregiving and health behavior (L. K. Wright, Chapter 13). In addition, future research should explore whether the motives that underlie caregiving vary across different population groups and the ways in which such differences affect the health behaviors of caregivers (L. K. Wright).

Origins and Development of Health Behaviors

Consistent with points made in Volume I (e.g., Gochman, Chapter 10; Lau, Chapter 3; Tinsley, Chapter 11) and integrating and building upon points made in this volume by Cowell and Marks (Chapter 4), O'Brien and Bush (Chapter 3), Prohaska and Clark (Chapter 2), and Rakowski (Chapter 5), there is a great need for research on the origins and development of health behaviors in young as well as in adult populations. Much research has been undertaken to shape and modify these behaviors, but few investigations have attempted systematically to explore their origins. Questions arise about the importance of a range of factors in the origins and development of such beliefs and behaviors: transitions; family, friends, peer groups, social relationships, and societal and cultural values and institutions. Basic research into the origins of health beliefs and actions and how they develop is thus an additional major challenge for future health behavior research.

Provider Issues

Provider issues represent a final component for future health behavior research. Demographic changes coupled with changing health policies will encourage providers to develop new "products," such as menopause management and different variants of managed care. Future research should explore the determinants of use of these services and whether patterns of use are determined by changes in needs, or by demographic or personal and social factors.

Future health behavior research should also determine whether interventions could be more effective if directed at changing behaviors or at changing the structure of system, including both health care and nonhealth institutions. These findings will be informative in the development of health care policy (J. D. Wright & Joyner, Chapter 10).

Future research should also examine provider barriers to health behavior in caregivers and whether these barriers vary across different population groups. Finally, future health behavior research should examine dimensions of professional roles to advise about making them optimally effective in relation to the management of chronic illness (Gallagher & Stratton, Chapter 11).

SUMMARY

A wide range of health behaviors can readily be seen to be influenced by a broad spectrum of personal and social factors in a number of diverse populations. Health behavior research on population groups has focused largely on needs for care and on the prevalence and determinants of risk behaviors. The relevance for health behavior of transitions within population groups, and the effects of stigma on several of these transitions, have been discussed. Identified methodological issues include obtaining data from hard-to-reach population elements and developing appropriate comparisons and controls. Among the important areas for future research, in addition to remedying methodological problems, are the different meanings attached to health and health behaviors for different population groups, the origins and development of health beliefs and health actions, and provider behaviors.

Concepts and Definitions
A Glossary for Health Behavior Research

With few exceptions, the definitions in this Glossary are either taken verbatim, paraphrased, or abstracted from this *Handbook*. Specific chapters and, where appropriate, sources cited herein are identified. Italicized terms within a definition denote additional Glossary entries.

Consistent with the focus of this *Handbook* on health *behavior*, the Glossary does not routinely define diseases or medical treatments. Space limitations preclude defining every "named" intervention or program, or every social or behavioral science model that is not especially focused on health behavior. A number of these programs and models, however, are listed in the Index.

acceptance See *adherence; compliance*.

access framework A conceptual refinement of the *health services utilization model* that predicts the use of and satisfaction with health care; basic components are health policy, the organizational and accessibility characteristics of the delivery system, and *predisposing, enabling*, and *need factors* (Aday & Andersen, 1974, in Aday & Awe, I, 8). See *utilization framework*.

action stage In the *transtheoretical model*, the phase in which persons have modified their behavior and are participating in the appropriate health practice (Prohaska & Clark, III, 2).

active coping In health contexts, a tendency or motivation to exercise personal control, reflecting preference for decision making in health care, preference for behavioral involvement, and low expectations that health care professionals can control one's health (Christensen, Benotsch, & Smith, II, 12).

active patient orientation See *mutual participation model*.

active prevention See *prevention, active*.

activities of daily living (ADL) Instrumental and basic behaviors necessary for everyday life (Prohaska & Clark, III, 2).

adherence Practice of following health care provider recommendations (Clark, II, 8; Chrisler, II, 17); "an interdependent network of regimen behaviors rather than a single behavior" (Wysocki & Greco, II, 9); following recommended screening procedures (Rimer, Demark-Wahnefried, & Egert, II, 15); congruence between patient behaviors and advice or instructions provided by health care providers; medical adherence: how closely a patient's medication-taking behaviors match instructions prescribed by a physician (Creer & Levstek, II, 7). The concept embraces total adherence and acceptance, as well as degrees thereof; in relation to smoking, it includes not only total cessation, but also participation in cessation activities, as well as the actions of change agents (Glasgow & Orleans, II, 19). It connotes active, voluntary behavior designed to produce a therapeutic effect (Chrisler, II, 17). See *compliance*.

ADL See *activities of daily living*.

affective behavior, physician's Comprises acts aimed at establishing a relationship with patients in which the physician accepts the patient as a human being whose anxiety-arousing problems cannot be alleviated by technical procedures; it involves the physician attributing therapeutic importance to, and engaging in warm, open relations with the patient; being attentive to problems that may not be related to disease; gathering information about personal and family problems and social relations; and explaining the rationale of the diagnosis and treatment (Ben-Sira, II, 2).

AIDS Acquired immunodeficiency syndrome: a condition in which exposure to the *HIV* (human immunodeficiency virus) leads to the destruction of the body's natural defenses against infection (Thomason & Campos, III, 8).

analytical framework for the study of child survival A conceptual model designed to understand morbidity and mortality in children in developing countries; basic components are maternal factors, environmental contamination, nutrient deficiency, and injury and personal illness control (Mosley & Chen, 1984, in Coreil, III, 9).

anthropology of medicine See *medical anthropology*.

appropriate interventions/care Lists of indications for use of procedures consensually generated by nationally recognized experts (Rand Corporation/McGlynn, Kosecoff, & Brook, 1990, in DiMatteo, II, 1). Compare *inappropriate/unnecessary care*.

attributable risk Amount of disease (disability or mortality) in a population group that could be eliminated if a risk factor were eliminated (Prohaska & Clark, III, 2).

authority, physician The physician's power over others (Haug, II, 3).

autonomy, physician The physician's power or ability to resist or withstand being compelled by others (Haug, II, 3).

autonomy, principle of A moral standard stressing the obligation to respect rights to self-determination (Nilstun, IV, 11).

autonomy, self-care See *self-care autonomy*.

availability bias A concept that explains safety and risk avoidance behaviors, denoting the inclination to be inordinately influenced by dramatic events that have low probabilities of happening but are vivid in memory; ease of recall being a function of saliency, recency, and emotional impact (Slovic, 1978, in Cohen & Colligan, II, 20).

behavioral epidemiology The study of the relationships between lifestyles and mortality and morbidity patterns in a population (Rakowski, III, 5).

behavioral model See *health services utilization model*.

beneficence, principle of A moral standard stressing the obligation to benefit others, especially not to harm them (Nilstun, IV, 11).

bruxism Spasmodic grinding of the teeth in other than chewing movements (Gift & White, IV, 7).

caregiver, informal Layperson who provides personal care to an older, ill family member or close friend (Wright, III, 13).

care-seeking behavior, theory of A conceptual framework in nursing, incorporating components of the *health belief model*, *theory of reasoned action*, and Triandis's theory of interpersonal behavior; designed to predict preventive rather than illness-related behaviors; basic components are affective arousal, perceived utility, *social norms*, and habits (Lauver, 1992a, in Blue & Brooks, IV, 5).

central place theory A conceptual framework based on land economics that is used to relate a hierarchy of levels of health care services to concentrations of population and distances (Scarpaci & Kearns, II, 5).

children's health belief model A conceptual framework for understanding children's health behaviors, incorporating components of the *health belief model*, environmental variables, and readiness factors (O'Brien & Bush, III, 3).

chronic Referring to an illness or condition that is incurable and lasts through a person's lifetime (Gallagher & Stratton, III, 11).

cognitive appraisal The process of intellectually evaluating and deciding on available options to engage in a particular behavior (Cowell & Marks, III, 4).

cognitive developmental theory A conceptual framework for understanding the development of children's thinking; assumes that children take an active rather than a passive role in constructing their own knowledge and understanding of health and illness and that they move through universally recognized sequences in doing so (O'Brien & Bush, III, 3).

cognitive representations Personal images or schemata of illness, disease, and being healthy, and the meanings attached to these images; persons develop their own individualized images or schemata in relation to symptoms and illness that are often different from the representations of physicians and the medical community (Lau, I, 3).

coming out Disclosure of nonheterosexual identity by a lesbian or a gay man (VanScoy, III, 7); can also mean self-recognition of such identity.

commonsense representation of illness The images or schemata of illness, disease, or symptoms held by a layperson; the images include an identity, a set of consequences, a time-line, a cause, and a cure or control (Lau, I, 3).

communication Exchange of meaning, either verbally or nonverbally, between people to establish a commonality of thought, attitude, feeling, and ideas (DiMatteo, II, 1).

communication campaign Use of mass media on a health topic, typically involving television, radio, newspaper, magazines, and other channels to convey health information or to provide motivation for health actions (Swinehart, IV, 18).

community A social entity or system made up of individuals together with formal organizations, such as local government, businesses, and educational institutions, and voluntary organizations, such as religious, fraternal, or service groups; informal social networks; and families. Critical to the concept is the premise that various components are related to each other and have the potential for being mobilized in relation to health promotion programs (Schooler & Flora, IV, 15).

community health promotion Interventions for effecting change in communities that involve social planning, social action, and locality development (Rothman, 1979, in Schooler & Flora, IV, 15).

community organization An intervention strategy designed to empower a community and to enhance its competence and problem-solving ability; of particular importance for increasing the success of a *health promotion* program (Schooler & Flora, IV, 15).

compadrazgo A system of selecting *comadres* (female friends) and *copadres* (male friends) for one's children; levels of perceived support from these friends are related to health status and health behavior (Dressler & Oths, I, 17).

competence gap The difference in health-related knowledge and skill between physicians and other health professionals and their patients or clients (Haug, II, 3).

compliance Degree of correspondence between the physician's prescription and the patient's behavior (Sackett & Haynes, 1976, in DiIorio, II, 11; Morisky & Cabrera, II, 14); congruence between medical recommendations and the degree to which a patient takes medicine, follows a diet, or changes lifestyle behaviors (Trostle, II, 6); an ideology that transforms a physician's theories about patients' behavior into research strategies and potentially coercive interventions that strengthen physicians' authority (Trostle, II, 6). See also *adherence*.

conscientiousness factor A theoretical personality dimension reflecting "will to achieve," "dependability," and "self-control" thought to be related to medication adherence in renal dialysis patients (Christensen et al., II, 12).

consciousness raising A component of the *transtheoretical model*, denoting a process by which people move from not being ready to initiate a behavior to being ready to initiate it (Rakowski, III, 5).

consumerism A framework for viewing physician–patient interactions that argues for patient autonomy and sole decision making as essential in combating physician paternalism (DiMatteo, II, 1), or in which an "activist" patient approaches health care as a problem-solving endeavor that requires active coping (Pratt, 1978, in Wiese & Gallagher, IV, 4).

contemplation In the *transtheoretical model*, the stage in which people are aware that a problem exists and are seriously thinking about overcoming it (Prohaska & Clark, III, 2).

contracting Use of a written document, resulting from the negotiation of a treatment plan between a patient and medical personnel, that identifies the reinforcements the patient will receive contingent on performing the behaviors stipulated in the treatment plan (Creer & Levstek, II, 7).

control beliefs See *locus of control*.

control demand model A conceptual framework developed to understand how workplace characteristics are related to health behaviors such as smoking, alcohol use, exercise, and self-protective behavior; basic components are levels of control over work, psychological demands, and social support (Eakin, I, 16).

control, perceived behavioral See *perceived behavioral control*.

convergence hypothesis A proposition that suggests that as gender roles become more similar, gender differences in health behavior decrease or disappear (Waldron, I, 15).

conversation model A conceptual framework for viewing physician–patient interactions in which the patient continually provides the physician information about values, preferences, and constraints and the physician engages in "thinking out loud" about possible courses of action, recommended interventions, and their implications, using language that is understood by the patient (DiMatteo, II, 1).

coping appraisal   Evaluation of adaptive responses to threat; a component of the *protection motivation theory* (Rogers & Prentice-Dunn, I, 6).

coping mode   Way of responding to threat messages (Rogers & Prentice-Dunn, I, 6). See *protection motivation theory*.

cue to action   A stimulus, either internal or external, that can trigger health-related cognitive processes or health actions (Strecher, Champion, & Rosenstock, I, 4).

cultural consensus model   A conceptual framework to assess the degree to which a body of information is shared within a social group; provides an estimate of shared beliefs related to health and illness (Dressler & Oths, I, 17).

culture   A set of interlocking cognitive schemata that literally construct much of what people do on a daily basis; the manner in which a social group stores and transmits information; a system of symbols or abstract elements that are learned and patterned socially (Dressler & Oths, I, 17).

damaging cycle   A chain of events in which a somatic disturbance leads to a detrimental appraisal of health, which then precipitates stress, which then increases the risk of further somatic disturbance (Ben-Sira, II, 2).

decisional balance theory   A conceptual framework for understanding how persons make specific choices, based on comparisons of perceived positive and negative aspects of a behavior, and including gains and losses to self and others and approval or disapproval of self and others (Janis & Mann, 1977, in Marcus, Bock, & Pinto, II, 18).

demography, health   See *health demography*.

deskilling   Transference of work functions once controlled exclusively by physicians or nurses to positions lower down on the occupational hierarchy (Salloway, Hafferty, & Vissing, II, 4).

developing country   A designation based on economic, demographic, and social/health indicators, given to a nation that is relatively poor, with a relatively young and fertile population and relatively scarce health and social resources (Coreil, III, 9).

developmental model of diabetes self-management   A conceptual framework for understanding

the responsibilities that patients and families can assume in monitoring, evaluating, and adjusting treatment for insulin-dependent diabetes mellitus; basic components include demographic factors, family functioning, psychological stress, and interactions with providers to acquire necessary skills (Wysocki & Greco, II, 9). See *self-management, childhood diabetes*; *self-regulation/self-regulatory skills*.

diagnosis   Naming of a condition by medical professionals; represents the interplay of social, institutional, and cultural factors together with personal symptoms through which time and location at which medical professionals and other parties determine the existence and legitimacy of a condition (Brown, 1995, in Gochman, IV, 20).

diagnosis related group/diagnostic related group (DRG)   One of 438 groupings of patient conditions that have been the basis for federal reimbursements to hospitals for Medicare patients since 1983 (Daugherty, IV, 10); hospitals are paid a fixed amount for a given DRG regardless of length of stay and services provided.

disease   A biological/organic abnormality; not identical to illness (Lau, I, 3); the measurable deviation of an organic system from some independently defined optimum (Dressler & Oths, I, 17).

doctrine of specific etiology   See *specific etiology, doctrine of*.

DRG   See *diagnosis related group*.

drinking culture   Group norms, particularly within work settings, that encourage and support consumption of alcohol; closely related to *occupational culture* (Eakin, I, 16).

ecological model   A conceptual framework that integrates five levels of personal and social systems: intrapersonal, interpersonal, organizational, community, and public policy in public health efforts (Buchanan, IV, 9).

edentulous   Without teeth; toothless (Gift & White, IV, 7).

effectiveness   Benefits of medical care measured by improvements in health (Aday & Awe, I, 8).

efficiency   A relationship between improvements in health and the resources required to produce them (Aday & Awe, I, 8).

elaboration likelihood model   A conceptual framework to predict attitude change; persuasion is proposed to be a function of the audience's active involvement in processing a message and the importance of the message's topic to the audience (Petty &

Cacioppo, 1986, in Rogers & Prentice-Dunn, I, 6; Wiese & Gallagher, IV, 4).

emic Denotes a way of knowing reflecting an internal or cultural "insider" perspective (Weidman, 1988, in Gochman, I, Part V); emic behavior is behavior that a person believes to be related to health, regardless of whether it is externally validated (Eakin, I, 16). Compare *etic*.

empowerment Enabling individuals, families, and communities to take control over their lives and their environment (e.g., Rappaport, 1984, in Schooler & Flora, IV, 15).

enabling factor A resource characteristic, such as family income or community availability, that predicts use of health services; a component of the *health services utilization model* (Aday & Awe, I, 8).

energized family A conceptual framework for understanding the family as a social system; basic components are regularity of interaction among members, contacts with the larger community, working together to advance members' interests, and coping with and mastering their lives. Energized families tend to encourage autonomy, rather than use "autocratic" parenting, and to socialization methods, resulting in children with better levels of health behaviors (Pratt, 1976, in Gochman, I, 10; Tinsley, I, 11).

epidemiology "Study of the distribution and determinants of diseases and injuries in human populations" (Inhorn, 1995, in Gochman, IV, 20).

epidemiology, behavioral See *behavioral epidemiology*.

epidemiology, psychosocial See *psychosocial epidemiology*.

equity The degree to which the benefits and burdens of medical care are fairly distributed in a population (Aday & Awe, I, 8); the degree to which participants (either patients or professionals) believe that the ratio of benefits received to their efforts and resources expended is equal or skewed in their favor (Daugherty, IV, 10).

etic Denotes a way of knowing reflecting an external or cultural "outsider" perspective (Weidman, 1988, in Gochman, I, Part V). Etic behavior is behavior that external observers believe to be related to health, independent of the behaving individual's beliefs (Eakin, I, 16). Compare *emic*.

eudaimonistic health A state of exuberant well-being (Lau, I, 3).

exercise Physical activity of moderate intensity (Marcus et al., II, 18).

explanatory model A cognitive framework of health processes based on both cultural knowledge and idiosyncratic experience that is used to understand health status, illness, and sickness; basic components include etiology, timing of onset of symptoms, pathophysiology, course of sickness, and treatment. Explanatory models exist at both lay and professional levels (Kleinman, 1980, & Kleinman, Eisenberg, & Good, 1978, in Dressler & Oths, I, 17).

facilitative environment An environment in which "nonsmoking cues and cessation information are persistent and inescapable" (Glynn, Boyd, & Gruman, 1990, in Glasgow & Orleans, II, 19).

familism Importance of family and relatives in a person's live, particularly in relation to care-seeking behavior (Geertsen, I, 13).

family aggregation A concept denoting intrafamilial similarities in health variables compared to nonfamilial similarities (Sallis & Nader, 1988, in Gochman, I, 10).

family code A system of norms for a family's behavior, including core assumptions, beliefs, family stories, myths, and rituals (Tinsley, I, 11).

family concordance Degree to which members of a family exhibit similarity in a specified health behavior (Baranowski, I, 9).

family, energized See *energized family*.

family health culture The unique combination of family experiences, beliefs, perceptions of symptoms, and reactions to the perceptions that influences the way in which families seek care or treatment (Black, 1986, in Gochman, I, 10).

fighting the illness A posture of gritty defiance as a way of dealing with a chronic illness (Gallagher & Stratton, III, 11).

fixed role hypothesis A proposition suggesting that men's more structured role obligations, compared with women's, may make it more difficult for men to engage in care-seeking behavior and thus accounts for women's greater use of health services (Marcus & Siegel, 1982, in Gochman, I, Part IV).

Flexner Report An analysis and recommendations relevant to United States medical education, prepared by Abraham Flexner in 1910, that became the basis for the reform of and standardization of medical training; remains a critical foundation for late 20th-century medical education (Weise & Gallagher, IV, 4).

folk illness A shared interpretation of a cluster of symptoms within a social group that is at variance with a biomedical framework (Dressler & Oths, I, 17).

framework of relationships model   A conceptual scheme for understanding compliance behavior, especially for epilepsy; basic components are the *health services utilization model*, the *health belief model*, and health education, with an emphasis on adequate financial and community resources (Di Iorio, II, 11).

gay   Without a gender qualifier, refers to a homosexual, a person who engages or desires to engage in sexual behavior with a person of the same gender (Kauth & Prejean, III, 6).

gay man   A male who engages or desires to engage in sexual behavior with another male; a homosexual (Kauth & Prejean, III, 6).

gender role   The social roles, behaviors, attitudes, and psychological characteristics that are more common, more expected, and more accepted for one sex or the other; includes a group of interrelated behaviors, attitudes, and psychological characteristics that influence a variety of risk and risk-taking behaviors as well as care-seeking behaviors (Waldron, I, 15).

GOBI   Acronym for *G*rowth monitoring, *O*ral rehydration, *B*reast-feeding and *I*mmunization, the four cornerstone child survival interventions in developing countries (Coreil, III, 9).

grazing   Snacking throughout the day (O'Brien & Bush, III, 3).

group ties   See *social ties*.

habit   A behavior that does not require conscious effort but is set in motion by situational cues (Schneider & Shiffrin, 1977, in Maddux & DuCharme, I, 7) and is less under the control of conscious cognitive processes and deliberate decisions.

healing   The social processes and actions brought to bear to deal with a condition of disease or illess (Fabrega, I, 2).

healing culture   The totality of institutions involved in treatment of disease, including biomedical and alternative approaches and the range of choices available, and the culture of medicine and its rituals and stresses (e.g., Foster & Anderson, 1978, in Gochman, IV, 20).

healmeme   A unit of symbolic cultural information that gives meaning to the domain of health, well-being, sickness, and healing; underlies and constitutes a society's health-related beliefs and behaviors (Fabrega, I, 2).

health   A state of being, almost impossible to define satisfactorily; includes components of physiological, psychological, and social functioning (Gochman I, 1; Lau, I, 3). What is considered to be health is appreciably determined by societal and cultural factors (Fabrega, I, 2). A continuous variable reflecting a capacity or ability to perform, as well as the use of that capacity to achieve expectations and to negotiate the demands of the social and physical environment (Tarlov, 1992, in Reed, Moore-West, Jernstedt, & O'Donell, IV, 2); "an individual or group capacity relative to potential to function fully in the social and physical environment" (Tarlov, 1992, in Flipse, IV, 3).

health behavior, formal   Actions taken for the prevention or treatment of a condition or for the maintenance or enhancement of health that involve the use of institutionalized services such as physicians and hospitals (Pol & Thomas, III, 1).

health behavior, informal   Actions taken for the prevention or treatment of a condition or for the maintenance or enhancement of health that do not involve the use of institutionalized services such as physicians and hospitals; these actions include self-care, tooth brushing, and use of over-the-counter medications (Pol & Thomas, III, 1).

health belief model   A conceptual framework designed to predict preventive actions and eventually used to predict illness and sick role behaviors; basic components of the model are perceived susceptibility to some illness, perceived severity or seriousness of that condition, perceived benefits of taking a specified action, and perceived barriers to taking such action (Strecher, Champion, & Rosenstock, I, 4).

health care management   See *management, health care*.

health care manager   See *manager, health care*.

health culture   A society's repertoire of patterns for cognition, affect, and behavior in relation to health, sickness, and well-being (Weidman, 1988, in Gochman, I, Part V).

health demography   Application of the content and methods of demography to the study of health-related phenomena; analyzes the influence of demographic factors such as age, marital status, and income on the health status and health behavior of poplations and the differential impact of health-related phenomena on demographic groupings; focuses on the implications of population change for health care (Pol & Thomas, III, 1). See *behavioral epidemiology*; *psychosocial epidemiology*.

health education   Efforts to change behavior in order to improve health (Glanz & Oldenburg, IV, 8); "any combination of learning experiences designed to facilitate voluntary adaptations of behavior conducive to health" (Green, Kreuter, Deeds, & Partridge, 1980, p. 7, in Glanz & Oldenburg, IV, 8).

health input–output model   See *input–output model, health.*

health maintenance organization (HMO)   A prepaid group practice for delivering comprehensive health care from a specific set of providers. See *managed care.*

health policy   Aggregate of federal, state, and local laws, rules, and regulations that govern the financing, regulation, and organization of health care (Aday & Awe, I, 8).

health-promoting self-care system model   A conceptual framework for nursing, integrating self-care deficit nursing theory, the *interaction model of client health behavior*, and the *health promotion model of nursing*, designed to predict individual autonomy and responsibility for health-promoting behaviors (Simmons, 1990a, in Blue & Brooks, IV, 5).

health promotion   "any combination of health education and related organizational, economic, and environmental supports for behavior of individuals, groups, or communities conducive to health" (Green & Kreuter, 1991, in Glanz & Oldenburg, IV, 8); "the science and art of helping people change their lifestyle to move toward a state of optimal health ... by a combination of efforts to enhance awareness, change behavior, and create environments that support good health practices" (O'Donnell, 1989, in Glanz & Oldenburg, IV, 8); "the process of enabling people to increase control over, and to improve, their health ... a commitment to dealing with the challenges of reducing inequities, extending the scope of prevention, and helping people to cope with their circumstances ... creating environments conducive to health, in which people are better able to take care of themselves" (Epp, 1986, in Glanz & Oldenburg, IV, 8). The term was seldom used prior to 1980.

health promotion model, nursing   A conceptual framework for nursing, similar to the *health belief model*, used to predict engaging in behaviors that maintain or improve well-being, rather than prevent disease; basic components are importance of health, perceived control of health, perceived *self-efficacy*, definition of health, perceived health status, *perceived benefits* of health-promoting behaviors, and *perceived barriers* to health-promoting behaviors (Pender, 1982, in Blue & Brooks, IV, 5).

health psychology   "The aggregate of the specific educational, scientific, and professional contributions of the discipline of psychology to the promotion and maintenance of health, the prevention and treatment of illness, the identification of etiologic and diagnostic correlates of health, illness and related dysfunction" (Matarazzo, 1980, p. 815, in Gochman, IV, 20); "any aspect of psychology that bears upon the experience of health and illness, and the behavior that affects health status" (Rodin & Stone, 1987, pp. 15–16, in Gochman, IV, 20).

health-seeking process model   A conceptual framework for understanding people's experiences with sickness holistically as natural histories of illness; basic components are symptom definition, illness-related shifts in role behavior, lay referral, treatment actions, and adherence (Chrisman, 1977, in Dressler & Oths, I, 17).

health service system   Arrangements for the potential rendering of care to consumers, including the volume and distribution of services and their accessibility and organization (Aday & Awe, I, 8). See *health services utilization model.*

health services utilization model   A conceptual framework designed to predict use of health care, such as visits to physicians and dentists and use of medications and clinical facilities; basic components are *predisposing*, *enabling*, and *need factors* (Aday & Awe, I, 8); sometimes referred to as the *behavioral model.*

heterosexism   An assumption, especially among health providers and institutions, that heterosexuality, or male–female sexual expression, is normative and superior to others (VanScoy, III, 7).

HIV   See *AIDS.*

HMO   Acronym for *health maintenance organization* (Daugherty, IV, 10). See *managed care.*

homeless assistance act, Stewart B. McKinney   A 1987 federal law that extended the National Health Care for the Homeless Initiative to a total of 109 cities (Wright & Joyner, III, 10).

homeless, literally   Persons who spend their nights either in outdoor locations, in temporary overnight shelters, or in other places not intended for human habitation (Wright & Joyner, III, 10).

homelessness   No agreed-upon definition (Wright & Joyner, III, 10). See *homeless, literally*; *housed, marginally.*

homophobia   An irrational fear of homosexuality (Eliason, Donelan, & Rundall, 1992, in Vanscoy, III, 7).

housed, marginally   Persons with a claim to some minimal housing, but who are at high risk of being *homeless* (Wright & Joyner, III, 10).

illness   The subjective experience of some biological/ organic/social/emotional abnormality; not identical to disease (e.g., Lau, I, 3); the social and psychological concomitants of putative physiological problems (Conrad, 1990, in Gochman, I, 1); incapacity for role performance (Gerhardt, 1989a, in Gochman, I, 1); motivated deviance (Segall, I, 14); the individual experience of suffering or distress, or disvalued states of being and functioning (Dressler & Oths, I, 17).

illusion of safety   Workers' practicing of safe behavior under supervision but of unsafe behavior, such as taking shortcuts and engaging in risky actions, in the absence of supervision; convinces management that it has done its job and that safety regimens are being followed when in reality they are not (Cohen & Colligan, II, 20).

image theory   A conceptual framework for decision making based on the fit between alternative choices and an individual's images, plans, or principles (Mitchell & Beach, 1990, in Rogers & Prentice-Dunn, I, 6).

inappropriate/unnecessary care   A medical intervention with risks that exceed the potential benefit to the patient (DiMatteo, II, 1). Compare *appropriate intervention/care*.

informal caregiver   See *caregiver, informal.*

information seeking   A generic process that underlies behavior change and comprises a cluster of behaviors including but not limited to reading articles about health, attending to media programs on health, and reading food package labels (Rakowski, III, 5; Swinehart, IV, 18).

information vigilance factor   A tendency or motivation to attend actively to threat-relevant information and sensory experiences related to health and treatment, reflecting *information seeking*, internal health *locus of control*, and monitoring of sensory information (Christensen et al., II, 12).

inoculation theory   A conceptual framework suggesting that providing persons in advance with information and counterarguments enables them to resist persuasive and pressuring appeals to engage in risk behaviors; sometimes termed "social inocula-

tion theory" (McGuire, 1968, in Kelder et al., IV, 14; Bruhn, IV, 1).

input–output model, health   A framework combining external factors such as the physical and community environments and the macrosocial structure with internal biological–genetic–psychic factors as predictors of role fulfillment and well-being (Tarlov, 1992, in Flipse, IV, 3).

inreach   Directing health promotion and prevention strategies at persons already in the health care system (Rimer et al., II, 15).

intention, behavioral   A person's subjective probability or prediction of performing a specified behavior; a basic component of the *theory of reasoned action*/theory of planned behavior. It has been inaccurately defined as what a person intends or plans to do and the degree to which a person has developed conscious plans to enact some behavior in the future (Maddux & DuCharme, I, 7). See *self-prediction*.

interaction model of client health behavior   A conceptual framework in nursing to explain and predict a range of health behaviors; basic components are elements of client singularity, such as background, motivation, cognitive appraisal, and affective responses, and elements of client–professional interactions, such as affective support, health information, decisional control, and professional competence (Cox, 1982, in Blue & Brooks, IV, 5).

interfamilial consensus   A concept denoting the degree of similarity in illness-related conceptions in randomly selected pairs of persons (Susman et al., 1982, in Gochman, I, 10).

intrafamilial transmission   A concept denoting the degree of similarity in illness-related conceptions found in parent–child pairs (Susman et al., 1982, in Gochman, I, 10).

justice as fairness   A conceptual framework applied to health issues that stipulates that each person has an equal right to liberty, that persons with similar abilities and skills should have equal access to services, and that social and economic institutions should be arranged to benefit maximally the least well off (Nilstun, IV, 11).

justice, principle of   A moral standard stressing the obligation to act fairly in the distribution of burdens and benefits, especially not to discriminate against anyone (Nilstun, IV, 11).

KAP (acronym for *Knowledge, Attitudes,* and *Practices*)   A standardized measure to assess knowledge of disease risk factors, use of a health service, and perceptions of therapeutic efficacy; used extensively in *developing countries* (Coreil, III, 9).

landscape, therapeutic A combination of physical and humanly imposed environmental characteristics of treatment settings that facilitate the healing process (Gesler, 1992, in Gochman, IV, 20).

language of distress Terminology as well as nonverbal cues that patients use to present their conditions to health professionals (Helman, 1991, in Gochman, IV, 20).

lay-intelligible cues An action on the part of the physician that serves as a basis for the patient's understanding of a condition and its treatment and for the patient's evaluation of the physician's treatment and competence (Ben-Sira, II, 2).

lay referral system The informal network of family members, friends, and community contacts who provide information and advice about the care-seeking process prior to use of a professional (Geertsen, I, 13).

learned resourcefulness Tendency to apply self-control skills in solving behavioral problems, e.g., use of strategies to delay gratification or tolerate frustration (Rosenbaum, 1980, in Christensen et al., II, 12).

lesbian A woman who engages or desires to engage in sexual behavior with another female; the preferred term is "lesbian identity," denoting a woman whose identity is defined by other women (VanScoy, III, 7).

lesbian epistemology A way of knowing the world that reflects a lesbian's own identity and constructions of reality, including of health and illness, in contrast to patriarchal, heterosexist constructions (VanScoy, III, 7).

lesbian invisibility The degree to which lesbian health issues or lesbian identity are hidden or ignored in health services and in the lesbian's interactions with the health care system (VanScoy, III, 7).

libertarianism A conceptual framework applied to health issues that emphasizes the liberty of all individuals to do what they please with themselves and their property, provided they do not interfere with the like liberty of others (Nilstun, IV, 11).

lifespan A framework for individual development that includes chronological age as well as biological and social role transitions (Prohaska & Clark, III, 2).

lifestyle Utilitarian social practices and ways of living adopted by an individual that reflect personal, group, and socioeconomic identities. A health lifestyle involves decisions to live or not to live healthfully; decisions about food, exercise, coping with stress, smoking, alcohol and drug use, risk of accidents, and physical appearance; and reflects social norms and values (Cockerham, I, 12).

lifestyle changes Modifications of behavior resulting from negotiated agreements rather than physician's orders (Chrisler, II, 17).

locality development A cooperative, broadly based approach to community health promotion interventions involving wide discussion and joint problem solving among many diverse groups (Rothman, 1979, in Schooler & Flora, IV, 15).

locational attributes Proximity, centrality, and convenience of health care facilities (Scarpaci & Kearns, II, 5).

locus of control, internal Beliefs that things that happen are a result of one's own ability to influence events as opposed to being the result of chance or fate or of powerful other forces; has been used to predict varied health behaviors (Reich, Zautra, & Erdal, I, 5).

managed care A form of delivering health services in which an organization assumes total responsibility and financial risk for its participants' health, providing all needed services and treatments on a prepaid, capitation basis; an outgrowth of *health maintenance organizations (HMOs)* (Daughtery, IV, 10).

management, health care Tasks of planning, organizing, directing, communicating, coordinating, and monitoring organizational functions in health settings by persons specifically designated and empowered to do so; execution of these tasks through an orderly institutional process carried out by persons designated as managers, regardless of their specific titles (Daugherty, IV, 10).

manager, health care An administrator, executive, director, or chief; anyone who has, or shares in, the legal authority and responsibility for the functions, direction, and achievements of a health organization (Daugherty, IV, 10).

media advocacy Use of mass media to advance a social or public policy objective (Pertschuk, 1988, in Schooler & Flora, IV, 15).

medical anthropology The study of cultural factors related to disease and its explanations, and to healing, treatment, responses to illness and interactions between healers and persons who are sick (Gochman, IV, 20).

medical geography   The study of physical, climatic, and locational factors related to disease and its explanations and to healing, treatment, responses to illness, and interactions between healers and persons who are sick (Barrett, 1993, in Gochman, IV, 20).

medical model   A framework for looking at illness that is based largely on the 19th-century linkages of germ theory and acute diseases and that accords physicians and medical institutions primacy in diagnosis and treatment; an overdependence on medical metaphors in dealing with behavioral variability and problems in living.

medical pluralism   Existence of a multiplicity of medical systems, usually biomedical plus varied indigenous ones, within a society; alternatively, a multiplicity of healing techniques, rather than of medical systems (Durkin-Longley, 1984, in Gochman, I, Part V; Stoner, 1986, in Gochman, IV, 20).

medical sociology   The study of social and societal factors related to disease and its explanations and to healing, treatment, responses to illness, and interactions between healers and persons who are sick (Gochman, IV, 20).

medicalization   Expansion of the jurisdiction of the profession of medicine to include many problems not previously defined as medical entities (Gabe & Calnan, 1989, in Gochman, I, Part IV).

medication event monitor system   A device attached to a medication bottle that records the date and time of every opening, for use in studying adherence (Di Iorio, II, 11).

medicocentrism   Practice of viewing health- and illness-related phenomena solely from the point of view of the physician, particularly in reference to *sick role* (Segall, I, 14).

meme   A unit of symbolic cultural information (Fabrega, I, 2). See *healmeme*.

mental illness, severe (SMI)   A diagnosis in the family of schizophrenic or any other psychotic disorders, or any bipolar disorder, as well as any other medical disorder that is of at least 2 years' duration and disables the patient in at least two major areas of life (Hawley, III, 12).

mutual participation model   A framework for physician–patient interaction in which the patient takes an active role in care and both parties share the goal of the patient's well-being (Szasz & Hollender, 1956, in DiMatteo, II, 1).

narrative representation   Presentation of materials in the context of a story about someone doing something, for some purpose, that results in specific consequences; used in interventions to increase safety and reduce injury (Cole, IV, 17).

narrative thinking   Translation of personal experiences into stories that integrate facts, perceptions, emotions, intentions, actions, and consequences into coherent meaning; involves knowing through stories lived and stories heard and told; contrasted with *paradigmatic thinking* (Howard, 1991, in Cole, IV, 17).

National Health Care for the Homeless   An initiative take in 1984 by the Robert Wood Johnson Foundation and the Pew Charitable Trusts to establish health care clinics for the homeless in 19 United States cities (Wright & Joyner, III, 10).

need factor   A characteristic such as health status or illness that predicts use of health services; a component of the *health services utilization model* (Aday & Awe, I, 8).

negotiating   An intervention to increase adherence that involves medical personnel and the patient jointly discussing and agreeing upon the treatment plan (Creer & Levstek, II, 7).

negotiating model of decision making   A framework for physician–patient interaction in which physician and patient belief systems and expectations are given equal value (Reed et al., IV, 2).

occupational culture   Group norms and practices within work settings that often shape the discourse on health, including how workers define situations of threat and danger, and influence risk behaviors such as smoking and alcohol use (Eakin, I, 16).

operational research model   A way of conducting investigations that begins with a practical, problem-focused question rather than with a conceptual framework; characteristic of research in international health (Coreil, III, 9).

oral rehydration therapy (ORT)   An intervention to treat diarrheal conditions in *developing countries* (Coreil, III, 9).

organizational barrier   A structural problem within the health care system that hampers a patient's perceptions of availability and accessibility of care; organizational barriers may include compromised quality of care, patient's perceptions of inhospitable facilities, distance and transportation problems, waiting time, inflexible hours, dearth or lack of bilingual or bicultural staff, and exclusionary policies (Morisky & Cabrera, II, 14).

organizational culture See *occupational culture.*

outcome expectancy A person's beliefs about the consequences of some behavior (e.g., Maddux & DuCharme, I, 7; Baranowski, I, 9); perceived value of the consequence of a given behavior (Di Iorio, II, 11).

pain A multifaceted noxious experience involving sensory, cognitive, and emotional dimensions (Gift & White, IV, 7).

paradigmatic thinking Cognitive processes concerned with the construction of context-free and abstract formal concepts and principles; both the goal and method of science, logic, and mathematics, in contrast to *narrative thinking* (Cole, IV, 17).

parochialism/cosmopolitanism A conceptual framework for understanding social ties within families and families' relationships to the larger community. Parochial families are presumed to demonstrate strong commitment to family (usually paternal) tradition and authority and to have enduring friendships primarily with persons whose backgrounds are similar to their own; cosmopolitan families demonstrate less commitment to family authority and expand their friendships over time, including persons with diverse backgrounds. This typology has guided some research into use of health services and attitudes toward health professionals, but its value has been limited (Suchman, 1965, in Geertsen, I, 13).

passive prevention See *prevention, passive.*

paternalism Characterizing an act by a person or a group, *P*, intended to avert some harm or promote some good for a person or a group, *Q*, where *P* has no reason to believe that the act agrees with the current preferences, desires, or dispositions of *Q*, and *P*'s act is a limitation of *Q*'s right to self-determination (Nilstun, IV, 11).

patient role The component of the sick role that involves interaction with health professionals and/or the formal health care system, in contrast to *self-care* and informal care behaviors (Segall, I, 14).

perceived barriers A person's belief that a specified health action has negative value, particularly in terms of impediments or costs; a component of the *health belief model* (Strecher et al., I, 4).

perceived behavioral control A person's belief in the relative ease or difficulty of performing a specified health action; importance increases as volitional control decreases (Maddux & DuCharme, I, 7); similar to *self-efficacy.*

perceived benefits A person's belief that a specified health action has positive value, particularly in reducing the threat of an illness or health condition; a component of the *health belief model* (Strecher et al., I, 4).

perceived health competence Belief in one's ability to influence one's personal health outcomes effectively (Christensen et al., II, 12).

perceived severity/seriousness A person's belief that an illness or health condition would have negative consequences; a component of the *health belief model* (Strecher et al., I, 4).

perceived social norm A person's belief about how other people view and evaluate a behavior (e.g., Maddux & DuCharme, I, 7).

perceived susceptibility A person's belief about risk for an illness or health condition; a component of the *health belief model* (Strecher et al., I, 4).

perceived threat A function of perceived susceptibility and perceived seriousness providing an impetus for taking some action; a component of the *health belief model* (Strecher et al., I, 4); also a component of *protection motivation theory.*

physician authority See *authority, physician.*

physician autonomy See *autonomy, physician.*

poverty An exceptionally low standard of living officially defined by the U.S. Bureau of the Census, based ultimately on cost of food and adjusted annually for inflation (Wright & Joyner, III, 10).

power, patient The degree to which patients exert control over encounters with physicians and other health care professionals; basic factors are the patient's age, gender, race, education and knowledge, and health status (Haug, II, 3).

power, physician Dominance of and control by the physician over patients and other health professionals; basic factors are the physician's age, gender, race, practice style, and social status (Haug, II, 3).

precaution adoption process model A conceptual framework to predict protective or risk-reducing behavior; identifies five basic stages—unaware, aware but not personally engaged, engaged but deciding on a course of action, planning to act but not yet doing so, and acting—plus a maintenance stage (Weinstein & Sandman, 1992, in Gochman, I, Part II). See *transtheoretical model.*

PRECEDE Acronym for part of a conceptual framework for developing and evaluating health education programs, denoting the basic terms: *P*redisposing, *R*einforcing, and *E*nabling *C*auses in *E*ducational *D*iagnosis and *Evaluation* (Green, Kreuter, Deeds, & Partridge, 1980, in Glanz & Oldenberg, IV, 8). See *PROCEED*.

precontemplation In the *transtheoretical model*, the stage at which there is no apparent intention to change behavior (Prohaska & Clark, III, 2).

predisposing factor A characteristic such as a health belief, family composition, or social position of family that predicts use of health services; a component of the *health services utilization model* (Aday & Awe, I, 8).

preparation In the *transtheoretical model*, the stage at which a person has taken small steps to engage in some behavior but has not yet taken effective action (Prohaska & Clark, III, 2).

PREPARED™ Acronymic name of a system of improving provider–patient communication and patient self-efficacy and satisfaction; denotes the basic components: recommended *P*rocedure, *R*eason for it, patient's *E*xpectations, *P*robability of achieving them, *A*lternative treatments, *R*isks, *E*xpenses, prior to making a *D*ecision (DiMatteo, II, 1).

prevention, active Individual actions to eliminate or reduce the likelihood of a negative health outcome, in contrast to *passive prevention* (Gauff & Miller, 1986, in Gochman, I, 1).

prevention, passive Societal, institutional, or governmental activities to eliminate or reduce the likelihood of a negative health outcome, in contrast to *active prevention* (Gauff & Miller, 1986, in Gochman, I, 1).

prevention/preventive behavior Any activity (medically recommended or not) undertaken to eliminate or reduce the likelihood of contracting a disease or incurring a negative health outcome, or of detecting a disease at an early, asymptomatic stage (Gochman, I, 1).

prevention, primary Reduction or elimination of risk factors (Last, 1987, in Buchanan, IV, 9).

prevention, secondary Asymptomatic detection of a disease in its early stages (Gochman, I, 1).

principle of justice See *justice, principle of.*

problem-based learning An approach to professional education in which curricular materials resemble problems that students will face as practitioners (Bruhn, IV, 1).

PROCEED Acronym for part of a conceptual framework for developing and evaluating health education programs, denoting the basic terms: *P*olicy, *R*egulatory, and *O*rganizational *C*onstructs for *E*du-

cational and *E*nvironmental *D*evelopment (Green et al., 1980, in Glanz & Oldenburg, IV, 8). See *PRECEDE*.

professional role See *role, physician/provider.*

protection motivation theory A conceptual framework to determine the effects of threatening health information on attitude and behavior change; basic components are internal and external sources of information, cognitive mediating processes of *threat appraisal* and *coping appraisal*, and adaptive or maladaptive coping modes (Rogers & Prentice-Dunn, I, 6).

psychosocial epidemiology Application of epidemiological methods to determine health-related personal and social characteristics in a population, e.g., people's perceptions of social support, religiosity, and health (Rakowski, III, 5).

public health Collective actions of society to assure the conditions for people to be healthy (Institute of Medicine, 1988, in Buchanan, IV, 9).

reactance Workers' tendency to be defiant about safety and risk behaviors as a way of maintaining their control when they believe their behavior is being manipulated (Cohen & Colligan, II, 20). See *illusion of safety*.

reciprocal determinism A concept expressing the constant interaction between a person, the person's behavior, and the person's family and social environment in the development and maintenance of health behaviors (Baranowski, I, 9; Baranowski & Hearn, IV, 16).

relapse In the *transtheoretical model*, the movement from one stage to a previous stage (Prohaska & Clark, III, 2); in the context of regimens of dental flossing and brushing for plaque removal, defined as *adherence* at less than 43% (McCaul, II, 16).

relapse prevention model A conceptual framework, derived from *social learning theory*, for understanding how and why people backslide from a path of behavior change (Marlatt & Gordon, 1985, in Marcus et al., II, 18).

relative risk Ratio of adverse health consequences of a specified behavior accruing to groups who do and do not perform that behavior (Prohaska & Clark, III, 2).

resource model of preventive health behavior A conceptual framework in nursing to predict health actions; basic components are health resources, including perceived health status, energy level, concern about health, feelings about taking care of one's health; and social resources, such as educational level and income (Kulbok, 1985, in Blue & Brooks, IV, 5).

response efficacy Belief that adopting a behavior will reduce some threat (Strecher et al., I, 4).

risk behavior, sexual Any behavior that increases the likelihood of a sexually transmitted disease (STD), including *AIDS*; such behaviors include sexual intercourse without latex protection, actions that expose open sores or cuts to infected bodily fluids, and sharing intravenous drug use apparatus (Thomason & Campos, III, 8).

risk, relative See *relative risk*.

role, physician/provider A set of normative expectations for the full-time professional activity of caring for the sick, involving the development of technical proficiency, affective neutrality, and objectivity and placing the welfare of the patient above that of the professional's personal interests (Parsons, 1951, 1975, in Salloway et al., II, 4).

role, sick See *patient role*; *sick role*.

safe sex Sexual behavior in which there is no chance of direct bloodstream access to infected blood, blood products, seminal fluid, vaginal fluid, or breast milk (Thomason & Campos, III, 8).

safer sex Sexual behavior that reduces the likelihood of exchange of bodily fluids (Thomason & Campos, III, 8).

secular trend Health behavioral changes in a community that are not attributable to health education or health promotion intervention (Glanz & Oldenburg, IV, 8).

selective survival Changes in the composition of a population due to the higher mortality rates at advancing age of individuals participating in risk behaviors (Prohaska & Clark, III, 2).

self-care A process whereby laypersons can function effectively on their own behalf in health promotion and prevention and in detecting and treating disease (Levin, 1976, in Gochman, I, Part IV); often used interchangeably with *self-management, self-regulation* (Di Iorio, II, 11). See *self health management*.

self-care agency An individual's capacity to gather information, make decisions, and perform skillfully the behaviors necessary to assume personal control in health promotion and maintenance as well as in the prevention and treatment of illness (e.g., Orem, 1985, in Blue & Brooks, IV, 5).

self-care autonomy Demonstrating the ability and skills necessary to self-manage a condition (Wysocki & Greco, II, 9).

self-care autonomy, appropriate Expecting a child to have the requisite ability and skills to manage a condition at a level appropriate to the child's maturity (Wysocki & Greco, II, 9).

self-care autonomy, constrained Expecting a child to have the requisite ability and skills to manage a condition at a level less than appropriate to the child's maturity (Wysocki & Greco, II, 9).

self-care autonomy, excessive Expecting a child to have the requisite ability and skills to manage a condition at a level greater than appropriate to the child's maturity (Wysocki, II, 9).

self-efficacy Belief or judgment about one's ability to execute some action successfully (Strecher et al., I, 4; Maddux & DuCharme, I, 7); confidence in one's ability to perform a particular behavior (Baranowski, I, 9). See *health belief model*; *perceived behavioral control*; *protection motivation theory*; *theory of reasoned action*.

self health management Undertaking of lay activities to promote health, to prevent illness, and to detect and treat illness when it occurs; includes a range of behaviors such as: health maintenance activities, illness prevention, symptom evaluation, self-treatment, and use of a variety of health resources such as lay network members as well as diverse health professionals (Segall, I, 14).

self-management, childhood diabetes Assumption of responsibility by a patient and the patient's family for monitoring, evaluating, and adjusting treatment; basic components include demographic factors, family functioning, psychological stress, and interactions with providers to acquire necessary skills (Wysocki & Greco, II, 9). See *self-regulation/self-regulatory skills*.

self-management, epilepsy Sum total of steps a person takes to control seizures and to control the effects of having a seizure disorder; common practices include taking medications at prescribed times, avoiding factors that trigger seizures, following safety precautions such as not driving when seizures are not under control, avoiding running out of medications, consulting with professionals about treatment or unexpected problems, and monitoring seizure frequency; often used interchangeably with *self-care, self-regulation* (Di Iorio, II, 11).

self-prediction What one states one will do in contrast to *behavioral intention*: what one predicts one will do (Maddux & DuCharme, I, 7). See *intention, behavioral; theory of reasoned action.*

self-regulation/self-regulatory skills   Ability to control or change one's health behavior, including goal setting, monitoring movement toward goals, exerting effort and skill to reach goals, and rewarding self for attaining goals (Baranowski, I, 9); used interchangeably with *self-care, self-management* (Di Iorio, II, 11); a conceptual framework designed to understand behavior change, particularly in relation to disease management; basic components include *self-efficacy, outcome expectancy,* monitoring feedback, role modeling, social support, and learning of necessary skills (Clark, II, 8).

sense of place   Personal and social meanings or particular significance that people attach to physical locations or settings, as distinct from the objective or physical space dimensions (Tuan, 1974, in Scarpaci & Kearns, II, 5; Gochman, IV, 20).

setting   The conventional "bricks and mortar" facilities in which health care takes place as well as the psychosocial implications of such places for provider–patient encounters (Scarpaci & Kearns, II, 5).

sex, safe   See *safe sex.*

sexism   In health care, a focus primarily on male health issues and on health roles for women that are subordinate to those of men (Elder, Humphreys, & Lakowski, 1988, in VanScoy, III, 7).

shared decision making model   A framework for physician–patient interaction in which the physician is obliged to present the patient with all available information without filtering it, and without giving advice, in order for the patient to be able to make the most informed decision about care (Wennberg, 1990, in Reed et al., IV, 2).

sick call   The processing of health complaints in correctional facilities, which requires that inmates sign up, have their requests reviewed and triaged, and then be seen by a provider; inmates have no choice of providers or of appointment time (Anno, III, 14).

sick role   A conceptual framework developed by Parsons (1951, in Segall, I, 14) for analyzing the behavior of a person who has been diagnosed as ill; basic components are the person's rights to be exempt from responsibility for the incapacity and from normal role and task obligations and the person's duties to seek professional care and to abide by professional advice and recover (Segall, I, 14).

sick role, alternative   Elaboration of the Parsonian

sick role model, adding the person's rights to make decisions about health care and to be dependent on lay others for care and social support and the person's duties to maintain health and overcome illness and to engage in routine self-management; assumes that members of the person's social network are prepared to take on added responsibilities and to function as caregivers as needed (Segall, I, 14).

sickness   A departure from being healthy, often defined through a combination of symptoms experienced, not feeling "right" or "normal," and consequences such as restricted activity (Lau, I, 3); the social side of illness (Gochman, I, 1); the social construction of an episode of illness, the way illness is dealt with in society (Fabrega, I, 2); a form of deviance (Segall, I, 14); the contextualized definition of dysfunction, a process by which signs and symptoms are given socially recognizable meanings (Dressler & Oths, I, 17).

social action   An approach to community health promotion interventions involving advocacy or conflict strategy that entails mass mobilization of low-power components and use of political pressure (Rothman, 1979, in Schooler & Flora, IV, 15).

social cognitive theory   A general social psychological conceptual framework adapted to understand the acquisition or health behaviors; basic components are *outcome expectancy, self-efficacy,* skills, and social evaluation of and feedback on behavior (Baranowski, I, 9; Di Iorio, II, 11; Marcus et al., II, 18).

social epidemiology   See *psychosocial epidemiology.*

social learning theory   A conceptual framework for understanding the acquisition of health behaviors; basic components are observation, modeling, and reinforcement in interpersonal contexts (Tinsley, I, 11; Marcus et al., II, 18).

social marketing   Use of merchandising and advertising techniques to increase the effectiveness of health-related campaigns, e.g., for immunizations and family planning; basic components are lowering the price; responding to market demands, such as needs; emphasizing relative advantages of the service or product; making the service or product accessible to the population; and using a full range of mass media to promote the service or product (Buchanan, IV, 9).

social network   A broad conceptual framework for examining social ties and social support; includes dimensions of structure (e.g., number and density of linkages, interaction (e.g., nature and quality), and function (e.g., provision of information, resources, and emotional support). Not identical to *social support*; networks may be unsupportive (Ritter, 1988, in Gochman, I, Part IV).

social norms Generally held beliefs about the appropriateness or desirability of some behavior.

social planning A technical approach to community health promotion interventions using rational empirical processes of data accumulation, and persuasion involving experts (Rothman, 1979, in Schooler & Flora, IV, 15).

social structure The organization or patterning of social ties; regularities in interpersonal linkages. *Parochialism/cosmpolitanism* has been a major typology of social structure relevant to health behavior research (Geertsen, I, 13).

social support Aggregate of social ties involving interpersonal relationships that protect people from negative experiences, including both structural (e.g., living arrangements, participation in social activities) and functional (e.g., emotional support, encouraging expression of feelings, provision of advice) dimensions (e.g., Ritter, 1988, in Gochman, I, Part IV); a range of interpersonal exchanges that include not only the provision of physical, social, and emotional assistance, but also the subjective consequences of making individuals feel that they are the subject of enduring concern by others (Pilisuk & Parks, 1981, in Morisky & Cabrera, II, 14).

social support, directive Assumption by others of responsibility for tasks or decisions in relation to *adherence* (Fisher et al., II, 10).

social support, nondirective Participation by others in cooperating, sharing, and expressing understanding of feelings in relation to *adherence* without attempts to control or alter tasks or decisions (Fisher et al., II, 10).

social ties Interpersonal linkages, including those with household members, relatives, and friends (Geertsen, I, 13).

sociology of medicine See *medical sociology.*

specific etiology, doctrine of An essentially mechanistic medical model that specified that for each illness there was a single, necessary, and sufficient causal agent or pathogen (Pasteur, 1873 [cited in Hamann, 1994], in Wiese & Gallagher, IV, 4).

stage models of adoption See *transtheoretical model.*

stages of change models See *transtheoretical model.*

stepped-care model A conceptual framework for increasing smoking cessation that matches intensity of treatment to stages of change (Glasglow & Orleans, II, 19).

stereotyping Physician's categorization of a patient as bad or undesirable, using the patient's behavior as a clue indicative of potential challenge to the physician's authority (Ben-Sira, II, 2).

support-mobilizing hypothesis A conceptual framework for understanding caregiver behavior, based on the assumption that stress will motivate the caregiver to elicit support (Bass, Tausig, & Noelker, 1988/1989, in Wright, III, 13).

t'ai chi An ancient Chinese system of exercise and meditation being introduced in selected religious communities as a health behavior intervention (Duckro, Magaletta, & Wolf, III, 15).

theory of planned behavior See *theory of reasoned action.*

theory of reasoned action A conceptual framework designed to predict intentions to engage in or change specified health behaviors (Maddux & DuCharme, I, 7); basic components are a person's attitudes toward a specified behavior and a person's perceptions of the social norms regarding the behavior. See *intention, behavioral; self-prediction.*

therapeutic landscape See *landscape, therapeutic.*

threat appraisal Evaluation of maladaptive responses (Rogers & Prentice-Dunn, I, 6). See *protection motivation theory.*

transtheoretical model A conceptual framework for predicting behavior change that assumes a progression of stages from *precontemplation* of change through *contemplation, preparation, action,* maintenance, and *relapse,* with different intervention approaches appropriate for each stage (Prohaska & Di Clemente, 1992, in Gochman, I, Part II; Rimer et al., II, 15; Glasgow & Orleans, II, 19); incorporates behavioral intentions, *decisional balance theory, self-efficacy,* and individual processes of behavioral change (Marcus et al., II, 18).

utilitarianism A conceptual framework applied to health issues that emphasizes the maximization of some desired state (Nilstun, IV, 11).

utilization framework A refinement of the *health services utilization model* designed to predict type and purpose of health care use; basic components are societal determinants such as technology and social norms, health service system resources and organizations, and *predisposing*, *enabling*, and *need factors* (Andersen & Newman, 1973, in Aday & Awe, I, 8).

value-based learning   An approach to professional education that places values, ethics, and moral issues at the curricular core (Bruhn, IV, 1).

wellness   Realization of the optimum health potential of an individual, family, or community; achieved by enhancing physical, psychological, and sociological well-being through activities aimed at the promotion of health (Blue & Brooks, IV, 5).

window of vulnerability   A period in the family life cycle when the strength of the family's influence on health behaviors has the potential for diminishing (Lau, Quadrel, & Hartman, 1990, in Gochman, I, 10).

worksite program   One or more health promotion activities conducted in an occupational setting (Schooler & Flora, IV, 15).

Contents of Volumes I–IV

VOLUME II.   PROVIDER DETERMINANTS

VOLUME III.   DEMOGRAPHY, DEVELOPMENT, AND DIVERSITY

VOLUME IV.   RELEVANCE FOR PROFESSIONALS AND ISSUES
FOR THE FUTURE

Index to Volumes I–IV

In addition to the entries in this Index, the reader is encouraged to look at the Contents of each volume and the Contents of Volumes I–IV that appears at the end of each volume, as well as at the Glossary contained in each volume. Space limitations precluded listing *every* intervention or program, government document, or disease or condition identified in the chapters. Similarly, passages dealing *solely* with etiologies, morbidity, mortality, and demographic correlates of diseases with no relevance for health behavior were not indexed.

ISBN 0-306-45445-9

90000